USMLE STEP 1

SECRETS

USMLE STEP 1

SECRETS

Third Edition

Thomas A. Brown, MD
Medical Director
Doctors Express Danbury
Danbury, Connecticut

Sonali J. Shah
MD/PhD Candidate
University of Connecticut School of Medicine
Farmington, Connecticut

SAUNDERS

ELSEVIER

1600 John F. Kennedy Blvd.
Ste 1800
Philadelphia, PA 19103-2899

USMLE STEP 1 SECRETS, THIRD EDITION   ISBN: 978-0-323-08514-4

Notices

Knowledge and best practice in this field are constantly changing. As new research and experience broaden our understanding, changes in research methods, professional practices, or medical treatment may become necessary.

Practitioners and researchers must always rely on their own experience and knowledge in evaluating and using any information, methods, compounds, or experiments described herein. In using such information or methods they should be mindful of their own safety and the safety of others, including parties for whom they have a professional responsibility.

With respect to any drug or pharmaceutical products identified, readers are advised to check the most current information provided (i) on procedures featured or (ii) by the manufacturer of each product to be administered, to verify the recommended dose or formula, the method and duration of administration, and contraindications. It is the responsibility of practitioners, relying on their own experience and knowledge of their patients, to make diagnoses, to determine dosages and the best treatment for each individual patient, and to take all appropriate safety precautions.

To the fullest extent of the law, neither the Publisher nor the authors, contributors, or editors assume any liability for any injury and/or damage to persons or property as a matter of products liability, negligence, or otherwise, or from any use or operation of any methods, products, instructions, or ideas contained in the material herein.

Library of Congress Cataloging-in-Publication Data
Brown, Thomas, 1972-
    USMLE step 1 secrets / Thomas A. Brown, Sonali J. Shah. – 3rd ed.
      p. ; cm. – (Secrets series)
    Includes bibliographical references and index.
    ISBN 978-0-323-08514-4 (pbk. : alk. paper)
    I. Shah, Sonali J. II. Title. III. Title: USMLE step one secrets.   IV. Series: Secrets series.
    [DNLM: 1. Clinical Medicine–Examination Questions. WB 18.2]
    LC classification not assigned
    610.76–dc23   2012015347

Senior Content Strategist: James Merritt
Content Development Specialist: Andrea Vosburgh
Publishing Services Manager: Patricia Tannian
Senior Project Manager: Sharon Corell
Design Direction: Steven Stave

Printed in the United States of America

Last digit is the print number: 9   8   7   6   5   4

Working together to grow
libraries in developing countries

www.elsevier.com | www.bookaid.org | www.sabre.org

ELSEVIER   BOOK AID
International   Sabre Foundation

CONTRIBUTORS

Thomas A. Brown, MD
Medical Director, Doctors Express Danbury, Danbury, Connecticut

Dana M. Carne
Fourth-Year Medical Student, Dartmouth Medical School, Hanover, New Hampshire; Dartmouth-Hitchcock Medical Center, Lebanon, New Hampshire

Bjorn I. Engstrom, MD
Intern, Department of Medicine, Beth Israel Deaconess Medical Center, Boston, Massachusetts

Raj Ganeshan
Third-Year Medical Student, University of Connecticut School of Medicine, Farmington, Connecticut

Nikki Goulet, MD
Resident, Department of Surgery, University of Connecticut School of Medicine, Farmington, Connecticut

Jessica M. Intravia, MHA
Third-Year Medical Student, University of Connecticut School of Medicine, Farmington, Connecticut

Douglas W. Jones
Fourth-Year Medical Student, Dartmouth Medical School, Hanover, New Hampshire

Khoshal Latifzai
Fourth-Year Medical Student, Dartmouth Medical School, Hanover, New Hampshire

Stephen B. Marko
Third-Year Medical Student, University of Connecticut School of Medicine, Farmington, Connecticut

Henry L. Nguyen
Research Associate, University of California, San Diego, La Jolla, California

Brandon Olivieri, MD
Internal Medicine Intern, Yale-New Haven Hospital, New Haven, Connecticut; Radiology Resident, Diagnostic Imaging, Mount Sinai Medical Center, Miami Beach, Florida

Anna Radwan
Third-Year Medical Student, University of Connecticut School of Medicine, Farmington, Connecticut

Allyson M. Reid
Third-Year Medical Student, University of Connecticut School of Medicine, Farmington, Connecticut

Eric B. Roth
Fourth-Year Medical Student, Dartmouth Medical School, Hanover, New Hampshire

David Austin Schirmer, III, MD
Resident, Department of Gynecology and Obstetrics, Emory University School of Medicine, Atlanta, Georgia

Sonali J. Shah
MD/PhD Candidate, University of Connecticut School of Medicine, Farmington, Connecticut

Jaime Stevens, MD, MPH
Resident, Department of Psychiatry, University of Miami/Jackson Memorial Hospital, Miami, Florida

J. Pedro Teixeira
Fourth-Year Medical Student, Dartmouth Medical School, Hanover, New Hampshire

Edmund Tsui
Third-Year Medical Student, Dartmouth Medical School, Hanover, New Hampshire

PREFACE

Preparing for the United States Medical Licensing Examination (USMLE) Step 1 can be an intimidating and nerve-wracking experience. For one thing, this score *actually* counts! Although for many of you the most important goal in taking Step 1 is passing this exam, we know that is not enough. Earning a spot in a competitive field or residency program requires you to do more than just pass in order to compete with other high-caliber students. Let us pause right here and take a moment to introduce ourselves. We are the authors of *USMLE Step 1 Secrets*, and we have one aim in writing this book: We are here to help you earn the *highest* score you possibly can on this exam.

How early should you begin studying for the USMLE?
Students frequently ask this question, but unfortunately there is no simple way to answer it. Students commonly allocate anywhere from 1 to 6 months to study for boards, but some take more time and a rare few may need less. The point is that each student should begin his or her preparations at a time that makes sense for that particular individual. When planninig your own study schedule, consider how busy you estimate you will be in the months leading up to your exam (do not neglect your coursework!), how many hours per day you are willing to dedicate to productive study time, and how well you think you retain information in the short term versus the long term. Most medical students will have figured out which study styles work best for them long before they even begin to think about boards. Do not drastically change your study habits for the USMLE if you have found methods that work well for you.

How will this book help you prepare for Step 1?
As you may have already figured out, there are hundreds of review books available to help you prepare for this exam. While the content in these books may overlap quite a bit, the way that material is presented can vary drastically from resource to resource. The trick to selecting good review books is to purchase a *few* that mesh well with your learning style and the actual format of the USMLE. The more books you have in front of you, the greater the potential for confusion and the less productive you will feel. In other words, an overabundance of resources eventually will become an impediment to your studying. The most efficient test takers are the students who consolidate their study materials as time goes by. Start with a fresh copy of the newest edition of *First Aid for the USMLE Step 1*. This will be your primary resource for the USMLE Step 1. Our book is designed to supplement the information that you learn in First Aid and help you place it into clinical context through a mix of basic-concept and case-based questions. The detailed answers we provide to our questions will offer you insight into the way that the USMLE will expect you to think through questions on test day. In addition, our book will provide you with dozens of valuable study tips (including tips from third- and fourth-year medical students who have earned competitive scores on the USMLE Step 1) to facilitate your studying.

We begin each chapter with an insider's guide that will provide you with our best study strategies for that particular subject. In addition, each chapter includes a number of "Step 1 Secrets" that will point out the highest-yield topics to focus on for boards. It is our mission to offer you the type of valuable information that you can really use to boost your score on test day, and you will find it exclusively in the third edition of *USMLE Step 1 Secrets*.

Now that you have selected your resources, how should you go about studying for the exam?

- Set up a study schedule as *early* as possible. Determine when you will begin studying, how much time you will dedicate to the exam each week or month, and when you would like to cover specific subject areas in your review process. Keep in mind that you will need the last few weeks before boards to review all of the content that you have studied.
- Make a *flexible* study schedule, especially early in your preparations. Give yourself some free time every day to enjoy other activities and relax your mind. This will increase the productivity of your study time.
- Purchase a copy of First Aid as soon as possible and casually review it when studying for your medical school exams, especially during your second year. There is no need to place your emphasis on studying for your board exam before you are ready, but at least familiarizing yourself with First Aid in advance will make you feel much more comfortable when beginning your USMLE studying.
- Annotate your copy of First Aid with notes from *USMLE Step 1 Secrets* and other high-yield resources. All of your notes will therefore be in one place in the weeks leading up to your exam date, and you will have a much easier time getting through all of the material during your final review phase.
- Begin using question bank software months before your exam date. Most students use Kaplan Qbank, USMLE World, USMLE Consult, or USMLERx. If you have the time and budget to do so, we recommend purchasing more than one product from the aforementioned list. You can use one program casually (tutor mode) and the other program more intensely (random questions, timed mode) to simulate actual exam conditions. No matter which mode you use, you will benefit from reading all of the answer explanations at the end. Consider marking questions with great learning points or excellent diagrams so that you can easily find them again. Keep in mind that you can download question bank applications for your Smartphone.
- The night before your exam, try to put your books away and get a good night's rest. Half of the battle will be keeping your focus through an intense, 8-hour exam day. If you feel the need to study the day before or morning of your exam as a "warm up" or to relieve some anxiety, we recommend going through the Rapid Review section at the end of First Aid or a few of your own notes. You may also consider answering a couple of practice questions, but be wary of looking at the answers at this time in case you get them wrong. Avoid cramming any information (new or old) right before your exam to prevent an anxiety attack.
- Most important, try not to worry too much about your score on Step 1. While your board score will be an important factor in your residency application, it is not the *only* factor. (On the other hand, keep in mind that a good Step 1 score will not make up for poor grades in school.) You would not have gotten into medical school if you were not competent enough to pass this exam. All you need to do is put in the time and effort.

When will I get my score?

Naturally, this is one of the most frequently asked questions among eager examinees who have completed the USMLE Step 1. Scores are typically made available on the NBME website 3 to 5 weeks after your exam date (lag time is determined by the number of students who have taken the exam during your window). On the morning that your score will be released, you will receive an email from NBME alerting you that your score will be made available that afternoon. Your score report will contain your numerical score and a brief outline of your performance in a broad array of areas. The information provided will be quite similar to the score report you receive if you elect to take a practice NBME exam through the NBME website.

Ten things students wish they had known prior to taking the USMLE Step 1:

1. Questions on the USMLE Step 1 are often slightly longer than those found in most question bank programs. Most students finish in time, but keeping on pace will be very important to your success on this exam.
2. Prior to the start of your exam, you will be given a small markerboard on which to scribble formulas and perform calculations during your exam. You may take a *few minutes* before you actually begin your exam to jot down some notes. Determine what you will write on your whiteboard during the final week of your review so as not to waste time during your exam.
3. Anatomy throws many students for a loop on Step 1 because they are often unsure how to prepare for this subject. Be sure to read our "Insider's Guide to Clinical Anatomy for the USMLE Step 1" in Chapter 26 of this book.
4. You should expect to have a small percentage of questions on topics that you have never before seen or studied. You may also get four to five questions on the same topic. If you do not know the answer, take your best guess and move on. Do not let yourself become flustered or frustrated because you may otherwise miss some easy questions.
5. You are allowed 45 minutes of break time during your exam, but you can gain an extra 15 minutes by skipping the tutorial (you can watch a similar tutorial on the NBME website before your exam date). Most students find an hour of break time to be adequate, but you should spend some time before your exam planning out how you will allot your time. Do not forget that you are expected to include lunch in your break time.
6. Bring snacks. You will be facing a long day. We suggest that you eat a small lunch and a few snacks in between blocks rather than one big lunch (some students will otherwise become lethargic during the afternoon). Be wary of selecting high-sugar snacks (the last thing you need while taking the USMLE is a sugar crash!).
7. While it is no secret that you should dress in comfortable clothing while sitting for your exam, students often do not know that they should wear as little jewelry and clothing with as few pockets as possible. To prevent the use of prohibited items, most testing centers will scan you with a metal wand and ask you to turn out your pockets each time you re-enter the examination room following a break. Not only is this a frustrating process, but also it is a waste of your break time. You will get through this inspection much more quickly with less jewelry and fewer pockets. Also remember to bring your ID and locker key with you every time you leave the test center.
8. All NBME forms are different! Do not be fooled by students who tell you that their questions were identical to those in the USMLE World, Kaplan Qbank, USMLE Consult, or USMLERx. There is no guarantee that your experience will be the same as theirs. The more questions you do, the better prepared you will be. We recommend that you reserve at least 1000 practice questions to answer in conditions that closely simulate the exam (blocks of 46 questions, random assortment, and timed mode).
9. When scheduling your exam date, keep in mind that having more time to study will not necessarily improve your performance. Every individual has a peak performance window, and trying to study past this window *may* hurt your score. For those of you who have more flexibility than your friends when planning your exam date, be careful about delaying boards for too long. It is possible that you will find it increasingly more difficult to concentrate on studying once your friends have moved past this stage. It is also not advisable to delay your exam too long after you have completed the second year of medical school because you may spend more time relearning the basics.
10. You should arrive at your testing center 30 minutes prior to your start time. If you speed through the registration process, you may be allowed to begin your examination early. This may be a good option for some students, particularly those who would otherwise spend the time building anxiety. Another good option for anxiety relief is to sign up for a practice examination at your testing site a few weeks before your actual exam date. In order to do this, you must request a permit from the NBME website.

One final note...

Although it will be a challenging task, studying for the USMLE Step 1 will also be a rewarding experience that will prepare you for a successful transition into your clinical years. Students often say that they feel incredibly accomplished (and intelligent!) after sitting for this examination. We guarantee that your score on the USMLE will greatly reflect the work you put into studying and your attitude about the experience, so aim high and keep your chin up. Before you know it, the USMLE Step 1 will be behind you and you will be well on your way to a wonderful career in medicine.

Wishing you the best of luck,

Thomas A. Brown and Sonali J. Shah

MORE SECRETS FOR SUCCESS ON THE USMLE STEP 1

The 6 to 8 weeks you spend studying for Step 1 is a unique time in your education. You are given this opportunity to solely dedicate yourself to acquiring a vast body of knowledge without any distracting write-ups, quizzes, or other tedious assignments. Embrace the task as an opportunity for self-improvement because if approached correctly, your endurance, maturity, and study skills will drastically sharpen. These skills will serve you well for the rest of your career, far after the details of embryological processes and biochemical nuances have faded. Actively seek and appreciate the moments when your mind feels stuffed with information; it will empower you. Studying for Step 1 was the best time of my life that I would never want to repeat.

SV, Medical Class of 2012

Although it seems intuitive, be sure to put in time doing practice questions in a variety of subject areas. DO NOT solely focus on areas in which you are already proficient or areas you really enjoy. Suffer through the sections that are the bane of your existence, and you will see marvelous results!

SAB, MD/PhD Candidate, Medical Class of 2012

While Step 1 is a hugely important exam and everyone around you may be freaking out about how to study for it, the most important thing to remember is that it is still just an exam. It is very important not to get caught up in how everyone around you is studying for the exam. Whatever techniques work for you in terms of studying for exams is the same way you should study for this exam. Changing your study techniques specifically for this exam can be very harmful. If you study best at home, then study at home; and if you study in the library with friends, then study in the library with friends. You don't have to have a study partner if that doesn't work for you even if other people suggest it.

SL, Medical Class of 2012

Each version of the exam is different. To score 99, it's important to know all topics really well, including the low-yield material. Most importantly, do as many questions as you can once you are done reviewing the materials. USMLE World and Kaplan Qbank are amongst the best ones available in the market. Do NBMEs to gauge your performance. Sleep well the night before the exam because it is a long exam, which will test not only your knowledge but also your endurance.

VP, Medical Class of 2013

Work out. Every day.

SM, Medical Class of 2013

I just read through Harrison's and Robbins throughout my second year. I know these books seem daunting, but if you read 20 pages a day, you can finish both books and learn the material from the best sources. The only review book that I used was First Aid. I realize that this method won't work for most people, but it worked for me and I ended up doing really well on the USMLE Step 1 boards.

AO, Medical Class of 2013

One of the most significant tools to prepare for the USMLE Step 1 is the question bank. I used both the Kaplan and USMLE World Question banks and found that the two were essential. Kaplan questions are good to use as a learning resource to help in going through the First Aid review book because they reference page numbers according to the topic of each question. The USMLE World questions, I thought, were very close to the actual questions presented on my exam. This question bank is a good tool to use daily in the last 2 months before the exam.

AG, Medical Class of 2013

One technique that really worked for me was to record all the questions I got wrong on USMLE World or Kaplan Qbank and all facts I commonly forgot as I went through studying First Aid and other books. I recorded brief facts (one or two lines) in a notebook as I studied and reviewed that list every day. Over the weeks of studying, that list of forgotten/incorrect facts grew to span many, many pages in my notebook, but by recording them in a separate location, I was able to have a central resource that was easy to review. I believe this really helped prevent getting the same things repeatedly wrong. I also remember getting questions on Step 2 correct specifically because I had written them down and read them over 20 to 30 times.

SL, Medical Class of 2012

There is no such thing as reading First Aid (and whatever other quality sources you choose to use) too many times. Every time you read material for a given disease you will find new meaning, especially after doing practice questions on that given topic. Seeing the same material from a different perspective (after getting questions wrong on that topic) hones you in on different aspects of what is stated.

SV, Medical Class of 2012

It's important to start early and pace yourself. Try to get into a habit early on of spending a few hours each night devoted to reading high-yield material and completing a few practice problems. Next, I'd suggest that you pick a study partner or a small group to meet with on a weekly basis to help solidify your knowledge in the various subject areas. Lastly, make time for study breaks! Take a day or two off every couple of weeks to just relax, catch up with family and friends, and take your mind off the USMLE. It will keep your mind refreshed, and you will be more effective in your studying. Good luck!

GR, Medical Class of 2013

Don't get overwhelmed by too many sources because they will start to confuse you. Stick to as few core sources as possible, and go over them multiple times.

CN, MD/PhD Candidate, Entering Class of 2008

Get the big physiologic concepts down before studying the minor details. Save biochemistry for last because it requires a lot of memorization. But perhaps the best thing to do is to purchase a question bank program early and use that to study for your classes throughout the year to reinforce the material. Go through as many questions as you can, but most importantly, do NOT study the night before your exam. Good luck.

WJM, Medical Class of 2012

Despite the constantly mounting anxiety and pressure of doing well as test day nears, do not forget to take some time to relax and vent. The last thing you want to do is crash and burn right before the big day.

CA, Medical Class of 2013

1) If you elect to take a practice exam through your testing center, you may find that it repeats a lot of the questions available through NBME online practice exams. 2) Do not forget your locker key when you go out for breaks. 3) Check out your testing site ahead of time to guarantee that there will not be construction going on while you are taking your exam.

RG, MD/MPH Candidate, Entering Class of 2009

Be sure to start early and form a study plan that makes sense. Start reviewing high-yield topics from the beginning and focus on concepts rather than minute details. Spend more time focusing on Qbank explanations rather than worrying about whether you get the questions right or wrong.

EA, Medical Class of 2013

Study the way you are used to studying. This is not the time to change your good study habits. Question banks are a good way to build your endurance for the big day. Start off with untimed exams to familiarize yourself with the format of the questions, then work your way up to the hour-long, timed exams. Don't be discouraged if your scores start off low. They will surely improve as you continue to do questions throughout the year. Give yourself some time off every once in awhile. Prevent burnout by going to the movies or cooking dinner with friends whenever you start to feel overwhelmed.

AR, Medical Class of 2013

Review your annotated copy of First Aid in its entirety within one week of your exam so you will feel confident that you have seen all of the material recently. There is no need to go in sequential order at this time; draw out a study schedule that allows you to cover all the topics comfortably and spread the work evenly over 7 days. The day before your exam, simply flip through every page of First Aid (in an hour or two, tops!) just to make yourself feel good about how much you know. Review high-yield pharmacology, including drug antidotes and common drug toxicities, one final time and you'll be ready to go!

SB, Medical Class of 2013

Step 1 of the boards can be intimidating to tackle at first. However, I found that using First Aid as my primary source and adding notes from other high-yield resources like Qbank, *USMLE Step 1 Secrets* and *Goljan Rapid Review Pathology* made studying much more manageable. It was especially nice to have one consolidated study resource (i.e., First Aid) to which I referred when doing practice questions a few weeks before my exam.

KP, Medical Class of 2013

Avoid unnecessary drama during this time (it's the last thing you will want to deal with while you are busy cramming for boards!) and keep your good friends and family close. You will inevitably go through periods of intense fear and anxiety, and there may even be days where you feel like giving up on studying entirely. There is no doubt that you will want and need people you trust to pull you through this stressful time.

SS, MD/PhD Candidate, Entering Class of 2009

Trust in your preparation and have faith in yourself. No one ever feels 100% prepared on test day, but if you consistently put in the work, you *will* be ready to go.

TB, Medical Class of 2013

CONTENTS

CHAPTER 1

CARDIOLOGY

Raj Ganeshan, Thomas A. Brown, MD, and Sonali J. Shah

INSIDER'S GUIDE TO CARDIOLOGY FOR THE USMLE STEP 1

Cardiology is a widely tested subject on the USMLE Step 1, so it is important to achieve a good understanding of both the physiology and pathology of the heart. Become well-versed in pressure-volume loops, the Wiggers diagram, murmurs, and heart sounds (you will likely get a few audio questions on the USMLE that will require you to identify valvular defects based on the qualities of the murmurs detected through a *movable* virtual stethoscope), action potentials of atrial and ventricular myocytes versus pacemaker cells, and common pathologic conditions of the heart (e.g., rheumatic fever, congestive heart failure, cardiomyopathies, endocarditis). Cardiac pharmacology is also a high-yield subject. The majority of cardiology questions on the USMLE will require you to apply concepts rather than facts, so working through the cases in this chapter will be of tremendous value in your preparation for this subject.

BASIC CONCEPTS—HEMODYNAMICS

1. **What are the mathematical determinants of the arterial blood pressure?**
   The mean arterial pressure (MAP) is determined by how much blood the heart pumps into the arterial system in a given time (the cardiac output [CO]) and how much resistance the arteries have to this input (total peripheral resistance [TPR]). Mathematically, this is expressed as MAP = CO × TPR. Consequently, all drugs that lower blood pressure work by affecting either the CO or TPR (or both).
   Note: The primary determinant of systolic blood pressure (SBP) is CO, whereas the primary determinant of diastolic blood pressure (DBP) is TPR. Because approximately one third of the cardiac cycle is spent in systole and two thirds in diastole, the MAP can be calculated as MAP = 1/3 SBP + 2/3 DBP.

2. **What are the primary determinants of cardiac output?**
   The CO is the amount of blood pumped by the ventricles per unit time. It is determined by the volume of blood ejected during each ventricular contraction (stroke volume [SV]) and how frequently the heart beats (heart rate [HR]), expressed as CO = HR × SV. The HR can be affected by a variety of factors but is principally under the control of the autonomic nervous system. Beta blockers can reduce CO by decreasing HR and contractility.
   Note: In addition to their negative inotropic effect, the more cardioselective (non-dihydropyridine) calcium channel blockers (verapamil, diltiazem) can also reduce HR by slowing impulse transmission through the atrioventricular (AV) node. They achieve part of their antihypertensive effect through this mechanism.

3. **What are the three main factors that affect stroke volume?**
   The determinants of SV are preload, contractility, and afterload.

4. **What is preload, and how does it affect stroke volume?**
   Preload is the degree of tension (load) on the ventricular muscle when it begins to contract. The primary determinant of preload is end-diastolic volume.

   The most widely accepted theory explaining the relationship of preload and SV is the Frank-Starling mechanism, which describes how an increased preload results in an increased SV. It states that stretching of ventricular muscle fibers occurs with increasing end-diastolic volumes, causing greater overlap between actin and myosin within sarcomeres. This results in a greater extent and velocity of myocyte shortening during contraction, which allows for a stronger ventricular contraction and larger SV. This mechanism allows the heart to maintain its ejection fraction in the face of increased preload. By decreasing intravascular volume, diuretics reduce preload and can be used to lower blood pressure. Venodilators also reduce preload and can therefore be used for similar purposes.

   In addition, a variety of positions or maneuvers can be tried to manipulate venous return (preload) to the heart. For example, both the Valsalva maneuver (expiration against a closed glottis) and standing will decrease preload, and both squatting and passive leg raising will increase preload. Having the patient perform these actions can be useful when distinguishing various murmurs from one another (Fig. 1-1).

   Note: Another theory to explain the Frank-Starling relationship proposes that cardiac troponin becomes increasingly sensitive to cytosolic calcium at greater sarcomere lengths, thereby resulting in increased calcium binding and increased force of muscle contraction. Note that beyond a certain point, increasing preloads will result in less efficient ventricular contraction and a smaller SV. This situation occurs in heart failure.

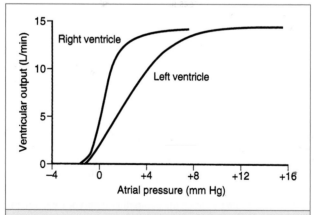

Figure 1-1. Increased ventricular output as a function of end-diastolic volume (reflected by atrial pressure). (From Guyton AC, Hall JE: Textbook of Medical Physiology, 11th ed. Philadelphia, WB Saunders, 2006, p 112.)

5. **What is contractility and how does it affect stroke volume?**
   Contractility is a measure of how forcefully the ventricle contracts at a given preload. Naturally, a more forceful contraction will eject a greater fraction of blood from the ventricle, thereby increasing the SV. Contractility is principally influenced by the activities of the sympathetic nervous system (β_1-adrenergic receptors) and parasympathetic nervous system (muscarinic [M_2] cholinergic receptors) on ventricular myocytes. By antagonizing this sympathetic input to

the myocardium, beta blockers exert part of their antihypertensive effects by reducing contractility, which reduces SV, CO, and oxygen demand. Contractility is also increased by increased concentrations of intracellular calcium (which is indirectly achieved by digitalis and decreased concentrations of extracellular sodium). This mechanism will be explained in further detail in the discussion regarding digitalis. In addition to beta blockade, contractility is decreased by systolic dysfunction, hypoxia, hypercapnia, calcium channel blockade, and acidosis (K^+ loss from cells secondary to H^+/K^+ exchange results in a more negative transmembrane potential that decreases myocyte excitability).

6. **What is afterload and how does it affect stroke volume?**

Afterload is the pressure or resistance against which the ventricles must pump blood, the primary determinant of which is systemic arterial pressure. For a given preload and contractility, increasing the afterload will decrease the SV. A simplified way of understanding this is to think of the time available for electrical and mechanical systole as finite. With increased afterload, more time is taken up by isovolumic contraction to build up to a pressure that exceeds the aortic pressure and allow the aortic valve to open. This step leaves less time for blood to enter the aorta from the ventricle (SV) during the rapid and slow ejection phases.

Note: In aortic stenosis, the stenotic aortic valve increases the afterload, which in the absence of compensatory changes such as ventricular hypertrophy tends to reduce SV and CO. Systemic hypertension also increases afterload by increasing the pressure against which the left ventricle must pump.

7. **What are the primary determinants of peripheral resistance?**

Total peripheral resistance (TPR) to blood flow is principally mediated by arteriolar diameter, which is modified by arteriolar vasoconstriction and dilation, respectively. Recall that resistance to blood flow through a vessel is inversely proportional to the fourth power of the radius. Hence, relatively small changes in arteriolar diameter (and thus radius) can have profound effects on blood flow.

The sympathetic nervous system promotes arteriolar vasoconstriction by stimulating α_1-adrenergic receptors, which increases calcium influx (via calcium channels) into arteriolar smooth muscle and stimulates their contraction. Consequently, α_1-adrenergic receptors and arteriolar calcium channels are two selective targets for antihypertensive drugs.

In all organs except for the lungs, arteriolar vasodilation is promoted by tissue hypoxia and accumulation of metabolic wastes, such as adenosine, that accumulate when oxygen demand increases (e.g., during exercise). This vasodilation allows supply to meet demand.

Note: In general, there is no direct parasympathetic innervation of the vasculature. However, vasodilation of arterioles can be caused by exogenous cholinomimetic administration. These drugs act on uninnervated muscarinic receptors (M_3-receptors) on endothelial cells and stimulate release of nitric oxide. Nitric oxide diffuses to the adjacent smooth muscle, resulting in vasodilation and decreased peripheral resistance.

8. **What is the mechanism by which the sympathetic nervous system responds to a reduction in blood pressure?**

When blood pressure drops, arterial baroreceptors located within the carotid sinus (afferent limb mediated by the glossopharyngeal nerve) sense decreased vessel stretch and fire less frequently. This response increases efferent sympathetic outflow and inhibits parasympathetic outflow, which helps restore the blood pressure by increasing heart rate and stimulating peripheral vasoconstriction. Conversely, if the blood pressure increases, baroreceptors in the carotid sinus or aortic arch (afferent limb mediated by the vagus nerve; responds only to increases in blood pressure) fire more frequently because they are being "stretched" more, which causes greater inhibition of the sympathetic outflow (Fig. 1-2).

Note: The aortic arch and carotid sinuses also have chemoreceptors, which should not be confused with the baroreceptors. Chemoreceptors work to maintain Po_2, Pco_2, and pH.

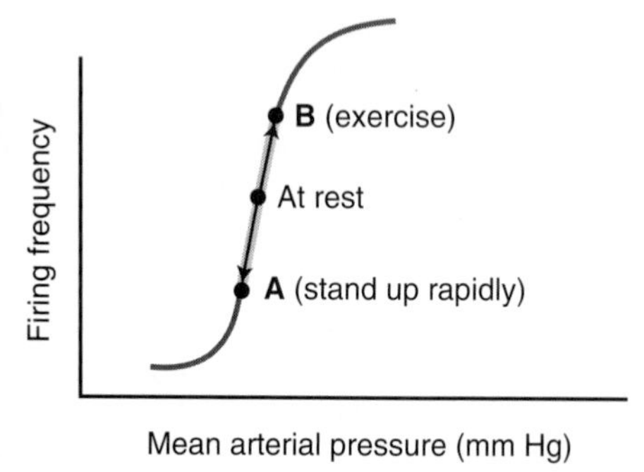

Figure 1-2. Control of blood pressure by the baroreceptor reflex. (From Brown TA: Rapid Review Physiology. Philadelphia, Mosby, 2007, p 144.)

9. **How do the α_1-receptor antagonists work?**

The α_1-receptor antagonists include the "zosins" (prazosin, terazosin, doxazosin) and antagonize peripheral vasoconstriction stimulated by the sympathetic nervous system (which is mediated by α_1-receptors). α_1-Receptors are located on vascular smooth muscle and coupled to G_q proteins. Antagonists cause decreased release of inositol triphosphate (IP_3) and subsequently prevent the release of calcium from intracellular stores, resulting in smooth muscle relaxation and arteriolar vasodilation.

α_1-Receptors are also responsible for contraction of the pupillary dilator muscle and intestinal/bladder sphincters. Thus, α_1-receptor antagonists can lead to miosis and bladder/bowel movement.

10. **How do the α_1-receptor antagonists cause orthostatic hypotension?**

Upon standing from a supine or sitting position, transient hypotension and lightheadedness (from cerebral hypoperfusion) might occur as a result of venous pooling in the lower extremities, which decreases venous return and MAP. This response is ordinarily compensated for by the baroreflex, which promotes peripheral venoconstriction and tachycardia. However, if the α_1-receptors are blocked in the peripheral venules, this reflex will be less effective at restoring the blood pressure. Nevertheless, a reflex tachycardia, which is mediated by β-receptors, will be maintained. This increase in pulse rate can be used in diagnosing orthostatic hypotension.

Note: Reflex tachycardia occurs to maintain CO. Recall that CO = HR × SV. Thus, if SV is reduced because of decreased venous return to the heart, HR must increase to maintain CO.

11. **What hemodynamic changes occur during exercise?**

Exercise requires more oxygen to be delivered to skeletal muscle to meet its increased metabolic demand. This delivery is accomplished mainly by an increase in CO secondary to increases in both SV and HR. Contraction of the lower limb muscles pushes blood toward the right atrium and increases venous return. MAP is only modestly increased during exercise despite the large increase in CO, because skeletal muscle vasodilation is mediated mostly by local cellular metabolites, which significantly decrease the SVR and allow skeletal muscle to receive up to 85% of the increased CO.

12. **Which clinical scenarios would shift the CO and venous return curves to the points labeled 1 to 4 on Figure 1-3?**

1. Exercise: Lower limb muscles push blood toward the right atrium and increase venous return. Sympathetic activity increases CO by increasing HR, SV, and contractility.
2. Arteriovenous fistulas: Increased venous return from an arteriovenous fistula will shift the venous return curve to the right. CO does increase but only because of the increased preload

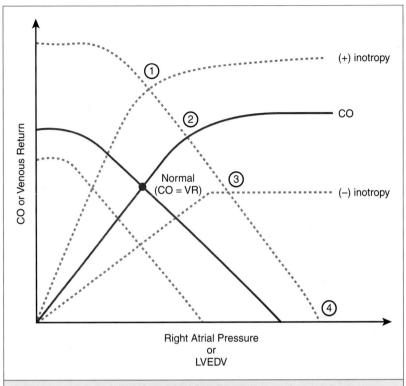

Figure 1-3. Cardiac output (CO) and venous return curves. LVEDV, left ventricular end-diastolic volume.

(Frank-Starling mechanism); this increase is therefore not due to a change in contractility (inotropy). If these arteriovenous anastomoses were much larger, the operating point of the heart would be shifted to (1) because it would cause a large decrease in SVR and stimulate the activity of the sympathetic nervous system, increasing inotropy; these large anastomoses are sometimes referred to as AV shunts.

3. Compensated heart failure: Patients with this condition have elevated right atrial pressures due to an increased volume status caused by the activity of the renin-angiotensin-aldosterone system (RAAS). Their cardiac function is decreased (decreased inotropy), but they can maintain a normal CO at rest with the increased volume (Frank-Starling mechanism).
4. Ventricular fibrillation: Ventricular fibrillation causes equalization of all pressures. Right atrial pressure increases to become equal to the mean systolic filling pressure. CO in ventricular fibrillation simply becomes equal to zero.

BASIC CONCEPTS—EXCITATION-CONTRACTION COUPLING

1. **What is the source of cytosolic calcium during ventricular systole?**
   During the plateau phase (phase 2) of the ventricular myocyte action potential, voltage-gated calcium channels allow calcium influx from the extracellular fluid into the cytosol, stimulating calcium release from the sarcoplasmic reticulum, a phenomenon referred to as *calcium-induced calcium release*. In fact, the majority of the cytosolic calcium comes from the sarcoplasmic

reticulum, not the extracellular fluid. This mechanism of calcium release is in contrast to release from skeletal muscle, in which depolarization of the cell membrane triggers sarcoplasmic calcium release without entry of extracellular calcium into the cytosol.

2. **What is the function of calcium in cardiac muscle contraction?**
   Cytosolic calcium binds to troponin C, resulting in a conformational change that removes tropomyosin from myosin-binding sites on actin to allow for the sliding filament mechanism of contraction. The force of contraction is proportional to the intracellular Ca^{2+} level. Note that unlike skeletal muscle, cardiac muscle is dependent on extracellular calcium influx for contraction to occur.

   The cardioselective calcium channel blockers (verapamil, diltiazem) reduce contractility by antagonizing extracellular calcium entry and the subsequent calcium-induced calcium release that occurs in heart muscle. In addition to decreasing heart rate, this action is another mechanism by which calcium channel blockers work to lower blood pressure.

3. **What is the mechanism by which β-adrenergic stimulation increases cardiac contractility?**
   β-Adrenergic stimulation results in an increase in cyclic adenosine monophosphate (cAMP), which promotes cAMP-dependent phosphorylation of a number of proteins via protein kinase A (PKA). Phosphorylation of L-type calcium channels results in increased calcium entry into the myocyte. In addition, β-adrenergic stimulation results in phosphorylation and inhibition of a protein called phospholamban, which normally serves as an inhibitor of the sarco/endoplasmic reticulum calcium adenosine triphosphatase, or ATPase (SERCA). Thus, inhibition of phospholamban allows for increased calcium entry into the sarcoplasmic reticulum and subsequent increase in calcium release during the next action potential, which augments myocyte contractility.

4. **What is the contribution of the sympathetic nervous system to ventricular relaxation?**
   In addition to stimulating calcium influx, the β-adrenergic pathway also stimulates calcium uptake by the ventricular sarcoplasmic reticulum due to phosphorylation of SERCA by PKA. This removal of cytosolic calcium into the sarcoplasmic reticulum is required for ventricular relaxation; so the more rapidly it is removed, the more rapidly the ventricles relax. Such rapid ventricular relaxation at elevated HRs is important to ensure adequate ventricular filling during the decreased period of diastole. Recall that HR is increased with sympathetic stimulation via direct binding of cAMP to special channels in the pacemaker cells that conduct the If current ("funny current"; this current is carried by sodium ions and allows the membrane potential to become progressively less negative during the repolarization phase of the pacemaker cell), which increases the probability of their open time, thereby promoting sodium influx and increasing the slope of phase 4 depolarization.

   Note: Calcium uptake into the sarcoplasmic reticulum is an energy-requiring process, and in ischemic heart disease the reduced oxygen delivery makes calcium uptake less efficient, thereby impairing ventricular relaxation and causing diastolic dysfunction.

BASIC CONCEPTS—ARRHYTHMIAS

1. **What is the relationship between the various phases of the ventricular myocyte action potential and the different ion fluxes across the cell membrane?**
   In phase 0 of the action potential, the sharp rise in membrane voltage is due to sodium influx. Phase 1 involves a brief repolarization that is due to the transient outward flow of potassium that follows sodium channel inactivation. In phase 2, the action potential plateaus are due to a balance between calcium influx and potassium efflux. During phase 3, there is rapid repolarization due to unopposed potassium efflux. Phase 4 is the resting potential, which is maintained predominantly through the opening of potassium channels. Intracellular

concentrations of K+ are maintained at high levels in cardiac myocytes because of the action of membrane-bound Na+K+-ATPase. Opening of potassium channels during phase 4 leads to potassium efflux (down its concentration gradient). Since the cell is permeable only to potassium at this time, negatively charged counter ions for K+ are unable to diffuse outward with potassium. As potassium leaves the cell, anions left behind cause the cell to become increasingly negative in charge. Therefore the effluxed potassium ions are attracted back toward the interior of the cell to maintain resting potential. Because phase 4 is dominated by potassium permeability, it therefore has a value close to the potassium reversal potential (-85 mV) (Fig. 1-4).

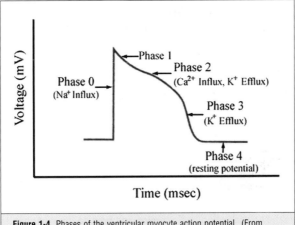

Figure 1-4. Phases of the ventricular myocyte action potential. (From Brown TA, Brown D: USMLE Step 1 Secrets. Philadelphia, Hanley & Belfus, 2004, p 77.)

Note: The antiarrhythmic agents all work by affecting one or more components of the action potential. Class I antiarrhythmics block sodium channels and antagonize phase 0. Class III antiarrhythmics work by blocking potassium channels, which prolongs phase 3 depolarization. Some class IA and all class III antiarrhythmics increase action potential duration as well as the QT interval. Toxicity of these agents can lead to torsades de pointes, which is associated with long QT syndrome.

2. **What is responsible for the drifting of the resting membrane potential in nodal cells?**
These cells are more permeable to sodium, so sodium influx during the "resting" membrane potential causes the membrane to gradually depolarize. Because nodal cells lack the fast voltage-gated sodium channels (I_{Na}) found in the rest of the myocardium, this is accomplished by the I_f sodium current, a unique "leaky" sodium channel that promotes the gradual depolarization of these cells through sodium influx. Eventually, when the membrane depolarizes to its "threshold,"; this state will activate slow calcium channels that engender an action potential (Fig. 1-5).
Note: The calcium channel blockers verapamil and diltiazem affect heart rate by antagonizing these slow calcium channels on the SA node. These drugs are considered class IV antiarrhythmics.

3. **Through what mechanism does sympathetic stimulation increase heart rate?**
The release of norepinephrine from sympathetic neurons causes activation of β_1-adrenergic receptors in nodal tissue. These receptors stimulate production of cAMP, resulting in an increase in I_f and a positive chronotropic effect on the heart. In essence, sympathetic stimulation increases

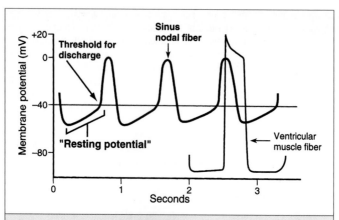

Figure 1-5. Rhythmic discharge of a sinus nodal fiber. The sinus nodal action potential is also compared with that of ventricular muscle fiber. (From Guyton AC, Hall JE: Textbook of Medical Physiology, 11th ed. Philadelphia, WB Saunders, 2006, p 117.)

the cellular influx of sodium ions and decreases the efflux of potassium ions, thus increasing the slope of the resting potential in the nodal cells. Beta blockers reduce heart rate by antagonizing this effect. **Note:** The beta blockers are considered class II antiarrhythmics.

4. **What are the classes of antiarrhythmics and how do their mechanisms of action and potential side effects vary?**
   See Table 1-1 for this information.

TABLE 1-1. ANTIARRHYTHMIC DRUGS

Drug Class	Mechanism of Action*	Prototype Agent(s)	Potential Side Effects
IA	Inhibits Na^+ and K^+ channels, prolongs QRS complex and QT interval, prolongs effective refractory period (ERP)	Quinidine, procainamide	Lupus-like syndrome (procainamide), torsades de pointes
IB	Inhibit Na^+ channels, shortens repolarization, ↓ QT interval	Lidocaine	
IC	Inhibit Na^+ channels, prolongs QRS complex	Flecainide	
II	↑ PR interval, ↓ automaticity (↓ slope of phase 4 depolarization in nodal cells)	Propranolol	

Continued

TABLE 1-1. ANTIARRHYTHMIC DRUGS—continued

Drug Class	Mechanism of Action*	Prototype Agent(s)	Potential Side Effects
III	Inhibits K^+ channels	Amiodarone	Pulmonary fibrosis, corneal deposits, gray man syndrome, hepatotoxicity, thyroid dysfunction
IV	Inhibits calcium channels, ↑ PR interval, ↓ automaticity	Verapamil, diltiazem	Flushing

*There is considerable overlap regarding the mechanisms of action of these antiarrhythmics. For the sake of simplicity, only the *primary* mechanism of action is considered in this classification.

CASE 1-1

A 60-year-old man presents for his third visit in 2 months with a blood pressure of approximately 155/95 mm Hg on each occasion. Physical examination is unremarkable. A 3-month trial of diet and exercise modifications fails to reduce his blood pressure.

1. **What are the types of hypertension and which does this patient most likely have?**
The two types of hypertension are essential (primary, idiopathic) hypertension and secondary hypertension. Essential hypertension is thought to account for approximately 90% of cases of hypertension and is most likely to be due to an inability of the kidney to properly excrete sodium at a given filtered load; this has been described through the *pressure natriuresis theory*. When approaching a patient with hypertension, it is important to first rule out secondary hypertension, which indicates additional pathologic changes. Treatment of secondary hypertension is aimed at addressing the underlying cause of the condition. Potential sources of secondary hypertension include renal artery stenosis, primary hyperaldosteronism, pheochromocytoma, coarctation of the aorta, chronic renal disease, excessive alcohol use, pregnancy, increased intracranial pressure, and various medications, such as monoamine oxidase inhibitors, oral decongestants, nonsteroidal anti-inflammatory drugs, and oral contraceptives. If causes of secondary hypertension are ruled out, then essential hypertension is diagnosed by exclusion.
    Note: The mechanisms involved in essential hypertension are poorly understood. A second theory proposes that people with essential hypertension have increased vascular resistance. This may be due to increased circulating vasoconstrictors, increased sensitivity to these substances, or a deficiency of the nitric oxide vasodilation pathway.

2. **How is hypertension defined and what are the potential complications?**
The Joint National Committee on Detection, Evaluation, and Treatment of High Blood Pressure guidelines (JNC 7) for defining hypertension are presented in Table 1-2.

TABLE 1-2. JOINT NATIONAL COMMITTEE ON DETECTION, EVALUATION, AND TREATMENT OF HIGH BLOOD PRESSURE GUIDELINES FOR DEFINING HYPERTENSION

Category	Blood Pressure Range (mm Hg)	
	Systolic	Diastolic
Normal	<120	<80
Prehypertension	120-139	80-89
Hypertension: stage 1	140-159	90-99
Hypertension: stage 2	≥160	≥100

Evidence suggests that the risk for complications in hypertensive disease is a continuum, increasing as blood pressure rises. It is also largely influenced by comorbid conditions. Major complications of hypertension include accelerated atherosclerosis, premature cardiovascular disease, diastolic (and to a lesser extent, systolic) heart failure, stroke, intracerebral hemorrhage, chronic renal insufficiency, end-stage renal disease, retinopathy, and acute hypertensive crisis.

3. **What are four classes of drugs that could be useful in treating this man's hypertension?**
   - Diuretics (e.g., thiazides, loop, potassium-sparing)
   - Inhibitors of the renin-angiotensin-aldosterone system (e.g., angiotensin-converting enzyme [ACE] inhibitors, angiotensin receptor blockers)
   - Vasodilators (e.g., direct-acting, calcium channel blockers)
   - Sympatholytics (e.g., clonidine)

CASE 1-1 continued:

Because this patient has received three elevated blood pressure readings in the past 2 months and is unresponsive to lifestyle modifications, he is started on metoprolol.

4. **What is the mechanism by which metoprolol will reduce blood pressure in this man?**
   Metoprolol is a relatively selective β_1-adrenergic receptor blocker. Antagonizing these receptors decreases heart rate and contractility, both of which reduce CO, thereby lowering blood pressure (recall that MAP = CO × TPR). Beta blockers also reduce blood pressure by blocking the renal secretion of renin. Both β_1- and β_2-adrenergic blockers appear to inhibit the renin-angiotensin-aldosterone system (RAAS) to some extent. For this reason, beta blockers might be more effective in hypertensive patients with elevated plasma renin levels as opposed to normal or low plasma renin levels.

5. **What pharmacologic property makes certain beta blockers more "cardioselective" than others?**
   Some beta blockers (atenolol, esmolol, nebivolol, and metoprolol) are more selective for the β_1-receptors on the heart, with less effect on the β_2-receptors that lead to smooth muscle relaxation in the bronchioles and skeletal muscle arterioles. Thus, specific β_1-antagonists have less affinity to inhibit catecholamine-mediated bronchodilation and peripheral muscle vasodilation.

6. **Caution should be used in prescribing beta blockers for patients with which comorbid conditions and why?**
   - Asthma: Risk of worsening bronchospasm by preventing β_2-mediated bronchodilation. (Even β_1- "selective" antagonists have some effect, especially at high doses.) For the purpose of the USMLE, remember that β_1-selective blockers should be used in patients with pulmonary disease.

- COPD (chronic obstructive pulmonary disease) patients for similar reasons.
- Peripheral arterial disease: Exacerbation of claudication. (Vasodilation in skeletal muscle arterioles is mediated by β_2-adrenergic receptors present on vascular smooth muscle cells.)
- First-degree atrioventricular (AV) block: Beta blockers decrease AV conduction and thus further lengthen the already prolonged PR interval on the electrocardiogram (ECG). This can result in excessive cardiac depression. (Beta blockers should not be given at all to patients with second- or third-degree AV block because they could delay AV conduction even further. Certain calcium channel blockers, such as verapamil and diltiazem, might also reduce AV conduction and, when used in combination with beta blockers, can produce a serious AV block.)
- Diabetes: Beta blockers reduce the normal symptoms of hypoglycemia (e.g., headache, confusion, slurred speech, anxiety, tremors, palpitations) that provide warning to diabetic patients prior to reaching dangerously low blood sugar levels.
- Because of their ability to reduce myocardial oxygen demand, beta blocker use has been shown to have a survival benefit in patients with congestive heart failure. However, caution should be used when placing patients on beta blockers, as they may initially exacerbate CHF symptoms (decompensated heart failure).
- Erectile dysfunction: beta blockers may inhibit b2 adrenergic receptor-mediated vasodilation.
- Depression: Mechanism of action is unclear, but presumably involves alterations in monoamine neurotransmitter signaling.

CASE 1-1 continued:

After a number of months, the patient returns to the office complaining of an impaired ability to keep up with his wife on their daily hikes. He feels that he gets tired more quickly, attributes this to the metoprolol, and plans to quit taking his medication.

7. **What might be occurring in this patient and how would you recommend he discontinue his medication?**
    Beta blockers are likely impairing his exercise tolerance by preventing the necessary increase in HR to meet his oxygen demand. Trying him on another class of antihypertensives would be reasonable, but his metoprolol should first be tapered because chronic beta blocker use substantially increases the sensitivity of the heart to catecholamines by upregulating beta receptors on cardiomyocytes. Consequently, sudden withdrawal of these drugs can lead to tachycardia, arrhythmias, and acute myocardial infarction. For this reason, patients should always be gradually weaned off beta blockers.

SUMMARY BOX: HYPERTENSION

- Essential hypertension is the most common type of hypertension.
- The most common causes of secondary hypertension are renal artery stenosis and primary hyperaldosteronism.
- Beta blockers lower blood pressure in part by reducing renin secretion from the kidneys (primarily a β_1-receptor–mediated effect).
- Beta blockers decrease atrioventricular (AV) conduction and therefore should be used cautiously in patients with first-degree heart block.

CASE 1-2

A 48-year-old man is newly diagnosed with both type 2 diabetes mellitus and hypertension. To help control his blood sugar, he is started on metformin.

1. **How would the fact that this patient also has diabetes influence treatment for his hypertension? Consider drug choice and aggressiveness of treatment.**
   Angiotensin-converting enzyme (ACE) inhibitors are the preferred first-line antihypertensives in diabetics. ACE inhibitors have been shown to reduce the progression of proteinuria (and the subsequent nephropathy) in diabetic patients. Although the mechanism behind the nephroprotective actions of ACE inhibitors remains unclear, it could be related to their ability to preferentially dilate the efferent arteriole and thereby reduce glomerular filtration pressures.

   Diabetes is a cardiovascular risk factor and predisposes patients to both microvascular and macrovascular damage. Tight blood pressure control is critical in diabetics to reduce the mortality risk from macrovascular disease (CAD, CVA, PVD). Additionally, it reduces the risk of microvascular complications such as retinopathy, nephropathy, and neuropathy.

2. **What are the mechanisms by which ACE inhibitors lower blood pressure?**
   These drugs prevent the conversion of angiotensin I to angiotensin II. Angiotensin II contributes to peripheral vasoconstriction, stimulation of thirst, renal sodium reabsorption in the proximal tubule, and aldosterone production, all of which are antagonized by ACE inhibitors (Fig. 1-6).

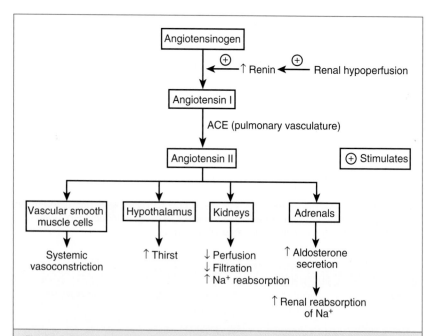

Figure 1-6. Enzymatic cascade in the renin-angiotensin-aldosterone system. Note diagrammatic representation of physiologic actions of angiotensin II. ACE, angiotensin-converting enzyme. (From Brown TA: Rapid Review Physiology. Philadelphia, Mosby, 2007, p 148.)

3. **Why might the use of beta blockers to control this man's hypertension not be an ideal choice (at least for the purpose of boards)?**
   These drugs could mask important signs of hypoglycemia, such as tremor and palpitations, that are mediated through the sympathetic nervous system. Beta blockers also antagonize epinephrine-stimulated hepatic gluconeogenesis and glycogenolysis, thereby contributing to hypoglycemia. However, hypoglycemia is much more of a concern with diabetics on second-generation sulfonylureas, dipeptidyl peptidase (DPP-4) inhibitors, or insulin.
   Note: Although beta blockers could mask many of the symptoms associated with hypoglycemia, they will not prevent the diaphoresis commonly seen in severe hypoglycemia, because sweat glands are innervated by sympathetic cholinergic nerves rather than sympathetic adrenergic nerves.

4. **What effect might starting a thiazide diuretic have on glycemic control in this patient?**
   Diuretics commonly worsen hyperglycemia in diabetics. Although the mechanism(s) remain uncertain, the hyperglycemia is likely related to a combination of hypokalemia and intravascular volume depletion that occurs with initiation of diuretic therapy. Hypokalemia can contribute to impaired glucose tolerance because it inhibits insulin secretion, stimulates insulin resistance, and impairs cellular glucose uptake (potassium is a necessary cotransporter for glucose uptake).
   The intravascular volume depletion resulting from diuresis reduces CO, which stimulates the sympathetic nervous system, thereby promoting insulin resistance and reduced glucose uptake by the liver and skeletal muscle.
   Whereas this is seldom seen clinically, for the purpose of boards you should note that thiazide diuretics should be used cautiously in diabetics because they may theoretically increase risk of hyperlipidemia and hyperuricemia.

CASE 1-2 continued:

The patient is started on lisinopril, which he initially tolerates well. After about a month he develops an annoying dry cough and wonders if it is somehow related to his new medication.

5. **What is the mechanism by which ACE inhibitors, such as lisinopril, can cause a cough?**
   Angiotensin-converting enzyme (ACE) is also known as kininase; it can degrade bradykinin in the blood. Accumulation of bradykinin with ACE inhibitors is believed to be the primary cause of the cough. It is thought that the accumulated bradykinin somehow stimulates nociceptors in the airways, thereby initiating the cough reflex. This undesirable side effect can be avoided by using angiotensin receptor blockers (ARBs) such as losartan.

6. **Cover the columns on the right side of Table 1-3, and for each antihypertensive drug in the left column, try to name the class of drug, mechanism of action, and primary side effects associated with its use.**

TABLE 1-3. ANTIHYPERTENSIVE DRUGS			
Drug	Drug Class	Primary Mechanism of Action	Primary Side Effects
Hydralazine	Arterial vasodilator	Unknown	Lupus-like syndrome Reflex tachycardia

Continued

ischemia promotes anaerobic respiration and the release of substances such as lactic acid that cause cardiac pain.

Note: Recall that visceral cardiac pain is sensed by sympathetic fibers that travel parallel to the coronary vessels and enter the spinal cord between C8 and T4. Be alert for "silent" cardiac ischemia in patients with autonomic neuropathy (e.g., diabetics) or patients who have received a heart transplant (in which the autonomic fibers have been severed).

CASE 1-3 continued:

The patient states that his episodes of chest pressure generally last around 5 minutes but never longer than 15 minutes. They often occur when he uses the push-mower to mow the lawn on the steep part of the yard or when he rides his bicycle up a hill, but not when he is walking, sitting, or sleeping. He thinks the severity and pattern of chest pain have stayed pretty much the same since he first noticed it 6 months ago.

2. **Does this patient have stable or unstable angina? How are they different, and which is more serious?**

   He has stable angina. In stable angina, a constant and predictable level of physical exertion elicits the chest pain or substernal discomfort. Stable angina usually lasts between 2 and 5 minutes, sometimes over 10 minutes, but rarely over 15 minutes or less than 1 minute. It is always promptly relieved by rest. In contrast, unstable angina is characterized by the development of chest pain at rest or after only mild exertion and can last longer than 15 minutes. Unstable angina is more serious because it indicates a disruption within the atheromatous plaque(s) in the coronary arteries that is causing ischemia. It may also involve the formation of a nonocclusive thrombus. When unstable angina develops, the patient should be emergently evaluated to rule out an impending myocardial infarction.

3. **How can angina occur in the absence of coronary atherosclerosis?**

   This angina occurs in Prinzmetal's (variant or vasospastic) angina, in which transmural cardiac ischemia occurs due to vasospasm of the coronary arteries. You should suspect Prinzmetal's angina in a patient who has anginal symptoms at rest or in the morning. Prinzmetal's angina is thought to be chemically mediated by an increased platelet production of thromboxane A_2 (TXA_2) or an increased production of endothelin-1 in damaged endothelial cells. Severe anemia could also theoretically produce angina because of reduced delivery of oxygen to the heart and an increased demand on the heart to pump more blood because there are fewer red blood cells in circulation. On rare occasions, patients with pheochromocytoma without coronary artery disease can experience severe coronary vasospasm resulting in cardiac ischemia and, at times, even myocardial infarction. Lastly, ventricular hypertrophy may cause subendocardial ischemia and angina because the increase in myocardial perfusion is usually not as great proportionally as the degree of myocardial hypertrophy.

4. **What are the principal physiologic determinants of myocardial oxygen supply?**

   Myocardial oxygen supply is dependent on coronary artery perfusion and the arterial oxygen-carrying capacity.

   - Myocardial perfusion is primarily dependent on diastolic time, diastolic perfusion pressure, thickness of the myocardium, and the vascular resistance of the coronary arteries.
   - Arterial oxygen-carrying capacity is largely dependent on the hemoglobin concentration and the efficiency of gas exchange at the lungs (oxygen saturation).

   Although severe anemia or hypoxemia can decrease myocardial oxygen supply substantially, supply is more often limited as a result of inadequate myocardial perfusion. This can result from tachycardia (decreased time spent in diastole, the period when the majority of left ventricular blood flow occurs), inadequate diastolic perfusion pressure resulting from hypotension, dehydration, valvular abnormalities such as aortic regurgitation, or an increased left ventricular end-diastolic pressure (LVEDP), which occurs in concentric and eccentric hypertrophy.

5. **What are the principal physiologic determinants of myocardial oxygen demand?**
Any factor that affects the hemodynamics of the cardiovascular system can affect myocardial oxygen demand. Thus, oxygen demand is increased as HR, contractility, afterload, and sympathetic activity increase. To compensate for elevated oxygen demand, the heart increases coronary blood flow, which in turn increases oxygen delivery. Recall that oxygen extraction from the coronary arteries is very efficient (assumed to be 100%), so the only way to increase oxygen delivery to the heart is to alter coronary blood flow.

6. **Which factors contribute to a myocardial oxygen demand that exceeds supply in this man?**
Demand is increased by the sympathetic mediated increase in HR as well as contractility in response to exercise. At the same time, supply is decreased because an elevated HR gives his sclerotic coronary arteries less time to increase blood flow to the myocardium by shortening the amount of time available for diastole.

7. **Why is nitroglycerin effective in eliminating anginal pain?**
Nitroglycerin is converted within endothelial cells to nitric oxide, which is also referred to as endothelium-derived relaxation factor (EDRF) because of its vasodilatory effects. Perhaps the most important reason nitroglycerin eliminates anginal pain is its effect on reducing myocardial oxygen demand secondary to venous dilation (decreasing preload) and arteriolar dilation (reducing afterload). For Step 1, however, it is important to know that the effect of nitroglycerin is much greater on reducing preload than afterload because it dilates veins more than arteries. In any case, decreasing preload and afterload reduces cardiac contractility and myocardial wall tension, which additionally allows greater myocardial perfusion during systole. Nitroglycerin and other organic nitrates also exert effects directly on the coronary vasculature, including vasodilation of the coronary arteries and relief of coronary artery spasm. The precise mechanisms by which nitrates reduce symptoms of anginal pain therefore will depend on which pathologic mechanism is responsible for the angina in a given patient (e.g., atherosclerotic occlusion, vasospasm).

   Note: High doses of nitrates can produce *reflex tachycardia*, which occurs in response to hypotension, and this can further exacerbate anginal pain by increasing myocardial oxygen demand. Because nitrates relax both vascular and nonvascular smooth muscle, they can relieve the pain of both angina and esophageal spasm, making it difficult to distinguish between these two conditions based solely on their response to nitrates. The compensatory tachycardia that develops because of nitroglycerin-mediated vasodilation can be prevented with beta blockers.

8. **What are the mechanisms by which beta blockers decrease myocardial oxygen demand and, therefore, the symptoms of angina?**
Beta blockers exert negative chronotropic and inotropic effects on the heart, producing a reduction in afterload, which reduces wall stress and myocardial O_2 demand, and increased myocardial perfusion as a result of increased time spent in diastole, when the myocardium is largely perfused. For these reasons beta blockers are helpful in preventing angina and in certain circumstances can also be used to treat angina.

CASE 1-3 continued:

An exercise stress test is performed to evaluate the possibility of coronary artery disease and to assess the patient's level of cardiopulmonary function. While he is on the treadmill, the ECG reveals cardiac ischemia (shown by ST-segment depression) when his heart rate and blood pressure have both increased ~50% above baseline.

9. How could a similar evaluation be made in a patient in whom an exercise stress is contraindicated (e.g., orthopedic condition or chronic lung disease)?
    Pharmacologic agents can be used to simulate the stress of exercise. Dobutamine (a synthetic catecholamine) has positive inotropic and chronotropic effects on the heart, so its administration is physiologically similar to physical exertion because both cause an increase in myocardial oxygen demand. However, adenosine (a potent coronary vasodilator with a short half-life) is more commonly used, along with positron emission tomography (PET) scanning to acquire an accurate image of coronary perfusion.

SUMMARY BOX: ANGINA

- The three main forms of angina are stable, unstable, and variant. Distinguishing among these patterns has important implications for prognosis and treatment.

- An imbalance between myocardial oxygen supply and demand underlies the pathophysiology of angina.

- Nitroglycerin's primary mechanism of action is dilation of peripheral veins, which reduces preload and therefore myocardial oxygen demand. It also has direct effects on the coronary arteries, so it can be useful for all three forms of angina.

CASE 1-4

A 52-year-old man presents to the emergency department for evaluation of a crushing substernal pressure sensation for the past hour. He is obese and diaphoretic. The pain radiates to his left arm and his jaw. He is concerned because he usually gets chest pain only after exercising, which is typically relieved by rest but this pain began at rest. Additionally, he feels nauseated, which is not something he noticed during past episodes.

1. What disorder is on top of the differential diagnosis list at this point and why?
    Myocardial infarction (MI), likely due to underlying coronary artery disease, is the probable diagnosis. The typical presentation involves crushing substernal pain for longer than 30 minutes that is not relieved by nitroglycerin. This diagnosis should be considered immediately because a timely intervention is essential to the patient's outcome. Acute MI is a leading cause of death in adults in the United States and has a high incidence rate in men between the ages of 40 and 65.

2. What are some common risk factors for myocardial infarction and cardiovascular disease in general?
    Male gender under age 65, family history of premature CAD, hypertension, diabetes mellitus, tobacco use, dyslipidemia (high low-density lipoprotein [LDL], low high-density lipoprotein [HDL], high triglycerides), and increased C-reactive protein (CRP) are just a few of the risk factors.

CASE 1-4 continued:

An ECG is performed immediately and reveals ST-segment elevation in two consecutive leads. A chest x-ray study does not show mediastinal widening or other abnormalities. The patient is administered morphine, oxygen, nitroglycerin, metoprolol, and aspirin. The consulting cardiologist decides that the patient is a suitable candidate for emergent angioplasty, and he is taken to the cardiac catheterization laboratory.

3. What kind of myocardial infarction is this patient experiencing?
He is experiencing an ST-segment elevation myocardial infarction (STEMI), the pathophysiology of which classically involves complete occlusion of a coronary artery resulting in transmural tissue infarction. Studies have shown that these patients are best treated emergently by angioplasty if this is available. On the other hand, subendocardial MIs (affect only a portion of the ventricular wall thickness,) lack ST-segment elevation, and are thus referred to as non-STEMI (NSTEMI). The subendocardium is particularly vulnerable to ischemia owing to exposure to high pressures and a relative lack of collateral circulation. NSTEMIs are typically caused by a near total occlusion of a coronary artery. Patients with NSTEMIs also have elevations in cardiac enzymes due to myocardial damage, and these patients may also benefit from cardiac catheterization.

4. In addition to analysis of the electrocardiogram, what serum tests could be ordered to confirm or rule out a myocardial infarction?
When a patient presents to the emergency department with an MI, an ECG is the gold standard to determine whether to send the patient to the catheterization laboratory or administer thrombolytics when a catheterization laboratory is not readily accessible. Levels of cardiac enzymes, which have leaked out of the necrotic myocardial tissue, may be more sensitive indicators of MI but may not elevate to diagnostic levels until several hours after the onset of chest pain. These enzymes include troponin I (TnI), creatine kinase MB fraction (CK-MB), aspartate transaminase (AST), and myoglobin, with each having unique specificities and different times for peak elevation. Myoglobin rises soon after onset of cardiac pain. Although it is a very early marker, it is nonspecific for MI. Troponin I rises after 4 hours and is the most specific among the markers; it also remains elevated for the longest period of time (7–10 days). CK-MB has good specificity and begins to rise with troponin. It does not remain elevated nearly as long as troponins do, but this pattern can be clinically useful in diagnosing a recurrent MI if CK-MB becomes elevated again after 72 hours. AST has poor specificity and peaks the day after an MI.
Because these enzymes remain elevated for some time, they may be more useful than an ECG (which provides only a snapshot of the heart for a moment in time) in someone who describes symptoms of an MI that occurred in the past few days (Fig. 1-7).

CASE 1-4 continued:

In the cardiac catheterization laboratory, the patient's angiogram shows a 95% narrowing of the left anterior descending coronary artery. Angioplasty is performed, and a bare metal stent is successfully placed, restoring patency to the vessel. After 6 days in the hospital, the patient is discharged with prescriptions for lisinopril, lovastatin, clopidogrel, and metoprolol in addition to the daily aspirin and as-needed nitroglycerin he was already taking.

5. What other treatment option is available besides angioplasty to restore coronary blood flow? What are the major contraindications to its use?
Thrombolytic therapy with tissue plasminogen activator (tPA) or streptokinase, which must be performed within a certain time frame to be effective. Thrombolytic therapy is contraindicated in patients at high risk for hemorrhage (e.g., recent major surgery, bleeding disorder, anticoagulant use, severe hypertension, recent hemorrhagic cerebrovascular accident [CVA]).

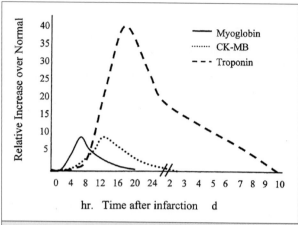

Figure 1-7. Myoglobin, creatine kinase MB fraction (CK-MB), and cardiac troponin increase after a myocardial infarction (MI). CK-MB peaks after about 16 to 24 hours and remains elevated for approximately 72 hours. Troponin peaks around 24 hours after an MI and remains elevated for 7 to 10 days. (From Henry JB: Clinical Diagnosis and Management by Laboratory Methods, 20th ed. Philadelphia, WB Saunders, 2001, p 297.)

Note: Bleeding caused by thrombolytic therapy can be treated with *aminocaproic acid*, which inhibits the activation of plasminogen.

STEP 1 SECRET

Knowing the antidotes for common drug overdoses will be useful for Step 1.

6. **What is the physiologic rationale for giving beta blockers to patients who have had heart attacks?**
As in angina, these drugs lower myocardial oxygen demand, making the heart less susceptible to infarction. Additionally, because infarction creates an area of fibrosis that can produce an arrhythmia, beta blockers are also useful for their antiarrhythmic properties. However, if the infarction involves the tissues of the conduction pathway and results in heart block, beta blocker use may be contraindicated. Overall, beta blockers have been shown to reduce mortality when given after an MI.

7. **How might a myocardial infarction result in the following short- and long-term abnormalities?**
A. Pulmonary edema?
    Pulmonary edema can result in two ways: (1) The weakened left ventricle (LV) might no longer be able to effectively pump blood into the aorta, resulting in a reduced ejection fraction. This is termed *systolic dysfunction*. (2) The left ventricle could still pump effectively but might become stiff (noncompliant) as a result of the infarct (and ongoing ischemia), thus necessitating increased ventricular filling pressures to achieve an adequate end-diastolic volume. This is termed *diastolic dysfunction*. Regardless of the precise cause (LV pump failure or

noncompliance), the increased left ventricular filling pressures result in increased left atrial and pulmonary hydrostatic capillary pressures, ultimately leading to transudation of fluid into the pulmonary interstitium and alveolar space.

Initially, this interstitial fluid is completely removed by the pulmonary lymphatics. However, when the pulmonary capillary hydrostatic pressure increases too much (typically >30 mm Hg), the ability of the lymphatics to remove excess fluid is overcome, and interstitial fluid and intra-alveolar fluid accumulate, resulting in pulmonary edema. Pulmonary edema reduces oxygen diffusion across the pulmonary membrane, causing hypoxemia, which further exacerbates the failing heart. This is one reason why oxygen therapy may be beneficial after a severe MI.

B. Arrhythmias?

Leakage of electrolytes from the necrotic myocardial cells results in electrolyte imbalances that can instigate arrhythmias. These arrhythmias are most common within a few days after the MI.

C. Murmur?

If the MI causes rupture of the ventricular septum or a papillary muscle, then the respective murmurs of a ventricular septal defect (VSD) or valvular regurgitation would be heard (both of which are holosystolic murmurs).

D. Ventricular rupture?

The inflammatory reaction in the infarcted site weakens the myocardial wall. Ventricular rupture typically occurs between 3 and 7 days after the infarct and can result in hemopericardium.

E. Pericarditis?

The inflammatory reaction to necrotic myocardium can also cause pericarditis (usually within the first week after the MI). Suspect this if the patient has a pericardial friction rub. Dressler's syndrome is a type of pericarditis that develops 1 to 10 weeks after an MI and is presumed to result from an autoimmune process that occurs secondary to leakage of intracellular proteins from necrotic myocardial cells. Consider this diagnosis whenever you see a patient who presents with pleuritic chest pain and symptoms of pericardial effusion several weeks after MI. Patients with this autoimmune pericarditis also typically experience fever.

8. **What is sudden cardiac death, and why are patients who have had myocardial infarctions predisposed to it?**

Sudden cardiac death is defined as death within 1 hour of onset of symptoms (usually due to a lethal arrhythmia). This is most commonly associated with nonocclusive clots, which usually cause subendocardial infarcts. Subendocardial infarcts are often referred to as non–Q wave MIs or NSTEMIs.

SUMMARY BOX: CORONARY ARTERY DISEASE

- Major modifiable coronary risk factors include hypertension, smoking, and dyslipidemia, and major nonmodifiable risk factors include age, male gender if under age 65, and family history of premature heart disease. Elevated C-reactive protein (CRP) and homocysteinuria are emerging as other important risk factors.

- Cardiac muscle enzymes such as creatine kinase MB fraction (CK-MB) and cardiac-specific troponins are sensitive indicators of myocardial infarction (MI) depending on when their blood concentrations are measured.

- Post-MI patients are at increased risk for another MI as well as a number of other complications, including pulmonary edema, ischemic myocardial rupture, pericarditis, arrhythmias, and sudden cardiac death.

CASE 1-5

A 72-year-old woman with a long history of poorly controlled hypertension and diabetes presents with a 1-month history of worsening fatigue and shortness of breath (dyspnea). Initially, she experienced difficulty breathing only with exertion, but recently it occurs even at rest. She admits to supporting herself with two pillows at night to help with breathing (two-pillow orthopnea).

1. **What disorder is at the top of your differential diagnosis list?**
    These symptoms are a classic presentation of heart failure, but causes such as myocardial ischemia, lung disease, anemia, and atrial fibrillation should be considered. Diagnosis of heart failure is largely based on a careful history and physical examination and supported by tests that assess cardiac function.

CASE 1-5 continued:

On examination she has distended neck veins, bibasilar pulmonary crackles, and bilateral lower extremity edema. Her apical impulse is displaced laterally past the midclavicular line, and an S_3 gallop is appreciated on auscultation. On chest x-ray, the cardiac silhouette appears slightly enlarged, and an echocardiogram reveals an ejection fraction of 38% and no valvular abnormalities. Plasma levels of brain natriuretic peptide (BNP) are substantially elevated.

2. **In pathophysiologic terms, what is heart failure?**
    Heart failure results from either (1) pathologically depressed CO or (2) normal CO that can only be maintained at elevated ventricular filling pressures, which pathologically increases venous hydrostatic pressures. It therefore follows that there are two major categories of symptoms seen in heart failure: those due to depressed CO and those due to fluid accumulation caused by increased filling pressures. Heart failure is also categorized according to the side of the heart that has failed to function. Left-sided heart failure results in a decrease in the inotropic ability of the heart to pump the necessary amount of blood to the rest of the body. It can be compensated for by the renin-angiotensin-aldosterone system (RAAS), which will increase intravascular volume, venous return, and contractility to maintain CO, or it can be decompensated with worsening heart failure and result in a decreased CO. Symptoms such as fatigue, lethargy, and weakness are due to inadequate CO and are worse on exertion.

    Whether the heart failure is compensated or decompensated, ventricular pressures become elevated, and varying degrees of pulmonary edema ensue, leading to dyspnea. If left-sided heart failure is not treated, the pulmonary pressures will remain elevated and can cause the right side of the heart to fail; this is called biventricular failure. This leads to a similar backup of blood in the venous circulation, resulting in jugular venous distention, hepatomegaly, and pitting edema.

    Heart failure that manifests with the symptoms listed previously is called congestive heart failure (CHF). Notice that this woman has signs of both left-sided and right-sided heart failure.

    Note: The most common cause of right-sided heart failure is left-sided heart failure. Other less common causes of right-sided heart failure include pulmonary hypertension, tricuspid regurgitation, pulmonary stenosis, and septal defects.

3. **What are the differences between systolic and diastolic heart failure? Which does this woman most likely have?**
    Heart failure can be broadly classified as systolic (pump) failure or diastolic (filling) failure. Systolic heart failure is characterized by insufficient contractility of the ventricles, with an ejection fraction below 40%. Diastolic heart failure is characterized by poor ventricular compliance, resulting in insufficient filling of ventricles during diastole; hence diastolic failure is also known as "heart failure with a preserved ejection fraction." It is estimated that approximately two thirds of

patients with heart failure have systolic failure and the remaining one third have diastolic failure. However, because most patients with systolic dysfunction have components of diastolic dysfunction as well, this classification scheme is characterized by substantial overlap.

This patient likely has systolic heart failure because of the reduced ejection fraction and S_3 heart sound. Although hypertension is a primary cause of diastolic heart failure, it is also a major risk factor for coronary artery disease, which may be the underlying cause of her systolic failure.

Note: The ejection fraction is defined as stroke volume divided by end-diastolic volume (SV/EDV) and is normally 55% to 75%.

4. **What is the etiology of heart failure?**
Systolic heart failure is associated with myocardial damage or ischemia as well as volume-overloaded states such as valvular regurgitation and kidney disease. Diastolic heart failure is usually associated with pressure overload (hypertension) and myocardial ischemia, but may also be caused by infiltrative diseases such as amyloidosis.

Note: The end result of coronary heart disease (if not properly managed) is an ischemic cardiomyopathy with components of both systolic and diastolic failure, because both systole and diastole are energy-requiring processes.

5. **The body's response to heart failure is initially helpful but becomes maladaptive with time. For each of the following physiologic responses observed in heart failure, describe both the adaptive *and* pathologic results.**
A. Increased sympathetic activity
Adaptive: Increased sympathetic outflow results in tachycardia and increased contractility of the heart, both of which increase CO. Interestingly, patients in heart failure secrete three to four times more norepinephrine a day than normal, healthy individuals. Recall that the determinants of cardiac output are given by the equation

$$CO = HR \times SV$$

Additionally, in the setting of reduced CO (such as systolic heart failure), vasoconstriction caused by elevated sympathetic outflow helps maintain sufficient arterial pressure to provide adequate perfusion to critical organs. Remember, the determinants of arterial pressure are CO and TPR:

$$MAP = CO \times TPR$$

Pathologic: The sympathoadrenal activation seen in the context of a failing heart results in a reduced amount of time spent in diastole. This decreases the time available for coronary perfusion (supply), in a setting where the load on the heart (demand) is already being increased by sympathetic activity. After time, the increased load results in cardiac remodeling and worsening cardiac function and is exacerbated by a decreased blood supply. Additionally, the sympathetically mediated chronic vasoconstriction in skeletal muscles that occurs during heart failure and the decreasing CO are largely responsible for the muscle fatigue observed in these individuals.
B. Fluid retention
Adaptive: The kidneys sense reduced CO through decreases in renal perfusion and glomerular filtration rate (GFR). They respond by activating the renin-angiotensin-aldosterone system to retain fluid and expand the plasma volume. This elevation in intravascular volume increases venous return to the heart and subsequently increases preload. This response has a positive inotropic effect on the heart via the Frank-Starling relationship and will increase CO.

Pathologic: The increased preload from fluid retention places an increased workload on the heart. This can precipitate symptoms of angina secondary to insufficient coronary perfusion. Excessive preloads stretch the myocardium to a point of suboptimal overlap of actin and myosin filaments in the sarcomeres, reducing contractility. Finally, fluid retention can also cause complications associated with excessive volume expansion, such as pulmonary edema.

Note: Because nitrates and diuretics both decrease preload (as well as afterload to some degree), they help alleviate the *symptoms* of CHF associated with excessive volume expansion.

C. Myocardial hypertrophy

Adaptive: The value of this process depends on the type of overload that occurs in heart failure. In a pressure-overloaded heart (from hypertension or aortic stenosis), there is concentric hypertrophy (circular thickening of the myocardium) that strengthens ventricular contractions in the setting of a significant afterload. In pressure-overloaded ventricles, the increased systolic wall stress causes addition of sarcomeres in parallel, which reduces the stress on each sarcomere according to the Law of Laplace (wall stress = pressure X radius/thickness). In a volume-overloaded heart, the increase in diastolic wall stress from increased end-diastolic volume causes poor alignment of sarcomere fibrils (past the adaptive point of the Frank-Starling relationship), so sarcomeres are added in series to expand the chamber volume and optimize fiber alignment.

Pathologic: Oxygen demand of the hypertrophied heart is increased, which might exacerbate an existing ischemic condition. In fact, the vascular supply to the heart often does not increase proportionately to the muscular hypertrophy. Additionally, the thickened myocardium requires a larger distance for oxygen to diffuse, which is already exacerbated by the elevated ventricular diastolic pressures of heart failure. This reduces the gradient for oxygen diffusion from the coronary arteries through the myocardium (see Case 1–3, question 4). Hypertrophy also reduces ventricular compliance, which can cause or worsen diastolic dysfunction. The sympathetic nervous system and angiotensin II are involved in mediating the ventricular remodeling found in hypertrophy as well as in ventricular dilation.

Note: If an adequate CO is restored by these compensatory mechanisms, the heart failure is said to be *compensated*. If these physiologic reflexes alone cannot restore adequate CO, the heart failure is said to be *decompensated*.

6. **Given the pathophysiologic adaptations in heart failure just noted, why might beta blockers be beneficial in heart failure?**
Beta blockers have many effects that additively decrease the overall cardiac workload and improve function of an ailing heart:
   1. Inhibit sympathetic activity
      - Decrease preload by preventing sympathetic mediated venoconstriction
      - Decrease contractility and heart rate
      - Decrease afterload
   2. Decrease renin secretion
      - Decrease fluid retention and afterload
   3. Decrease cardiac remodeling

7. **How is digitalis, which is used in heart failure, believed to increase cardiac contractility?**
Similar to skeletal muscle fibers, cardiac muscle fibers contract when the intracellular calcium levels rise. Digitalis increases the intracellular calcium by an indirect mechanism involving ion exchanges. By inhibiting the sodium/potassium pump, digitalis increases intracellular sodium. However, it is the extracellular/intracellular sodium gradient that drives the sodium/calcium

exchanger. Consequently, in the presence of high intracellular sodium less calcium is pumped out of the cell, increasing intracellular calcium and contractility.

Note: In contrast to drugs such as ACE inhibitors and beta blockers, which have been shown to extend life, digitalis has been shown to improve cardiac performance and quality of life without an improvement in mortality risk. It is not a first-line agent in the treatment of heart failure.

STEP 1 SECRET

Digitalis is a high-yield drug for Step 1. In addition to its mechanism of action, it is important to know common side effects of digitalis. These effects include cholinergic effects (e.g., diarrhea, vomiting, increased PR interval), arrhythmias, and blurry yellow vision. Digitalis/digoxin toxicity is treated by stopping the medication and administering potassium, magnesium, and anti-digoxin Fab fragments. Lidocaine is given for digoxin-induced arrhythmias.

8. In Table 1-4, cover the right-hand column and attempt to give the mechanism of action for each of the listed drugs used in CHF.

TABLE 1-4. DRUGS USED FOR CONGESTIVE HEART FAILURE

Drug	Drug Class	Mechanism of Action
Digitalis	Cardiac glycoside	↑ inotropic effect, ↓ chronotropic effect, ↑ ejection fraction
Metoprolol	Beta blocker	↓ chronotropic effect, ↓ inotropic effect, ↓ myocardial demand
Captopril	ACE inhibitor	↓ aldosterone, ↓ plasma volume, ↓ actions of ATII
Losartan	ATII receptor antagonist	Inhibits actions of ATII

ACE, angiotensin-converting enzyme; ATII, angiotensin II.

OTHER RELATED QUESTIONS

9. **What is "high-output" heart failure?**

High-output heart failure refers to the *inability* of the heart to *maintain an elevated cardiac output* in pathologic situations that demand it, for example, in hyperthyroidism, arteriovenous malformations, anemia, and sepsis.

Note: In the case of arteriovenous malformations, the drastic drop in TPR when going from a high-pressure arteriole to a low-pressure venule demands an increase in CO to maintain MAP. The high CO causes an increased load on the heart, which when maintained for a long time can cause the function of the heart to eventually deteriorate.

SUMMARY BOX: HEART FAILURE

- Heart failure is a complex clinical syndrome that represents a final common pathway for a variety of pathologic processes that impair cardiac function.

- Heart failure is classified by two general types: systolic (pump) and diastolic (filling) dysfunction, with considerable overlap.

- The initially adaptive physiologic responses (increased sympathetic activity, fluid retention, and myocardial hypertrophy) become maladaptive when prolonged, leading to progressive deterioration of cardiac function and eventual death.

- When thinking about heart failure, categorize the findings according to whether they suggest left-sided versus right-sided heart failure, preserved versus reduced ejection fraction, and compensated versus decompensated cardiac output.

CASE 1-6

A 50-year-old man presents complaining of chest pain that occurs at gradually diminishing levels of physical exertion, as well as two recent episodes of syncope while golfing. Cardiovascular examination reveals a blood pressure of 120/90 mm Hg, a loud crescendo-decrescendo systolic murmur best appreciated at the upper right sternal border (with radiation to both carotid arteries), and a weak and delayed carotid upstroke. An ECG reveals left ventricular hypertrophy, and an echocardiogram reveals a bicuspid aortic valve with reduced valvular orifice (<1 cm^2).

1. **What is the diagnosis?**
   Aortic stenosis, a common valvular disorder in which excessive narrowing of the aortic valve increases afterload, is the likely diagnosis. If left untreated, aortic stenosis may result in angina, exertional syncope, dyspnea from heart failure, and increased cardiovascular mortality. Symptoms are often, but not always, seen when the area of the aortic orifice is less than 1 cm^2 (normal area is 3 cm^2).

2. **What likely predisposed this patient to developing aortic stenosis?**
   Stenosis generally occurs only in elderly patients secondary to calcification, which is referred to as senile calcific aortic stenosis. However, congenitally bicuspid or even unicuspid valves (as opposed to the normal tricuspid aortic valve) calcify and narrow at an earlier age, usually in the late 40s or in the 50s, as happened with this man.

3. **What causes heart murmurs and why does this patient have one?**
   Murmurs are caused by turbulent flow, which occurs at elevated flow velocities. In this case, the stenotic aortic valve forces the heart to contract more forcefully, which generates a significant pressure gradient between the left ventricle and the aorta, creating high-flow velocities across the aortic valve. The murmur of aortic stenosis decreases in intensity when preload is decreased, such as what occurs when standing still. The murmur increases in intensity when preload is increased, which occurs with inspiration and Valsalva maneuver, for example.
   Note: Carotid bruits are due to the same mechanism as murmurs, with the stenotic lumen causing increased flow velocities and a resulting turbulent blood flow that can be auscultated.

4. **What compensatory left ventricular changes occur as a result of aortic stenosis?**
Cardiomyocytes respond to pressure and volume overload stressors differently. In response to volume overload (e.g., aortic regurgitation), sarcomeres within myocytes are added in series, which has the effect of increasing ventricular lumen volume—an adaptive response termed *eccentric hypertrophy*. Aortic stenosis, however, is characterized by a pathologically elevated afterload, and thus leads to pathophysiologic changes that resemble those observed with systemic hypertension. The myocardium responds to an increased afterload by adding sarcomeres in parallel, resulting in a hypertrophied myocardium that is better able to eject blood against increased resistance. This adaptive response is termed *concentric hypertrophy*. One of the drawbacks of both forms of myocardial hypertrophy is that the thickened myocardium is typically less compliant, requiring increased filling pressures and predisposing to dyspnea and pulmonary edema.

5. **Why does this patient have a weak, delayed carotid upstroke with a narrowed pulse pressure on physical examination? Think about how the left ventricular pressure-volume loop changes in aortic stenosis.**
In aortic stenosis, a significant proportion of cardiac work is devoted to generating sufficient force to overcome the valvular resistance. Consequently, a smaller proportion of cardiac work is used to eject blood, resulting in decreased stroke volume (SV) and pulse pressure. This is also affected by the amount of time available for ejection because more time, of the finite amount available for systole, is consumed by isovolumic contraction. Additionally, ventricular hypertrophy can impair diastolic filling, reducing preload. Recall that elevated preload. . . normally compensates for decreased SV via the Frank-Starling mechanism.

A LV pressure-volume loop comparing changes in LV pressure and volume throughout the cardiac cycle in a normal heart and one with aortic stenosis is shown in Figure 1-8. Note that in aortic stenosis, higher pressures must be generated during isovolumic contraction (phase II) because of the increased afterload. This leaves correspondingly less energy and time available for the ejection phase (phase III), and therefore the SV in aortic stenosis (uncompensated) is reduced. This reduced SV explains the weak and delayed carotid upstroke (pulsus parvus et tardus) and the decreased pulse pressure evident on physical examination.

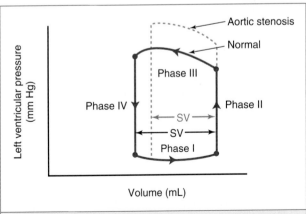

Figure 1-8. Pressure-volume changes in aortic stenosis. SV, stroke volume. (From Brown TA: Rapid Review Physiology. Philadelphia, Mosby, 2007, p 128.)

STEP 1 SECRET

You should practice interpreting diagrams depicting pressure-volume loops in relation to the events in the cardiac cycle.

6. **As a result of aortic stenosis, do ventricular myocytes spend more time in isotonic or isometric (isovolumic) contraction?**

Myocytes spend more time in isometric (isovolumic) contraction to overcome the increased afterload caused by the stenotic aortic valve. Because the time available for electrical and mechanical ventricular systole is finite, this results in a shortened isotonic ejection phase.

7. **Explain the cause of this patient's presenting complaints. What is most likely causing his episodes of syncope? His chest pain?**

Patients with stenotic aortic valves have left ventricular outflow obstruction that limits their ability to augment cardiac output. This particularly occurs in the setting of exercise, when widespread peripheral vasodilation necessitates increased cardiac output, resulting in relative cerebral hypoperfusion and symptoms of syncope. Thus, the syncope experienced by this patient while golfing results from his inability to meet the required increase in cardiac output. His chest pain is due to the accumulation of byproducts of anaerobic respiration in cardiomyocytes. Anaerobic metabolism occurs and is due to the myocardial ischemia resulting from the increased myocardial demand caused by the work required to pump against a stenotic valve as well as a decreased coronary supply secondary to a reduced SV.

8. **What are some causes of increased myocardial oxygen *demand* in aortic stenosis?**

The increased left ventricular mass requires more oxygen for normal contractile function. In addition, the increased left ventricular pressures that develop to overcome the outflow obstruction increase the workload on the left ventricle, further increasing the myocardial volume of oxygen (MVo_2) demand. Additional time spent in systole to eject the blood also increases the myocardial oxygen demand. Finally, inadequate CO in aortic stenosis activates the sympathetic nervous system and increases contractility, which further elevates myocardial oxygen demand.

9. **What are some causes of decreased myocardial oxygen *supply* in aortic stenosis?**

As heart rate increases to compensate for a depressed CO, less time is spent in diastole (which is when the majority of coronary perfusion occurs). Additionally, owing to decreased compliance, left ventricular diastolic pressure increases, which further reduces perfusion. Finally, aortic pressure is reduced because of the decreased SV, which decreases coronary blood flow (Fig. 1-9).

10. **Why is atrial fibrillation a particularly dangerous complication in aortic stenosis (aside from the risk of embolic stroke)?**

Aortic stenosis often results in elevated left atrial pressures and subsequent dilation of the left atrium. Dilation of the left atrium compresses the conducting fibers, thereby predisposing patients to atrial fibrillation.

Normally the "atrial kick," the additional ventricular filling that atrial contraction normally provides, does not provide a significant percentage of the cardiac output (CO). However, in situations in which the CO is impaired, such as aortic stenosis, this extra filling is essential to

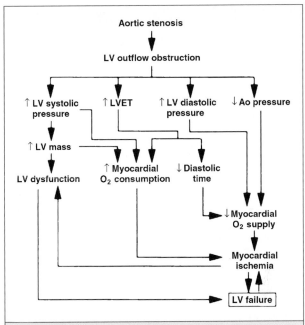

Figure 1-9. Causes of increased myocardial oxygen demand and decreased myocardial oxygen supply. Ao, aortic; LV, left ventricular; LVET, LV ejection time. (From Boudoulas H, Gravanis MB: Cardiovascular Disorders: Pathogenesis and Pathophysiology. St. Louis, Mosby, 1993, p 64.)

sustain an adequate CO. Because his CO is already compromised, atrial fibrillation would remove the atrial kick's contribution to CO and could precipitate severe heart failure.

11. **Describe the murmur of aortic stenosis**
   Aortic stenosis is characterized by a systolic crescendo-decrescendo ejection murmur best appreciated at the upper right sternal border. It may radiate to the carotid arteries.
   The murmur of aortic stenosis is enhanced by increased preload (squatting, passive leg raising) and expiration. As a general rule of thumb, left-sided murmurs increase on exhalation and right-sided murmurs increase on inspiration.
   If aortic stenosis results in the formation of a noncompliant ventricle, an S_4 heart sound may be heard. Atrial fibrillation will prevent the S_4 heart sound from developing.

STEP 1 SECRET

Murmur characteristics are a favorite topic for Step 1. Be sure that you can distinguish murmurs according to location, characteristic symptoms, and maneuvers used to alter their sounds. Remember to practice listening to audio files of the most testable murmurs. These murmurs include those accompanying aortic/pulmonary stenosis, aortic regurgitation, mitral/tricuspid regurgitation, mitral/tricuspid regurgitation, mitral valve prolapse, hypertrophic cardiomyopathy, ventricular septal defects, and patent ductus arteriosus.

SUMMARY BOX: AORTIC STENOSIS

- Aortic stenosis most commonly presents as a crescendo-decrescendo systolic murmur heard loudest at the upper right sternal border and radiating to both carotid arteries. A delayed carotid upstroke and narrowed pulse pressure are associated findings.

- Decreased cardiac output (in decompensated states) and increased myocardial oxygen demand are important consequences of aortic stenosis. It follows that the natural history of this condition leads to angina, syncope, heart failure, and premature death.

CASE 1-7

A 56-year-old moderately obese, postmenopausal woman with type 2 diabetes is evaluated during her annual examination. Examination is significant for abdominal obesity as well as a curvilinear patch of darkly pigmented skin around her neck. Blood work reveals an elevated low-density lipoprotein (LDL) cholesterol, low high-density lipoprotein (HDL) cholesterol, markedly elevated triglycerides, and a fasting plasma glucose level of 145 mg/dL.

1. **This patient's constellation of symptoms is consistent with what syndrome, and what is its significance?**
   These symptoms are consistent with the metabolic syndrome (insulin resistance syndrome, syndrome X). This syndrome is highly prevalent and increasing in the United States and is significant because it identifies patients at increased risk of premature death from cardiac causes. Metabolic syndrome is particularly common in postmenopausal women and may affect up to a quarter of the people currently living in the United States. As defined by the 2001 National Cholesterol Education Program (ATP III), the metabolic syndrome is diagnosed by the presence of at least three of the following five features:
   - Central obesity (waist circumference >35 inches in women, >40 inches in men)
   - Triglyceride levels ≥150 mg/dL
   - HDL cholesterol <50 mg/dL in women, <40 mg/dL in men)
   - Fasting blood glucose ≥110 mg/dL
   - Blood pressure ≥130/85 mm Hg

   It is clear that patients who fulfill criteria for the metabolic syndrome are at significant risk for increased morbidity and mortality associated with cardiovascular disease and diabetes. Hence the diagnosis of metabolic syndrome can help identify patients who should be treated with stringent cardiovascular risk factor modification strategies, despite the fact that these factors may not individually indicate to do so. Management of the metabolic syndrome consists of controlling each of the component factors individually, aiming for weight control, improved lipid profiles, increased insulin sensitivity, and decreased blood pressure.

2. **Part of this woman's presentation is dyslipidemia, a disorder of lipoprotein metabolism. What is the structure of a lipoprotein, where are lipoproteins synthesized, and what are the major types of lipoproteins?**
   Lipoproteins are macromolecular structures composed of an inner core of cholesterol esters and triglycerides (the latter may also be referred to as triacylglycerols) and an outer core of apolipoproteins, phospholipids, and unesterified free cholesterol. The major types of lipoproteins include chylomicrons, very low-density lipoproteins (VLDLs), intermediate-density lipoproteins (IDLs), LDL, and HDL. Chylomicrons are synthesized within intestinal enterocytes, whereas VLDL is synthesized within the liver. IDL and LDL are both formed within the circulation via VLDL catabolism. HDL is synthesized by the liver and intestine.

3. **What are the functions of the various forms of lipoproteins? How are they removed from the circulation?**

Chylomicrons: delivery of dietary triglycerides to adipose tissue, skeletal muscle, and cardiac muscle; cholesterol-rich chylomicron remnants are then taken up by the liver.

VLDL: delivery of liver-synthesized triglycerides to adipose tissue, skeletal muscle, and cardiac muscle; removed by intravascular conversion to IDL and ultimately LDL.

LDL: delivery of cholesterol to cells throughout the body; removed by internalization via LDL receptor (principally in the liver).

> **Note:** Defects in LDL receptor or internalization of LDL receptor cause *familial hypercholesterolemia*.

HDL: return of excess cholesterol from cells to the liver for biliary excretion; can remove cholesterol from atheromatous plaques.

CASE 1-7 continued:

The patient decides to try lifestyle modifications, focusing on a low-fat, low-cholesterol diet and walking for 45 minutes 4 days a week. After 3 months, her follow-up visit reveals that her weight and lipid profile are largely unchanged. As a result, she is prescribed simvastatin. Before she takes her first dose, her liver enzymes are checked, and she is told that this test will need to be repeated periodically.

4. **What is the mechanism of action of simvastatin (and other statins)?**

Statins inhibit the hepatic synthesis of cholesterol by inhibiting 3-hydroxy-3-methylglutaryl (HMG) CoA reductase, which is the enzyme that catalyzes the rate-limiting step in cholesterol synthesis. Not only do these drugs reduce cholesterol synthesis, but they stimulate cells to respond to decreased intracellular cholesterol levels through upregulation of LDL receptors on their surfaces, which promotes cholesterol intake and further lowers cholesterol levels in the blood. Statins are the most potent pharmacologic agents for lowering cholesterol contained in LDL. They also cause a modest reduction of triglycerides but have only a small effect on increasing high-density lipoprotein cholesterol (HDL-C).

5. **In addition to liver tests, which other enzymes might be monitored when using a statin? With these toxicities in mind, adding which other class of cholesterol-lowering drugs to her regimen should only be done with great caution?**

Because statins and fibrates can independently cause muscle damage (myositis) and liver damage (hepatotoxicity), these risks are increased when the two classes are used together. Just as hepatotoxicity is evaluated by periodically monitoring hepatic enzymes, such as alanine transaminase (ALT) and aspartate transaminase (AST), myopathy and rhabdomyolysis can be evaluated by monitoring creatine phosphokinase (CPK) levels.

6. **What are the cause and clinical significance of this woman's hypertriglyceridemia?**

Triglycerides come from two places: those consumed in the diet (dietary) and those synthesized by the liver (nondietary). Dietary triglycerides are broken down in the gut and then re-formed in intestinal enterocytes, where they are packaged in chylomicrons. Chylomicrons enter the lymphatics and eventually drain into the venous circulation via the thoracic duct. Nondietary triglycerides are primarily synthesized in the liver and enter the bloodstream packaged in VLDLs.

Recent meta-analyses suggest that elevated triglycerides are an independent risk factor for coronary vascular disease. One theoretical mechanism for this finding may be attributed to the transfer of triglycerides to HDL by cholesterol ester transfer protein (CETP). Triglyceride-rich HDL is rapidly catabolized by lipoprotein lipase, which results in a decrease in HDL levels whenever triglycerides are elevated.

7. **What enzymatic mechanism clears triglycerides from the circulation?**
Lipoprotein lipase (present on the luminal surface of capillary endothelial cells in adipose tissue, skeletal muscle, and cardiac muscle) releases fatty acids from triglycerides present in chylomicrons and VLDL. The released fatty acids then diffuse into the cells.
   Note: Insulin stimulates lipoprotein lipase protein synthesis. If this enzyme concentration is low as in type 1 diabetes, then triglycerides accumulate in the circulation and hasten the development of atherosclerosis.

8. **What is the clinical significance of elevations in LDL levels?**
Such abnormalities have been shown to be associated with a number of pathophysiologic conditions, including atherosclerosis, chylomicronemia, obesity, Alzheimer's disease, xanthomas, and dyslipidemia associated with diabetes, insulin resistance, and infection.

9. **What is the clinical significance of this patient's low HDL-C?**
Low HDL-C is another risk factor for coronary heart disease. HDL-C is involved in reverse cholesterol transport, in which excess cholesterol is transported from peripheral tissues and atheromatous plaques to the liver for conversion into bile salts or unaltered excretion in the bile. Recall that biliary excretion is the only major mechanism for cholesterol removal from the body. Additionally, there is growing evidence to support a role for HDL-C in preventing LDL oxidation. This could be an important finding because oxidized LDL is the atherogenic form (e.g., macrophages do not phagocytose normal LDL but only oxidized LDL, and are then transformed into foam cells).
   Note: Unlike normal LDL, oxidized LDL can be taken up by scavenger receptors, thus promoting pathologic cholesterol accumulation and atherosclerosis.
   Plasma HDL levels can increase with exercise, moderate alcohol consumption, and pharmacologic agents such as niacin (most notably), fibric acids, and statins (generally modest effect).
   Note: A ratio of total cholesterol to HDL cholesterol can be used to predict coronary vascular disease (CVD) risk. An optimal ratio is ≤ 3.5. A person with total cholesterol of 180 mg/dL but an HDL of only 30 mg/dL would have a ratio of 6, which would place that person at high risk for developing CVD.

10. **What is the mechanism of action of the lipid-lowering fibrates/fibric acid derivatives (e.g., gemfibrozil, fenofibrate)?**
These agents are PPAR-alpha (peroxisome proliferator-activated receptor-alpha) agonists that lead to increased synthesis of lipoprotein lipase, causing a significant reduction in triglyceride level. They also increase the expression of enzymes involved in fatty acid oxidation, which results in a decrease in the availability of triglycerides for VLDL synthesis. Lastly, they increase levels of apo A-I and apo A-II, both of which promote increased HDL levels. Fibrates have little effect on LDL directly.
   Side effects of fibrates include hepatotoxicity, gallstones, and myositis.

11. **How does niacin influence the lipid profile, and what is the unique pharmacologic feature of niacin in managing lipid levels?**
Niacin (nicotinic acid) is a water-soluble B vitamin that has multiple beneficial effects on the overall lipid profile. It increases HDL-C by 25% to 35%, reduces LDL by 15% to 25%, and significantly reduces triglycerides (TGs). Mechanisms of action include promotion of LPL activity to enhance TG clearance from circulating VLDL (thus reducing LDL) and decreased hepatic uptake of apo A-I (which decreases clearance of HDL from circulation). Niacin is unique among the hypolipidemic agents in that it is the most potent agent for increasing HDL levels.
   Note: A major side effect of niacin is facial and upper body flushing (niacin rush). Taking aspirin or another type of nonsteroidal anti-inflammatory drug (NSAID) prior to the niacin to reduce the synthesis of vasodilatory prostaglandins can minimize this

flushing. Do not confuse this reaction with the flushing observed with vancomycin, which causes red man syndrome that can be relieved with antihistamine use prior to administration.

12. **How do the bile-sequestering resins (e.g., cholestyramine, colestipol) lower LDL cholesterol levels?**

The bile-sequestering resins bind bile acids in the intestine and prevent their reuptake in the distal ileum. This stimulates increased hepatic synthesis of bile acids. Because these acids are formed from cholesterol, increasing their synthesis will increase cholesterol catabolism, upregulate LDL receptors on hepatocytes, and decrease serum cholesterol levels.

Note: These drugs impair the bile-mediated emulsification, digestion, and absorption of fats, fat-soluble vitamins (vitamins A, D, E, and K), and certain drugs. Consequently, adverse effects of bile-sequestering resins commonly include bloating, flatulence, abdominal pain, steatorrhea, deficiencies of fat-soluble vitamins, and inadequate oral bioavailability of some drugs including warfarin, thiazides, and select statins. Decreased bile acid reabsorption also promotes the formation of cholesterol gallstones, which is enhanced by co-administration with fibrates.

OTHER RELATED QUESTION

13. **What is the cause of the disorder of lipid metabolism known as abetalipoproteinemia?**

Abetalipoproteinemia is an autosomal recessive genetic disorder characterized by the absence of apolipoprotein B, resulting in a deficiency of chylomicrons (apo B-48), VLDL (apo B-100), and LDL (apo B-100). Since chylomicrons cannot be produced and secreted without apo B-48, intestinal biopsy will reveal large, lipid-vacuolated enterocytes, and blood tests will reveal markedly decreased (or even absent) plasma chylomicrons. Symptoms include steatorrhea, weight loss, potential anemia, and malabsorption of fat-soluble vitamins. A deficiency in vitamin E can specifically present with neurologic symptoms due to spinocerebellar and corticospinal degeneration.

SUMMARY BOX: THE METABOLIC SYNDROME AND DYSLIPIDEMIAS

- The metabolic syndrome is characterized by abdominal obesity, dyslipidemia, insulin resistance, and hypertension. It is a marker for increased cardiovascular risk.

- Treatment of the metabolic syndrome consists of treating each of its components with lifestyle modifications and pharmacologic agents to control weight, improve lipid profiles, heighten insulin sensitivity, and lower blood pressure.

- Cholesterol-lowering medications include statins (most potent for lowering LDL-C), niacin (most potent for increasing HDL-C), fibrates, and bile-sequestering resins.

CHAPTER 2

PULMONOLOGY

Jessica M. Intravia, MHA, Thomas A. Brown, MD, and Sonali J. Shah

INSIDER'S GUIDE TO PULMONOLOGY FOR THE USMLE STEP 1

Pulmonology is a favorite subject for Step 1 because it provides a lot of opportunity to integrate across disciplines. Therefore, you should expect to find pulmonology questions on related subjects such as microbiology, cardiology, and clinical anatomy (we especially recommend spending some time with an anatomy atlas to refamiliarize yourself with chest x-ray films). However, this does not mean that USMLE test makers will forget to include questions regarding pulmonary physiology and pathology. In fact, many pulmonology questions on Step 1 will require you to apply conceptual knowledge of pathophysiology. In other words, avoid memorizing a ton of detailed information for this subject. Instead, focus on reasoning through the pathophysiology of various conditions as they relate to the lung (e.g., *why* compliance increases with emphysema, *why* altitude changes alter pH, *why* certain diseases alter $AaDo_2$). You will notice that the key point is to constantly ask yourself "why?" when studying for this subject!

BASIC CONCEPTS—MECHANICS OF BREATHING

1. **What are the driving forces for the following:**
   A. Inspiratory airflow?
   A negative intrapleural pressure (i.e., the pressure outside the lungs) is created by the opposing tendencies of the chest wall to expand and the lung to collapse. This negative intrapleural pressure is transmitted to the alveoli such that there is a pressure gradient between alveolar air spaces and the external environment, resulting in airflow into the lung.
   Muscles involved in forced inspiration include the diaphragm, external intercostals, innermost intercostals, and scalene and sternocleidomastoid muscles.
   B. Expiratory airflow?
   An increase in intrapleural pressure (i.e., becomes less negative) is created by relaxation of the diaphragm and elastic recoil of the lungs and chest wall. Contraction of the abdominal muscles (rectus abdominis, internal and external obliques, transversus abdominis) during forced expiration can also increase the intrapleural pressure. The internal intercostals are also involved in forced expiration.

2. **What are the forces of resistance for the following:**
   A. Inspiratory airflow
   Airway resistance, compliance resistance, and tissue resistance are the forces of resistance for inspiration; collectively, these forces determine the overall work of breathing.

Airway resistance is generated by the friction between rapidly moving air molecules and the walls of the airways. It is typically a small component of the work of breathing. Airway resistance is greater in the large airways because they are *arranged in series,* whereas the small airways are *arranged in parallel.*

The total resistance (R_T) of a specific number (n) of resistors in series is equal to the sum of their individual resistances such that

$$R_T = R_1 + R_2 + R_3 \cdots + R_n$$

By contrast, the total resistance (R_T) of a specific number (n) of resistors in parallel is calculated as

$$1/R_T = 1/R_1 + 1/R_2 + 1/R_3 \cdots + 1/R_n$$

Compliance resistance is generated as the lungs inflate and overcome the intrinsic elastic recoil of the lungs. The work to overcome this resistance (compliance work) normally accounts for the largest proportion of the work of breathing. Note that compliance work is reduced in obstructive lung disease and increased in restrictive lung disease.

Tissue resistance is generated as the pleural surfaces slide over each other during respiration. This resistance is normally minimal because of the presence of pleural fluid. Note that tissue resistance can increase markedly in conditions in which the pleural surfaces become adherent to each other, as may occur with an empyema (Fig. 2-1).

B. Expiratory airflow

Reduction in airway diameter associated with increased intrathoracic pressures affect resistance during expiration. Expiration is typically a passive process because this resistance is small and is easily overcome by the energy provided by elastic recoil of the lung and chest wall. However, in certain conditions in which airway diameter is pathologically reduced (e.g., asthma) or the forces of elastic recoil of the lung are reduced (e.g., emphysema), expiration may become an active process requiring use of accessory muscles.

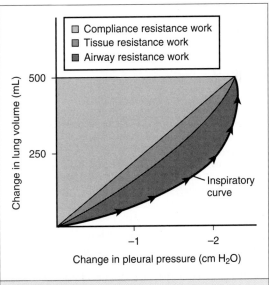

Figure 2-1. Relative contributions of the three types of resistance to the total work of breathing. (From Brown TA: Rapid Review Physiology. Philadelphia, Mosby, 2007.)

3. **What does pulmonary compliance measure?**
Compliance is a measure of lung distensibility. Compliant lungs are easy to distend. Compliance (C) can be measured as the change in volume (ΔV) required for a fractional change in pressure (ΔP):

$$C = \Delta V / \Delta P$$

The properties of compliance and elastance (tendency of the lung to recoil inward; see question 5) are inversely proportional to one another. In conditions in which elastance decreases (e.g., emphysema), compliance will automatically increase.

4. **With respect to the compliance curve of the lungs, how might breathing at an elevated functional residual capacity in chronic obstructive pulmonary disease result in less "efficient" breathing?**
Figure 2-2 shows a compliance curve of the lungs. Note that the lungs are most compliant in the midportion of the inspiratory curve (steepest slope). Breathing at an elevated functional residual capacity (as patients with chronic obstructive pulmonary disease [COPD] are prone to do for a variety of reasons) is less efficient and requires more work.

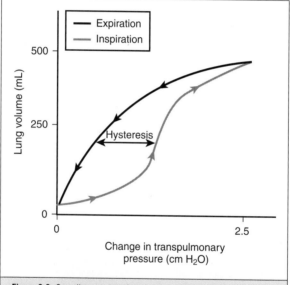

Figure 2-2. Compliance curve of the lungs: lung volume plotted against changes in transpulmonary pressure (the difference between pleural and alveolar pressure). (From Brown TA: Rapid Review Physiology. Philadelphia, Mosby, 2007.)

5. **What does pulmonary elastance measure? How is pulmonary elastance altered in restrictive and obstructive lung diseases and why?**
Elasticity is the property of matter that makes it resist deformation. As elasticity increases, increasingly greater pressure changes will be required to distend the lungs. Pulmonary elastance (E) can be calculated as the change in pressure (ΔP) divided by the change in volume (ΔV):

$$E = \Delta P / \Delta V$$

In restrictive lung diseases such as silicosis and asbestosis, which are characterized by parenchymal fibrosis, pulmonary elastance increases. In COPD, which is characterized by parenchymal destruction, elastance decreases.

6. **How does surfactant affect alveolar surface tension?**
Water molecules lining the surface of alveoli are attracted to each other and are repelled by the hydrophobic air molecules. The attractive force between water molecules generates surface tension, which in turn produces a *collapsing pressure* that promotes alveolar collapse. Surfactant is composed of phospholipids (mainly lecithin and sphingomyelin) that reduce the collapsing pressure by minimizing the interaction between alveolar fluid and alveolar air (Fig. 2-3).

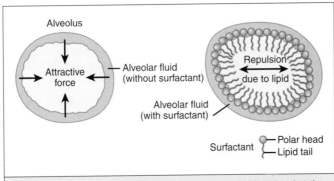

Figure 2-3. Role of surfactant in reducing alveolar surface tension. Note the orientation of the hydrophilic "head" in the alveolar fluid and the hydrophobic "tail" in the alveolar air. (From Brown TA: Rapid Review Physiology. Philadelphia, Mosby, 2007.)

7. **Why are smaller alveoli more prone to collapse, and how is this relevant to neonatal respiratory distress syndrome?**
Laplace's law states that the collapsing pressure (P) is directly proportional to surface tension (T) and inversely proportional to the alveolar radius (R), such that smaller alveoli will experience a larger collapsing pressure:

$$P = 2T/R$$

The combination of small alveoli and inadequate surfactant production in premature infants contributes to respiratory failure in the neonatal respiratory distress syndrome.
Fetal amniotic fluid can be measured for lecithin and sphingomyelin content, the ratio of which can serve as an indicator of fetal lung maturity. A ratio of <1.5 is a strong predictor of neonatal respiratory distress syndrome. Maternal steroids can be given if the fetus is less than 35 weeks old in order to increase fetal lung maturity before delivery.

8. **What is the minute ventilation?**
Minute ventilation is the total volume of air that enters and exits the lung each minute. The normal (resting) minute ventilation is a function of tidal volume and respiratory rate:

$$Minute\ ventilation = Respiratory\ rate \times Tidal\ volume$$

Example:

$$= 12\ breaths/min \times 500\ mL/breath$$
$$= 6\ L/min$$

9. **What is "dead space"? What is the difference between anatomic dead space and physiologic dead space?**

Dead space refers to lung volume that is ventilated but not perfused by deoxygenated blood, such that there is no potential for gas exchange in this space. The anatomic dead space is lung volume that receives ventilation, but in which there are no pulmonary capillaries available for gas exchange. This anatomic dead space includes the nasal cavity, pharynx, larynx, trachea, bronchi, and conducting bronchioles, often referred to as the *conducting airways*. The physiologic dead space includes both the anatomic dead space and the alveoli that are ventilated but not perfused (alveolar dead space), so no gas exchange occurs in them either.

The majority of physiologic dead space can be attributed to the apex of the lung due to poor perfusion at the apex compared with the base. Exercise decreases physiologic dead space by improving perfusion to the entire lung.

10. **Why is the alveolar minute ventilation a much better representation of *functional* ventilation?**

Alveolar minute ventilation is the volume of air that enters and exits the alveoli per minute. To calculate this rate, the anatomic dead space has to be taken into account and subtracted from the tidal volume. The typical anatomic dead space is about 150 mL.

$$\text{Alveolar ventilation} = \text{Respiratory frequency} \times (\text{Tidal volume} - \text{Anatomic dead space})$$
$$= 12 \text{ breaths/min} \times (500 \text{ mL/breath} - 150 \text{ mL})$$
$$= 4.2 \text{ L/min}$$

The alveolar ventilation is a much better representation of *functional* ventilation because the alveoli are where gas exchange occurs.

STEP 1 SECRET

You are expected to know basic formulas such as those listed in the preceding questions. They will not be provided to you on the USMLE. A computerized calculator will be available for your use.

BASIC CONCEPTS—VENTILATION-PERFUSION MATCHING

11. **What does the ventilation/perfusion ratio measure, and what is its approximate value? What is an "ideal" value for this ratio?**

The ventilation/perfusion ratio (V̇/Q̇) measures how well pulmonary perfusion and pulmonary ventilation are matched, indicating how efficiently oxygenation of blood is occurring in the pulmonary capillaries. Normally, the lungs receive close to the entire cardiac output (~5 L/min), and the prototypical 70-kg man has an alveolar ventilation rate of roughly 4 L/min (as shown in question 10). A ventilation rate of 4 L/min and a pulmonary perfusion rate of 5 L/min yield a V̇/Q̇ ratio of 0.8, which implies suboptimal matching of pulmonary ventilation and perfusion. A V̇/Q̇ ratio of 1 is ideal, and represents optimal matching of pulmonary ventilation and perfusion.

The V̇/Q̇ ratio can be applied to the lungs as a whole, or to separate areas of the lungs, and is a measure of the efficiency of ventilation in those separate areas as well. Regional differences in ventilation and perfusion exist across various zones of the lungs because of the force of gravity. In an upright subject, both blood flow and perfusion are decreased at the apex of the lung and increased at the base of the lung. However, the decrease in perfusion is greater than the decrease in ventilation at the apex of the lung, leading to an increased V̇/Q̇ ratio. Likewise, the

$\dot{V}/\dot{Q}$ ratio at the base is decreased because the increase in perfusion is greater than the increase in ventilation. This difference leads to an apical $\dot{V}/\dot{Q}$ ratio of 3, while the basal $\dot{V}/\dot{Q}$ ratio is closer to 0.6.

During exercise, the greater increase in alveolar ventilation and lesser increase in cardiac output lead to a more uniform $\dot{V}/\dot{Q}$ ratio from apex to base that more closely approximates the ideal $\dot{V}/\dot{Q}$ ratio of 1.0.

12. **What conditions cause an increase in the $\dot{V}/\dot{Q}$ ratio?**
The $\dot{V}/\dot{Q}$ ratio increases whenever pulmonary ventilation is proportionately greater than pulmonary perfusion. As just discussed, exercise is a normal situation in which ventilation increases proportionally more than perfusion, and in this case it optimizes the $\dot{V}/\dot{Q}$ ratio. A pathologic condition that increases the $\dot{V}/\dot{Q}$ ratio is a pulmonary embolus. In this condition, patients are often tachypneic (respiring rapidly), which increases ventilation. The clot in the lungs also reduces pulmonary perfusion, so both of these processes increase the $\dot{V}/\dot{Q}$ ratio. In fact, the $\dot{V}/\dot{Q}$ ratio in the blocked segment would theoretically approach infinity because blood flow to that region is completely blocked ($\dot{Q} = 0$). The pathologic consequence of an increased $\dot{V}/\dot{Q}$ ratio is that ventilation is "wasted" in lung areas that are not adequately perfused.

13. **What causes a decrease in the ventilation/perfusion ratio?**
Generally, any lung disease in which the process of ventilation itself is compromised will decrease the amount of oxygen that the pulmonary blood flow receives, predisposing the patient to hypoxemia. This is deleterious because less oxygen diffuses into the blood that flows through the lungs. Additionally, less carbon dioxide can be "blown off," predisposing to hypercapnia. An example is asthma, in which the bronchoconstriction that occurs impairs ventilation and reduces the $\dot{V}/\dot{Q}$ ratio.

Patients with decreased $\dot{V}/\dot{Q}$ ratio will respond to oxygen administration. However, a $\dot{V}/\dot{Q}$ ratio of 0 generally implies an obstructed mainstem bronchus and will not respond to oxygen.

14. **What effect does chronic obstructive pulmonary disease usually have on the ventilation-perfusion ratio?**
Airway obstruction in COPD can reduce ventilation relative to perfusion, decreasing the $\dot{V}/\dot{Q}$ ratio. However, pulmonary capillary loss in COPD can increase ventilation relative to perfusion, causing an increased $\dot{V}/\dot{Q}$ ratio. In fact, if these two processes are occurring in the same patient, this patient can have a normal $\dot{V}/\dot{Q}$ ratio despite severe ventilation/perfusion mismatches in different parts of the lung!

15. **What is the difference between an anatomic shunt and a physiologic shunt?**
Most anatomic shunts occur within the heart when deoxygenated blood from the right side of the heart crosses the septum and mixes with oxygenated blood from the left side of the heart. This mixture results in varying degrees of hypoxemia that cannot be improved with the administration of 100% O_2.

In a physiologic shunt, deoxygenated blood bypasses the gas-exchanging unit. Atelectasis can occur in many lung diseases including pneumonia. In atelectasis, ventilatory obstruction to the gas-exchanging unit leads to a subsequent loss of volume and a $\dot{V}/\dot{Q}$ ratio of 0.

BASIC CONCEPTS—GAS EXCHANGE

16. **What influences the diffusion of gases from the alveoli into the pulmonary capillaries, and vice versa?**
Gas diffusion across a membrane (the pulmonary membrane in this case) is described by Fick's law of diffusion:

$$V_{gas} = \frac{A \times D\ (P_1 - P_2)}{T}$$

where V_{gas} is the volume of gas that traverses the membrane per unit time, A is the surface area of the membrane, D is the diffusivity of the particular gas in the particular membrane, $P_1 - P_2$ is the partial pressure difference of the specific gas across the membrane, and T is the thickness of the membrane.

It is important to recognize that all pulmonary diseases that create respiratory dysfunction affect one or more of the parameters in the diffusion equation. For example, in asthma, the impaired ventilation reduces the pressure gradient for oxygen across the membrane. In emphysema, ventilation is impaired (reducing the pressure gradient) and the surface area of the pulmonary membrane is reduced from loss of alveoli.

Note: The *diffusing capacity* of the pulmonary membrane is defined as the volume of gas (typically measured using carbon monoxide) that can diffuse across the pulmonary membrane per mm Hg pressure difference across the membrane. It can be seen from Fick's law that the diffusing capacity is dependent on the surface area, gas diffusivity, and membrane thickness.

17. **What is the alveolar-arterial oxygen gradient and what is the clinical significance of its magnitude?**
The alveolar-arterial oxygen gradient ($P_{AO_2} - P_{aO_2}$, sometimes designated AaD_{O_2}) is a measure of the difference in oxygen tension, or partial pressure, between the alveoli and arterial blood. In a healthy person, a typical alveolar oxygen tension (P_{AO_2}) might be roughly 110 mm Hg, whereas the arterial oxygen tension (P_{aO_2}) might be roughly 100 mm Hg. In such a healthy person, this slight 10 mm Hg difference in the partial pressure of oxygen between these two "compartments" reflects the highly efficient diffusion of oxygen across the pulmonary membrane. AaD_{O_2} increases by 3 mm Hg with every decade of life past the age of 30, but should never exceed 25 mm Hg. A high alveolar-arterial oxygen gradient implies the presence of pulmonary disease that is causing impaired diffusion of alveolar oxygen across the pulmonary membrane, resulting in hypoxemia. In contrast, AaD_{O_2} can appear normal in a patient who is hypoventilating.

18. **How is the alveolar-arterial oxygen gradient calculated?**

$$AaD_{O_2} = \text{Alveolar oxygen partial pressure} - \text{Arterial oxygen partial pressure}$$

where

$$\text{Alveolar oxygen partial pressure} = \frac{F_{IO_2}(PB - PH_2O) - P_{ACO_2}}{R}$$

where F_{IO_2} = the fraction of inspired oxygen (usually 0.21), PB is barometric pressure (usually 760 mm Hg), PH_2O is water vapor pressure (usually 47 mm Hg), P_{ACO_2} = alveolar pressure of carbon dioxide, which equals the arterial pressure of carbon dioxide due to rapid diffusion across the alveolar membrane, and R = the respiratory quotient (usually 0.8).

19. **What are the primary determinants of respiratory drive?**
Respirations do not occur without input from the nervous system, which comes from the medullary respiratory center (or from conscious drive). The respiratory center responds to input from central and peripheral chemoreceptors. Hypoxia, hypercapnia, and acidemia stimulate peripheral chemoreceptors that then transmit to and stimulate the respiratory center to increase the rate and depth of respirations. Central chemoreceptors are stimulated by hypercapnia by way of CO_2 diffusing across the blood-brain barrier and dissolving to form carbonic acid, thereby

lowering the pH of the central nervous system (CNS). Central chemoreceptors do not respond directly to hypoxia.

Note: The predominant mechanism of respiratory suppression of the barbiturates, benzodiazepines, opioids, and general anesthetics is to make the medullary respiratory center less responsive to increases in P_{aCO_2}.

20. **How does increasing or decreasing the arterial P_{CO_2} affect pH?**
When CO_2 dissolves in water, the following reaction occurs:

$$CO_2 + H_2O \overset{CA}{\leftrightarrow} HCO_3^- + H^+$$

where CA is carbonic anhydrase.

If additional CO_2 is added, the reaction shifts to the right, creating more hydrogen ions, which decrease the pH of the solution. Conversely, removal of CO_2 pushes the reaction to the left, resulting in removal of H^+ from solution, with an overall increase in pH. It is this reaction that the lungs exploit to compensate for alterations in arterial pH.

By increasing or decreasing ventilation, and thereby affecting the arterial P_{CO_2} levels, the pH can be raised or lowered.

21. **What is respiratory acidosis? Respiratory alkalosis?**
In respiratory acidosis, the lungs are not ventilating well, and the CO_2 that builds up shifts the equation in question 20 to the right, lowering the pH to an abnormal level. In respiratory alkalosis, the lungs are blowing off too much CO_2, shifting the same equation to the left and raising the pH to an abnormal level. In both cases, the respiratory rate and depth are pathologically mismatched to the physiologic demands/needs.

The kidneys attempt to compensate for respiratory acidosis by retaining bicarbonate, or for respiratory alkalosis by increasing bicarbonate excretion, exploiting the other side of this chemical reaction. Unlike the process of respiratory compensation, renal compensation is slow and can take several days to be complete.

STEP 1 SECRET

Recognizing various acid-base disorders not only is a USMLE favorite but will be a very useful skill during your clinical years!

22. **What are the forced expiratory volume and the FEV_1/FVC ratio?**
The forced expiratory volume (FEV_1) is the maximum amount of air that can be expired *in 1 second* following a full inspiration. The forced vital capacity (FVC) is the total amount expired following a full inspiration. The FEV_1/FVC ratio is therefore the percent volume of air that can be expired in 1 second relative to the maximum expiration.

23. **What is the principal difference between "restrictive" and "obstructive" lung disease with respect to the FEV_1/FVC ratio?**
In restrictive lung disease (e.g., pulmonary fibrosis), decreased pulmonary compliance limits *inspiratory* volumes. Although expiration is not impaired, the limited inspiratory volumes result in smaller FEV_1 and FVC volumes. Furthermore, the increased pulmonary elastic recoil results in a smaller decrease in FEV_1 than in FVC, resulting in a normal or modestly increased FEV_1/FVC ratio.

In obstructive lung disease, *expiratory* airflow is impaired secondary to airway narrowing, and from decreased pulmonary elastic recoil in emphysematous COPD. FEV_1 is decreased proportionally more than FVC, resulting in a reduced FEV_1/FVC ratio.

Table 2-1 lists some examples of obstructive and restrictive lung diseases.

TABLE 2-1.   OBSTRUCTIVE AND RESTRICTIVE LUNG DISEASES

Obstructive Lung Diseases	Restrictive Lung Diseases
Chronic bronchitis	Neuromuscular diseases (poliomyelitis, myasthenia gravis,
Emphysema	Duchenne muscular dystrophy, Guillain-Barré syndrome)
Asthma	Acute respiratory distress syndrome (ARDS)
Bronchiectasis	Neonatal respiratory distress syndrome
Cystic fibrosis	Sarcoidosis
	Idiopathic pulmonary fibrosis
	Goodpasture's syndrome
	Wegener's granulomatosis
	Drug toxicity
	Pleural diseases

STEP 1 SECRET

You may be asked to interpret spirometry readings and flow volume diagrams on the USMLE. It is important to know how to determine the FEV_1/FVC ratio from one of these diagrams to identify the category of pulmonary disease a patient may have. You should often be able to tell this from the shape of the diseased curve compared with a normal curve.

CASE 2-1

A 23-year-old woman is evaluated for a chronic cough and episodes of dyspnea and chest tightness. The cough is worse at night and often wakes her from deep sleep. She denies ever smoking but does complain of seasonal allergies when pollen levels are high. Her respiratory symptoms also tend to worsen during this time.

1. **What disorder do you suspect?**
Chronic cough in a young adult, particularly a cough that worsens at night and is associated with dyspnea and chest tightness, is classic for asthma. However, gastroesophageal reflux disease and myocardial ischemia (though the latter is unlikely) need to be considered as well.

CASE 2-1 continued:

Examination while the patient is asymptomatic is entirely unremarkable. Pulmonary function testing is initially normal, but in response to a methacholine challenge, she experiences moderate respiratory distress and her FEV_1/FVC ratio drops to 55%. Her symptoms resolve and her FEV_1/FVC ratio normalizes following treatment with an albuterol inhaler.

2. **What is the diagnosis? How is this condition classified?**
   The diagnosis is asthma, which can be classified as extrinsic (allergic, type I) or intrinsic (nonallergic, type II) asthma. Extrinsic asthma commonly begins in children from families with allergic histories, whereas intrinsic asthma usually begins in adult life and can be associated with chronic bronchitis, exercise, or cold air. The distinction between intrinsic and extrinsic, although useful from a pathophysiologic perspective, is of limited value clinically, as most patients present with a spectrum of overlapping characteristics, including elevated IgE levels in those with nonallergic asthma.

3. **What is the pathophysiologic process causing symptoms in this woman?**
   This patient likely has extrinsic (i.e., allergic) asthma because she complains of seasonal allergies. Allergic asthma is initiated by a type I hypersensitivity reaction. Antigens from the environment enter the lungs and bind IgE antibodies on mast cells and basophils. This stimulates cross-linking of membrane-bound IgE antibodies, resulting in cellular degranulation and release of cytokines. Histamine (via G_q-linked H_1 receptors) and other proinflammatory mediators cause *reversible* bronchoconstriction and airway obstruction, leading to respiratory symptoms. Her symptom of chest tightness is likely related to this diffuse bronchoconstriction.

4. **About 5% of asthmatics are sensitive to aspirin, and some may even develop fatal bronchospasm from ingesting aspirin. What is currently believed to be the biochemical basis of this?**
   Aspirin inhibits cyclooxygenase (COX) and therefore prevents the synthesis of prostaglandins, while shunting substrates into the leukotriene pathway in some inflammatory cells. Pulmonary leukotrienes are potent bronchoconstrictors and therefore may exacerbate bronchospasm in asthmatics (and even nonasthmatics).
   Note: Asthmatics who also suffer from rhinitis and nasal polyps seem to be particularly sensitive to this effect of aspirin, and may need to avoid aspirin altogether. Many of these patients have a similar reaction to ibuprofen and naproxen. They should be instructed to take acetaminophen for analgesia.

5. **What is exercise-induced asthma?**
   Patients who suffer from exercise-induced asthma become short of breath during aerobic exercise. Unlike other forms of asthma, exercise-induced asthma is not associated with airway hyperresponsiveness or with airway remodeling. The exact mechanism of the condition is unknown. Patients find some relief with bronchodilator use prior to the onset of exercise.

6. **What is the explanation for the decreased FEV_1/FVC ratio in this woman?**
   This ratio is reduced in asthma because bronchoconstriction increases airway resistance and impairs the *rate* of expiratory airflow. Mediators include leukotrienes, cytokines (IL-4, IL-13) histamine, and eosinophils. Epithelium becomes fragile, and there is thickening of the basement membrane. Glucocorticoids inhibit this inflammation.

7. **Why does methacholine cause her FEV_1/FVC ratio to decrease?**
   The common denominator in the different types of asthma is *hyperreactivity of the tracheobronchial tree*, especially to inflammatory mediators. Methacholine is a direct cholinergic agonist that can cause bronchoconstriction via muscarinic receptor–mediated effects. Patients with asthma will respond to lower doses of methacholine than the general population. Often, a bronchodilator such as albuterol is administered prior to a repeat methacholine challenge. The degree of reversibility of decreased FEV_1/FVC ratio can be useful in distinguishing asthma from other causes of obstructive lung disease such as COPD.

8. **What is the residual lung volume and how is it affected in an asthma attack?**
   Residual lung volume is the volume of air left in the lung after a maximal expiration. The elevated resistance to expiratory airflow that develops during bronchoconstriction does not allow normal expiration of the usual percentage of alveolar gas at typical intrathoracic pressures, resulting in an increased residual volume. This increase in residual volume is typical of obstructive airway diseases. (**Note:** The increase in residual volume in emphysema is caused by *air trapping* in the smaller airways, not hypertrophy or bronchoconstriction as in asthma.)

9. **Why is wheezing generally heard most during expiration in asthma?**
   During expiration, the increase in intrathoracic pressure further decreases the diameter of airways that are already narrowed from bronchoconstriction, making it more difficult for air to flow, creating a turbulent and noisy airflow. Note that in acute asthmatic attacks, both inspiratory and expiratory wheezes are caused by bronchospasm.
   The pathophysiology of wheezing is different in COPD, in which bronchospasm rarely occurs. Rather, extensive parenchymal destruction promotes airway collapse during expiration because of the higher intrathoracic pressures, resulting in more of an expiratory wheeze.

10. **With respect to the pathophysiology of asthma, what are the two mechanistic targets of pharmacologic intervention?**
    Because bronchoconstriction and pulmonary inflammation play such an important etiologic role in asthma, pharmacotherapy in asthma is primarily aimed at stimulating bronchodilation (or preventing bronchoconstriction) and at inhibiting the pulmonary inflammatory process. We will discuss the specific drugs employed for these purposes later.

11. **Quick review: Cover the two columns on the right side of Table 2-2 and identify the class of drug and mechanism of action for the listed antiasthmatic drugs.**

TABLE 2-2.   DRUGS USED FOR TREATMENT OF ASTHMA

Agent(s)	Drug Class	Mechanism of Action
Albuterol, salmeterol	β_2-Agonist (short- and long-acting, respectively)	Bronchodilation
Cromolyn sodium	Mast cell stabilizer	Prevents release of histamine and other proinflammatory substances
Ipratropium	Anticholinergic (short-acting)	Inhibition of bronchoconstriction
Monteleukast	Leukotriene receptor antagonist	Inhibits activity of proinflammatory leukotrienes
Zileuton	5-Lipoxygenase inhibitor	Inhibits synthesis of leukotrienes
Beclomethasone Fluticasone	Glucocorticoid	Anti-inflammation via inhibition of synthesis of wide variety of proinflammatory agents

12. **Why are albuterol and salmeterol preferable to isoproterenol in treating asthma?**
    Although all three of these drugs are β-agonists, only albuterol and salmeterol are selective β_2-agonists, the adrenergic receptor type present in the lungs that mediates bronchodilation. Isoproterenol has both β_2- and β_1-agonist activity and can therefore stimulate cardiac β_1-receptors, resulting in tachycardia and palpitations.

Note: Beta blockers should generally be avoided in asthmatics because they can precipitate or exacerbate bronchospasm. If use of a beta blocker is warranted, selective β_1-receptor blockers (e.g., atenolol, esmolol, metoprolol, nebivolol) should be administered because they have less effect on respiratory function.

13. **This patient was put on a combination inhaler that contained a β_2-agonist and a corticosteroid. A month or so later she noticed a white cheesy exudate on her soft palate and pharynx. What probably happened?**
The patient likely developed oropharyngeal candidiasis (causative agent is *Candida albicans*); this infection is due to glucocorticoid-mediated suppression of the local immunologic response. For this reason, it is suggested that patients rinse their mouths after taking inhaled corticosteroids.

14. **Why are cromolyn sodium and nedocromil useful in the prevention but not treatment of asthmatic attacks?**
Cromolyn sodium and nedocromil inhibit mast cell degranulation and the release of histamines and prostaglandins that occurs in an allergic response asthmatic attack. However, once the mast cells have degranulated (i.e., following an acute asthma attack), these agents have no significant effects on the activity of the inflammatory mediators that are released. So, essentially, it is too late to use these drugs once symptoms have developed.

15. **What histologic changes would be expected in the bronchial smooth muscle and mucosa if a biopsy were performed in this patient?**
    1. *Smooth muscle hypertrophy* secondary to recurrent bronchoconstriction
    2. *Mucosal edema* (with a relative *eosinophilia*) secondary to a chronic subacute inflammatory process
    3. *Curschmann's spirals* (whorls of desquamated epithelium found in the mucus of asthmatics)
    4. *Charcot-Leyden crystals* (degranulated eosinophil membranes found in the mucus of asthmatics)

16. **What is theophylline and what are some of the drawbacks of its use?**
Theophylline is a methylxanthine derivative (meaning it has a structure similar to caffeine and purine bases) that can be used in the treatment of asthma. Its effectiveness is due to its bronchodilatory and anti-inflammatory actions, although the precise mechanisms by which it mediates these actions are beyond the scope of this book. Because theophylline is such an inexpensive drug, it remains the drug of choice in the treatment of asthma in many nonindustrialized countries, and is still occasionally used in the United States for the treatment of asthma that has been refractory to β-agonists, steroids, and other newer agents. Unfortunately, theophylline has a low therapeutic index and can precipitate seizures, cardiac arrhythmias, and even death. Plasma levels therefore have to be monitored regularly. Theophylline toxicity is treated with beta blockers.

SUMMARY BOX: ASTHMA

- Symptoms: Wheezing, cough (that is often worse late at night or early in the morning), chest tightness, and dyspnea. Symptoms are often triggered or worsened by exercise, cold air, or inhaled noxious particles. A history of prolonged upper respiratory tract infections is also characteristic of asthma.

- Pathology: Smooth muscle hypertrophy secondary to recurrent bronchoconstriction and mucosal edema (with a relative eosinophilia) secondary to a chronic subacute inflammatory process. Curschmann's spirals and Charcot-Leyden crystals are found in the mucus of asthmatics.

■ Diagnosis: Disproportionate decrease in the FEV_1/FVC ratio in response to methacholine.

■ Management: Effective agents include steroids, β_2-agonists, mast cell stabilizers, anticholinergics, leukotriene receptor antagonists, 5-lipoxygenase inhibitors, and theophylline.

CASE 2-2

A 36-year-old man who works on a farm is evaluated for a several-month history of worsening dyspnea with exertion. He is diagnosed with asthma and given an albuterol inhaler to be used when symptomatic. The patient has now returned to your office upset that his inhaler "doesn't do a darned thing!"

1. **What are some potential causes of this man's symptoms?**
   He may have asthma but be using the inhaler incorrectly. He may also have COPD, hypersensitivity pneumonitis, congestive heart failure (CHF), coronary artery disease, pulmonary hypertension, or anemia. More information is needed.

CASE 2-2 continued:

At the next visit he continues to inform you: "Doc, I don't understand it. I just bought this farm a month ago, and every time I go out there I get short of breath after only a few hours. I've never had trouble breathing this badly before. I can hardly work outside at this point."

2. **What is the most likely diagnosis at this time?**
   Acute attacks of dyspnea with a clear exposure history and lack of response to albuterol is suggestive of hypersensitivity pneumonitis (also known as extrinsic allergic alveolitis).

3. **What is the pathophysiology of this disorder and why doesn't albuterol help?**
   Hypersensitivity pneumonitis is an acute inflammatory disease of the alveoli; it results from an allergic reaction to a wide variety of allergens, and causes acute shortness of breath. It subsumes a wide variety of diseases with the same underlying etiology and pathogenesis, but can be due to exposure to different allergens (e.g., farmer's lung, pigeon handler's lung, humidifier lung). Unlike in asthma, the bronchioles are not affected, explaining why albuterol may not be helpful. Note that the "allergic" reaction is *not* IgE-mediated.

4. **How is hypersensitivity pneumonitis treated?**
   The most crucial aspect of treatment is avoidance of exposure to allergens. If there is continuous exposure to the offending allergen and continual alveolar inflammation (alveolitis), the chronic inflammation can ultimately result in irreversible pulmonary fibrosis.

SUMMARY BOX: HYPERSENSITIVITY PNEUMONITIS

■ Symptoms: Wheezing and dyspnea. Symptoms are often triggered or worsened by a variety of antigens including occupational exposures (as noted in the text).

■ Diagnosis: Diffuse infiltrates seen on chest x-ray film with appropriate symptoms and, if disease course is progressive, restrictive patterns on pulmonary function tests (PFTs) from eventual fibrosis.

- Pathology: Biopsy may show poorly formed, noncaseating granulomas or mononuclear cell infiltrates.

- Treatment: Most often reversible if diagnosed early and offending agent removed. Otherwise, progresses to pulmonary fibrosis.

CASE 2-3

A 37-year-old man with a known history of allergic asthma is evaluated in the emergency department for respiratory distress and low-grade fever. His albuterol inhaler has not been alleviating his symptoms in recent days. A chest x-ray study shows diffuse pulmonary infiltrates and laboratory workup reveals a marked eosinophilia and elevated IgE levels.

1. **What is the suspected diagnosis?**
   This presentation of fever, eosinophilia, and pulmonary infiltrates is classic for allergic bronchopulmonary aspergillosis (ABPA), a hypersensitivity response to the fungus *Aspergillus fumigatus*. ABPA occurs predominantly in patients with asthma.
   Note: Several other fungi can also cause identical clinical and laboratory findings but do so less commonly than *Aspergillus*.

2. **What other tests can be done to more confidently establish this diagnosis?**
   Skin sensitivity tests to the fungus *Aspergillus fumigatus*, as well as *Aspergillus*-specific serum IgE tests, may be performed.

3. **What is causing the pulmonary infiltrate?**
   There is marked infiltration of the pulmonary parenchyma with eosinophils in this disease, which is why this disease is known as one of the "eosinophilic pneumonias."
   Note: The eosinophilic pneumonias encompass a spectrum of diseases of different causes, all of which have in common eosinophilic infiltration of the lung and, often, peripheral blood eosinophilia, as in this patient. Allergic bronchopulmonary aspergillosis (ABPA) and other eosinophilic pneumonias are treated with corticosteroids.

SUMMARY BOX: ALLERGIC BRONCHOPULMONARY ASPERGILLOSIS

- Allergic bronchopulmonary aspergillosis typically occurs in asthmatics and manifests with dyspnea, fever, eosinophilia, and infiltrates on a chest x-ray study.

- Corticosteroids are the mainstay of treatment.

CASE 2-4

A 70-year-old man presents to the office with complaints of fever, cough, and fatigue for the past 3 days. Upon further questioning, you determine that his cough produces a "rusty"-colored sputum. Prior to this episode he reports that he has been "as healthy as can be expected" and denies smoking and drinking alcohol. His blood work shows an increased white blood cell count, while chest x-ray shows a right upper lobe infiltrate.

1. **What is the most likely diagnosis in this patient?**
   The patient's fever, increased white blood cell count, and chest x-ray appearance are all suggestive of lobar (typical) pneumonia. *Streptococcus pneumoniae* is a gram-positive organism often associated with lobar pneumonia in this age group. *Klebsiella pneumoniae* is another cause of lobar pneumonia, but is less likely in this patient. For the purpose of boards, *Klebsiella* pneumonia will likely present with red currant jelly sputum in an alcoholic or diabetic patient.

2. **How would your differential diagnosis change if the patient presented with a 2-week history of low-grade fever, cough, and diffuse patchy infiltrates seen on chest x-ray film?**
   This presentation is more typical of atypical (interstitial) or walking pneumonia. It typically follows a more indolent course than for lobar pneumonia and is often seen in adolescents and adults. Often, chest x-ray appearance is much worse than might be expected from the patient's symptoms. Bacterial causes of atypical pneumonia include *Mycoplasma, pneumoniae, Chlamydia pneumoniae,* and *Legionella pneumophila.* Viral causes include respiratory syncytial virus (RSV) and adenovirus.

3. **What are some common causes of pneumonia in different age groups?**
   See Table 2-3.

TABLE 2-3. COMMON CAUSES OF PNEUMONIA

Neonates (<4 wk)	Children (4 wk–18 yr)	Adults (18-40 yr)	Adults (40-65 yr)	Elderly
Group B streptococci *Escherichia coli*	Viruses (respiratory syncytial virus) *Mycoplasma Chlamydia pneumoniae Streptococcus pneumoniae*	*Mycoplasma C. pneumoniae S. pneumoniae*	*S. pneumoniae Haemophilus influenzae* Anaerobes Viruses *Mycoplasma*	*S. pneumoniae* Influenzavirus Anaerobes *H. influenzae* Gram-negative rods

CASE 2-5

A 75-year-old woman with a long history of smoking is evaluated for gradually worsening dyspnea over many years.

1. **What is the differential diagnosis?**
   Given her smoking history, this sounds like COPD, but other diagnoses to consider include restrictive lung diseases such as pulmonary fibrosis as well as nonpulmonary conditions such as CHF and anemia. A long history of smoking and worsening dyspnea could also be suggestive of lung cancer. We need more information.

CASE 2-5 continued:

Examination reveals a cachectic elderly woman who is unable to speak in complete sentences because of difficulty catching her breath. A prolonged expiratory phase is noted.

Lung fields are hyperresonant on percussion. A chest x-ray study shows hyperinflation of the lungs with flattening of the diaphragm. Pulmonary function tests (PFTs) reveal an FEV_1/FVC ratio of 45%. An electrocardiogram (ECG) indicates right ventricular hypertrophy. Blood work reveals an elevated hemoglobin and hematocrit.

2. **What is the diagnosis?**
   All of the preceding findings are suggestive of emphysema (COPD), an obstructive lung disease associated with exposure to cigarette smoke. Expiration is normally a passive process, but because of parenchymal destruction in COPD, the lungs lose their elastic recoil, and expiration becomes inefficient and prolonged, resulting in "air-trapping" and pursed-lip breathing. The reduced FEV_1/FVC ratio also suggests an obstructive process and argues against the other diagnostic possibilities. Finally, even the elevated hemoglobin would be an expected physiologic compensation for the hypoxemia associated with emphysema.

3. **What is the pathophysiologic explanation for the decreased FEV_1/FVC ratio in this woman?**
   The widespread destruction of alveolar septa and alveolar elastin in emphysema causes decreased elastic recoil of the alveoli, which is one of the major forces for expiratory airflow. This compromised expiratory airflow in COPD decreases both FEV_1 and FVC, with a particularly greater effect on FEV_1. Therefore the ratio of FEV_1 to FVC is decreased. Decreased FEV_1 to FVC ratio is the hallmark of an obstructive lung disease.

4. **What was the most likely cause of emphysema in this woman?**
   Chronic cigarette smoking is the most common cause of emphysema. Smoking is thought to damage the respiratory bronchioles and alveoli, resulting in chronic activation of alveolar macrophages and neutrophils. These cells release large amounts of elastase and other proteases, which degrade alveolar elastin and collagen, resulting in alveolar destruction and loss of elastic recoil during expiration. Cigarette smoke is also thought to directly inhibit alveolar elastin synthesis and to inhibit the activity of α_1-antitrypsin, a protease inhibitor synthesized and secreted by the liver.

5. **What histopathologic changes would a biopsy of this woman's lung likely reveal?**
   The destruction of alveolar elastin that occurs in emphysema results in permanent abnormal enlargement of the airspaces distal to the terminal bronchiole. This is accompanied by destruction of their alveolar walls, but without obvious fibrosis. This process causes the hyperlucency or darkness on chest x-ray film because the beam penetrates the tissue more (Fig. 2-4).

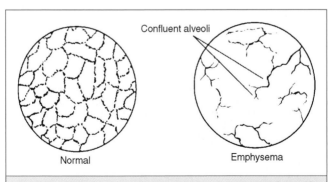

Confluent alveoli

Normal   Emphysema

Figure 2-4. Pulmonary changes in pneumonia and emphysema. (From Guyton AC, Hall JE: Textbook of Medical Physiology, 10th ed. Philadelphia, WB Saunders, 2000.)

6. **How do centriacinar and panacinar emphysema differ in terms of morphology and etiology?**

   Centriacinar emphysema is much more common than panacinar emphysema and is typically acquired secondary to a long history of cigarette smoking. In centriacinar emphysema, respiratory bronchioles are abnormally enlarged, whereas the distal alveoli are spared. Panacinar emphysema is associated with α_1-antitrypsin deficiency and involves abnormal enlargement of the distal alveoli, alveolar ducts, and respiratory bronchioles. This disease should be suspected in any adults with symptoms of emphysema but minimal exposure to cigarettes.

7. **Why may administration of large volumes of concentrated O_2 to this woman cause hypoventilation?**

   Due largely to the reduction in alveolar surface area available for gas exchange, patients with COPD may have become adjusted to abnormally high levels of plasma CO_2 (hypercapnia), such that ventilatory drive in these patients is maintained only by low plasma O_2 levels (hypoxemia). In theory, O_2 therapy may remove this ventilatory stimulus, causing hypoventilation and possibly respiratory failure, although this result is rarely seen clinically.

8. **How does emphysema cause the right ventricular hypertrophy seen on this patient's electrocardiogram?**

   First, recall that the pulmonary vessels respond to hypoxia by constricting and diverting blood flow from poorly ventilated to well-ventilated regions of the lung. This is normally an appropriate adaptive response. However, in COPD, the widespread hypoxia results in diffuse vasoconstriction, thereby pathologically elevating pulmonary arterial pressures. This can lead to right ventricular hypertrophy. A further mechanism contributing to the development of right ventricular hypertrophy involves emphysematous destruction of the alveolar septa and walls. This reduces the number of pulmonary capillaries, which forces increased blood flow through remaining blood vessels, further increasing pulmonary pressures.

RELATED QUESTIONS ON CHRONIC OBSTRUCTIVE PULMONARY DISEASE

9. **Why is an individual with α_1-antitrypsin deficiency at increased risk for developing emphysema?**

   α_1-Antitrypsin is a protein secreted by the liver which inhibits the activity of various proteolytic enzymes in the serum. Some of these enzymes, such as neutrophil elastase, degrade alveolar elastin. Widespread alveolar elastin degradation in the lungs then produces early-onset emphysema throughout the entire acinus (panacinar emphysema). Generally, this disease should be suspected in a nonsmoker who develops emphysema at an early age.

   Note that α_1-antitrypsin deficiency is not a true deficiency state; rather than being secreted by the liver, α1-antitrypsin accumulates in PAS (periodic acid-Schiff)-positive granules in the hepatocytes. This can eventually lead to hepatocellular carcinoma. Consider this diagnosis whenever you see a patient with symptoms of emphysema who also demonstrates symptoms of liver failure.

10. **Why do patients with emphysema breathe through pursed lips?**

    Normally, the equal pressure point (EPP) (point at which intrapleural pressure and alveolar pressure are equal) falls in the cartilaginous airways close to the mouth, preventing bronchial collapse (cartilage resists collapse). In patients with emphysema, alveolar pressure falls as a result of decreased elastic recoil pressure. The pressure in the alveolus (P_A) is defined by the relationship

$$P_A = P_{el} + P_l$$

where Pel = elastic recoil pressure and PL is the pressure across the lung. Decreased alveolar pressure shifts the equal pressure point into small, noncartilaginous airways, which are prone to collapse on expiration. Breathing through pursed lips elevates alveolar pressure and pushes the equal pressure point back toward the mouth to prevent expiratory airway collapse.

11. **What pharmacologic agents are used to treat chronic obstructive pulmonary disease?**
See Table 2-4.

TABLE 2-4. DRUGS USED FOR TREATMENT OF CHRONIC OBSTRUCTIVE PULMONARY DISEASE		
Drug	**Mechanism of Action**	**Clinical Use**
Albuterol	Dilation of airways	Relief of acute symptoms
Ipratropium	Prevention of bronchoconstriction	Prophylaxis
Glucocorticoids	Reducing inflammation	Relief of acute symptoms and occasionally prophylaxis

SUMMARY BOX: EMPHYSEMA

- Symptoms: Progressive insidious dyspnea. Note that emphysema and chronic bronchitis fall on a continuum for patients with chronic obstructive pulmonary disease, so there may be overlapping symptoms, and most often patients have characteristics of both diseases.

- Examination: Hyperresonance of the chest, decreased breath sounds bilaterally, prolonged expiratory phase, and pursed lip breathing. Pulse oximetry on room air at rest or with minimal exertion may be decreased.

- Diagnosis: Chest x-ray may show hyperinflation and hyperlucency of the lungs, increased anteroposterior diameter ("barrel chest"), and flattening of the diaphragm. Pulmonary function tests (PFTs) yield a FEV_1/FVC ratio <75%, with minimal improvement following the administration of bronchodilators. Patients are often hypoxemic, and this results in a modest polycythemia.

- Pathology: Destruction of lung parenchyma from pathologic activation of proteases. The destruction of alveolar elastin results in permanent abnormal enlargement of the air spaces distal to the terminal bronchiole. This is accompanied by destruction of their alveolar walls, but without obvious fibrosis.

- Treatment: Short acting beta-agonists such as albuterol for acute symptoms, ipratropium, and glucocorticoids for longer-term both acute treatment and chronic prophylaxis. Supplemental oxygen is the only treatment shown to improve survival.

- Potential complications: Right ventricular hypertrophy with pulmonary hypertension, hypoxemia necessitating supplemental oxygen, and (rarely) spontaneous pneumothorax from rupture of a surface bleb.

CASE 2-6

A 55-year-old man who is not closely followed by the medical community presents to the walk-in clinic with complaints of a chest cold, noting daily morning productive cough for the past 2 years. He has smoked a pack a day since the age of 20.

1. **What is the likely diagnosis?**
   He most likely has chronic bronchitis. Chronic bronchitis can be diagnosed in patients with a productive cough for at least 3 months in 2 consecutive years and history of chronic pulmonary infections. A history of smoking is typical.

2. **Why may cigarette smoking predispose to chronic lung infections?**
   The toxins in cigarette smoke paralyze the mucociliary tract, resulting in impaired mucus clearance from the airways. Furthermore, pseudostratified, ciliated cells are replaced with goblet cells. This "preneoplastic" condition is true squamous metaplasia, creating an environment susceptible to infection.

CASE 2-6 continued:

The patient notes that the cough produces whitish phlegm and that about 3 weeks ago he developed a runny nose, sore throat, and fever. He has also noted chest tightness and worsening shortness of breath. His physical examination is notable for wheezing, bibasilar crackles on inspiration, and cyanotic appearance.

3. **What is the pathogenesis of chronic bronchitis?**
   Chronic bronchitis is caused by chronic irritation of the airways by inhaled substances (e.g., cigarette smoke) and repeated infections of the airways. Histopathologically, there is hypertrophy of submucosal glands and goblet cells, resulting in mucus hypersecretion in both large and small airways, which reduces their diameters and makes expiration more difficult. Mucus hypersecretion is reflected by an elevated Reid index (normal Reid index is less than 40%; generally >50% in chronic bronchitis), which is defined as gland depth/total thickness of the bronchial wall between the epithelium and underlying cartilage. It objectively measures smooth muscle hypertrophy.

4. **What is the basis of the reduced FEV_1/FVC ratio in chronic bronchitis?**
   Hypertrophy of mucus-secreting glands and mucus hypersecretion lead to reduction of airway diameter. These changes are the principal causes of expiratory airflow limitation, with minimal effect on elastic recoil of the alveoli. This leads to a decreased FEV_1 with smaller changes in FVC, thus resulting in a reduced FEV_1/FVC ratio.
   The bronchial wall biopsy specimen from a normal patient (Fig. 2-5A) shows normal pseudostratified columnar epithelium with scattered goblet cells overlying smooth muscle and a submucosal gland. The bronchial wall biopsy specimen from a patient with chronic bronchitis (Fig. 2-5B) shows hyperplastic epithelium with mucous cell metaplasia overlying a hypertrophied submucosal gland.

5. **What is an acute exacerbation of chronic obstructive pulmonary disease? What classes of medications should be avoided or prescribed with great caution in these situations?**
   An acute exacerbation entails the acute onset of significantly greater dyspnea, as well as alterations in blood gases such as worsening hypoxemia or hypercapnia. These exacerbations are usually due to respiratory infections such as acute bronchitis or pneumonia. Drugs that suppress respiration, such as the opioid analgesics, benzodiazepines, and barbiturates, should be avoided in these patients. Beta blockers, which inhibit catecholamine-mediated bronchodilation, should also be avoided.

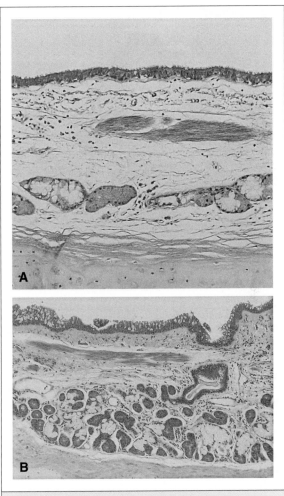

Figure 2-5. A, Bronchial wall from normal patient. **B,** Bronchial wall from a patient with chronic bronchitis. (From Cohen J, Powderly WG, Berkley SF, et al: Infectious Diseases, 2nd ed. Edinburgh, Mosby, 2004.)

6. **What acid-base abnormality is commonly found in chronic obstructive pulmonary disease patients and what is its origin?**

    Because of the depressed ventilation, hypercapnia ensues, which causes a respiratory acidosis. As a compensatory response, the kidneys excrete additional hydrogen ions and reabsorb increased amounts of bicarbonate (metabolic compensation), thereby restoring the pH toward normal.

7. **How might mechanical ventilation lead to respiratory alkalosis?**

    If tidal volumes and respiratory rate are set too high, this may "float" the patient to the other end of the spectrum, causing him to blow off too much CO_2 and go into respiratory alkalosis. The kidneys will attempt to compensate for this by excreting more bicarbonate to lower the pH back to normal.

    Note: Respiratory acidosis or alkalosis can develop rapidly, over minutes to hours. However, renal compensation occurs more slowly, and can take several days for complete compensation.

SUMMARY BOX: CHRONIC BRONCHITIS

- Symptoms: Productive cough, cyanosis, crackles, and wheezing.

- Diagnosis: Productive cough for 3 months in at least 2 consecutive years. Pulmonary function tests (PFTs) yield a FEV_1/FVC ratio <75%, with only slight improvement following the administration of bronchodilators. Patients are often hypoxemic and hypercapnic.

- Pathology: Hypertrophy of submucosal glands and goblet cells, resulting in mucus hypersecretion in both large and small airways, which reduces airway diameter and obstructs expiratory airflow. The Reid index (gland depth/total thickness of bronchial wall) objectively measures smooth muscle hypertrophy.

- Treatment: Bronchodilators and corticosteroids are mainstays of treatment. Antibiotics may be necessary for acute exacerbations of chronic bronchitis, which are often triggered by an infection. Drugs that suppress respiration, such as the opioid analgesics, benzodiazepines, and barbiturates, should be used very cautiously in these patients.

- Potential complications: May ultimately lead to right ventricular hypertrophy and right-sided heart failure.

CASE 2-7

A 50-year-old man who works in a shipyard and has a 40-pack-year history of smoking is evaluated for a several-year history of gradually worsening dyspnea. He denies orthopnea, paroxysmal nocturnal dyspnea, and edema.

1. **What is the likely diagnosis?**
   This patient may have either pulmonary fibrosis from asbestos exposure (asbestosis) or COPD from cigarette exposure. We need more information.

CASE 2-7 continued:

PFTs show an FVC < 50% of predicted for his age, height, and gender and an FEV_1/FVC ratio of 85%. His chest x-ray study is as shown in Figure 2-6.

2. **What is the diagnosis?**
   Given his elevated FEV_1/FVC ratio, he likely has a restrictive ventilatory defect, which is consistent with restrictive lung disease. Given his exposure history, he presumably has asbestosis. The chest x-ray study in Figure 2–6 shows a pleural plaque (with well-defined and angled margins), which is commonly seen in asbestosis.

3. **What are asbestos, asbestosis, and the pneumoconioses?**
   Asbestos is a fibrous derivative of silica that was commonly used as an insulator because of its fire-resistant properties, thereby placing insulation, shipyard, and construction workers at risk. Asbestosis is an interstitial lung disease that results in pulmonary fibrosis. Asbestos exposure also predisposes to malignancies (see next question). The pneumoconioses are a group of lung diseases caused by the inhalation of various types of dust particles in different occupational settings. The dust particles set off an inflammatory alveolitis, which, if the exposure continues, may lead to pulmonary fibrosis. Steroids may offer some relief in the early inflammatory stage but is of no benefit in the later fibrotic stage. Asbestosis is a type of pneumoconiosis.

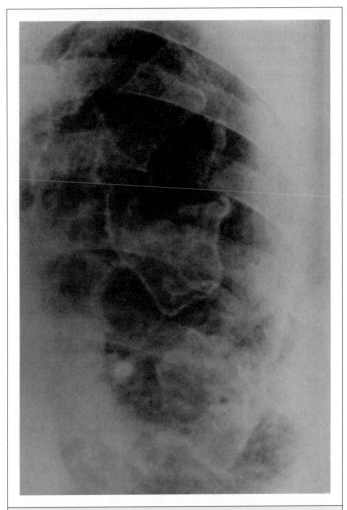

Figure 2-6. Centriacinar versus panacinar emphysema. (From Kumar V, Abbas K, Fausto N: Robbins and Cotran: Pathologic Basis of Disease, 7th ed. Philadelphia, WB Saunders, 2005.)

4. **To which malignancies does asbestosis predispose?**
   Asbestosis predisposes to mesothelioma and bronchogenic carcinoma. Smoking markedly increases the risk for developing asbestos-related bronchogenic carcinoma but *does not* increase the risk for developing asbestos-related mesothelioma. The incidence of bronchogenic carcinoma is greater than that of mesothelioma.

5. **What are some other common causes of pulmonary fibrosis?**
   A great variety of factors may cause pulmonary fibrosis, including silicosis, granulomatous diseases of the lung (e.g., sarcoidosis), connective tissue diseases (e.g., lupus, rheumatoid arthritis), and certain medications (e.g., amiodarone, bleomycin, methotrexate). It is also commonly idiopathic.

6. **What is the pathophysiologic explanation for the reduction in forced vital capacity in this man?**

   In pulmonary fibrosis, the fibrosis of the alveolar walls and septa makes the alveoli less compliant. The alveoli therefore do not expand as well for a given drop in intrathoracic pressure during inspiration, resulting in a reduced inspiratory volume, which translates to a reduced expiratory volume and reduced FEV_1 and FVC values. However, unlike obstructive disorders, the effect on FVC is much greater than the effect on FEV_1, and thus FEV_1/FVC ratio is normal or even increased (>80%; normal is 70–75%).

7. **What lung biopsy finding may be present in this patient that is unique to asbestosis?**

   Ferruginous bodies (or asbestos bodies), which are fibers of asbestos lined by hemosiderin deposits, may be seen. These yellow to brown, rod-shaped bodies stain positively with Prussian blue. You should be able to recognize an asbestos body in a histopathology image.

SUMMARY BOX: ASBESTOSIS

- Symptoms: Exertional dyspnea; with advanced disease, dyspnea at rest, dry cough, chest pain, and recurrent respiratory tract infections.

- Diagnosis: Look for history of exposure, chronically worsening dyspnea, and classic changes on chest X ray (e.g. pleural plaques).

- Pathology: Ferruginous bodies (or asbestos bodies), which are fibers of asbestos lined by hemosiderin deposits. These yellow to brown, rod-shaped bodies stain positively with Prussian blue.

CASE 2-8

A 45-year-old woman complains of chronic fatigue, as well as shortness of breath with exertion. Her history is significant for rather heavy menstrual bleeding (menorrhagia). She has never smoked. She shows no signs of cyanosis, and the only notable finding on physical examination is conjunctival pallor. Laboratory tests show hemoglobin (Hb) of 7.5 g/mL (normal range is 12–15 g/dL). Blood work reveals low plasma iron, ferritin, and increased total iron-binding capacity.

1. **What is the likely cause of this woman's dyspnea?**

   The patient is suffering from severe iron deficiency anemia, probably secondary to heavy menstrual flows.

2. **What is the difference between the Pao_2 and the arterial oxygen content?**

   The Pao_2 is the partial pressure of oxygen *dissolved* in arterial blood, also referred to as oxygen tension. The partial pressure of arterial oxygen is principally mediated by adequate ventilation and gas exchange and is unrelated to the hemoglobin concentration. Therefore, even in severe anemia, the Pao_2 can be completely normal if respiratory function is normal.

   The arterial oxygen content, on the other hand, is a measure of the total quantity of oxygen in a given volume of blood, and it is dependent upon the concentration of hemoglobin in the blood. The hemoglobin does not affect the partial pressure of oxygen in arterial blood but does mediate the amount of oxygen that is carried in blood at a given partial pressure of oxygen. Because each gram of Hb can bind approximately 1.34 mL of O_2 at normal Pao_2, the average person with [Hb] of 15 g/dL has an arterial O_2 concentration of 20% (i.e., 15 g Hb/dL × 1.34 mL O_2/g Hb = 20 mL O_2/dL, or 20 mL O_2/100 mL). In anemia, the reduced hemoglobin level will clearly reduce the arterial oxygen content (see Table 2-5).

TABLE 2-5. PULMONARY AND RESPIRATORY TERMINOLOGY

P_{AO_2} (mm Hg)	Partial pressure of alveolar oxygen
Pa_{O_2} (mm Hg)	Partial pressure of dissolved oxygen in arterial blood
Arterial Oxygen Content (mg/dL)	Total quantity of oxygen bound to hemoglobin in volume of arterial blood
Oxygen Capacity (Saturation) (%)	Percentage of oxygen-binding sites on hemoglobin with oxygen bound

You should know the formula for total oxygen content:

$$O_2 \text{ content} = [Hb] \times 1.34 \text{ mL } O_2/g \text{ Hb} \times \%Hb \text{ saturation} + 0.003 \text{ mL } O_2/100 \text{ mL blood/mm Hg} \times 100 \text{ mg Hg}$$

As you can see, Pa_{O_2} directly contributes very little to total oxygen content. However, Pa_{O_2} heavily influences Hb saturation, which does have a large effect on total oxygen content.

CASE 2-8 continued:

Arterial O_2 saturation by pulse oximetry on room air is 99%.

3. **What does arterial oxygen saturation measure?**
   Arterial oxygen saturation is a measure of the percentage of oxygen-binding sites on hemoglobin that have oxygen bound to them. As mentioned previously, it is determined by the Pa_{O_2}, with higher Pa_{O_2} values associated with greater oxygen saturation.
   Note that many factors other than the Pa_{O_2} can influence the affinity of hemoglobin for oxygen See Fig. 2-7 for examples of factors that can contribute to "leftward shift" and "rightward shift" of the oxygen dissociation curve.

4. **Why doesn't this woman's anemia make her cyanotic?**
   Cyanosis is caused by the presence of at least 5 g/dL of arterial *deoxy*hemoglobin, which occurs at low Pa_{O_2} values with reduced arterial oxygen saturation. As long as the Pa_{O_2} is normal in anemia, and it should be normal in the absence of respiratory disease, there should be good oxygen saturation and minimal deoxyhemoglobin. Note that this woman's O_2 saturation is 99%, indicating good respiratory function. Nevertheless, because the oxygen-carrying capacity of the blood is reduced secondary to decreased hemoglobin concentration, she still suffers the symptoms of anemia (e.g., fatigue).
   Note: Methemoglobinemia is another potential cause of cyanosis. In conditions such as pyruvate kinase deficiency or glucose-6-phosphate dehydrogenase (G6PD) deficiency or following exposure to oxidizing drugs such as benzocaine, the mechanisms that defend against oxidative stress within the red blood cells (RBCs) are overwhelmed, and the ferrous ion (Fe^{2+}) of the heme moiety of hemoglobin is oxidized to the ferric state (Fe^{3+}). This converts hemoglobin to methemoglobin, which is unable to bind oxygen.

5. **How is the anemia contributing to this woman's dyspnea?**
   The peripheral chemoreceptors cannot "sense" the low arterial oxygen content; they can only sense the Pa_{O_2}, which is normal because ventilation is unimpaired. However, the low oxygen content promotes anaerobic respiration, which lowers arterial pH and increases respiratory drive, causing dyspnea.

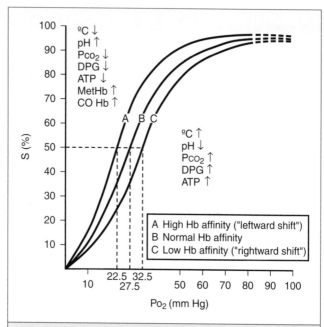

Figure 2-7. Curve B is from a normal adult at 38° C, pH 7.40, and Pco₂ 35.0 mm Hg. Curves A and C illustrate the effect on the affinity for oxygen (P₅₀) of variations in temperature(°C), pH, Pco₂, 2,3-diphosphoglycerate (DPG), adenosine triphosphate, methemoglobin, and carboxyhemoglobin. Curve A is of the newborn. (From Duc G: Assessment of hypoxia in the newborn: Suggestions for a practical approach. Pediatrics 48:469–481, 1971.)

RELATED QUESTIONS

6. **What are typical values for arterial and venous Po₂ and what do they represent with respect to the hemoglobin dissociation curve?**
At a normal arterial Po₂ of 100 mm Hg, hemoglobin is fully saturated. This corresponds to the "loading" portion of the hemoglobin dissociation curve, which occurs in the pulmonary capillaries (Fig. 2-8). In the peripheral capillaries, O₂ diffuses rapidly from the blood to the tissues, such that the Po₂ in venous blood drops to approximately 40 mm Hg, corresponding to hemoglobin that is only ~75% saturated (i.e., bound to three molecules of O₂).

STEP 1 SECRET

Know how to interpret oxygen dissociation curves and what factors shift the curve to the left or to the right. This is a commonly tested principle on the USMLE.

7. **Would exposure to carbon monoxide be expected to affect the Pao₂? Explain.**
No. Carbon monoxide exhibits its effect by binding to hemoglobin and preventing oxygen from dissociating from hemoglobin (leftward shift), but will not affect the amount of oxygen dissolved in plasma. Therefore, exposure to carbon monoxide should not alter Pao₂, although the O₂ *saturation* will decrease.

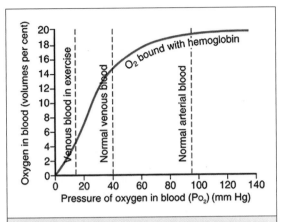

Figure 2-8. CXR of patient in Case 2-7. (From Grainger RG, Allison D, Adam A, et al: Grainger & Allison's Diagnostic Radiology: A Textbook of Medical Imaging, 4th ed. London, Churchill Livingstone, 2001.)

8. **Differentiate between external and internal respiration. Which is affected by anemia?**

Gas exchange between the alveoli and blood in the pulmonary capillaries is referred to as external respiration, whereas the exchange of gases between capillary blood and the interstitial fluid is referred to as internal respiration. Cellular respiration refers to the exchange of gases between the cells and the interstitial fluid. External respiration may be compromised by low atmospheric oxygen (e.g., high altitude) or poor alveolar ventilation (e.g., pneumonia). Internal and cellular respiration, by contrast, will be affected by anemia because less oxygen will be transferred from the capillary blood to the interstitium and cells.

SUMMARY BOX: ANEMIA

- Classic features include: Tachycardia, fatigue, dyspnea on exertion, and conjunctival pallor on physical examination without other obvious signs of cyanosis.

- Pa_{O_2} is the partial pressure of oxygen dissolved in arterial blood; it is also known as the oxygen tension. The PA_{O_2} is the alveolar oxygen tension.

- The arterial oxygen content measures the total amount of oxygen in blood and is primarily determined by the concentration of hemoglobin.

- The arterial oxygen saturation reflects the extent of hemoglobin saturation with oxygen. It is determined by the Pa_{O_2}, with a higher Pa_{O_2} causing greater oxygen saturation, although many other factors (e.g., temperature, 2,3-diphosphoglycerate [DPG]) can influence the affinity of hemoglobin for O_2.

- Cyanosis is caused by the presence of at least 5 g/dL of deoxyhemoglobin. Severely anemic patients are not typically cyanotic if their Pa_{O_2} is normal.

- Methemoglobinemia results from conditions associated with impaired ability of red blood cells (RBCs) to defend against oxidative stressors, such as pyruvate kinase and glucose-6-phosphate dehydrogenase (G6PD) deficiency or exposure to oxidizing agents such as benzocaine.

- Carbon monoxide binds hemoglobin avidly and prevents oxygen from dissociating from hemoglobin. It therefore does not typically cause cyanosis or alter the Pa_{O_2}.

CASE 2-9

A 35-year-old male victim of multiple blunt trauma is in shock because of splenic rupture. The patient is operated on and sent to the intensive care unit (ICU). The next day, he becomes acutely short of breath. A chest x-ray study shows diffuse, bilateral pulmonary infiltrates, and arterial blood gas analysis reveals severe hypoxemia. A Swan-Ganz catheter threaded through his superior vena cava (SVC), right atrium, and right ventricle and into his pulmonary artery shows a normal pulmonary capillary "wedge" pressure.

1. **What is the anticipated diagnosis?**
   He most likely has acute respiratory distress syndrome (ARDS), also known as adult respiratory distress syndrome. ARDS is the final common pathway reaction to various serious injuries to the lung. ARDS is diagnosed by the presence of acute-onset respiratory failure, bilateral diffuse pulmonary infiltrates, severe hypoxemia, and the coexistence of a disease known to cause it.

2. **What are the etiology and pathogenesis of this disease?**
   ARDS occurs secondary to a wide variety of diseases, including sepsis, shock, severe pancreatitis, gastric aspiration, and near drowning. The common link in all these conditions is widespread pulmonary capillary endothelial damage. This leads to inflammation and fluid extravasation into the alveoli and interstitium, resulting in significant alveolar and interstitial edema and, consequently, severe hypoxemia.

3. **How is this condition managed?**
   Supportive therapy with a ventilator to maintain oxygenation and treatment of the underlying disease that is causing it. Unfortunately, this condition can be very challenging to treat, in part because delivering a high F_{IO_2} (percent inspired oxygen) via a ventilator can produce damaging free radicals that further exacerbate the condition.

4. **What is the diffusion equation and which parameter is influenced most by the high concentration of inspired oxygen?**
   Recall that the diffusion equation relates an increase in diffusion rates to increases in the partial pressure gradient of a gas across the membrane, increased solubility of the gas, or an increased surface area available for diffusion. The high F_{IO_2} increases the partial pressure gradient of oxygen across the pulmonary membrane, which attenuates the reduction in diffusion that occurs because of the increased membrane thickness (from edema).

5. **Both congestive heart failure and acute respiratory distress syndrome can cause significant pulmonary edema. How does the cause of pulmonary edema differ in these two settings?**
   In CHF, increased hydrostatic pressure from fluid backing up in the pulmonary system causes pulmonary edema. Note that in this situation, the pulmonary capillary wedge pressure would be elevated from the fluid backup (typically as a result of a "stiff" left ventricle). In contrast, in ARDS, increased capillary permeability is the basis for the edema, so the increased pulmonary capillary wedge pressure should be normal.

6. **Why is it necessary to be particularly cautious in giving fluids to this patient?**
   Excessive fluids can push someone into CHF. The resulting increase in pulmonary edema can seriously compromise already inadequate respiratory function (increased edema makes the diffusion barrier even thicker).

RELATED QUESTION

7. Using the diffusion equation, explain why each of the conditions in Table 2-6 is associated with hypoxemia:

$$D = \frac{A \times S \, (P_1 - P_2)}{T}$$

SUMMARY BOX: ACUTE RESPIRATORY DISTRESS SYNDROME

- ARDS is respiratory distress with progressive hypoxemia despite oxygen therapy.

- Causes: Pancreatitis, pulmonary embolism, sepsis, gastric aspiration, and near drowning.

- Treatment: Supportive care (e.g. mechanical ventilation) and treatment of the underlying condition.

CASE 2-10

A 75-year-old woman with a 90-pack-year history of cigarette smoking complains of a 6-month history of hemoptysis, shortness of breath, fatigue, and an unintentional 30-lb weight loss. Chest x-ray reveals increased anteroposterior (AP) diameter and flattening of the diaphragm, but also reveals a large mass in her right upper lobe. Biopsy establishes that the mass is malignant. Laboratory tests show plasma sodium of 125 mEq/L (normal range is 135–145 mEq/L) and urine osmolarity of 450 mOsm.

1. What type of lung cancer does this woman likely have?
   Small cell (oat cell) carcinoma of the lung is most likely. Various paraneoplastic syndromes, including the syndrome of inappropriate secretion of antidiuretic hormone (SIADH), are commonly observed in small cell lung carcinoma. This woman's hyperosmolar urine in a setting of hyponatremia are consistent with SIADH, which makes small cell carcinoma more probable.

TABLE 2-6. CONDITIONS CAUSING HYPOXEMIA	
Condition	Explanation for Hypoxemia
Neuromuscular respiratory insufficiency	Decreased ventilation reduces ΔP
Pulmonary edema	Increased thickness of pulmonary membrane/ diffusion barrier
Emphysema	Reduced surface area of pulmonary membrane from alveolar degradation
	Reduced pressure gradient from impaired ventilation

Continued

TABLE 2-6. CONDITIONS CAUSING HYPOXEMIA—continued

Condition	Explanation for Hypoxemia
Pneumonia	Decreased oxygen diffusion due to pulmonary edema (i.e., T increases in diffusion equation) and reduced "available" surface area of pulmonary membrane
Asthma	Reduced pressure secondary to ventilatory insufficiency
Neonatal respiratory distress syndrome	Reduced surfactant increases surface tension in alveoli, causing alveoli to collapse, impairing ventilation (ΔP) and reducing surface area of pulmonary membrane
Acute respiratory distress syndrome (i.e., diffuse alveolar damage)	Presence of diffuse pulmonary infiltrates increases thickness of pulmonary membrane

ΔP, change in pressure.

STEP 1 SECRET

The USMLE loves paraneoplastic syndromes, especially those related to lung cancers! Be sure that you can recognize symptoms of paraneoplastic syndromes caused by various malignancies.

2. **If a patient with small cell carcinoma develops bilateral ptosis (droopy eyelids) as well as neuromuscular weakness, what paraneoplastic syndrome should be suspected?**
Lambert-Eaton syndrome occurs quite frequently in small cell carcinoma. It results from antibodies that attack the voltage-gated calcium channels on the terminal bouton of presynaptic motor neurons.

3. **If a lung tumor is growing at the apex of the lung and compressing the cervical sympathetic chain on that side, what manifestations might one see?**
The cervical sympathetic chain supplies the superior tarsal muscle (which elevates the eyelid), the dilator pupillae, and the sweat glands of the face. Therefore, cutting off this nerve supply results in ipsilateral ptosis, miosis, and anhydrosis (i.e., Horner syndrome). Note the distinction from Lambert-Eaton syndrome, in which the ptosis is bilateral.
   Note: Tumors in the apex of the lung are known as Pancoast tumors. They are most commonly seen with squamous cell carcinoma of the lung. Another commonly seen complication of lung tumors is superior vena cava syndrome (often associated with small cell carcinoma), in which the superior vena cava is compressed by the growing tumor. This impairs venous drainage from the head and upper limbs, resulting in swelling and purple discoloration of the arms and face.

4. **Although there are several different histologic types of lung cancer, what are the two principal classifications and why do they exist?**
    Small cell lung cancer (SCLC) and non–small cell lung cancer (NSCLC) are the two principal classifications. The therapeutic and prognostic considerations do not differ for subtypes of non–small cell cancers, and all are generally treated with surgery. Small cell carcinomas, however, both readily metastasize and are very susceptible to radiation therapy. Radiation therapy is therefore generally the first line of treatment. (See Case 10–4 from Chapter 10, Oncology, for more information.)

5. **Why are radon levels routinely measured before homes are purchased?**
    Excessive exposure to radon is another cause of lung cancer.

6. **How can squamous cell carcinoma cause hypercalcemia without any bony metastases?**
    This type of lung cancer is known to release parathyroid hormone-related peptide (PTHrP), which stimulates bone resorption in much the same fashion as parathyroid hormone (PTH) does.

DIFFERENTIAL DIAGNOSIS

7. **If a patient with small cell carcinoma has hypertension, hypernatremia, hypokalemia, abdominal striae, and a "buffalo hump," what should be suspected?**
    One should suspect Cushing syndrome due to ectopic adrenocorticotropic hormone (ACTH) production, another common paraneoplastic syndrome in small cell carcinoma.

SUMMARY BOX: SMALL CELL CANCER OF THE LUNG

- Symptoms: Dyspnea, rapid, unexplained weight loss, and any symptoms caused by a paraneoplastic syndrome.

- Diagnosis: Chest x-ray study, computed tomography (CT) scan, and biopsy. Various paraneoplastic syndromes such as syndrome of inappropriate secretion of antidiuretic hormone (SIADH) are associated with small cell carcinoma.

- Pathology: Cells are generally small, have little cytoplasm, and are round or oval, often resembling lymphocytes. Small cell cancer of the lung is also called oat cell cancer because of its appearance.

- Treatment: Small cell cancers often metastasize quickly and are, therefore, not amenable to resection. They are, however, responsive to radiation.

CASE 2-11

A 38-year-old black woman presents for evaluation of a several week history of nonproductive cough and shortness of breath with exertion. She also complains of generalized fatigue, night sweats, and unintentional weight loss. Physical examination reveals erythematous cutaneous nodules on the lower extremities and mild hepatosplenomegaly. A chest x-ray shows bilateral hilar lymphadenopathy. Blood work reveals hypercalcemia.

1. **What must be included in the differential diagnosis?**
    Both lymphoma and sarcoidosis must be included in the differential diagnosis.

CASE 2-11 continued:

These findings prompt the physician to request a mediastinal lymph node biopsy, which reveals noncaseating granulomas.

2. **Now what is the most likely diagnosis?**
   Sarcoidosis, a systemic granulomatous disease of unknown cause, is the most likely diagnosis.

3. **Why was the lymph node biopsy performed?**
   Bilateral hilar lymphadenopathy is quite characteristic of sarcoidosis, suggesting the diagnosis. A lymph node biopsy will confirm the diagnosis by showing noncaseating granulomas, a finding that is characteristic of sarcoidosis and not lymphoma.

STEP 1 SECRET

Sarcoidosis is a commonly tested topic for Step 1. Be able to recognize the symptoms of sarcoidosis and the appearance of granulomas on an image.

4. **How can sarcoidosis cause cor pulmonale (right ventricular failure)?**
   As an inflammatory pulmonary disease, sarcoidosis can cause widespread pulmonary fibrosis, with obliteration of the pulmonary vascular bed, resulting in significant pulmonary hypertension. The pulmonary vasoconstriction that occurs in hypoxemia from pulmonary fibrosis may also contribute to this process.

5. **How is pulmonary hypertension defined?**
   Normal pulmonary artery pressure is between 10 and 14 mm Hg. In pulmonary hypertension, the pulmonary artery pressure increases to greater than 25 mm Hg at rest or 35 mm Hg during exercise. This increase in the pulmonary artery pressure can cause atherosclerosis, medial hypertrophy, and intimal fibrosis of the pulmonary arteries.

6. **What is the difference between primary and secondary pulmonary hypertension?**
   Primary pulmonary hypertension is due to an inactivating mutation in the *BMPR2* gene. The *BMPR2* gene normally acts to inhibit vascular smooth muscle proliferation. Primary pulmonary hypertension is often observed in young women.
   Secondary pulmonary hypertension, on the other hand, is a consequence of chronic lung disease that is distinct from pulmonary hypertension itself. Examples include the destruction of lung parenchyma seen in COPD, the increase in pulmonary resistance seen in mitral stenosis, the decrease in cross-sectional area of the pulmonary vasculature bed seen with recurrent thromboemboli or hypoxic vasoconstriction, and the inflammation and medial hypertrophy seen with certain autoimmune diseases (e.g., sarcoidosis).

7. **How can sarcoidosis cause a restrictive cardiomyopathy?**
   Granulomatous infiltration of the myocardium can cause fibrosis and consequently reduced ventricular compliance. This is fairly similar to the pathogenesis of restrictive cardiomyopathy that develops from infiltration in amyloidosis and hemochromatosis.
   Note: Because elevated levels of angiotensin-converting enzyme (ACE) are frequently associated with sarcoidosis, the diagnostic workup often includes a measurement of serum ACE. The hypercalcemia that develops in sarcoidosis is due to increased production of 1,25-dihydroxyvitamin D_3 by the macrophages in granulomas. Sarcoidosis is also associated with Bell's palsy.

SUMMARY BOX: SARCOIDOSIS

- Symptoms: May be generalized or focused depending upon the organ(s) involved. With lung involvement, dyspnea on exertion and wheezing may be present. Skin changes including erythema nodosum, plaques, maculopapular eruptions, and subcutaneous nodules appear commonly. Anterior uveitis and polyarthritis may also be present.

- Diagnosis: Based on clinical (see symptoms), radiologic (bilateral hilar lymphadenopathy), and histologic findings (noncaseating granulomas).

- Pathology: Noncaseating granulomas that can involve almost any organ system.

- Treatment: Glucocorticoids are the first-line treatment followed by chemotherapeutic agents based upon the organ system and extent of involvement.

CASE 2-12

A 27-year-old man who is stabbed in the chest in a bar fight is taken to the emergency room by ambulance. He is conscious with rapid breathing (tachypnea), hypotension, and pleuritic chest pain. There is tracheal deviation to the left, jugular venous distention, right-sided hyperresonance to percussion, and decreased breath sounds over the right lung. A chest x-ray shows decreased vascular markings on the right side. A needle thoracostomy is performed immediately to decompress the lung, and then a chest tube is inserted to stabilize breathing.

1. **What is the diagnosis?**
   Pneumothorax. More specifically, because this patient has tracheal deviation to the opposite side of the affected lung he likely has a tension pneumothorax. Note that spontaneous pneumothorax normally causes tracheal deviation to the same side of the collapsed lung to fill the pleural space now unused by the lung. Tension pneumothorax is typically caused by penetrating injuries to the chest wall that cause defects in either parietal or viscera pleura, allowing air into the pleural cavity during inspiration. In a tension pneumothorax, the defect serves as a one-way valve, allowing air to enter but not exit. This causes intrathoracic pressures to increase to supra-atmospheric levels. This increased intrathoracic pressure results in mediastinal shifting and compression of the superior vena cava and inferior vena cava (reducing venous return), explaining the signs of tracheal deviation, jugular venous distention, and hypotension, respectively.

2. **Why should the chest tube be inserted immediately superior to the lower rib in the intercostal space in which it is inserted?**
   This position is necessary to avoid the neurovascular bundle (from top to bottom: vein, artery, nerve) that runs on the inferior aspect of each rib.

3. **What is the pressure inside the pleural cavity (intrapleural space) normally?**
   The pleural pressure is normally negative, which helps maintain the lungs in expanded form. When either the visceral or parietal pleura is punctured, the influx of air under atmospheric pressure abolishes the vacuum and results in a positive intrapleural pressure, which collapses the lung.

4. **How does hypoxia-induced vasoconstriction help compensate, to some extent, for the respiratory dysfunction caused by pneumothorax?**
   The blood that would ordinarily go to the collapsed (hypoxic) lung gets shunted to the opposite lung, where it can get oxygenated and reduce the level of hypoxemia that develops.

5. **Is this patient more likely to be experiencing respiratory acidosis or respiratory alkalosis? Explain.**

   Decreased effective ventilation secondary to a collapsed lung will cause hypercapnia and respiratory acidosis.

   Note: A pneumothorax can cause a *mixed* respiratory and metabolic acidosis because of both impaired ventilation, which increases plasma CO_2 levels, and increased anaerobic metabolism in the tissues from reduced oxygen delivery, which increases plasma levels of acids such as lactic acid.

6. **What effect will a pneumothorax have on the serum ionized calcium level?**

   It will increase it because acidosis causes displacement of calcium from binding sites on albumin (via increased competition with hydrogen ions for these binding sites). In contrast, alkalosis leads to the ionized form of albumin, which can bind free calcium and reduce serum ionized calcium concentrations. Hypoalbuminemia also results in low levels of serum ionized calcium secondary to increased affinity of albumin for calcium.

SUMMARY BOX: PNEUMOTHORAX

- Symptoms: Sudden onset of severe dyspnea with sharp pain in one's side.

- Diagnosis: The trachea and mediastinum will shift away from the side of the pneumothorax. Physical signs include a distended unilateral chest, hyperresonance, and absence of breath sounds.

- Pathology: Commonly associated with emphysema, asthma, connective tissue disorders such as Marfan syndrome, and trauma, so the pathologic features vary according to the cause.

- Treatment: Insert chest tube, stabilize breathing, and treat underlying cause.

CHAPTER 3

NEPHROLOGY

Thomas A. Brown, MD, and Sonali J. Shah

INSIDER'S GUIDE TO NEPHROLOGY FOR THE USMLE STEP 1

Nephrology can be a tricky subject for many medical students, especially because mastering renal physiology requires comfort with and even manipulation of several formulas. Luckily, the scope of nephrology-related questions on the USMLE tends to be rather limited. Focus heavily on the subjects listed in First Aid and then use the cases in this chapter to then test your understanding of the material. Be sure to understand detailed principles regarding nephron function and activation of the renin-angiotensin-aldosterone system. With regard to renal pathology, the most commonly tested subjects include renal failure, glomerulonephritis, urinary tract infections (UTIs), and renal stones.

CLINICAL RENAL DISEASE

CASE 3-1

A 78-year-old man comes to the emergency room because of inability to urinate for the past 2 days and is experiencing lower abdominal pain. He admits to urinary difficulties over the last few years, including difficulty initiating his stream, a weak stream, nocturia, and dribbling after voiding. He denies taking any tricyclic antidepressants, antipsychotics, antihistamines, or sympathomimetic agents. On physical examination his bladder seems palpably enlarged, and a digital rectal examination reveals an enlarged prostate. Microscopic urine examination shows no hematuria or crystalluria. Routine laboratory tests show significantly elevated blood urea nitrogen (BUN) and creatinine and a high-normal prostate-specific antigen (PSA) of 3.8. An abdominal ultrasound reveals a markedly distended bladder and enlargement of the renal pelves.

1. **What is the probable cause of this patient's problems?**
   This patient has acute urinary retention, most likely secondary to occlusion of the bladder neck by benign prostatic hyperplasia (BPH). BPH will generally result in a mild elevation of PSA, but typically not high enough to prompt evaluation for prostate cancer (which is traditionally undertaken for PSA levels >4). Although total PSA levels are elevated in both BPH and prostate cancer, free PSA levels will only be elevated with BPH. The elevated BUN and creatinine strongly suggest that this patient also has acute renal failure.

2. **What are the three etiologic classifications of acute renal failure?**
   Renal failure is classified as prerenal, renal (intrinsic), or postrenal (obstructive). This man's renal failure clearly has an obstructive etiology. Acute bladder distention caused by long-standing BPH has resulted in bilateral hydronephrosis (dilated renal pelves) and acute renal failure. Figure 3-1 shows severe hydronephrosis from long-standing obstruction, with marked dilatation of the renal pelvis and calyces and loss of cortical parenchyma.

3. **How is glomerular filtration rate (GFR) calculated?**
   The GFR can be calculated using the following formula:

$$GFR = K_f \times (P_G - P_B - \Pi_G + \Pi_B)$$

   where
   K_f = filtration coefficient, a constant
   P_G = hydrostatic pressure in the glomerular capillaries
   P_B = hydrostatic pressure in Bowman's capsule
   Π_G = oncotic pressure in the glomerular capillaries
   Π_B = oncotic pressure in Bowman's capsule, typically 0

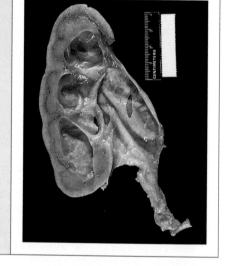

Figure 3-1. Hydronephrosis of the kidney, with marked dilation of the pelvis and calyces and thinning of the renal parenchyma. (From Kumar V, Abbas AK, Fausto N: Robbins and Cotran Pathologic Basis of Disease, 7th ed. Philadelphia, WB Saunders, 2005.)

4. **Why is the absence of hematuria on urinalysis important in establishing the diagnosis?**
   Urinary calculi (stones) can cause urinary tract obstruction and are often associated with hematuria or microscopic crystals in the urine. Stones can uncommonly cause obstructive renal failure, but usually only if they are present in the ureters bilaterally. Tumors of the bladder or ureters (either primary urothelial tumors or tumors that invade or compress the urinary tract) can also cause lower tract obstruction with renal failure and hematuria.

   Broadly speaking, obstructive renal failure is usually caused by obstruction at the level of the bladder neck or the ureters. Other causes of obstruction at the level of the bladder include neurogenic bladder and medication effects. Another classic (albeit uncommon) cause of ureteral obstruction is encasement of the ureters by retroperitoneal fibrosis.

5. **Why was it important to ask this patient about tricyclic antidepressants, antipsychotics, antihistamines, and sympathomimetics?**

These classes of drugs can all cause urinary retention secondary to cholinergic blockade, which inhibits contraction of the detrusor muscle.

Tricyclic antidepressants (e.g., amitriptyline, imipramine); the phenothiazine antipsychotics, which include low-potency "typical" antipsychotics such as chlorpromazine and thioridazine; and first-generation antihistamines such as diphenhydramine (Benadryl) are all older "dirty" agents that act on a multitude of receptor types, including muscarinic acetylcholine receptors. Hence, common side effects of these drugs include various anticholinergic actions such as dry mouth, constipation, and urinary retention. Recall that the detrusor muscle of the bladder is stimulated to contract by parasympathetic (cholinergic) innervation. The anticholinergic agent atropine has a similar effect. The anticholinergic effects of the widely used agents oxybutynin (Ditropan) and tolterodine (Detrol) are used therapeutically to control urge incontinence.

The sympathomimetics, on the other hand, can cause urinary retention by increasing the tone of the internal urethral sphincter.

Opiates (i.e., narcotics) have many anticholinergic-like side effects and (in addition to constipation, dry mouth, pupillary constriction, etc.) can cause acute urinary retention when given in high doses.

SUMMARY BOX: OBSTRUCTIVE ACUTE RENAL FAILURE

- The causes of acute renal failure (ARF) are divided into three groups: prerenal, renal (intrinsic), and postrenal (obstructive).

- Common causes of postrenal failure include benign prostatic hyperplasia (BPH) or prostate cancer, bladder tumors, and urinary retention (due to neurogenic bladder or anticholinergic, opiate, or sympathomimetic drugs). Unless present bilaterally, renal stones rarely lead to obstructive kidney failure.

- The diagnosis of obstructive renal failure is made, in part, by detection of hydronephrosis (pelvicalicectasis) on renal ultrasound.

CASE 3-2

A 68-year-old man experienced a ruptured abdominal aortic aneurysm and was rushed to the hospital and into the operating room (OR). During surgery, the surgeons had to clamp the abdominal aorta at a level superior to the renal arteries for a little over an hour. Although the patient survived the operation, the next morning he was found to have a severe acute decline in his renal function with a BUN of 75 mg/dL and creatinine of 3.2 mg/dL. His calculated GFR was depressed to ~10 mL/min, his urine output diminished to ~200 mL in 24 hours (despite his being normotensive), and a urine microscopy revealed "muddy brown" granular casts.

1. **What is the probable diagnosis?**

The likely diagnosis is acute tubular necrosis (ATN), secondary to prolonged ischemia during the operation.

2. **What is the pathophysiology of acute tubular necrosis?**

In ATN, the renal tubular epithelial cells are damaged and sloughed off from the tubular basement membrane. These sloughed cells can be formed by the tubules into epithelial cell casts. Such casts can sometimes be seen in the urine of patients with ATN. More commonly, the epithelial cell casts have been degraded somewhat into pigmented "muddy brown" granular casts that, like the epithelial cell casts, are highly suggestive of ATN. In some cases, the urine sediment will reveal nonpigmented transparent hyaline granular casts; such casts can be formed from further degradation of "muddy brown" casts, but they can also be formed from other processes as well and so are not specific for ATN.

ATN can be ischemic or toxic. That is, the tubular epithelium can be damaged by either ischemia (as in this patient) or by nephrotoxins such as the chemotherapeutic agent cisplatin, aminoglycoside antibiotics, the antifungal amphotericin B, intravenous radiographic contrast media, heavy metals (Fanconi syndrome), and the heme pigments myoglobin and hemoglobin.

3. **What is the cause of the decreased glomerular filtration rate and oliguria seen in acute tubular necrosis?**
The sloughed tubular epithelial cells block the lumen of the renal tubules, impeding urine flow. Additionally, the denuded areas of basement membrane allow back-leakage of filtered fluid. Although this back-leakage does not change the amount of fluid filtered across the glomerular membrane, it does change the amount of waste products that are excreted, which consequently changes the *calculated* GFR.

Both the obstruction to flow and the back-leakage explain why overall urine output is frequently reduced in ATN.

4. **What are the three phases of acute tubular necrosis?**
In the initiation phase, the injurious agent or condition is present, but the deterioration of renal function has not yet begun or is just beginning. In the maintenance phase, GFR is reduced and oliguria persists; it is at this time that uremic complications are likely to manifest. Finally, in the recovery phase, renal tubular epithelial cells proliferate and repopulate the denuded areas, and urine output normalizes.

5. **Other than the presence of "muddy brown" casts, how can prerenal azotemia due to ischemia be differentiated from ischemic acute tubular necrosis?**
In clinical practice, this is a very important distinction to make, because prerenal azotemia (by definition) will respond to fluid resuscitation, whereas ischemic ATN will not.

In prerenal azotemia, inadequate renal perfusion reduces GFR, but the reduced perfusion is not so severe as to cause cellular damage. The kidneys therefore function normally in response to the hypoperfusion by retaining Na^+. This typically results in a decreased fractional excretion (FE) of Na^+ (FENa$^+$) to below 1%. FENa$^+$ is simply the ratio of urine sodium to plasma sodium, but with each value normalized according to (i.e., divided by) the corresponding creatinine concentration:

$$FENa^+ = C_{Na}/GFR = (U_{Na} \times V/P_{Na})/(U_{Cr} \times V/P_{Cr}) = (U_{Na} \times P_{Cr})/(P_{Na}/U_{Cr})$$

where
C_X = clearance of substance X; volume of plasma from which substance X is cleared per unit time
U_X = excretion rate of substance X
V = urine volume
P_X = plasma concentration of substance X
Cr = creatinine

If the hypoperfusion is severe enough, prerenal azotemia will progress, resulting in the ischemic damage to the tubular epithelium that is characteristic of ATN. In ATN, because many of the tubular cells are no longer functional, the kidney is unable to retain Na^+ as it should in the setting of decreased GFR. As a result, the FENa$^+$ in ATN is typically >2%.

In addition to the FENa$^+$, the BUN/creatinine ratio can sometimes be useful in distinguishing between prerenal azotemia and ATN. Urea is primarily reabsorbed in the proximal tubule. In the setting of low extracellular volume (ECV), the increased Na^+ reabsorption in the proximal tubule (as stimulated by angiotensin II, the sympathetic nervous system, and intrinsic glomerular processes) will tend to pull additional urea out of the filtrate through bulk flow. Thus, BUN can be used as a marker for proximal Na^+ reabsorption. Creatinine, in contrast, is less affected by Na^+ reabsorption (recall that creatinine is a useful marker for GFR because it is not significantly reabsorbed). Specifically in prerenal azotemia, one expects a BUN/Cr ratio elevated to >20. In ATN, in which the reabsorption of Na^+ is impaired, this ratio is often <10 (damage to the renal tubules impairs urea reabsorption, so the BUN/Cr ratio is decreased). Although the BUN/Cr ratio is more readily available (as it requires only standard blood tests instead of both urine and blood), it is significantly less accurate than the $FENa^+$ and can change independently of renal function. A classic example is a gastrointestinal (GI) bleed in which large amounts of the protein hemoglobin are broken down in the GI tract into urea that is extensively reabsorbed into the circulation, elevating the BUN level and the BUN/Cr ratio in a manner that is completely independent of renal function.

RELATED QUESTION

6. **What is rhabdomyolysis and how can it cause acute tubular necrosis?**
Rhabdomyolysis is acute extensive destruction of skeletal muscle cells; it can occur with trauma (especially prolonged crush injuries), drugs (such as statins), and a host of other scenarios. With muscle injury, large amounts of the O_2 storage molecule myoglobin are released into the circulation and, upon arrival to the kidneys, lead to renal failure via multiple mechanisms. First, myoglobin is directly toxic to renal tubular epithelial cells. In addition, myoglobin can cause severe renal vasoconstriction (for poorly understood reasons), resulting in an ischemic component to the ATN. Finally, the released myoglobin can precipitate in the renal tubules and cause obstruction.

Contrast-induced ATN is similar to myoglobin-induced ATN in that it involves both direct toxic and vasoconstrictive/ischemic components, though the primary mechanism occurs through vasoconstriction. Contrast-induced ATN can be prevented with *N*-acetylcysteine, which is also used for cystic fibrosis treatment and acetaminophen toxicity.

SUMMARY BOX: ACUTE TUBULAR NECROSIS

- ATN is the most common cause of instrinsic renal failure.

- ATN can be ischemic or toxic. Toxins capable of causing ATN include cisplatin, aminoglycosides, vancomycin, amphotericin, intravenous contrast agents, and myoglobin.

- Ischemic ATN is distinguished from prerenal azotemia by the presence of "muddy brown" casts in the urinary sediment and an $FENa^+$ >2%. Prerenal azotemia, in contrast, is characterized by a bland sediment, by a $FENa^+$ <1%, and (less reliably) by a blood urea nitrogen/creatinine (BUN/Cr) ratio >20.

CASE 3-3

A 53-year-old white female patient develops mediastinitis following coronary bypass surgery. She becomes septic with multiorgan failure, requiring intensive care unit (ICU) admission, intubation, pressor support, and hemodialysis. Her sternal wound is surgically débrided, and intraoperative cultures grow methicillin-sensitive *Staphylococcus aureus*. After 1 week, she is discharged home on long-term intravenous nafcillin. Ten days after discharge, she returns to the emergency department complaining of several days of fever, nausea, malaise, and rash. On examination, she is febrile to 38.7° C, and she has a full body, intensely erythematous maculopapular rash. Initial laboratory findings are most notable for an elevated creatinine of 3.9 mg/dL; her creatinine had completely normalized prior to discharge. Her white blood cell (WBC) count is also moderately elevated at 12 units, with a differential of 62% neutrophils, 22% lymphocytes, 12% eosinophils, and 4% monocytes.

1. **What is the most likely cause for her acute renal failure?**
   This presentation is most consistent with acute interstitial nephritis (AIN) caused by nafcillin. AIN is most commonly an allergic reaction to a drug. Common culprits include antibiotics, particularly β-lactams (especially penicillins and cephalosporins) and sulfonamides; nonsteroidal anti-inflammatory drugs (NSAIDs); cimetidine; and proton pump inhibitors (PPIs), such as omeprazole and pantoprazole. AIN is less commonly caused by infections and is rarely a manifestation of an autoimmune disease (such as sarcoidosis).

   In a setting of ARF, the triad of fever, rash, and peripheral eosinophilia following initiation of new medication is highly suggestive of AIN, but all three of these nonrenal manifestations are present in only a minority of patients. Urine microscopy may show WBCs, WBC casts, and red blood cells. Urine eosinophils are highly suggestive, but may not be present in all cases. When the diagnosis of AIN is unclear, biopsy can be performed, but often empiric therapy with corticosteroids is attempted first.

2. **What are the three major types of NSAID-induced renal toxicity?**
   NSAIDs can cause a bewildering array of renal side effects.

   In addition to interstitial nephritis, NSAIDs can also cause nephrotic syndrome. This typically manifests as minimal change disease in an adult taking NSAIDs, but other types of glomerular processes (such as membranous nephropathy) are possible as well.

   The most common renal toxicity of NSAIDs is hemodynamically mediated acute renal failure. In the normal kidney, vasodilatory prostaglandins, such as PGI_2 (prostacyclin) and PGE_2, are produced to help maintain adequate renal perfusion. The enzyme cyclooxygenase (COX) is required for prostaglandin production. NSAID administration and the resultant inhibition of cyclooxygenase-1 or -2 by NSAIDs can result in vasoconstriction of the renal arterioles, renal hypoperfusion, and a dramatic decrease in GFR. Risk factors for NSAID-induced renal failure include age >65 years, baseline renal dysfunction, and intravascular volume depletion (e.g., diuretic use and cirrhosis). This is in part because such patients with renal dysfunction or volume depletion depend more heavily than normal on prostaglandin production to maintain adequate renal perfusion.

STEP 1 SECRET

Nonsteroidal anti-inflammatory drug (NSAID)-induced decrease in glomerular filtration rate (GFR) is an important concept to know for Step 1. In general, you should be aware of all of the mechanisms by which GFR and filtration fraction can be altered. You are likely to be asked a question on this topic.

STEP 1 SECRET

Remembering the most common conditions that cause eosinophilia can be helpful. These conditions include helminthic infections, asthma and allergic disorders, drug-induced acute interstitial nephritis (AIN), and certain forms of malignancy (e.g., Hodgkin's lymphoma).

SUMMARY BOX: ACUTE INTERSTITIAL NEPHRITIS ✔

- Acute interstitial nephriyis (AIN) is classically characterized by the triad of fever, rash, and peripheral eosinophilia in a setting of ARF after introduction of a new drug. Urine eosinophils, although often not present, are also highly suggestive of AIN.

- Agents associated with AIN include penicillins, cephalosporins, sulfonamides, nonsteroidal anti-inflammatory drugs (NSAIDs), and PPIs.

- NSAIDs can cause AIN, nephrotic syndrome, and most commonly, hemodynamic renal failure from inhibition of vasodilatory prostaglandins. Patients with advanced age, renal dysfunction, or low effective circulating volume (e.g., congestive heart failure [CHF]) are at highest risk for NSAID-induced acute renal failure (ARF).

CASE 3-4

A 65-year-old African-American woman with a long history of poorly controlled hypertension is evaluated for an elevated plasma creatinine that has been noted on routine laboratory tests over the past 6 months. Additional laboratory findings include hyperkalemia, hypocalcemia, hyperphosphatemia, and a metabolic acidosis. Hemoglobin A_{1c} and fasting glucose values are both normal. Urine microscopy does not reveal any hematuria or casts.

1. **What is most likely causing her blood urea nitrogen and creatinine elevation?**
   She has renal failure resulting from a long history of poorly controlled hypertension. Hypertension is the second most common cause of chronic kidney disease. Renal failure from hypertension is particularly common in African Americans.
   The pathologic changes associated with longstanding hypertension are termed *hypertensive nephrosclerosis* (also known as benign nephrosclerosis or hyaline arteriolar nephrosclerosis). As shown in Figure 3-2, hyaline arteriosclerosis is associated with hyaline deposition, marked thickening of the walls, and a narrowed lumen.

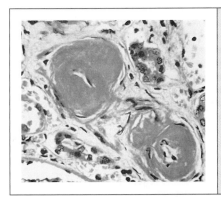

Figure 3-2. Hyaline arteriolosclerosis. High-power view of two arterioles with hyaline deposition, marked thickening of the walls, and a narrowed lumen. (Courtesy of Dr. M.A. Venkatachalam, Department of Pathology, University of Texas Health Sciences Center, San Antonio, TX.)

2. **What is the value of the normal fasting glucose and hemoglobin A_{1c} levels in the differential diagnosis?**
   This finding essentially rules out a component of diabetic nephropathy, the most common cause of chronic renal failure (CRF).

3. **What is the difficulty in establishing that this patient's renal failure was definitely due to hypertension, even if no other specific disease processes can be identified on renal biopsy?**

   The difficulty stems from the fact that hypertension is both a potential cause and a potential result of renal disease. Furthermore, if renal failure is chronic, renal biopsy findings can be nonspecific and may fail to distinguish between other precipitating insults. For example, her renal failure may have been due to a bout of glomerulonephritis that permanently damaged the kidneys, and her hypertension could have resulted from the kidney damage. Nevertheless, hypertension, regardless of its cause, contributes to progressive loss of renal function.

4. **How does this woman's renal failure explain her hypocalcemia?**

   In general, renal dysfunction leads to the accumulation of the various electrolytes that are normally excreted by the kidneys, resulting in hyperkalemia, hyperphosphatemia, and acidosis typical of renal failure. Calcium is rather unusual in that its serum levels may be *decreased* in renal failure. Keep in mind that in clinical practice, true hypocalcemia with chronic renal failure is rare due to the rapid compensatory increase in serum PTH levels that is mediated by the parathyroid glands.

   When it does occur, hypocalcemia results from several processes. First, the kidney is the site of 1,25-dihydroxyvitamin D (i.e., calcitriol) synthesis from 25-hydroxyvitamin D, via the activity of renal α_1-hydroxylase in the proximal tubule. Since the 1,25-dihydroxy form of vitamin D is the active form that stimulates intestinal calcium absorption, loss of renal parenchyma reduces synthesis of this compound and reduces intestinal calcium absorption. Second, as GFR declines, renal phosphate excretion declines and leads to hyperphosphatemia. This elevated serum phosphate can complex with serum calcium and reduce free ionized calcium levels. In addition, the increased phosphate, through negative feedback, also inhibits the synthesis of 1,25-dihydroxyvitamin D. (Recall that 1,25-dihydroxyvitamin D tends to increase serum levels of *both* Ca^{2+} and phosphate as it promotes the intestinal absorption of both substances. Parathyroid hormone [PTH], on the other hand, increases serum calcium levels while promoting phosphate excretion at the level of the kidney.)

   Note: There are two forms of vitamin D: plant-derived vitamin D_2 (ergocalciferol) is acquired in our diets; vitamin D_3 is made endogenously in our skin in a reaction that is catalyzed by ultraviolet (UV) rays (i.e., sunlight). In order to become biologically active, both vitamin D_2 and D_3 must be hydroxylated twice. The first hydroxylation is unregulated and occurs in the liver to produce the 25-hydroxyvitamin D diol form. The second step, which is impaired in renal failure, is highly regulated and produces the 1,25-dihydroxyvitamin D triol form (hence the name calci*triol*).

5. **Would parathyroid hormone levels be increased or decreased in this patient?**

   Because PTH is released in response to hypocalcemia (or hyperphosphatemia), PTH levels are increased in renal failure.

   Because this increase in PTH is reactive in nature (i.e., an appropriate response to the hypocalcemia and hyperphosphatemia of renal failure), it is termed secondary hyperparathyroidism. Patients in early renal failure will often have a high PTH level with relatively normal serum calcium. However, in severe renal failure, as both 1,25-hydroxyvitamin D levels decrease and phosphate levels increase to a greater extent, the progressively elevated PTH levels are unable to compensate, and progressively severe hypocalcemia develops.

   Note: Primary hyperparathyroidism, in which an abnormality of the parathyroid gland (typically glandular hyperplasia or an adenoma) results in increased PTH levels as a primary disturbance, causes *hypercalcemia* rather than hypocalcemia.

6. **How does parathyroid hormone normally act to regulate serum Ca^{2+}? How are parathyroid hormone levels normally regulated?**

   The various actions of PTH act overall to increase serum Ca^{2+} while maintaining serum phosphate levels.

   First of all, PTH stimulates bone reabsorption, which releases Ca^{2+} and phosphate into circulation. It also stimulates activation of vitamin D by stimulating the activity of

α_1-hydroxylase in the proximal tubule. The active 1,25-dihydroxyvitamin D then increases intestinal absorption of Ca^{2+} and phosphate and (at high levels) promotes bone resorption, again acting to increase serum levels of both Ca^{2+} and phosphate. Finally, PTH stimulates Ca^{2+} reabsorption at the level of the kidney while strongly promoting *phosphate excretion*.

Thus, PTH acts directly and indirectly at bone, the GI tract, and the kidneys to increase plasma Ca^{2+}. However, because the phosphate released from bone and absorbed from the GI tract is excreted in the kidneys, the combination of PTH and vitamin D activation tends to have no net effect on serum phosphate.

In general, PTH release is stimulated by low Ca^{2+} levels, whereas its release is inhibited (in a negative feedback mechanism) by the active 1,25-dihydroxy form of vitamin D (Fig. 3-3).

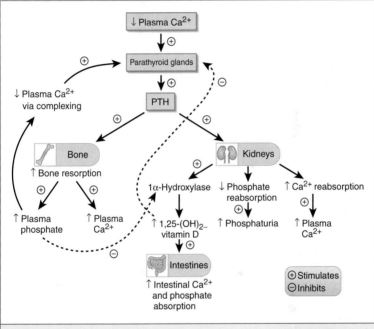

Figure 3-3. Parathyroid hormone (PTH) overview. (From Brown TA: Rapid Review Physiology. Philadelphia, Mosby, 2007, p 128.)

7. **What are the potential pathologic manifestations of the hyperparathyroidism that develops in renal failure?**
Although the elevated PTH seen in renal failure is an appropriate response to hypocalcemia, it has a negative impact on *bone metabolism*. The *chronically* high PTH levels stimulate chronic bone resorption, which can result in osteoporosis as well as abnormal cysts in areas of demineralized bone (*osteitis fibrosa cystica*).

In the chronic management of renal failure, in addition to the maintenance of relatively normal calcium and phosphate concentrations, a relatively normal PTH level is also an important therapeutic goal that often requires specific drug therapy. The agents used include active vitamin D analogs (that have negative feedback on PTH release) as well as newer agents that suppress PTH release by mimicking the action of calcium on the parathyroid gland.

STEP 1 SECRET

Parathyroid hormone (PTH) and vitamin D are routinely tested topics on the USMLE. It is very important to understand the difference between primary and secondary hyperparathyroidism and to know which conditions elevate levels of PTH and vitamin D.

8. **Why is this patient also predisposed to osteomalacia?**
   Osteomalacia is a disease of adults resulting from activated vitamin D deficiency in which there is *impaired mineralization* of newly deposited osteoid matrix in bone, making the bones more malleable (malacia). If this vitamin D deficiency and impaired mineralization occur in prepubertal children, prior to closure of the epiphyseal plates, it is referred to as rickets.

   Renal osteodystrophy includes the spectrum of bony changes that result from renal failure, and includes the osteitis fibrosa cystica caused by secondary hyperparathyroidism, osteomalacia from impaired vitamin D synthesis and decreased mineralization, and bone loss resulting from the need to buffer the metabolic acidosis that accompanies renal failure.

9. **How could this woman's renal failure explain the following findings?**
   A. Metabolic acidosis
   The kidneys normally excrete a large quantity of nonvolatile acids, including both inorganic acids (such as ammonium and hydrogen ions) and organic acids (such as sulfate and phosphate). Thus, a mixed anion gap and non–anion gap metabolic acidosis occurs in renal failure as these acids accumulate in the body.
   B. Hyperkalemia
   Normally, aldosterone drives the secretion of excess potassium (in exchange for sodium) in the distal tubule. Chronic renal failure predisposes to hyperkalemia, both because there are fewer nephrons capable of engaging in potassium secretion and because as GFR decreases, less potassium is filtered.
   C. Anemia. Would you expect a microcytic, normocytic, or macrocytic anemia?
   Renal erythropoietin synthesis is likewise compromised in severe renal failure, resulting in anemia. We would expect a normocytic anemia, because lack of erythropoietin will simply reduce the rate of erythropoiesis. Insufficiencies of iron or folate/vitamin B_{12} would cause microcytic or macrocytic anemias, respectively.

10. **Is this woman suffering from azotemia or uremia?**
    Azotemia refers to increased BUN and creatinine in an asymptomatic person. If this woman had symptoms from her renal failure, she would be described as suffering from uremia (i.e., she would be uremic).

    In other words, uremia is not defined by laboratory values. Instead, it is a *clinical syndrome* consisting of a constellation of symptoms or complications attributable to renal failure. Possible manifestations include nausea, pruritus, malaise, seizures, confusion (uremic encephalopathy), bleeding (from uremia-induced platelet dysfunction), pericarditis, and fluid overload.

11. **If she were uremic, and a friction rub was detected on physical examination, what might you suspect?**
    Uremic pericarditis, characterized by a fibrinous exudate within the pericardial space, would be likely. You can spot pericarditis by the presence of a friction rub on examination and chest pain that is relieved by sitting forward (as leaning forward elevates the heart from the diaphragmatic portion of the pericardium).

SUMMARY BOX: CHRONIC RENAL FAILURE

- Hypertension is both a major cause and a major complication of chronic renal failure (CRF).

- CRF is characterized by normocytic anemia (due to loss of renal erythropoietin production), hyperkalemia, mixed anion gap/non–anion gap metabolic acidosis, hypocalcemia, and hyperphosphatemia.

- Azotemia refers to the accumulation of renally cleared nitrogenous toxins in an asymptomatic individual.

- Uremia is a *clinical syndrome* of specific symptoms or complications attributable to renal failure such as nausea, pruritus, malaise, seizures, confusion, bleeding pericarditis, and fluid overload.

- Hypocalcemia in CRF is due to (1) decreased synthesis of the *active* form of vitamin D (1,25-dihydroxyvitamin D) in the proximal tubule, (2) complexing of free calcium by elevated phosphate levels, and (3) further inhibition of active vitamin D synthesis by the elevated phosphate.

- CRF results in *secondary* hyperparathyroidism. Elevated parathyroid hormone (PTH), in turn, can cause abnormal bone formation (osteitis fibrosa cystica), whereas deficiency of activated vitamin D can (in adults) lead to osteomalacia. The full spectrum of bony changes resulting from high PTH, low Ca^{2+}, and chronic acidosis is called renal osteodystrophy.

CASE 3-5

A 32-year-old woman with a history of hypertension presents for evaluation of right-sided flank pain. She denies urinary symptoms such as dysuria, urgency, and frequency. Examination is unremarkable, but laboratory workup reveals an elevated creatinine level and RBCs and protein in her urine. A renal ultrasound shows enlarged kidneys with numerous cysts bilaterally. The patient then recalls that her mother had some kind of kidney disease.

1. **What is the diagnosis?**
   She has autosomal dominant (adult) polycystic kidney disease (ADPKD). Note the diffuse, bilateral distribution of cysts in ADPKD shown in Figure 3-4. Be familiar with this high-yield image for Step 1.

2. **What is the primary complication of this disease?**
   End-stage renal failure is the primary complication.

3. **Why must urinary tract infections be treated aggressively in patients with this disease?**
   Patients with ADPKD are treated aggressively to prevent pyelonephritis, which can be remarkably difficult to treat in these patients. This is because the cysts are essentially urine cesspools that do not drain, providing an excellent breeding ground for bacteria.

4. **If this patient suddenly develops a severe headache, what vascular abnormality must be suspected?**
   Intracranial (berry) aneurysms are associated with ADPKD. Rupture of a berry aneurysm classically results in acute onset of a severe "worst-of-my-life" headache. Presumably, the

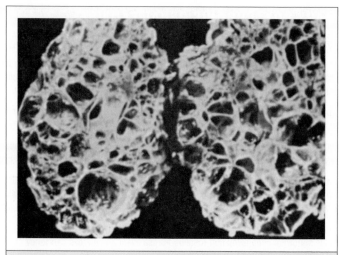

Figure 3-4. Autosomal dominant polycystic kidney disease (ADPKD) on cut section. Note diffuse, bilateral distribution of cysts. (Courtesy of F.E. Cuppage, Kansas City, KS.)

mutations in the polycystin gene that causes tissue to separate in the kidneys and form cysts also make it easier for vascular connective tissue to separate and form aneurysms.

STEP 1 SECRET

The relationship between berry aneurysm formation and autosomal dominant (adult) polycystic kidney disease (ADPKD) is a commonly tested Step 1 principle.

5. **How does autosomal dominant polycystic kidney disease differ from autosomal recessive polycystic kidney disease (other than the pattern of inheritance)?**
   Autosomal recessive (*infantile*) polycystic kidney disease typically presents in infancy, although there are less severe childhood and adolescent forms. It is always associated with liver abnormalities, including hepatic cysts and congenital hepatic fibrosis. In many patients, the congenital fibrosis leads to portal hypertension and liver dysfunction.
   Hepatic cysts (and less commonly, cysts in other organs such as the pancreas and lungs) do occur in ADPKD, but they are *not* associated with liver fibrosis or organ dysfunction.

6. **What is tuberous sclerosis and how can it be differentiated from ADPKD?**
   Tuberous sclerosis is a genetic disease that is also inherited in an autosomal dominant manner. In this disease, multiple cysts (and tumors) form in the kidneys, but the disorder is additionally characterized by a variety of central nervous system (CNS) abnormalities, including mental retardation and seizures (resulting from cerebral "tuber" formation), as well as a variety of characteristic dermatologic lesions such as ash-leaf macules, adenoma sebaceum (i.e., angiofibromas), shagreen patches (connective tissue nevi), and subungual and periungual fibromas. Tuberous sclerosis is associated with a variety of tumors including astrocytomas, renal angiomyolipomas, retinal hamartomas, and cardiac rhabdomyomas.

7. **What is von Hippel-Lindau syndrome and how can it be differentiated from ADPKD?**
Like ADPKD, autosomal recessive (infantile) polycystic kidney disease (ARPKD), and tuberous sclerosis, von Hippel-Lindau (VHL) syndrome is characterized by multiple cysts in both kidneys. It is an autosomal dominant disorder characterized by a tendency to form multiple types of neoplasms and hamartomas. In addition to cysts of the kidneys and other organs, affected patients develop hemangioblastomas of the CNS (Lindau tumors) and of the retina, pheochromocytomas, and pancreatic tumors. The renal cysts are often complicated by development of renal cell carcinoma, frequently bilateral.

STEP 1 SECRET

In addition to type I and II neurofibromatosis, tuberous sclerosis and von Hippel-Lindau disease are high-yield topics for Step 1. Be able to identify the various tumors associated with these conditions.

8. **What is medullary cystic disease and how can it be differentiated from ADPKD?**
In medullary cystic disease, the cysts are confined to the medulla; the cysts are not present throughout the kidney as in ADPKD. This rare cystic disease is also characterized by severe renal dysfunction.

9. **Quick review: Cover the far right column in Table 3-1 and give the characteristic features of each of the cystic kidney diseases.**

10. **Why is medullary sponge kidney not included in Table 3-1?**
True cysts do not form in medullary sponge kidney. Rather, segments of the collecting tubules become abnormally dilated in the medulla at the tips of the renal papillae. The primary complication of these dilations is a predisposition to nephrolithiasis and pyelonephritis. Isolated hematuria or urinary tract infections (UTIs) can also occur. This disorder is seen primarily in adults and, compared with medullary cystic disease, is relatively common.

11. **What is the most common cause of renal cysts?**
Most renal cysts are *incidental* non-neoplastic simple cysts that are not associated with a particular disease. Such simple cysts are more common with increasing age, occurring in up to 33% of people older than 50 years.

   Cysts are particularly common in patients on hemodialysis, increasing in incidence, size, and number with duration of dialysis. Dialysis-associated cysts are also generally asymptomatic, but can be complicated by hematuria.

TABLE 3-1. CYSTIC KIDNEY DISEASES				
Disease	Site of Cysts in Kidney	Mode of Inheritance	Age at Onset	Key Associated Features
ADPKD	Throughout	AD	Adulthood	Intracranial berry aneurysm and asymptomatic hepatic cysts

Continued

TABLE 3-1. CYSTIC KIDNEY DISEASES—continued

Disease	Site of Cysts in Kidney	Mode of Inheritance	Age at Onset	Key Associated Features
ARPKD	Throughout	AR	Infancy	Hepatic cysts and congenital hepatic fibrosis with possible portal hypertension and liver dysfunction
Tuberous sclerosis	Throughout	AD	Childhood	Mental retardation, seizure disorder, renal angiomyolipomas, cardiac rhabdomyomas, dermatologic lesions
von Hippel-Lindau disease	Cortex	AD	Teens to young adulthood	CNS and retinal hemangioblastomas, bilateral renal cell carcinoma
Medullary cystic disease	Medulla		Childhood	

AD, autosomal dominant; ADPKD, autosomal dominant polycystic kidney disease; AR, autosomal recessive; ARPKD, autosomal recessive polycystic kidney disease; CNS, central nervous system.

SUMMARY BOX: CYSTIC KIDNEY DISEASE

- Autosomal dominant (adult) polycystic kidney disease (ADPKD) is the most common cystic renal disease and is characterized by colicky abdominal or flank pain, hematuria, early-onset hypertension, and, ultimately, end-stage renal disease.

- ADPKD is associated with increased risk of pyelonephritis, intracranial (berry) aneurysms, and asymptomatic hepatic cysts.

- The less common autosomal recessive (infantile) polycystic kidney disease (ARPKD) is associated with cysts in the liver, pancreas, and lungs as well as liver dysfunction due to congenital hepatic fibrosis.

- Other cystic kidney diseases include tuberous sclerosis, von Hippel-Lindau syndrome, and medullary cystic disease. True cysts do not form in medullary sponge kidney.

- Most renal cysts are asymptomatic simple cysts *not* associated with any disease or neoplasm. Such cysts are common in persons older than 50 years.

- Hemodialysis is associated with asymptomatic cysts that tend to increase in incidence, size, and number with duration of dialysis.

CASE 3-6

A 5-year-old boy is brought to the clinic by his parents, who are concerned because he has been lethargic recently and appears "swollen" to them. Marked whole body edema (anasarca) is noted on physical examination. Laboratory tests reveal hyperlipidemia and hypoalbuminemia. Urinalysis reveals the presence of proteins and lipids in the urine, but no RBCs. Urine microscopy reveals the structure shown in Figure 3-5.

1. **What is the likely diagnosis in this child and why?**
   This child likely has nephrotic syndrome, characterized by massive proteinuria (>3 g/24 hours), hypoalbuminemia resulting in severe edema, and hyperlipidemia. Due to lipiduria and subsequent cholesterol precipitation, urine microscopy may show the presence of fatty casts (Maltese crosses), as shown in Figure 3-5. The massive proteinuria can make urine appear foamy or frothy. Although slight hematuria is sometimes seen in the nephrotic syndrome, it is typically transient and much less severe than that associated with the nephritic syndrome.

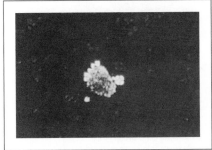

Figure 3-5. Urine microscopy for patient in Case 3-6. (From Henry JB: Clinical Diagnosis and Management by Laboratory Methods, 20th ed. Philadelphia, WB Saunders, 2001, Plate 18-12.)

The cause of the hyperlipidemia is unclear, but is believed to relate to increased protein synthesis by the liver. In response to the loss of serum proteins, the synthesis of many types of serum protein by the liver is increased. In fact, elevated lipoprotein synthesis is often responsible for the onset of hyperlipidemia. Although the synthesis of procoagulant (e.g., tissue factor, Factor VIII) and anticoagulant (e.g., antithrombin III) proteins is also increased, it happens that the balance is shifted towards procoagulants such that nephrotic syndrome is associated with an increased risk of clotting (particularly venous thromboembolism). In general, however, thrombotic complications of nephrotic syndrome are rare in children and tend to occur in adults with other risk factors for clotting.

2. **What is the likely cause of nephrotic syndrome in this patient?**
   Minimal change disease (also known as nil disease or lipoid nephrosis) is the most common cause of nephrotic syndrome in children and commonly occurs following infections.

3. **Assuming minimal change disease as the underlying pathologic condition, what would you expect gross histologic examination to reveal if a renal biopsy were performed?**
   The kidney would be *normal* or nearly normal on light microscopy. This is the reason for the term *minimal change* disease. The pathologic diagnosis is generally made using electron microscopy, which demonstrates diffuse flattening ("effacement") of the glomerular foot processes, resulting in increased permeability of the glomerular membrane and substantial proteinuria.
   Note: Focal segmental glomerular sclerosis (FSGS), another important cause of nephrotic syndrome, would also show diffuse effacement of the glomerular foot processes on electron

microscopy. However, light microscopy would reveal areas of sclerosis in some (but not all) glomeruli (i.e., focal sclerosis). FSGS is unlikely in a young child but is the most common cause of primary nephrotic syndrome in African-American adults. It is also associated with human immunodeficiency virus (HIV) infection, obesity, and heroin use (Fig. 3-6 and Table 3-2).

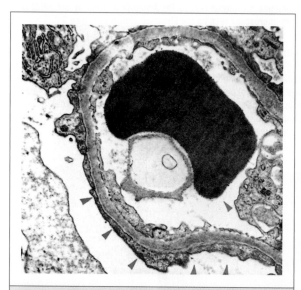

Figure 3-6. Fusion of the podocytes. Arrowheads show fusion of the podocytes, which should be separated by slit pores. This finding occurs in all glomerular diseases that present with the nephrotic syndrome. (From Goljan EF: Rapid Review Pathology, 2nd ed. Philadelphia, Mosby, 2007, p 406.)

4. **Why might this boy be susceptible to infections while suffering from this illness?**
Hypogammaglobulinemia occurs as a result of loss of immunoglobulins (along with other proteins, such as albumin) into the urine, thus predisposing this patient to infection.

5. **How should this boy be managed? Should a renal biopsy be performed?**
Nephrotic syndrome caused by minimal change disease (MCD) typically responds *extremely* well to steroids (i.e., prednisone). Because a majority of nephrotic syndrome cases in children are caused by MCD (roughly 80%), a renal biopsy is generally *not* needed. However, if this boy does not respond well to steroids, a renal biopsy would be necessary to determine the precise cause of the nephrotic syndrome.

  In contrast, FSGS characteristically responds *poorly* to steroids. Thus, FSGS should be suspected in any patient (particularly any older patient) with presumed MCD that does not respond rapidly to steroids.

6. **What are other major causes of nephrotic syndrome?**
There are five major causes of nephrotic syndrome. Three are primary renal diseases; two are systemic diseases capable of producing nephrotic syndrome. Although they all cause nephrotic syndrome, some have nephritic characteristics. In other words, there is a spectrum between nephrotic and nephritic syndrome.

TABLE 3-2. SUMMARY OF PRIMARY RENAL DISEASES THAT MANIFEST AS IDIOPATHIC NEPHROTIC SYNDROME				Membranoproliferative Glomerulonephritis	
	Minimal Change Nephrotic Syndrome	Focal Segmental Sclerosis	Membranous Nephropathy	Type I	Type II
Frequency*					
Children	75%	10%	<5%	10%	10%
Adults	15%	15%	50%	10%	10%
Clinical Manifestations					
Age (years)	2-6, some adults	2-10, some adults	40-50	5-15	5-15
Nephrotic syndrome	100%	90%	80%	60%	60%
Asymptomatic proteinuria	0	10%	20%	40%	40%
Hematuria	10-20%	60-80%	60%	80%	80%
Hypertension	10%	20% early	Infrequent	35%	35%
Time to progression to renal failure	Does not progress	10 years	50% in 10–20 years	10-20 years	5-15 years
Laboratory findings	Manifestations of nephrotic syndrome	Manifestations of nephrotic syndrome	Renal vein thrombosis, cancer, SLE, hepatitis B	None	Partial lipodystrophy
	↑ BUN in 15-30%	↑ BUN in 20-40%	Manifestations of nephrotic syndrome	Low C1, C4, C3-C9	Normal C1, C4, low C3-C9

Continued

TABLE 3-2. SUMMARY OF PRIMARY RENAL DISEASES THAT MANIFEST AS IDIOPATHIC NEPHROTIC SYNDROME—continued

	Minimal Change Nephrotic Syndrome	Focal Segmental Sclerosis	Membranous Nephropathy	Membranoproliferative Glomerulonephritis	
				Type I	Type II
Light microscopy	Normal	Focal sclerotic lesions	Thickened GBM, spikes	Thickened GBM, proliferation	Lobulation
Immunofluorescence	Negative	IgM, C3 in lesions	Fine granular IgG, C3	Granular IgG, C3	C3 only
Electron microscopy	Foot process fusion	Foot process fusion	Subepithelial deposits	Mesangial and subendothelial deposits	Dense deposits
Response to steroids	90%	15-20%	May slow progression	Not established	Not established

Modified from Goldman L, Ausiello D: Cecil Textbook of Medicine, 22nd ed. Philadelphia, WB Saunders, 2004.
↑, elevated; BUN, blood urea nitrogen; C, complement; GBM, glomerular basement membrane; HLA, human leukocyte antigen; Ig, immunoglobulin; SLE, systemic lupus erythematosus.
*Approximate frequency as a cause of idiopathic nephrotic syndrome. About 10% of cases of adult nephrotic syndrome are due to various diseases that usually manifest with acute glomerulonephritis.

The primary renal diseases are MCD (the most common cause of nephrotic syndrome in children), FSGS (the most common cause in African-American adults), and membranous nephropathy (the most common cause of nephrotic syndrome in white adults).

FSGS, of the three, is the most nephritic; in other words, it is most likely to be associated with some degree of hypertension, hematuria, or renal dysfunction (see Case 3-7 for more on nephritic syndrome). MCD, in contrast, is completely nephrotic.

Membranous nephropathy is usually idiopathic but can be associated with hepatitis B infection, autoimmune disease (particularly lupus), and malignancy (particularly carcinomas), or drugs. Light microscopy reveals basement membrane thickening and electronic microscopy shows characteristic dense deposits on the epithelial side of the basement membrane (Fig. 3-7).

The systemic diseases are diabetes and amyloidosis. Although diabetes is a major cause of nephrotic syndrome (because diabetes is so common), nephrotic syndrome is rather uncommon among diabetics. Amyloidosis is the least common of the five.

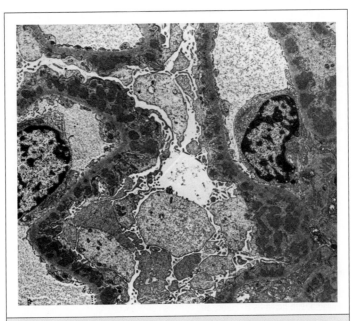

Figure 3-7. Membranous glomerulopathy. On ultrastructural examination, there are numerous, closely apposed epimembranous electron-dense deposits separated by basement membrane spikes (uranyl acetate, lead citrate stain; original magnification × 2500). (From Goldman L, Ausiello D: Cecil Textbook of Medicine, 22nd ed. Philadelphia, WB Saunders, 2004.)

STEP 1 SECRET

As mentioned in the Insider's Guide to Nephrology for the USMLE Step 1, glomerulonephritic syndromes are a favorite topic for the test makers. In addition to differentiating between nephritic and nephrotic syndrome and knowing which syndromes are associated with which diseases (e.g., hepatitis B and C associated with membranoproliferative glomerulonephritis type I), you should be able to identify each type of glomerulonephritis by light microscopy, electron microscopy, and immunofluorescence (if applicable).

SOME DIFFERENTIAL DIAGNOSIS CONCEPTS

7. **What condition might you suspect in a 6-year-old girl who presents with abdominal pain, joint pain, hematuria (or melena) and proteinuria, and a palpable purpura on her buttocks and lower extremities?**

Henoch-Schönlein purpura (HSP) is a small vessel vasculitis of children that commonly follows an upper respiratory tract infection. Presumably, the mucosal immune stimulation caused by the upper respiratory tract infection stimulates the production of IgA; thus, this disease is characterized by IgA deposition in small vessels of the gastrointestinal tract, glomeruli, joints, and skin; In addition to hematuria and proteinuria, the renal involvement can progress to hypertension and, uncommonly, acute renal failure. Likewise, the characteristically colicky abdominal pain can be accompanied by significant GI bleeding and, rarely, even intussusception.

Note: *Palpable* purpura always suggests a *vasculitic* process because inflammation of the small vessels of the skin allows RBCs to extravasate (i.e., leak) into the dermis and form the palpable lesion. In HSP, the rash tends to be present on the buttocks and lower extremities in a "waist-down" distribution.

SUMMARY BOX: GLOMERULAR DISEASE

- Nephrotic syndrome is characterized by massive proteinuria (>3 g/24 hours), hypoalbuminemia, edema (often anasarca), hyperlipidemia, and lipiduria, and (in adults) increased risk of venous thromboembolism.

- The nephritic syndrome is characterized by modest proteinuria (<3 g/24 hours), hematuria, renal insufficiency, hypertension, and urinary dysmorphic red blood cells (RBCs) and/or RBC casts on urine microscopy.

- The most common cause of nephrotic syndrome in children is minimal change disease, which is named for its normal appearance on light microscopy (LM). It usually responds rapidly to steroids.

- Focal segmental glomerular sclerosis (FSGS) is associated with human immunodeficiency virus (HIV) and heroin use, is frequently accompanied by nephritic complications, and tends to respond poorly to therapy.

- Membranous nephropathy is the most common cause of nephrotic syndrome in white adults; it is associated with hepatitis B, lupus, and various carcinomas.

- Henoch-Schönlein purpura is a small vessel vasculitis of children caused by IgA immune complexes and affects the glomeruli, the skin (with "waist-down" palpable purpura), joints (resulting in arthritis), and gastrointestinal (GI) tract (with abdominal pain or GI bleeding).

CASE 3-7

A 42-year-old man comes in for a pre-employment physical examination. He has no current complaints but mentioned that he has recovered only 1 to 2 weeks ago from a bad sore throat. Physical examination is significant for mild hypertension. Blood work reveals elevated BUN and creatinine, and urinalysis is significant for hematuria and microscopic proteinuria. Antistreptolysin O (ASO) and anti-DNase B titers are markedly elevated. Laboratory tests from a previous visit 3 months ago revealed normal BUN and creatinine levels.

1. **What is the likely diagnosis?**
   This man has acute nephritic syndrome (i.e., acute glomerulonephritis) characterized by a relatively sudden onset of *mild to moderate proteinuria* (i.e., <3 g/24 hours), *hematuria, renal insufficiency* (with elevated creatinine), and *hypertension.*
   Urine microscopy will also often show dysmorphic RBCs and RBC casts in glomerulonephritis (Fig. 3-8).

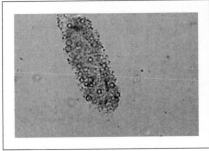

Figure 3-8. Erythrocyte cast (×200). (From McPherson RA, Pincus MR: Henry's Clinical Diagnosis and Management by Laboratory Methods, 21st ed. Philadelphia, WB Saunders, 2006.)

2. **What segment of the nephron is involved in acute nephritis? How does this compare with the nephrotic syndrome?**
   The glomerulus is damaged in glomerulonephritis. The presence of dysmorphic RBCs (which are deformed by passage through the damaged glomeruli) or RBC casts (which form within the renal tubules) indicate that hematuria is of a *glomerular* origin.
   The glomerulus is also the primary site of injury in nephrotic syndrome, but in general, different sides of the glomeruli are damaged. In nephrotic syndrome the foot processes and glomerular basement membrane are most damaged (exemplified by the foot process effacement seen in MCD or FSGS), whereas the endothelium and basement membrane are typically more involved in glomerulonephritis. It is the endothelial damage that allows for the leakage of RBCs through the glomerulus that is typical of glomerulonephritis.
   Again, realize that nephrotic and nephritic syndromes are two ends on the spectrum of glomerular disease. Certain diseases are very characteristically nephrotic (i.e., MCD), others are very nephritic (i.e., rapidly progressive or crescentic glomerulonephritis), and most others fall somewhere in between.

3. **What was the likely cause of this man's sore throat and what is its relationship to the renal dysfunction?**
   The patient likely had streptococcal pharyngitis, caused by group A β-hemolytic streptococcus (i.e., *Streptococcus pyogenes*), and is now suffering from poststreptococcal glomerulonephritis (PSGN). This condition is caused by antibody-antigen complex deposition in the glomerulus, resulting in inflammatory destruction of the glomerulus (primarily mediated via complement activation). For boards, look for subepithelial humplike deposits along the capillary basement membranes, as depicted by the straight arrow in Figure 3-9.
   In some patients, in whom the history of a prior infection may be difficult to elicit, antibody evidence of recent streptococcal infection can help make the diagnosis. The two most common antibodies tested for are those directed against the streptococcal antigens streptolysin O (diagnostic but not prognostic) and DNase B. The immune complex formation also results in consumption of complement, which is reflected in a decrease in serum complement levels.

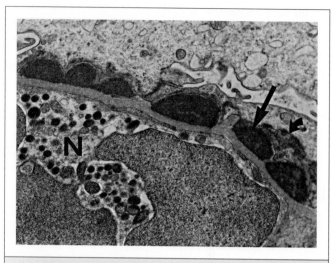

Figure 3-9. Electron micrograph of a portion of a glomerular capillary from a patient with acute poststreptococcal glomerulonephritis (PSGN) showing subepithelial dense deposits (*straight arrow*), condensation of cytoskeleton in adjacent epithelial cytoplasm (*small curved arrow*), and a neutrophil (*N*) marginated against the basement membrane with no intervening endothelial cytoplasm (magnification × 5000). (From Brenner BM: Brenner and Rector's The Kidney, 7th ed. Philadelphia, WB Saunders, 2004.)

4. **If the patient had recently suffered from cellulitis rather than pharyngitis, would it alter the diagnosis of his renal disorder?**
   No. Streptococcal infections of the skin and soft tissue can also cause a PSGN. **Note:** This contrasts with acute rheumatic fever, which is a postinfectious complication that exclusively follows streptococcal pharyngitis.

5. **What is the treatment for poststreptococcal glomerulonephritis?**
   The treatment is *supportive*. Hypertension must be controlled with medications and salt restriction. In general, steroids or immunosuppressive agents (used in many other glomerular diseases) are *not* used. Prognosis is generally much better in children than in adults.
   Note: Again in contrast with rheumatic fever, the incidence of PSGN is *not* decreased by antibiotic administration.

6. **How would the diagnosis change if a renal biopsy revealed "glomerular crescents"?**
   Glomerular crescents are the hallmark of crescentic or rapidly progressive glomerulonephritis (RPGN), which, as the name suggests, is a form of rapidly evolving glomerular disease that frequently responds poorly to treatment and progresses to renal failure.
   Crescents are formed by clusters of rapidly proliferating parietal epithelial cells and infiltrating leukocytes (Figs. 3-10 and 3-11).
   The major types of RPGN are distinguished using immunofluorescence. Pauci-immune glomerulonephritis is the most common cause of RPGN. Its name derives from the fact that on renal biopsy, immune complexes are *not* seen on immunofluorescence. Pauci-immune glomerulonephritis is commonly associated with vasculitic conditions such as Wegener's granulomatosis and the similar disorder microscopic polyangiitis. These conditions are in turn commonly associated with positive antineutrophil cytoplasmic antibodies (ANCA); Wegener's granulomatosis is usually c-ANCA positive (with a diffuse cytoplasmic staining pattern), whereas

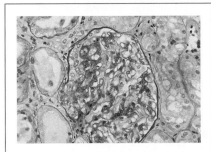

Figure 3-10. Normal glomerulus. (From Damjanov I: Pathology for the Health-Related Professions, 2nd ed. Philadelphia, WB Saunders, 2000.)

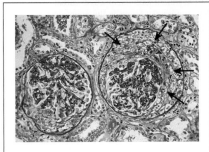

Figure 3-11. Crescentic glomerulonephritis. Arrows point to a proliferation of parietal epithelial cells in Bowman's capsule, occupying approximately 50% of the entire urinary space. The cells encase and compress the glomerular tuft. (From Kumar V, Abbas AK, Fausto, N: Robbins and Cotran Pathologic Basis of Disease, 7th ed. Philadelphia, WB Saunders 2005, p 977, Fig. 20-17.)

microscopic polyangiitis tends to be p-ANCA positive (with a *perinuclear* cytoplasmic pattern). Wegener's granulomatosis usually presents with a triad of glomerulonephritis and involvement of both the lower and upper respiratory tracts. The respiratory disease is usually in the form of oralulcers or purulent or bloody nasal discharge along with pulmonary nodules, infiltrates, or cavities.

Goodpasture syndrome is another form of RPGN caused by antibodies directed against the glomerular basement membrane (GBM). These anti-GBM antibodies form immune complexes that can be seen on immunofluorescence as *linear* deposits of IgG and C3. These anti-GBM antibodies can also react with the alveolar basement membrane of the lungs to cause pulmonary hemorrhage in addition to glomerulonephritis.

RPGN can also represent the end stage of many other forms of immune complex–mediated glomerulonephritis. In such a case, immunofluorescence typically reveals "lumpy-bumpy" granular (i.e., nonlinear) deposition along the glomeruli.

STEP 1 SECRET

Wegener's granulomatosis presents with upper respiratory symptoms but Goodpasture syndrome does not. Goodpasture syndrome involves linear deposits along the glomerular basement membrane (GBM) but Wegener's granulomatosis does not. You will be given at least one of these two pieces of information on your examination if the question requires you to distinguish the two diagnoses from one another.

7. **What is the most common cause of nephritis worldwide?**
IgA nephropathy (i.e., Berger's disease) is overall the most common primary glomerular disease (nephritic or nephrotic).

This disorder is in several ways similar to HSP but without any extrarenal manifestations. It is commonly seen a few days after a viral upper respiratory or GI illness. Renal biopsy typically shows immune complex deposition (composed of primarily IgA) within the mesangium (the same mesangioproliferative picture seen on biopsy in HSP).

The patients often present with chronic asymptomatic microscopic hematuria and trace proteinuria, with exacerbations characterized by *gross hematuria* occurring after viral infections. IgA nephropathy is a good example of disorder that can present with features of both nephrotic and nephritic syndromes.

8. **What syndrome do you suspect in a 13-year-old boy with microscopic hematuria and hearing loss?**

Alport syndrome (i.e., hereditary nephritis), although much less common, is clinically similar to IgA nephropathy in that it often presents with asymptomatic microscopic hematuria. It is caused by various mutations in type IV collagen normally found in the glomerular basement membrane and elsewhere. It is usually inherited in an X-linked manner (can be both dominant and recessive). The major clue to its diagnosis is the association with abnormal hearing and vision (i.e., sensorineural hearing loss and lens abnormalities). The presence of collagen IV in the skin allows for the diagnosis to be usually made by skin biopsy. Renal biopsy, if performed, typically shows fragmentation of the basement membrane in a "basket weave" pattern.

As an aside, there are only a few medications that can cause both ototoxicity and nephrotoxicity. These drugs include loop diuretics (such as furosemide), vancomycin, cisplatin, and aminoglycosides.

DIFFERENTIAL DIAGNOSIS

9. **Quick review: Cover the right column in Table 3-3 and attempt to diagnose the cause of the glomerulonephritis based on the laboratory findings and history provided in the left column.**

TABLE 3-3. DIFFERENTIAL DIAGNOSIS FOR GLOMERULONEPHRITIS

Findings on Laboratory Tests and History	Likely Cause of Glomerulonephritis
Anti-GBM antibodies, hematuria, and hemoptysis	Goodpasture syndrome (i.e., anti-GBM disease)
c-ANCA–positive with a history of bloody nasal discharge and hemoptysis	Wegener's granulomatosis
Defect in type IV collagen with congenital hearing and ocular impairment	Alport syndrome
Massive proteinuria and edema in an adult with hepatitis B	Membranous nephropathy
Hematuria, episodic abdominal pain, joint pain, and a lower extremity purpuric rash	Henoch-Schönlein purpura

c-ANCA, cytoplasmic antineutrophil cytoplasmic antibodies; GBM, glomerular basement membrane.

SUMMARY BOX: POSTSTREPTOCOCCAL GLOMERULONEPHRITIS ✓

- Poststreptococcal glomerulonephritis is an acute nephritic syndrome occurring 1 to 2 weeks after streptococcal sore throat or skin/soft tissue infection; antistreptolysin O (ASO) or anti-DNase B titers can be used to document recent infection. It typically resolves without specific therapy.

- Crescentic or rapidly progressive glomerulonephritis is a form of glomerulonephritis with rapid onset and poor prognosis. The three types are distinguished by immunofluorescence: (1) pauci-immune (i.e., antineutrophil cytoplasmic antibody–associated) disease (Wegener's granulomatosis or microscopic polyangiitis), (2) anti–glomerular basement membrane syndromes (e.g., Goodpasture syndrome), and (3) end-stage immune complex–mediated diseases.

- Both IgA nephropathy and Alport syndrome frequently present with asymptomatic microscopic hematuria. IgA nephropathy is the most common primary glomerular disease worldwide. Alport syndrome is caused by inherited defects in collagen IV and is often accompanied by hearing loss.

CASE 3-8

A 45-year-old man is evaluated in the emergency room (ER) for a several-hour history of severe left flank pain that radiates into his groin. He reports some mild nausea with the pain, but denies vomiting, diarrhea, or abdominal pain. He is writhing in pain but abdominal exam is largely unrevealing. Urine microscopy reveals gross hematuria without RBC casts, dysmorphic RBCs, or WBC casts. Routine laboratory tests done in the ER also show hypercalcemia.

1. **What is the diagnosis?**
   The severe flank pain (i.e., renal colic) and urologic (i.e., nonglomerular) hematuria suggest the diagnosis nephrolithiasis, which is confirmed by computed tomography (CT) scan. This stone is most likely secondary to chronic hypercalcemia.

2. **What are the most common causes of nephrolithiasis?**
   The vast majority of kidney stones are calcium stones (calcium oxalate or calcium phosphate); struvite stones (magnesium ammonium phosphate) are next most common, followed by uric acid stones and cystine stones. The most common causes include dehydration, hypercalcemia (calcium oxalate stones), infection (struvite stones), hyperuricosuria (uric acid stones), and impaired absorption of basic amino acids (cystine stones) (Figs. 3-12 to 3-14).

3. **How can nephrolithiasis cause renal failure?**
   If a ureter or ureteral pelvis is completely obstructed, this increases the hydrostatic pressure in the ureters and ultimately in the renal tubules. The increased hydrostatic pressure substantially diminishes the net filtration pressure at the glomerulus, causing an acute decline in the GFR. However, if, as is usually the case, the other kidney is intact and healthy, it can compensate for the decreased GFR in the obstructed kidney.

   Recall that obstruction of urine flow out of a kidney causes hydronephrosis (pelvicalicectasis), in which the renal pelvis and calyces dilate significantly. Hydronephrosis is usually detected on renal ultrasound or CT scan.

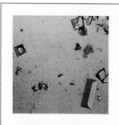

Figure 3-12. Coffin lid crystals of magnesium ammonium phosphate (struvite). (From Johnson RJ, Feehally J: Comprehensive Clinical Nephrology. London, Mosby, 2000.)

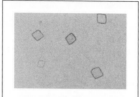

Figure 3-13. Uric acid crystals (×160). (From McPherson RA, Pincus MR: Henry's Clinical Diagnosis and Management by Laboratory Methods, 21st ed. Philadelphia, WB Saunders, 2006.)

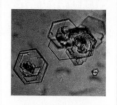

Figure 3-14. Hexagonal cystine crystals, which indicate cystinuria (×400). (From Piccoli G, Varese D, Rotunno M: Atlas of Urinary Sediments: Diagnosis and Clinical Correlations in Nephrology. New York, Raven, 1984.)

4. **What are the most common causes of hypercalcemia among both outpatients and inpatients?**

    Primary hyperparathyroidism is the predominant cause in the community, whereas malignancy-induced hypercalcemia predominates in hospitalized patients. Together, these two conditions account for over 90% of hypercalcemia cases.

    Recall that primary hyperparathyroidism is usually caused by either a parathyroid adenoma (in the majority of cases), hyperplasia (in about 10% of cases), or (rarely) by carcinoma. A popular mnemonic for the complications of hyperparathyroidism is "stones, bones, moans, and groans," referring to the increased risk for renal calculi, peptic ulcers (presumably from increased gastric acid secretion), and pathologic fractures as well as the possible symptoms of vague bone pains, muscle aches or weakness, malaise, fatigue, and depression. Any form of hypercalcemia (analogous to hyperglycemia) can cause polydipsia and polyuria from osmotic diuresis, while constipation and hypertension can occur from increased smooth muscle tone.

    Hypercalcemia is the most common metabolic derangement that complicates malignancy, occurring in 10% to 20% of cancer patients. Malignancies such as breast cancer and multiple myeloma can produce hypercalcemia by metastasizing to bone and causing lytic destruction; others, such as squamous cell cancer of the lung (and other organs) and renal cell carcinoma, secrete an ectopic hormone known as parathyroid hormone–related peptide (PTHrP).

    Note: Granulomatous diseases, such as sarcoid, and a subset of malignancies, particularly lymphomas, can produce hypercalcemia via excess formation and activation of *endogenous* vitamin D (i.e., calcitriol) by activated macrophages, presumably the same macrophages found within the granulomas or lymphomatous lesions that histologically characterize these diseases. Other causes of hypercalcemia include *hypervitaminosis D* (vitamin D intoxication) and the milk-alkali syndrome, in which excess calcium and absorbable alkali (such as the calcium carbonate of Tums) are ingested, resulting in alkalosis, hypercalcemia, and renal insufficiency.

    A commonly-used mnemonic for causes of hypercalcemia is **CHIMPANZEES**: excess **C**alcium ingestion, **H**yperparathyroidism or **H**yperthyroidism, **I**atrogenic (i.e., drug-induced, as from thiazide administration) or **I**mmobilization, **M**yeloma, **P**aget's disease of bone, **A**ddison's disease, **N**eoplasm, **Z**ollinger-Ellison syndrome (typically in association with multiple endocrine neoplasia type I syndrome), **E**xcess vitamin D, **E**xcess vitamin A, **S**arcoid and other granulomatous diseases. Note that many of these conditions, although potential causes of hypercalcemia, are more commonly associated with normal, rather than elevated, serum calcium.

5. **Why is hypercalcemia secondary to hyperparathyroidism less likely to cause renal calculi formation than other causes of hypercalcemia?**
Generally, the risk of calcium oxalate stone formation in the urine is proportional to the *urine* calcium concentration (rather than serum calcium concentration). Although primary hyperparathyroidism increases urine calcium concentration as in most other causes of hypercalcemia, it does so to a lesser extent, because PTH, in addition to promoting GI uptake of calcium and calcium release from bone, promotes hypercalcemia by stimulating renal tubular calcium reabsorption.

RELATED QUESTIONS

6. **How does urinary tract infection with bacteria such as *Proteus mirabilis* predispose to struvite stone formation?**
Struvite stones, which consist of magnesium ammonium phosphate, precipitate at *higher* urinary pH. *Proteus* species and other urinary pathogens elaborate the enzyme urease into the urinary tract, which cleaves urea to form ammonia and carbon dioxide. The ammonia released both increases the urinary pH and, within basic urine, forms the ammonium that can precipitate as part of the struvite stones. Struvite stones, like calcium oxalate stones, are radiopaque.
   Note: Struvite stones are often large, at times occupying all the renal calyces to form characteristic "staghorn" calculi.

7. **How does urinary pH influence the precipitation of uric acid stones?**
Uric acid, as a weak acid, is *less* soluble in its (neutral, protonated) uric acid form than in the (unprotonated, negatively charged) urate form. Thus, decreasing the urinary pH increases the concentration of the less soluble uric acid form, thereby facilitating crystallization.
   Because the diuretic acetazolamide increases urinary pH (as inhibition of carbonic anhydrase prevents bicarbonate reabsorption and results in increased urinary bicarbonate concentration), it can also be used to help dissolve uric acid stones.
   Uric acid stones are associated, like gout, with hyperuricemia and, most specifically, with hyperuricosuria. Thus, in addition to increased fluid intake (as used with all stone types) and urine alkalinization, allopurinol can be used to prevent recurrence of uric acid stones by decreasing uric acid synthesis (via inhibition of the enzyme xanthine oxidase).

8. **What is cystinuria and how does it lead to cystine stones?**
This is a genetic disease in which renal tubular reabsorption of cystine (and several other amino acids) is impaired. Specifically, there is a defect in the transporter responsible for the absorption of the *basic* amino acids cystine, ornithine, lysine, and arginine. Because cystine is not as soluble as these other amino acids, it precipitates selectively in this disease.
   Cystinuria is distinct from the disease homocystinuria. In the latter case a genetic defect in homocysteine catabolism causes extreme elevations in plasma and urine homocysteine concentrations.
   Also note that cystine and uric acid stones are both "organic stones," which are typically radiolucent, and so they cannot be visualized using x-rays but can be seen with CT scan. This contrasts with most calcium-containing stones, which are radiopaque and can be visualized using x-rays.

9. **How does Crohn's disease lead to an increased risk of kidney stones?**
Crohn's disease very frequently involves the terminal ileum, which is the primary site of bile salt reabsorption. Thus, Crohn's ileitis can cause bile salt malabsorption. As bile salts normally extensively bind calcium, the increased levels of bile salt in the intestinal lumen decrease the levels of free calcium in the gut. Less free calcium is therefore available to bind oxalate, which in turn, is then left unbound and free to be absorbed from the gut. As a result, patients with Crohn's

disease tend to hyperabsorb oxalate. This oxalate must eventually be excreted in urine, and the high urinary oxalate concentration predisposes to calcium oxalate stone formation.

Interestingly, by disrupting the solubility of bile, the bile salt malabsorption that occurs in Crohn's disease also increases the risk of gallstone formation.

SUMMARY BOX: NEPHROLITHIASIS

- Nephrolithiasis presents with "renal colic" and urologic (i.e., nonglomerular) hematuria, is usually diagnosed by computed tomography (CT), and can cause obstruction and (if bilateral) renal failure.

- Kidney stones are composed of (in order of decreasing incidence) calcium, struvite, uric acid, or cystine.

- The most common cause of hypercalcemia in hospitalized patients is malignancy, whereas primary hyperparathyroidism (caused by parathyroid adenoma or hyperplasia) is most common in outpatients.

- Mechanisms of hypercalcemia include direct lysis of bone (as in myeloma or breast cancer), ectopic production of parathyroid hormone (PTH)–related peptide (as in squamous cell lung cancer), and excess production of activated vitamin D by macrophages (by lymphomas or granulomatous diseases).

- Other, less common causes of hypercalcemia include exogenous calcium ingestion, milk-alkali syndrome, hypervitaminosis D or A, prolonged immobilization, drug effect (e.g., thiazides), Paget disease, and (uncommonly) endocrine disorders (i.e., Addison's disease or hyperthyroidism).

- Primary hyperparathyroidism is caused by adenomas (most commonly), by hyperplasia (in ~10%), and (rarely) by carcinoma. Possible symptoms and complications include kidney stones, pathologic fractures, peptic ulcers, vague muscle and bone pains, polydipsia, constipation, and hypertension.

- Struvite stones consist of magnesium ammonium phosphate and precipitate at a high urinary pH. As a result, they often complicate infections caused by urease-producing (i.e., urea-cleaving and ammonia-releasing) organisms like *Proteus*. "Staghorn" calculi are usually composed of struvite.

- Uric acid stones precipitate at *lower* urine pH and, as a result, the carbonic anhydrase inhibitor acetazolamide can be used to dissolve them.

- Cystinuria is a defect in tubular basic amino acid reabsorption that results in recurrent cystine stones.

- Crohn's disease leads to bile acid malabsorption, which in turn predisposes to both gallstones and kidney (calcium oxalate) stones.

CASE 3-9

A 38-year-old woman complains of sudden-onset urinary symptoms, including burning urination, frequent urination, urgency, and a feeling of incomplete bladder emptying, as well as nausea, vomiting, and right-sided back pain. On examination she has a fever of 102.5° and right-sided costovertebral angle tenderness. Urinalysis reveals numerous WBCs, bacteria, and WBC casts. She is admitted to the hospital and prescribed ciprofloxacin. She is also told to drink plenty of fluids.

1. **What is the most likely diagnosis?**
   She most likely has acute pyelonephritis.
   Although they can be seen with other causes of renal parenchymal inflammation (such as acute interstitial nephritis), WBC casts in the setting of such urinary symptoms are essentially pathognomonic for acute pyelonephritis.

2. **What is the most common source of infection in pyelonephritis?**
   In the vast majority of cases, these infections are the result of ascending infection from the bladder and urinary tract, whereas in a minority, the infection is from hematogenous dissemination. The most common infectious agents are fecal flora that have colonized the vaginal introitus. *Escherichia coli*, in particular, is the predominant pathogen. In sexually active young women, infection with *Staphylococcus saprophyticus* (a type of coagulase-negative staphylococcus distinct from *Staphylococcus epidermidis*) is second most common. Among the relatively uncommon cases of hematogenous seeding of the renal parenchyma, coagulase-positive *S. aureus* is the most common pathogen.
   Note: Unlike the gram-negative organisms that are common causative agents of UTI, *S. saprophyticus* tests esterase-positive and nitrite-negative (gram-negative organisms are positive for both markers).

3. **Why are pregnant women with asymptomatic bacteriuria treated more aggressively than nonpregnant women with the same condition?**
   Although asymptomatic bacteriuria (bacteria in the urine without symptoms or other evidence of infection) rarely causes problems in nonpregnant women, a significant percentage of pregnant women with this condition will go on to develop pyelonephritis. Aside from the obvious dangers of developing bacteremia and sepsis, pyelonephritis also increases the risk of premature delivery.

4. **Why are pregnant women with bacteriuria more susceptible to pyelonephritis?**
   Pregnancy results in relaxation of the basal tone of the ureteral smooth muscle. This ureteral dilation or physiologic hydronephrosis increases urine pooling and, in turn, the risk of ascending infection. This ureteral relaxation is believed to be a result of increased progesterone levels of pregnancy, similar to the relaxation of GI smooth muscle that results in the constipation that is also characteristic of pregnancy.

5. **What is acute interstitial nephritis and how does it differ from acute pyelonephritis?**
   AIN, like pyelonephritis, is characterized by inflammation of the renal interstitium. However, rather than infection, it is caused by an allergic reaction, most commonly a drug hypersensitivity. Although infectious agents (less commonly than drugs) can also precipitate AIN, the infectious process itself is minimally involved in the pathogenesis, whereas the immunologic hypersensitivity to the infectious agent is paramount. AIN can also be a manifestation of autoimmune disorders such as sarcoid (albeit rarely).
   See Case 3-3, question 1, for a review of AIN as a cause of intrinsic acute renal failure.

6. **Why are urinary tract infections in men younger than 50 often evaluated aggressively?**
   These infections are usually due to urologic abnormalities, because ordinarily younger men are quite resistant to urinary tract infections (with the exception of sexually transmitted diseases

[STDs]). Women are presumably more predisposed to UTIs because of the shorter length of the female urethra and the proximity of the vagina and perineum to the urethral meatus.

7. **Why are men older than 50 predisposed to urinary tract infection?**
The benign prostatic hyperplasia (BPH) that commonly develops in this group causes greater urinary retention and stasis of bladder urine, which facilitates bacterial overgrowth.

SUMMARY BOX: ACUTE PYELONEPHRITIS

- Acute pyelonephritis can result in urinary tract infection (UTI) symptoms, fever, and nausea and vomiting. Costovertebral angle tenderness on examination and white blood cell (WBC), bacteria, and WBC casts in the urine are highly suggestive.

- Pyelonephritis usually results from ascending urinary infection caused by fecal flora, most commonly *Escherichia coli*. In young women, *Staphylococcus saprophyticus* is second only to *E. coli*. Hematogenous infection of the kidneys is most commonly caused by *Staphylococcus aureus*.

- Pregnancy predisposes to ascending urinary infection; thus, asymptomatic bacteriuria in pregnancy is treated to prevent pyelonephritis (and the subsequent risk of sepsis and preterm delivery).

- Men older than 50 years are predisposed to UTI from benign prostatic hyperplasia–related urine retention and stasis. Likewise, adult men under 50 with a UTI should be evaluated for sexually transmitted diseases (STDs) or urinary anomalies.

FLUID AND ELECTROLYTES

Thomas A. Brown, MD, and Sonali J. Shah

CHAPTER 4

INSIDER'S GUIDE TO FLUID AND ELECTROLYTES FOR THE USMLE STEP 1

Many of the important concepts that were touched upon in Chapter 3 are further explored in Chapters 4 and 5, on fluid and electrolytes and acid-base balance, respectively. Concepts relating to fluid and electrolytes make up a large portion of the renal physiology and pharmacology material tested on Step 1. You will soon see that this is *not* a section that requires memorizing lots of small details. Instead, it demands a thorough understanding of the mechanisms of action of various hormones and drugs involved in regulating fluid and electrolyte balance. Know which segments of the nephron are affected by these individual hormones and drugs. If applicable, it is a good idea to categorize how each hormone or drug affects glomerular filtration rate (GFR), renal plasma flow (RPF), filtration fraction, etc. For those of you who do not have a strong background in renal physiology, you may need to read through the discussion in this chapter a few times to fully grasp all of the material.

BASIC CONCEPTS—RENAL FILTRATION AND TRANSPORT PROCESSES

1. **What forces govern the glomerular filtration rate at the level of the glomerulus?**
   These forces are the same forces that affect fluid movement in the systemic capillaries. Forces that drive fluid across the glomerular membrane include the hydrostatic pressure in the glomerular capillaries and the oncotic pressure in Bowman's space (Fig. 4-1). Because there is usually very little protein in Bowman's space, the contribution from the filtrate's oncotic pressure is typically negligible. Forces that oppose fluid movement across the glomerular membrane are the hydrostatic pressure in Bowman's space and the plasma oncotic pressure.

   Glomerular hydrostatic pressure and, in turn, glomerular filtration rate (GFR), is altered by constriction or dilation of the afferent and efferent arterioles. Because the glomerulus is located between the afferent and efferent arterioles, changes in the caliber of the arterioles tend to have opposite effects on the glomerulus. Either dilation of the afferent arteriole or constriction of the efferent arteriole will increase glomerular pressure and filtration. Likewise, constriction of the afferent arteriole or dilation of the efferent arteriole will decrease glomerular pressure and GFR.

   Note: Most circulating vasoconstricting and vasodilating agents act on the afferent arteriole. An important exception, however, is angiotensin II, which acts preferentially to vasoconstrict the *efferent* arteriole. Thus, angiotensin II works to preserve GFR in a setting of decreased renal perfusion. Angiotensin-converting enzyme (ACE) inhibitors decrease GFR by inhibiting the *formation* of angiotensin II on the efferent arteriole (see question 2).

   In addition to the oncotic and hydrostatic pressures, the surface area and integrity of the glomerular membranes are also important determinants of GFR. Mathematically, these factors are represented through a filtration constant. These factors are most relevant in disease states in which the glomeruli are damaged. The formula for calculating GFR is given in Chapter 3.

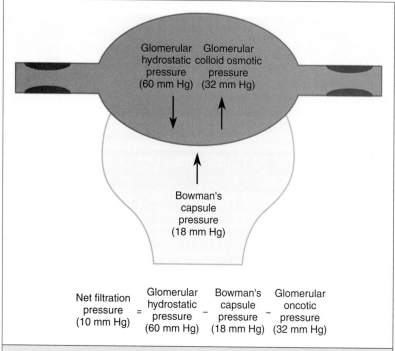

Figure 4-1. Summary of forces causing filtration by the glomerular capillaries. The values shown are estimates for healthy humans. (From Guyton AC, Hall JE: Textbook of Medical Physiology, 11th ed. Philadelphia, WB Saunders, 2007.)

2. **How do angiotensin-converting enzyme inhibitors and angiotensin receptor blockers affect glomerular filtration rate?**

   ACE inhibitors and angiotensin receptor blockers (ARBs) tend to decrease GFR acutely. Blocking the action of angiotensin II results in vasodilation of the efferent arteriole, which decreases intraglomerular pressure and, in turn, decreases filtration.

   Although ACE inhibitors and ARBs usually produce a decrease in GFR (manifesting as an increase in plasma creatinine) in the short term, they have an important beneficial effect on preserving renal function in individuals with diabetes and other chronic kidney diseases. This benefit likely results from the fact that a decrease in glomerular pressure, despite acutely decreasing GFR, may over the long term decrease the "wear" on the glomeruli. Because of this benefit, a certain degree of creatinine elevation is tolerated when starting an ACE inhibitor or ARB.

3. **What is meant by the term *filtration fraction* and how will increasing the glomerular capillary oncotic pressure (without changing anything else) affect the filtration fraction?**

   The filtration fraction is the percent of plasma passing through the glomerular capillaries that is actually filtered by the glomerulus. It can be calculated as shown here:

   $$\text{Filtration fraction (FF)} = \frac{\text{Glomerular filtration rate}}{\text{Renal plasma flow}}$$

   Normally, this fraction is about 20%. Because the glomerular capillary oncotic pressure opposes filtration, increasing it will decrease the net filtration pressure and decrease the filtration fraction.

4. **What are the three layers of the glomerular "filter" and how do they contribute to the process of renal filtration at the glomerulus?**

The three components of the glomerular filter include the *endothelial cells* of the glomerular capillaries, the underlying *basement membrane*, and the *glomerular epithelial cells*. These components all contribute to renal filtration in distinct ways.

The endothelium of the glomerular capillaries is fenestrated. Along with the high hydrostatic pressure present in the glomerular capillaries, the fenestration of these capillaries allows for the filtration of large volumes of plasma across the capillary bed.

The underlying basement membrane is negatively charged, which helps prevent filtration (and subsequent loss in the urine) of large negatively charged plasma proteins. Importantly, these negatively charged proteins include albumin, which is why loss of albumin and hypoalbuminemia can occur in various types of glomerular disease (particularly in nephrotic syndromes).

The glomerular epithelial cells or podocytes compose the final layer of the glomerular filter. These specialized cells have cytoplasmic extensions called foot processes, with intervening slit-pores, that together envelop the glomerular capillaries and form a final barrier for filterable molecules to traverse prior to entering the capsular space of the glomerulus.

Note: The glomerulus also contains macrophage-like mesangial cells and mesangial matrix interspersed between these layers (Fig. 4-2). The function of the mesangium is not very well understood (though it may serve both a structural role and a housekeeping role). Regardless, the mesangium can be an important site of glomerular disease.

5. **What is the significance of the creatinine clearance and how is it measured?**

The clearance of any substance is defined as the volume of plasma that is "cleared" of that substance per unit of time. For example, a creatinine clearance rate of 125 mL/min implies that, every minute, creatinine is being completely removed and excreted (by the kidneys) from 125 mL of plasma. As shown by the following equation, the clearance of a substance can be calculated by dividing the rate of urinary excretion of a substance by the substance's plasma concentration. The rate of urinary excretion of a substance can be determined from its concentration in urine and the urine flow rate.

$$C = \frac{\text{Urinary flow rate (mL/min)} \times \text{Urinary creatinine concentration}}{\text{Plasma creatinine concentration}}$$

$$= \frac{V \times U_{cr}}{P_{cr}}$$

You can easily derive this formula by recalling that all creatinine that appears in the urine is a result of the removal of creatinine from plasma:

$$\text{Rate of creatinine removal from plasma} = \text{Rate of creatinine excretion in urine}$$

$$P_{cr} \times C = V \times U_{cr}$$

$$C = \frac{V \times U_{cr}}{P_{cr}}$$

Because creatinine is (for the most part) neither reabsorbed nor secreted, its clearance rate very closely approximates the actual GFR, and it is therefore an important indicator of renal function.

Clinically, a single plasma creatinine level is frequently used, along with a patient's weight, age, and gender (and in some equations, race and serum albumin as a measure of nutrition status), to estimate creatinine clearance and GFR. These additional factors are included to estimate the rate of creatinine production, which depends on one's muscle mass (creatinine is a byproduct of the muscle energy storage molecule creatine). Note that these equations (such as the Cockroft-Gault equation and the more sophisticated modification of diet in renal disease [MDRD] equation)work well only when the patient's renal function is at a steady state. They work poorly when it is rapidly changing, as in acute renal failure.

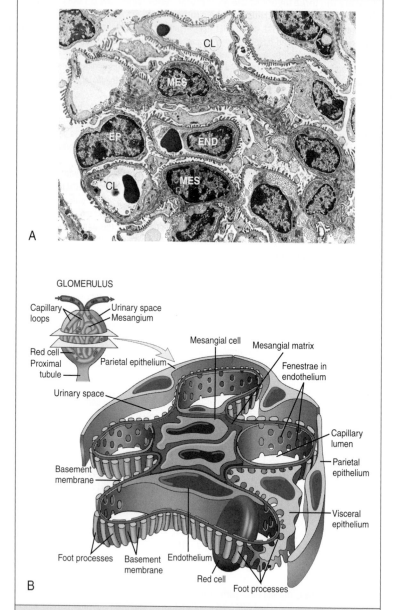

Figure 4-2. A, Low-power electron micrograph of renal glomerulus. CL, capillary lumen; END, endothelium; EP, visceral epithelial cells with foot processes; MES, mesangium. **B**, Schematic representation of a glomerular lobe. (Courtesy of Dr. Vicki Kelley, Brigham and Women's Hospital, Boston, MA.)

SUMMARY BOX: GENERAL CONCEPTS IN RENAL FILTRATION AND TRANSPORT PROCESSES

- The determinants of glomerular filtration rate (GFR) include the hydrostatic and oncotic pressures within the glomerular capillaries, the hydrostatic and oncotic pressures of Bowman's space, and the collective glomerular surface area and integrity (i.e., filtration constant).

- The hydrostatic pressure within the glomerular capillaries is regulated by vasoconstriction and vasodilation of the efferent and afferent arterioles.

- Most circulating vasoactive substances act to constrict or dilate the afferent arteriole. Angiotensin II is unique in that it acts primarily to constrict the *efferent* arteriole.

- Angiotensin-converting enzyme (ACE) inhibitors and angiotensin receptor blockers (ARBs) may acutely decrease GFR, but their effect on lowering glomerular pressure helps preserve renal function over the long term in patients with chronic kidney disease.

- The three components of the glomerular filter are (1) the capillary endothelial cells, (2) the basement membrane, and (3) the epithelial cells, or podocytes, and the intervening mesangium.

- Creatinine clearance is an important indicator of GFR. Clinically, it is usually estimated from a single measurement of serum creatinine concentration. However, recall that numerous variables (e.g. age, gender, muscle mass) can affect the creatinine concentration.

- Estimates of creatinine clearance are *inaccurate* in the setting of a rapidly changing GFR (i.e., acute renal failure).

BASIC CONCEPTS—RENAL CONTROL OF ACID–BASE BALANCE

1. **Why is net renal acid excretion necessary to maintain acid-base homeostasis?**
   Daily metabolism generates a large quantity of nonvolatile acids (e.g., lactate, sulfate, phosphate) that cannot be excreted by the lungs. These nonvolatile acids must be excreted by the kidneys to prevent the development of a metabolic acidosis.
   Nonvolatile acids are derived primarily from the metabolism of dietary proteins in meat and other foods. In contrast, metabolic breakdown of carbohydrates and fats yields largely carbon dioxide, which is easily excreted by the lungs. Vegetarians, for example, typically generate less dietary acid for their kidneys to excrete and, as a result, on average tend to have less acidic urine.

2. **What mechanisms does the kidney use to maintain acid-base balance despite this acid load?**
   In general, the kidney acts to prevent acidosis from developing by secreting acid into the urine while reabsorbing base.
   More specifically, the kidneys (1) efficiently reabsorb *filtered* bicarbonate in the proximal tubule (through a mechanism that is coupled with hydrogen ion secretion into the tubular fluid), (2) synthesize de novo both bicarbonate (HCO_3^-) to be retained and the acid ammonium (NH_4^+) to be secreted, (3) secrete titratable buffers such as ammonia and phosphate (which bind hydrogen ions and increase the acid excretory capacity of the urine without causing a precipitous drop in urinary pH), and (4) actively pump acid (in the form of hydrogen ions) into the tubular fluid at the distal tubule.

3. **How do the kidneys reabsorb filtered bicarbonate?**

   Hydrogen ions that are secreted into the lumen of the proximal tubule (primarily via countertransport with Na^+) react with bicarbonate in the filtrate to form carbonic acid, which rapidly dissociates into carbon dioxide and water, both of which can then diffuse back into the cell (Fig. 4-3). In the cell, the reverse reaction takes place. Thus, carbon dioxide reacts with water to generate bicarbonate and a proton (hydrogen ion). The bicarbonate is ultimately returned to the venous circulation, whereas the hydrogen ion is secreted back into the tubular lumen.

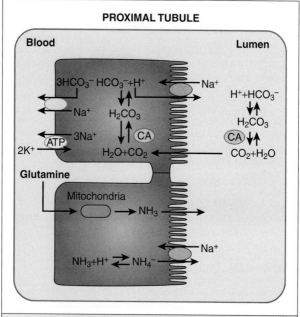

Figure 4-3. Proximal tubule. (From Goldman L, Ausiello D: Cecil Textbook of Medicine, 22nd ed. Philadelphia, WB Saunders, 2004.)

4. **What effect does the diuretic acetazolamide have on the acid-base balance of the body? In what clinical conditions might it be used?**

   Acetazolamide is an inhibitor of carbonic anhydrase, an enzyme present in the proximal tubule of the nephron (the enzyme is actually anchored to the luminal surface of the plasma membrane of tubular epithelial cells). This enzyme normally catalyzes the rapid dissociation of carbonic acid in the tubular fluid into CO_2 and H_2O, an essential step in the reabsorption of bicarbonate (as described previously). The net effect, therefore, of inhibiting carbonic anhydrase is increased urinary excretion of bicarbonate. Because this negatively charged bicarbonate must be excreted with some accompanying sodium, acetazolamide is also a diuretic (albeit a weak one).

   This pharmacotherapeutic mechanism of action essentially mimics the pathophysiology seen in proximal (type II) renal tubular acidoses, in which bicarbonate reabsorption by the tubular epithelium is impaired. The result of decreased bicarbonate reabsorption is a mild metabolic acidosis. This ability of acetazolamide to create a metabolic acidosis can be utilized therapeutically in the treatment or prevention of respiratory alkaloses that develop at elevated altitudes (i.e., mountain sickness). It is also useful to treat conditions such as cystinuria (alkalinizes urine to prevent stone formation) and glaucoma (decreases aqueous humor secretion).

5. **How are bicarbonate and ammonium generated de novo by the kidney?**

The deamination of glutamine in the proximal tubule generates two ammonium (NH_4^+) molecules and two bicarbonate (HCO_3^-) molecules. The ammonium molecules (which essentially consist of acidic protons being carried by ammonia) are secreted into the tubular lumen, whereas the basic bicarbonate molecules are reabsorbed into the systemic circulation (Fig. 4-4).

Glutamine deamination is stimulated by increased levels of H^+ ions or CO_2 within the cells of the proximal tubule. Thus, this mechanism appropriately increases the renal synthesis of bicarbonate (to be retained) and ammonium (to be secreted) in acidotic conditions.

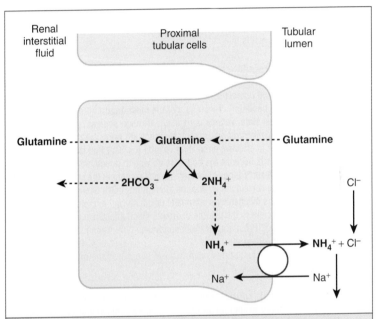

Figure 4-4. Production and secretion of ammonium ion (NH_4^+) by proximal tubular cells. Glutamine is metabolized in the cell yielding NH_4^+ and bicarbonate. The NH_4^+ is actively secreted into the lumen by means of a sodium-NH_4^+ pump. For each glutamine molecule metabolized, two NH_4^+ are produced and secreted and two HCO_3^- are returned to the blood. (From Guyton AC, Hall JE: Textbook of Medical Physiology, 11th ed. Philadelphia, WB Saunders, 2007.)

SUMMARY BOX: RENAL CONTROL OF ACID-BASE BALANCE

Metabolism generates a large quantity of nonvolatile acids that must be excreted by the kidneys. This is accomplished by several mechanisms:

- The reabsorption of filtered bicarbonate in the proximal tubule via a mechanism requiring the activity of carbonic anhydrase

- The de novo synthesis of bicarbonate (to be retained) and ammonium (to be secreted)

- The secretion of titratable buffers (e.g., ammonia, phosphate to increase the acid-carrying capacity of urine)

- The secretion of acid via a proton pump in the distal tubule

For more information on the regulation of acid-base balance, see Chapter 5.

BASIC CONCEPTS—RENAL CONTROL OF EXTRACELLULAR FLUID BALANCE

1. **What are the extracellular fluid compartments of the body and how do their relative sizes compare to the intracellular fluid compartment?**

   The extracellular fluid (ECF) consists of the interstitial fluid and plasma.

   Overall, total body water in a healthy young man is roughly 60% of body weight (whereas in a female subject it is about 50%). For an "average" 70-kg man, total body water is 42 L (recall that 1 L of water weighs 1 kg). About two thirds of the total body water is found within cells; the other one third makes up the ECF volume. Thus, a 70-kg man has about 14 L of ECF: $(70 \times 0.6) \times 1/3$. Plasma volume accounts for about one third to one fourth of the ECF (about 4 L or so in a 70-kg individual), whereas the rest is interstitial fluid.

2. **How do the kidneys regulate extracellular fluid volume?**

   The kidneys regulate ECF *volume* by adjusting the rate of excretion of *sodium*. In contrast, the kidneys regulate body fluid *osmolarity* and *sodium concentration* by altering the excretion of *free water* (water without sodium). This is one of the most important concepts in renal physiology: In the normal state, *volume* is regulated through *sodium balance,* whereas *osmolarity* and *sodium concentration* are regulated through *water balance*.

   To be more precise, it is effective circulating volume (or ECV) that is regulated by the body, not the ECF volume. This is because the body has no way to directly follow ECF volume levels. Instead, various pressure and volume detectors located throughout the circulatory system (in the atria, the aortic arch, the carotid sinus, and the afferent arterioles of the kidney) monitor the ECV and, through various mechanisms, stimulate or inhibit Na^+ excretion. ECV is *not* a measurable volume. It refers to the volume of arterial blood effectively perfusing tissue. ECV is generally proportional to ECF, but notable exceptions occur during congestive heart failure (CHF), cirrhosis, and nephrotic syndrome.

   The renin-angiotensin-aldosterone system (RAAS) is possibly the most important of these mechanisms.

3. **What is the normal role of the renin-angiotensin-aldosterone system?**

   The RAAS acts to maintain an appropriate plasma volume and blood pressure in order to ensure adequate organ perfusion.

   RAAS is activated in response to decreased ECV. Specifically, reduced renal blood flow is sensed by a group of specialized smooth muscle cells located in the wall of the afferent arterioles (part of the juxtaglomerular apparatus). This sensing mechanism allows for decreased arteriolar perfusion to stimulate renin secretion.

   Renin enzymatically cleaves the serum precursor protein angiotensinogen into angiotensin I, which, in turn, is cleaved in the lungs and elsewhere by the endothelial enzyme ACE into the physiologically active peptide angiotensin II. Angiotensin II is a potent vasoconstrictor that acts to increase blood pressure; in fact, it is the most potent physiologic vasoconstrictor known. Angiotensin II also has a direct effect to promote Na^+ reabsorption in the proximal tubule. A third action of angiotensin II is stimulation of aldosterone release from the adrenal cortex. Aldosterone stimulates the reabsorption of Na^+ (coupled to the secretion of K^+ or H^+) in the distal tubule of the nephron. This retained Na^+ (more specifically the fluid volume that accompanies it) helps restore ECV toward normal.

4. **What is the role of the sympathetic nervous system in maintaining effective circulating volume?**

   In addition to helping maintain blood pressure via systemic vasoconstriction, the sympathetic nervous system (which is also activated by low ECV) stimulates Na^+ retention in several ways. First, sympathetically mediated afferent arteriolar vasoconstriction decreases GFR, which indirectly promotes sodium retention through RAAS activation. The sympathetic fibers to the afferent arteriole also directly stimulate renin release. Finally, the sympathetic nervous system (like angiotensin II) promotes Na^+ reabsorption in the proximal tubule.

5. **How does the antidiuretic hormone regulate extracellular fluid volume?**
Under normal conditions, antidiuretic hormone (ADH) does *not* work to regulate ECF volume. Instead, ADH normally functions to regulate the reabsorption of free water in the collecting duct in response to changes in body fluid *osmolarity*.

However, when ECV is severely compromised (decreased by 5-10% of normal), the secretion of ADH by the posterior pituitary is stimulated. Thus, with significant hypovolemia, the function of ADH changes to help preserve volume rather than osmolarity.

This ability of ADH to sacrifice osmolarity to help maintain ECV is an exception to the preceding rule stating that water balance is regulated to maintain osmolarity and sodium balance is regulated to maintain volume. When volume is low enough, the body abandons this usual division of labor and retains sodium *and* water regardless of osmolarity. This change is illustrated by disease states such as CHF, nephrotic syndrome, and cirrhosis. Because these three diseases are characterized by decreased ECV, hyponatremia commonly occurs in all of them as a result of chronically high ADH levels.

CASE 4-1

A 78-year-old woman is evaluated for refractory hypertension. Her current antihypertensive regimen includes a thiazide diuretic, an ACE inhibitor, a beta blocker, and an α_1-receptor antagonist. Examination is significant for a blood pressure of 184/105 mm Hg and an abdominal bruit. A renal angiogram reveals a 95% occlusion of the left renal artery. Renal angioplasty is performed to relieve the occlusion, and her blood pressure subsequently normalizes.

1. **What disease did this patient have and what is its underlying cause?**
This elderly lady had renovascular hypertension (or renal artery stenosis), which is most commonly due to atherosclerosis of the renal arteries. Fibromuscular dysplasia of the renal arteries, a less common disease that primarily affects middle-aged women, also produces renovascular hypertension by occluding the lumen of the renal arteries.

2. **How does the renin-angiotensin-aldosterone system contribute to renovascular hypertension?**
If one kidney is significantly hypoperfused because of renal artery narrowing, it will release abnormally high levels of renin. This will increase systemic angiotensin II and aldosterone levels, which will cause widespread vasoconstriction and significant salt and water retention by both the normal and the abnormal kidneys. Both of these actions result in increased blood pressure. In essence, renovascular hypertension results when the kidneys are "misinformed" about the pressure and volume status of the body.

3. **How do the kidneys regulate blood pressure independently of the renin-angiotensin-aldosterone system?**
Along with renin, angiotensin II, aldosterone, ADH, and the sympathetic nervous system as described earlier, additional mechanisms for regulating ECV and blood pressure exist.

At higher arterial pressures, the kidneys are better perfused, which directly results in increased GFR. Increased GFR alone increases the volume of urine that is produced, thereby reducing the ECF volume and blood pressure. This phenomenon is referred to by some as a "pressure natriuresis." At lower arterial pressures the reduced perfusion reduces GFR and increases tubular reabsorption of salt and water ("glomerulotubular balance"), helping to expand ECF volume and restore the blood pressure.

Atrial natriuretic peptide (ANP) is yet another hormonal agent that helps regulate ECV and blood pressure. High ECV stimulates the cardiac atria to release ANP, which, as its name suggests, promotes natriuresis (i.e., sodium excretion) by the kidneys and thereby decreases ECV. In the setting of low ECV, ANP release is inhibited.

4. **If angiotensin II promotes vasoconstriction, why doesn't the angiotensin II released during hypovolemic states reduce glomerular filtration rate?**
   The preferential action of angiotensin II on the *efferent* (rather than the afferent) arteriole elegantly allows it to maintain GFR despite causing widespread vasoconstriction and reduced renal perfusion. Although vasoconstriction of efferent arteriole reduces renal blood flow, it also increases the hydrostatic pressure of the glomerulus, which increases the net filtration pressure and maintains the GFR.

STEP 1 SECRET

If it has not become apparent yet, it is critical to know that angiotensin II maintains glomerular filtration rate (GFR) by preferentially constricting the efferent arteriole. Recall that angiotensin II will also increase filtration fraction (FF), because GFR is increased and renal plasma flow (RPF) is reduced:

$$FF = GFR/RPF$$

It is unlikely that GFR is increased simply because angiotensin II is produced only in a setting of relative renal hypoperfusion, but it's fair to say that angiotensin II acts to preserve GFR.

5. **Why should angiotensin-converting enzyme inhibitors (or angiotensin receptor blockers) be avoided in patients with bilateral renal artery stenosis?**
   The normal role of angiotensin II in maintaining GFR in the face of hypovolemia is even more pronounced in the setting of bilateral renal artery stenosis (RAS).
   Kidneys with bilateral RAS are dependent on angiotensin II–mediated constriction of the efferent arteriole to maintain glomerular filtration pressure and GFR. This tonic angiotensin-mediated constriction of the efferent arteriole is driven by high plasma levels of angiotensin II. An ACE inhibitor (or an ARB) in this setting will cause the efferent arteriolar vasoconstriction to abruptly cease, and GFR in both kidneys may drop precipitously, possibly resulting in acute renal failure.

SUMMARY BOX: RENAL CONTROL OF EXTRACELLULAR FLUID BALANCE

- Total body water is about 60% of body weight in men and 50% in women. About two thirds of this is intracellular and one third is extracellular. Plasma accounts for about one third to one fourth of extracellular fluid (ECF) volume.

- Under normal conditions, ECF volume or, more precisely, *effective circulation volume* (ECV) is regulated by adjusting the rate of *sodium* excretion. Likewise, *osmolarity* is regulated by adjusting the rate of *free water* excretion. The body will always attempt to maintain sodium balance before water balance.

- ECV and blood pressure are regulated by the renin-angiotensin-aldosterone system, the sympathetic nervous system, atrial natriuretic peptide, and intrinsic renal mechanisms.

- When ECV is decreased by 5% to 10% of normal, antidiuretic hormone (ADH) release is stimulated, helping maintain volume while potentially sacrificing osmolarity.

- Renal artery stenosis (RAS) leads to hypertension, in part, via chronic activation of the renin-angiotensin-aldosterone system. RAS is most commonly caused by atherosclerosis, but, in younger women, may be caused by fibromuscular dysplasia.

- Angiotensin-converting enzyme (ACE) inhibitors and angiotensin receptor blockers (ARBs) should be avoided in patients with bilateral RAS due to dependence on high levels of angiotensin II for maintenance of glomerular filtration rate (GFR).

RENAL CONTROL OF EXTRACELLULAR FLUID OSMOLARITY

CASE 4-2

A 48-year-old man was admitted to the hospital for an elective cholecystectomy, and a presurgical workup reveals a serum sodium level of 125 mEq/L (normal 135–145 mEq/L). He complains of some fatigue, anorexia, and very mild confusion. Vital signs are all within normal limits, as is his physical examination. Urinalysis reveals a urine osmolarity of 620 mOsm/kg.

1. **What is the most likely diagnosis and what is its cause?**
   Unexplained hyponatremia in the setting of increased urine osmolarity strongly suggests the syndrome of inappropriate secretion of antidiuretic hormone (SIADH).
   In this disorder, excess release of the posterior pituitary hormone ADH causes excess free water retention in the collecting duct of the nephron. This additional water dilutes the plasma (resulting in decreased osmolarity and hyponatremia) and *inappropriately* concentrates the urine (as opposed to the *appropriate* concentration of urine in a setting of hypovolemia).

CASE 4-2 continued:

Further questioning reveals a 60-pack per year history of smoking. He denies any recent vomiting or diarrhea, has a normal albumin level, and shows no signs of heart failure. He denies taking diuretics or other medications. A chest x-ray film reveals a 3-cm, spiculated pulmonary nodule near the hilum of the right lung.

2. **What syndromes are associated with syndrome of inappropriate secretion of antidiuretic hormone ?**
   SIADH is associated with a myriad of diseases and disorders. For Step 1, ectopic secretion of ADH by small cell carcinomas of the lung is the classic cause of SIADH. In addition to this paraneoplastic syndrome, SIADH can be seen in a variety of nonmalignant diseases of the lung, including tuberculosis, pneumonia, pneumothorax, chronic obstructive pulmonary disease (COPD), and asthma.
   SIADH can also occur from lesions or tumors of the pituitary or hypothalamus and in the setting of other types of intracranial pathology such as head trauma, stroke and intracranial bleeds, and infection. It has also been associated with pain, nausea, and the postoperative state.

Importantly, SIADH also occurs as a medication side effect, particularly with psychotropic medications such as antiepileptics, antipsychotics, and antidepressants (including selective serotonin reuptake inhibitors [SSRIs]).

3. **What is the function of antidiuretic hormone?**

ADH (previously known as vasopressin) has two primary functions that correspond to its two names: the maintenance of plasma osmolarity and the maintenance of plasma volume and blood pressure.

To maintain plasma osmolarity, ADH is secreted in response to increased plasma osmolarity and reduces the osmolarity by increasing free water reabsorption in the collecting ducts of the kidneys. It does so by stimulating the insertion of water channels (aquaporins) into the luminal membranes of the collecting ducts. This is the antidiuretic function of the hormone.

As described earlier, ADH helps maintain plasma volume and blood pressure in the setting of dramatically decreased ECV. In addition to increasing water reabsorption to expand ECV, it works to maintain blood pressure through arterial vasoconstriction; hence the older term *vasopressin*.

4. **Why is the antidiuretic hormone release in SIADH "inappropriate"?**

The excess ADH release seen in SIADH is considered "inappropriate" because the ADH release is not occurring in response to appropriate physiologic stimuli, that is, increased osmolarity and hypovolemia. Rather, the ADH secretion occurs in an unregulated autonomous fashion.

In general, patients with SIADH are either euvolemic or only mildly hypervolemic. This seemingly unnatural phenomenon occurs because despite the elevated ADH levels, the body's other mechanisms for regulating volume status are preserved. In particular, the increased ADH-stimulated water reabsorption is countered by decreased activity of the renin-angiotensin-aldosterone and sympathetic nervous systems and increased levels of BNP, such that ECV and ECF volume are maintained near normal.

Euvolemia in spite of elevated ADH levels is important for two reasons. First, it reinforces the notion that *volume* is regulated through *sodium balance* whereas *osmolarity* and *sodium concentration* are regulated through *water balance*. Second, it helps distinguish SIADH from other causes of hyponatremia that are generally associated with pronounced hypovolemia or hypervolemia (more specifically, a reduced effective circulating volume [e.g., profuse diarrhea, CHF, nephrotic syndrome]).

5. **What is the result of inadequate antidiuretic hormone release?**

An inadequate level of ADH is the characteristic feature of central diabetes insipidus (DI), in which the posterior pituitary does not secrete sufficient ADH. DI is marked by excessive renal loss of free water, resulting in dilute urine, increased plasma osmolarity, and *hypernatremia*. Note that the production of concentrated urine in a setting of hypernatremia is also *inappropriate*.

DI can be generally divided into two major categories: central DI or nephrogenic DI. The inadequate ADH release of central DI is seen with head trauma, surgery, or other intracranial processes such as infection, tumor, or stroke. Central DI is treated with a synthetic analog of ADH called desmopressin (or DDAVP). This drug binds specifically to vasopressin-2 (V2) receptors on the collecting duct that mediate the renal effects of ADH.

Nephrogenic DI results from the inability of the kidneys to respond to ADH and is caused by drug toxicity (e.g., lithium), hypercalcemia, and various other conditions. Nephrogenic DI, by definition, will *not* respond to DDAVP. The underlying cause of nephrogenic DI must be corrected, although salt restriction and thiazide diuretics (to block renal diluting ability) may be helpful.

STEP 1 SECRET

Distinguishing central diabetes insipidus (DI) from nephrogenic DI is high yield for Step 1. Remember that nephrogenic DI will respond poorly to synthetic analogs of antidiuretic hormone (ADH), whereas central DI will show a full response to treatment.

6. **How does hyponatremia result in the central nervous system symptoms (fatigue, anorexia, and confusion) seen in this patient?**
   Sodium is the primary determinant of plasma and interstitial fluid osmolarity. Hyponatremia thus results in an osmotic shift of extracellular fluid into cells, including brain cells. This can result in cerebral edema and a wide variety of neurologic effects. If hyponatremia is severe, coma and convulsions may occur.

7. **Why must the hyponatremia be corrected slowly in this patient?**
   Overly rapid correction of hyponatremia (>12 mEq/24 hours) is thought to place patients at high risk for the development of central pontine myelinolysis (CPM), a disorder that can result in flaccid quadriplegia, dysphagia, facial weakness, and in some cases, coma. A rare but classic manifestation of pons destruction in CPM is the "locked-in syndrome," in which a conscious patient demonstrates paralysis of all muscles except those involved in eye-opening and vertical gaze. The pathophysiology of CPM is believed to involve overly rapid shift of fluid back out of brain cells in response to a rapid increase in plasma osmolarity, resulting in the death of myelin-producing oligodendrocytes and loss of myelin in the pons and other regions of the brain. In fact, magnetic resonance imaging (MRI) studies have shown that multiple areas of the brain are damaged with the overly rapid correction of hyponatremia, leading to symptoms such as cognitive and psychiatric dysfunction. Thus, the term *osmotic demyelination syndrome* is perhaps a better descriptor of the pathophysiology than the classic term *central pontine myelinolysis*. This disorder is classically seen in alcoholics who seem to be predisposed on the basis of malnutrition.
   Overly rapid correction of *hypernatremia* also leads to serious central nervous system (CNS) toxicity, but in the form of *cerebral edema* rather than CPM. Again, it is prudent to avoid correcting faster than 0.5 mEq/L/hour.

8. **Why was it important to ask about vomiting, diarrhea, or diuretic use?**
   These are all causes of sodium wasting that can result in hyponatremia. Note that in these cases there are significant fluid (i.e., volume) losses also, resulting in *hypovolemic* hyponatremia. In contrast, SIADH is associated with a euvolemic or mildly hypervolemic hyponatremia (see question 4 earlier).
   Other causes of hypovolemic hyponatremia include salt wasting from mineralocorticoid deficiency (i.e., adrenal insufficiency) or "third-spacing" events (e.g., severe burns, pancreatitis, or bowel obstruction).
   Note: In this setting, the ADH release is *appropriate* (i.e., stimulated by the hypovolemia and decreased ECV).

9. **Why was it important to examine the albumin level and look for evidence of heart failure?**
   Hypoalbuminemia (from liver disease or nephrotic syndrome) and heart failure both cause fluid retention and hyponatremia, resulting in *hypervolemic* hyponatremia.
   In this setting, ADH release is appropriate because despite total body hypervolemia, these conditions are characterized by decreased ECV.

10. **How would levels of plasma antidiuretic hormone, plasma osmolarity, and serum osmolarity be expected to differ between syndrome of inappropriate secretion of antidiuretic hormone, diabetes insipidus, and psychogenic polydipsia?**
   These features are compared in Table 4-1.

SUMMARY BOX: RENAL CONTROL OF EXTRACELLULAR FLUID OSMOLARITY

- Antidiuretic hormone (ADH, vasopressin) has two primary effects: (1) increased free water reabsorption in the collecting ducts (the antidiuretic function) and (2) systemic vasoconstriction (the pressor function).

- Under normal conditions, ADH is released in response to increased osmolarity. ADH release is also stimulated by a large decrease (i.e., drop of 5% to 10% or more) in effective circulating volume (ECV). Release of ADH that is not caused by either stimulus is considered "inappropriate."

- The classic cause of hyponatremia due to syndrome of inappropriate secretion of antidiuretic hormone (SIADH) is ectopic ADH secretion by a small cell carcinoma of the lung. Other causes include pituitary or hypothalamic lesions, various other lung and central nervous system (CNS) diseases, drug side effects, pain, nausea, and the postoperative state.

- Hyponatremia and high ADH levels can occur in congestive heart failure (CHF), cirrhosis, or nephrotic syndrome. Other causes of hyponatremia include sodium wasting via the gastrointestinal (GI) tract (i.e., from vomiting and diarrhea) or kidneys (i.e., from diuretic use). In these diseases, ADH release is considered "appropriate" due to the reduced effective circulating volume.

- Inadequate ADH results in diabetes insipidus (DI) with free water wasting and hypernatremia. DI is either central (inadequate ADH release) or nephrogenic (inability of the kidney to respond to ADH, think lithium exposure).

PHARMACOLOGY OF DIURETICS

1. **How do diuretics work to lower extracellular fluid volume?**
   All diuretics act to inhibit the reabsorption of sodium and thereby increase the rate of excretion of sodium and lower ECF volume. In other words, all diuretics are natriuretics.

   However, the effect of all diuretics is ultimately limited in that the decrease in ECF volume achieved results in less sodium delivery to the nephrons, such that the rate of sodium excretion eventually decreases back to baseline (i.e., equal to the rate of sodium intake). A new steady state is achieved at a lower ECF volume. Continued administration of the diuretic is required to maintain the lower ECF volume.

2. **What percentage of the filtered sodium is reabsorbed under normal conditions (i.e., in the absence of diuretics)?**
   The majority of sodium is reabsorbed in the proximal tubule, and each subsequent segment reabsorbs progressively less. The actual amounts are listed in Table 4-2.

   Notice that about 99% of filtered sodium is normally reabsorbed. In general, the proximal tubule and ascending loop of Henle are relatively permeable and reabsorb large amounts of sodium (and water with it) via relatively low-energy-requiring mechanisms, whereas the

TABLE 4-1. ADH LEVELS IN SIADH, DIABETES INSIPIDUS, AND PSYCHOGENIC POLYDIPSIA

Syndrome	Plasma ADH	Plasma Osmolarity	Urine Osmolarity	Pathophysiologic Explanation	Classic Step I Association
SIADH	High	Low	Inappropriately high	ADH causes excess water reabsorption by the kidneys, creating an inappropriately concentrated urine in the setting of low plasma osmolarity	Small cell carcinoma of the lung
Central diabetes insipidus	Low	High	Low	Lack of hypothalamic ADH secretion causes wasting of free water in excess of sodium, resulting in hyperosmolar plasma	Head trauma (disruption of the pituitary stalk)
Nephrogenic diabetes insipidus	High	High	Low	Inability of the kidneys to respond to ADH results in wasting of free water and hyperosmolar plasma	Lithium toxicity
Psychogenic polydipsia	Low	Low	Maximally dilute (about 50 mOsm)	Enormous free water intake overwhelms ability of normal kidneys to excrete free water despite creating a maximally dilute urine	Schizophrenia or other psychiatric disease

ADH, antidiuretic hormone; SIADH, syndrome of inappropriate antidiuretic hormone [secretion].

TABLE 4-2. SODIUM REABSORPTION ALONG THE NEPHRON	
Segment	Percentage
Proximal tubule	60
Loop of Henle	25
Distal tubule	10
Collecting duct	4

subsequent segments tend to be impermeable and use higher energy mechanisms to actively "extract" increasingly small amounts of sodium remaining against progressively higher concentration gradients.

These percentages are important in that the potency of each type of diuretic depends not only on the amount of sodium reabsorption that can be potentially inhibited in each region, but also on the resorptive capacity of the nephron segments *distal* to the site of diuretic action. These distal segments tend to compensate for the inhibition of proximal Na^+ reabsorption by increasing reabsorption. For example, although one might predict that inhibition of proximal tubular sodium reabsorption (by, for example, carbonic anhydrase inhibitors) would result in the greatest diuresis, it tends to produce only a small diuresis because the downstream nephron segments respond to increased sodium delivery with increased reabsorption.

Diuretics that act in the distal tubule and cortical collecting duct (i.e., the K^+-sparing diuretics) are also weak diuretics because they can influence, at most, only 10% to 15% of the filtered sodium load. Loop diuretics are the most potent diuretics, in part because a large amount of sodium is reabsorbed in the loop of Henle *and* the distal tubule and collecting duct downstream are limited in their ability to compensate. Note, however, that the primary reason why loop diuretics are the most potent diuretics is that they impair the generation of the medullary interstitial osmotic gradient that allows for urine concentration (see question 3, next).

3. **In which region of the nephron does each of the major diuretic types (carbonic anhydrase inhibitors, osmotic diuretics, loop diuretics, thiazides, and K^+-sparing diuretics) act? What are their mechanisms of action and their major uses?**

The details of renal sodium transport and the mechanisms of each diuretic type are best learned in conjunction with to regions of the nephron.

Carbonic anhydrase inhibitors (CAIs), such as acetazolamide, effectively act to inhibit $NaHCO_3$ (sodium bicarbonate) reabsorption in the proximal tubule (their mechanism is previously reviewed in detail in "Renal Control of Acid-Base Balance", question 4). CAIs are not commonly used as diuretics, in part because, as mentioned earlier, they have a weak diuretic effect due to their proximal site of action. Furthermore, because the metabolic acidosis that develops from CAI administration decreases the amount of filtered bicarbonate that is potentially reabsorbed, this small diuretic effect is rapidly lost. In addition to the treatment/prevention of altitude sickness, CAIs are used to treat open-angle glaucoma, as carbonic anhydrase is involved in the synthesis of aqueous humor of the eye.

Osmotic diuretics also act primarily in the proximal tubule. Osmotic diuretics are substances that are freely filtered at the glomerulus but are poorly reabsorbed. They inhibit sodium and water reabsorption by increasing the osmolarity of the tubular fluid and counteracting the normal small osmotic gradient responsible for reabsorption of water and sodium in the proximal tubule. Osmotic diuretics are not often clinically used for their diuretic effects. The most commonly used pharmacologic osmotic diuretic is mannitol, which can be used in the acute treatment of cerebral edema/elevated intracerebral pressure or elevated intraocular pressure (as in acute closed-angle glaucoma). Certain endogenous substances (such as glucose, urea, and calcium) can act as osmotic diuretics when present at very high serum levels (e.g., glucose in diabetes or urea in renal failure).

The *loop diuretics*, such as furosemide (Lasix), block the $Na^+/K^+/2Cl^-$ cotransporter present on the luminal surface of the thick ascending limb of the loop of Henle. In addition to their site of action, loop diuretics are the most potent diuretics currently available because their inhibition of sodium transport in the loop of Henle abolishes the countercurrent mechanism used to generate the concentrated medullary interstitium required to excrete maximally concentrated urine. In addition to impairing concentrating ability, they also block the nephron's diluting ability because they act to block the reabsorption of sodium in the water-impermeable thick ascending limb. Loop diuretics are first-line agents in treatment of fluid overload caused by cardiac, hepatic, or renal disease (i.e., CHF, cirrhosis, nephrotic syndrome). They are particularly useful in treatment of acute cardiogenic pulmonary edema because loop diuretics also have rapid venodilator effects that effectively decrease cardiac preload.

Thiazide diuretics, such as hydrochlorothiazide, act to block the Na^+/Cl^- cotransporter on the luminal surface of the early distal tubule (i.e., the cortical diluting segment). Again, because they inhibit sodium reabsorption at a water-impermeable segment of the nephron, thiazides impair the nephron's diluting ability; unlike loop diuretics, however, they do not alter concentrating ability. They are relatively potent diuretics. Their major use is in the treatment of isolated mild to moderate hypertension; in fact, they are considered first-line agents for this use because they are very inexpensive and were shown in the largest antihypertensive trial to date (ALLHAT Study) to effectively reduce cardiovascular mortality relative to calcium-channel blockers, ACE inhibitors, and alpha-blockers.

There are two subtypes of K^+-*sparing diuretics*. They all inhibit, either directly or indirectly, the activity of a specific type of Na^+ channel (the amiloride-sensitive channel) on the luminal surface of the principal cells of the late distal tubule and cortical collecting duct (Fig. 4-5). The expression of these surface channels is normally increased by the activity of aldosterone. Amiloride and triamterene act by directly blocking these Na^+ channels (aldosterone-independent action), whereas spironolactone and eplerenone act by blocking the mineralocorticoid receptor upon which aldosterone normally acts (aldosterone-dependent action). Because sodium reabsorption in the distal tubular cells is linked (via the basolateral Na^+/K^+-ATPase) to K^+ excretion, inhibition of Na^+ reabsorption results in retention of K^+ as well. K^+-sparing diuretics are the weakest diuretics; as such, they are typically used as adjuncts to other diuretics in the treatment of fluid overload and hypertension. They are particularly useful in preventing hypokalemia caused by other diuretics. The two aldosterone antagonists also have an important role in the treatment of CHF, for which they have been documented to have a mortality risk benefit (similarly to beta blockers and ACE inhibitors). The aldosterone antagonists are also particularly useful in the treatment of fluid overload related to cirrhosis, which, like CHF, is characterized by low ECV and high aldosterone levels. They can also be used in the specific treatment of other causes of hyperaldosteronism.

4. **How does each major diuretic type affect the concentrations of serum electrolytes?**

All diuretics increase K^+ secretion except, of course, for K^+-sparing diuretics. Hypokalemia is particularly common with the stronger loop and thiazide diuretics. There are multiple mechanisms for diuretic-induced hypokalemia. First, proximally acting diuretics increase the flow rate of fluid past the principal cells of the late distal tubule, which lowers the K^+ concentration of the tubular fluid and thereby promotes K^+ secretion. Similarly, proximally acting diuretics increase distal delivery of Na^+ which also promotes K^+ secretion by increasing the rate of exchange of Na^+ for K^+ (see Fig. 4-5). Diuretics also indirectly promote hypokalemia by decreasing ECV, which leads to increased aldosterone levels and aldosterone-stimulated K^+

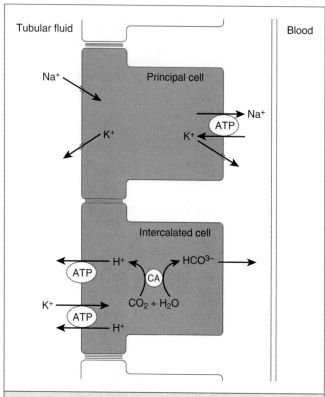

Figure 4-5. Transport pathways in principal cells and H$^+$-secreting intercalated cells of the distal tubule and collecting duct. CA, carbonic anhydrase. (From Koeppen BM, Stanton BA: Renal Physiology, 4th ed. Philadelphia, Mosby, 2007.)

secretion. CAIs also promote hypokalemia via induction of a metabolic acidosis. In the late distal tubule, K$^+$ and H$^+$ are secreted in exchange for reabsorbed Na$^+$ such that increased distal delivery of H$^+$ results in a decrease in H$^+$ secretion and a concomitant increase in K$^+$ secretion (see Chapter 5, Acid-Base Balance, for more on the interaction between K$^+$ levels and acid-base balance).

Hyponatremia can occur as a side effect of either loop or thiazide diuretics. Both of these diuretic types impair the nephron's diluting ability (i.e., the nephron's ability to separate water and sodium). Diuretic-induced hyponatremia occurs particularly with thiazides in elderly patients (whose kidneys tend to have a decreased diluting ability at baseline).

The effects of diuretics on Ca^{2+} and Mg^{2+} balance are relatively complicated and involve, among other mechanisms, changes in the luminal voltage gradients. However, the most clinically relevant effects are the dramatic *increase* in Ca^{2+} excretion caused by loop diuretics and the unique ability of thiazides to *decrease* Ca^{2+} excretion. Loop diuretics are frequently used with intravenous fluids in the treatment of severe or symptomatic hypercalcemia (such as hypercalcemia of malignancy). Thiazides have unique effects on calcium balance because the distal tubule is the only segment of the nephron in which calcium reabsorption does *not* occur in parallel with sodium reabsorption. Because thiazides tend to cause hypercalcemia by decreasing urinary calcium concentration, they can be used in the prevention of calcium kidney stone formation. Recall that elevated serum calcium predisposes to calcium stone formation only by promoting elevated *urinary* calcium.

In contrast with the differing effects on calcium, loop and thiazide diuretics can *both* cause clinically relevant hypomagnesemia.

Finally, each of the major diuretic types has a predictable effect on acid-base balance. CAIs, by inhibiting bicarbonate excretion, tend to promote metabolic acidosis. The stronger thiazide and loop diuretics, by producing decreased ECV, tend to promote a contraction alkalosis. Contraction alkalosis refers to an increase in bicarbonate reabsorption that occurs with fluid loss and subsequent sodium reabsorption. K^+-sparing diuretics tend to promote (a generally mild) acidosis by promoting H^+ retention in a manner similar to their ability to promote K^+ retention (i.e., inhibition of Na^+ reabsorption in the late distal tubule inhibits the secretion of K^+ and H^+ in exchange for Na^+).

See Chapter 5, Acid-Base Balance, for more on the effects of diuretics on acid-base balance.

5. **What are the other relatively common or important side effects of diuretics?**
One of the most common side effects of diuretics is a direct extension of their therapeutic effect: overdiuresis and hypovolemia. Prerenal azotemia from overdiuresis is by far the most common type of diuretic-induced nephrotoxicity.

Multiple commonly used diuretics can cause hypersensitivity reactions associated with the sulfonamide residues they contain. These diuretics include acetazolamide, thiazides, and multiple loop diuretics (including furosemide). Similarly, loop diuretics and thiazides can cause allergic interstitial nephritis (albeit rather uncommonly). Ethacrynic acid is unique among the loop diuretics in that it does not contain a sulfonamide residue and hence would have no allergic cross-reactivity with other loop diuretics or sulfonamides.

The potent loop diuretics have the most potential for volume depletion and electrolyte abnormalities. Loop diuretics also tend to promote hyperuricemia, which, along with diuretic-induced hypovolemia, can aggravate or trigger gout. Loop diuretics can also cause ototoxicity (particularly ringing in the ears or hearing loss), but generally only with large, rapidly administered intravenous doses. Ototoxicity is rare in the doses commonly used in clinical practice today.

Thiazides are similar to loop diuretics in their potential to exacerbate hyperuricemia and gout. Thiazides can also somewhat exacerbate hyperlipidemia or hyperglycemia (though generally not to a clinically relevant degree).

Spironolactone is a relatively nonspecific inhibitor of corticosteroid receptors, with significant antiandrogen effects in addition to its antimineralocorticoid effects. These effects on sex steroids can manifest as gynecomastia and erectile dysfunction in men and hirsutism or breast tenderness in women. These nonspecific effects of aldosteronism can be clinically useful in the treatment of acne vulgaris and hirsutism (i.e., spironolactone may both cause and treat hirsutism). In contrast, eplerenone selectively blocks only the mineralocorticoid receptors and therefore does not have these antiandrogen effects.

STEP 1 SECRET

Mechanisms of action, uses, and side effects of diuretics and angiotensin-converting enzyme (ACE) inhibitors are extremely important to focus on when studying for Step 1. This importance is probably no secret to you at this point. The detailed discussion in this chapter speaks for itself!

SUMMARY BOX: PHARMACOLOGY OF DIURETICS

- All diuretics lower extracellular fluid volume by inhibiting the tubular reabsorption of sodium.

- The potency of each diuretic depends both on the capacity for sodium reabsorption of the segment upon which the diuretic acts and upon the resorptive capacity of the downstream segments capable of compensating for the proximal inhibition of sodium reabsorption.

- Carbonic anhydrase inhibitors and osmotic diuretics act primarily in the proximal tubule.

- Loop diuretics, the most potent diuretics, act by blocking Na^+ reabsorption in the thick ascending limb and abolishing the nephron's concentrating ability. They are first-line agents in the treatment of fluid overload due to cardiac, hepatic, or renal disease.

- Thiazide diuretics block Na^+ reabsorption in the early distal tubule and are first-line agents in the treatment of isolated mild to moderate hypertension.

- K^+-sparing diuretics either directly block Na^+ reabsorption in the late distal tubule or cortical collecting duct or do so indirectly by blocking the activity of aldosterone upon mineralocorticoid receptors.

- All diuretics, except for K^+-sparing diuretics, tend to increase K^+ excretion and cause hypokalemia.

- Loop diuretics can dramatically increase calcium excretion, whereas thiazides increase calcium reabsorption.

CHAPTER 5

ACID-BASE BALANCE

Bjorn I. Engstrom, MD, Thomas A. Brown, MD, and Sonali J. Shah

BASIC CONCEPTS

1. **How is extracellular hydrogen ion concentration regulated?**
   The hydrogen ion concentration $[H^+]$ in the extracellular fluid is very tightly controlled and is regulated by the respiratory system, the kidneys, and various buffers. The very close relationship between the $[H^+]$, P_{CO_2}, and $[HCO_3^-]$ can be expressed as follows:

   $$[H^+] = 25 \times (P_{CO_2}/[HCO_3^-])$$

   A process that raises $[H^+]$ is called an acidosis whereas a process that lowers $[H^+]$ is called an alkalosis. If these processes lead to an alteration in blood pH to <7.36 or >7.44, there is metabolic derangement that can be described as an acidemia or an alkalemia, respectively. However, in everyday language these terms are used rather loosely, and -osis is often used when -emia is really what is meant.

2. **How does a change in HCO_3^- or in P_{CO_2} affect pH?**
   A change in HCO_3^- of 10 mEq/L up or down causes pH to increase or decrease by 0.15 unit, respectively. Acutely, a change in P_{CO_2} of 10 mm Hg up or down causes pH to decrease or increase by 0.08 unit, respectively. A chronic change in P_{CO_2} levels alters blood pH by 0.03 unit per 10 mm Hg of P_{CO_2} (due to renal compensation; see Case 5-2 for details).

   The first step in interpretation is to determine the primary disorder. Figure 5-1 can be used for this purpose. Normal values for $[HCO_3^-]$ and P_{CO_2} are 22 to 28 mEq/L and 35 to 45 mm Hg, respectively.

CASE 5-1

An older woman has had diarrhea for 2 days. She is tachypneic on examination. Her laboratory values are as follows:
   pH: 7.2
   P_{CO_2}: 19 mm Hg
   $[HCO_3^-]$: 7 mEq/L
   $[Cl^-]$: 120 mEq/L
   $[Na^+]$: 140 mEq/L

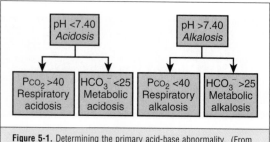

Figure 5-1. Determining the primary acid-base abnormality. (From Piccini JP, Nilsson KR: The Osler Medical Handbook, 2nd ed. Baltimore, Johns Hopkins University, 2006.)

1. **What is the primary acid-base disorder?**

   The laboratory results reveal acidemia (more specifically, metabolic acidosis with normal anion gap), which is consistent with the history of diarrhea for 2 days.

   Note: If you had trouble arriving at this diagnosis, we will attempt to walk you through it here. The first thing you must do is look at the pH and realize that it is abnormally low. This number tells us our patient has an acidemia. Next, determine whether the acidemia is the result of respiratory or metabolic causes. Bicarbonate and P_{CO_2} are both low. Bicarbonate is a base, and decreased levels of bicarbonate will result in metabolic acidosis. CO_2, on the other hand, is an acid. Low levels of CO_2 thus result in an alkalosis. In this situation, the body tries to correct for the decreased pH of metabolic acidosis through hyperventilation and loss of CO_2. Therefore, this patient has a metabolic acidosis with respiratory compensation. In contrast with metabolic compensation by the kidneys, respiratory compensation occurs immediately.

   Anion gap (AG) can be assessed using the formula:

   $$AG = \text{Unmeasured anions} - \text{Unmeasured cations}$$
   $$= \text{Measured cations} - \text{Measured anions}$$
   $$= [(Na^+ + K^+)] - [(Cl^- + HCO_3^-)]$$

   Because potassium concentration is generally small in comparison to the other electrolytes in the formula, it is normally discounted from the formula. Note that the anion gap is normally positive because unmeasured anions (primarily serum proteins) far outnumber unmeasured cations.

   Therefore, $AG = [Na^+] - [(Cl^- + HCO_3^-)]$. In this patient, AG is 13 mEq/L (normal range = 8-16 mEq/L). In the normal state, these unmeasured anions consist primarily of albumin and phosphate.

STEP 1 SECRET

You must know all of the causes of anion gap and non–anion gap metabolic acidosis. These causes are discussed later in the chapter.

2. **What are the mechanisms involved in metabolic acidosis due to diarrhea?**

   Diarrhea essentially represents the loss of bicarbonate-rich fluid. Intestinal fluid is fairly rich in bicarbonate, but normally much of this bicarbonate is reabsorbed via a Cl^-/HCO_3^- exchange process in the colon. Diarrhea shortens intestinal transit time, limiting the opportunity for colonic Cl^-/HCO_3^- exchange and thereby increasing the concentration of bicarbonate in the stool. This loss of bicarbonate is thus electrically balanced by an increase in serum Cl^-

concentration. As mentioned in the preceding note, the AG remains unchanged. A similar process of Cl^- retention occurs in all non-AG acidoses. This is why a non-AG metabolic acidosis can alternatively be described as a hyperchloremic metabolic acidosis.

3. **What else is considered in the differential diagnosis for non–anion gap metabolic acidosis?**

Non-AG metabolic acidoses can be roughly divided into renal and nonrenal causes. In the setting of an acidemia, the appropriate response of the kidney is to excrete excess acid as NH_4^+. This NH_4^+ is generally paired with Cl^- to maintain electrical neutrality. As such, the urine excretion of Cl^- can be measured to determine renal NH_4^+ excretion. This calculation is specifically done using the equation for the urine anion gap (UAG):

$$UAG = \text{unmeasured anions} - \text{unmeasured cations}$$
$$= \text{measured cations} - \text{measured anions}$$
$$= [(U_{Na} + U_K) - U_{Cl}]$$

Note that urine HCO_3^- is excluded from this equation because, due to the acidity of urine, its concentration is typically negligible. A negative UAG signifies an appropriate renal response since NH_4^+ makes up a large portion of the unmeasured cations in the equation, and, likewise, urine Cl^- concentration will be increased due to pairing with NH_4^+. A failure to excrete ammonium during an acidemia will give a positive UAG.

An acidosis resulting from such a failure by the kidney to excrete NH_4^+ is called a renal tubular acidosis (RTA). See Table 5-1 for a description of the three types of renal tubular acidoses.

A negative UAG in the setting of a non-AG acidosis most often indicates diarrhea as the nonrenal cause. However, other causes include ureteral-colonic fistulas, exogenous acid ingestion or administration (consider parenteral nutrition in a hospitalized patient), posthypocapnic acidosis, early renal failure, and "dilutional acidosis." In the case of ureteral-colonic fistulas, urine rich in Cl^- enters the colon, where the Cl^- is reabsorbed in exchange for HCO_3^-, resulting in HCO_3^- loss in a mechanism similar to diarrhea. Posthypocapnic acidosis is a result of persisting renal compensation to a chronic respiratory alkalosis (see Case 5-2, question 2). Acidosis in early renal failure can result from loss of the ability to generate ammonia; late renal failure, in contrast, generally results in a mixed AG/non-AG acidosis (see next question). Dilutional acidosis, which is commonly seen in hospitalized patients, is a result of excess normal saline administration; normal saline represents a large Cl^- load (specifically, 154 mEq/L of Cl^-), which results in increased bicarbonate excretion to maintain electrical neutrality.

4. **Is there appropriate compensation or is there a mixed disorder in this patient?**

An appropriate compensation for metabolic acidosis is to decrease P_{CO_2}, that is, excrete volatile acid, through hyperventilation. Such respiratory compensation is virtually immediate. Using the equation in Table 5-2, the expected change in $P_{CO_2} = 1.2 \times (25 - 7) = 21.6$. The actual change in this case is $(40 - 19) = 21$, reflecting appropriate compensation.

In looking at Table 5-2, it is apparent that the lungs, in responding to metabolic acid-base disturbances, can more readily excrete CO_2 than retain it. This response is both rather intuitive (severe hypercapnia can be quite dangerous, rapidly leading to mental status changes and coma) and useful in remembering that the degree of respiratory compensation for metabolic acidosis is greater than the compensation. **Note:** Compensation during any acid-base disturbance is never complete.

5. **What would it mean if, in the same patient, appropriate compensation was not present and P_{CO_2} was instead 30 mm Hg?**

This value would mean that there is a mixed disorder, that is, more than one primary disorder occurring at the same time. A P_{CO_2} of 30 mm Hg in this case would represent inappropriate retention of CO_2, indicating a respiratory acidosis in addition to the metabolic acidosis.

TABLE 5-1. CLASSIFICATION OF RENAL TUBULAR ACIDOSIS (RTA)

Type	Pathophysiology	Urine pH	Degree of Acidosis	Serum [K^+]	% HCO_3^- Excretion (After Bicarbonate Load)
I (distal RTA)	Inability to secrete H^+ in distal tubule	>5.3	Severe (serum HCO_3^- often <10 mEq/L)	Decreased	<3%
II (proximal RTA)	Deficit of carbonic anhydrase and HCO_3^- reabsorption in proximal tubule, can begin to reabsorb bicarbonate after pH decreases below a threshold level May lead to impaired proximal tubular reabsorption of other nutrients (e.g., glucose, phosphate, amino acids)	<5.3	Modest (serum HCO_3^- 12-16 mEq/L)	Decreased	>15%
IV (hyperkalemic RTA)	Hypoaldosteronism or aldosterone resistance	<5.3	Mild (serum HCO_3^- 14-20 mEq/L)	Increased	<3%

TABLE 5-2.	RESPIRATORY COMPENSATION FOR METABOLIC ACID–BASE DISTURBANCES	
Condition	**Primary Change**	**Expected Compensation**
Metabolic acidosis	Decreased HCO_3^-	Decreased $P_{CO_2} = 1.2 \times \Delta HCO_3^-$
Metabolic alkalosis	Increased HCO_3^-	Increased $P_{CO_2} = 0.7 \times \Delta HCO_3^-$

SUMMARY BOX: ACID-BASE DISTURBANCES, METABOLIC ACIDOSIS

- First determine the primary disturbance using pH, P_{CO_2}, and HCO_3^-.

- Then determine if the degree of compensation is appropriate or if there is a mixed disorder.

- It is "easier" for the body to blow off CO_2 than to retain it, that is, greater compensation for metabolic acidoses than for metabolic alkaloses.

- For a metabolic acidosis, first determine the anion gap (AG).

- $AG = [Na^+] - [(Cl^- + HCO_3^-)]) = $ unmeasured anions − unmeasured cations; normal anion gap is ~ 10.

- If a non-AG metabolic acidosis exists, search for clues in the history (e.g., diarrhea, rapid infusion of normal saline) and determine the urine anion gap (UAG).

- $UAG = (U_{Na} + U_K) - U_{Cl} = $ unmeasured anions − unmeasured cations.

- If the UAG is negative, the kidneys are working normally (i.e., are excreting NH_4Cl).

- If the UAG is positive, renal tubular acidosis (RTA) is likely; look at urine pH, serum pH, serum potassium, and the fractional excretion of HCO_3^- after a bicarbonate load to determine which type.

CASE 5-2

You are called to consult on an intensive care unit patient who has developed sudden-onset tachypnea and tachycardia. His laboratory values follow:
pH: 7.5
P_{CO_2}: 20 mm Hg
$[HCO3^-]$: 20 mEq/L

1. **What is the primary acid-base disorder?**
Following Figure 5-1, we see that the primary disorder is a respiratory alkalosis.

2. **What is the differential diagnosis in this patient?**
Intensive care unit (ICU) patients are at increased risk for pulmonary embolism (PE) because they are immobile and more often have serious diseases such as congestive heart failure (stasis), recent surgery (injury to endothelium), or cancer (hypercoagulable state). Therefore, a PE is the most likely cause of his condition (particularly given the sudden onset of his vital signs changes). Pleuritic chest pain, mild fever, or hemoptysis would also support a diagnosis of PE, but signs and symptoms of PE in an ICU patient are often much more subtle.

Hypoxia from a PE leads to hyperventilation and respiratory alkalosis. However, hypoxia and hyperventilation can occur in virtually any form of lung disease, including pneumonia, pulmonary edema (as caused by congestive heart failure [CHF] or acute respiratory distress syndrome [ARDS]), or restrictive lung disease. Pain, anxiety, and various central nervous system (CNS) disorders are common causes of respiratory alkalosis in the ICU that occur in the absence of hypoxia. Asthma patients are interesting because although they can develop hypoxia, these patients very dramatically hyperventilate during asthma attacks such that a degree of respiratory alkalosis develops that is out of proportion to the hypoxia.

It is important to note that if hyperventilation persists, respiratory muscle fatigue can arise, leading to CO_2 accumulation and respiratory acidosis (a process referred to as hypercapnic respiratory failure).

STEP 1 SECRET

Step 1 loves to ask questions about pulmonary embolism (PE) because it is such a common diagnosis. Many students are tricked by the fact that PE more commonly produces respiratory alkalosis rather than respiratory acidosis. Remember that PE patients are tachypneic; hyperventilation leads to excess removal of CO_2 from the bloodstream.

3. **Is there appropriate compensation or is this a mixed disorder?**
   Because the full effect of renal compensation for respiratory disturbances is not immediate, for acid–base disturbances with a respiratory cause, one must first determine if the disturbance is acute or chronic. In this patient, the respiratory alkalosis is acute. The appropriate compensation for any respiratory alkalosis is to decrease serum HCO_3^- through increased renal excretion. Using the equation in Table 5-3, the appropriate acute change in $HCO_3^- = 0.2 \times \Delta Pco_2 = 0.2 \times 20 = 5$. The actual change in this case is $25 - 20 = 5$; therefore, there is appropriate acute compensation.

TABLE 5-3. **RENAL COMPENSATION FOR RESPIRATORY ACID–BASE DISTURBANCES**

Condition	Primary Change	Expected Compensation
Acute respiratory acidosis	Increased Pco_2	Increased $HCO_3^- = 0.1 \times \Delta Pco_2$
Chronic respiratory acidosis	Increased Pco_2	Increased $HCO_3^- = 0.35 \times \Delta Pco_2$
Acute respiratory alkalosis	Decreased Pco_2	Decreased $HCO_3^- = 0.2 \times \Delta Pco_2$
Chronic respiratory alkalosis	Decreased Pco_2	Decreased $HCO_3^- = 0.5 \times \Delta Pco_2$

STEP 1 SECRET

It is not likely that the USMLE will ask you to calculate the degree of renal or pulmonary compensation for an acute or chronic acid–base disorder using the formulas listed in Tables 5-2 and 5-3. However, these are important formulas to know for your clinical years, particularly because they can help you spot mixed disorders.

4. **Does the degree of compensation allow you to draw any conclusions as to the duration of the condition?**

Yes. Even if the history of an acute process was not available in this patient, we could conclude from his laboratory values that his respiratory alkalosis is acute. If this were a more chronic presentation, as occurs at high altitude or in pregnant women (progesterone-induced increase in tidal volume), the kidneys would have responded by excreting more bicarbonate. The decrease in HCO_3^- would have been $0.5 \times \Delta P_{CO_2} = 10$. Because it takes a couple of days for the kidneys to fully adjust to an alkalosis, we know that the duration of this condition is much shorter.

If you are attempting to remember the preceding numbers, it is useful to realize that the kidneys more easily and more rapidly excrete HCO_3^- than retain HCO_3^- when responding to respiratory acid-base disturbances. Thus, renal compensation for respiratory alkaloses is both more complete and more rapid than the compensation for respiratory acidoses (see Table 5-3 and Fig. 5-2).

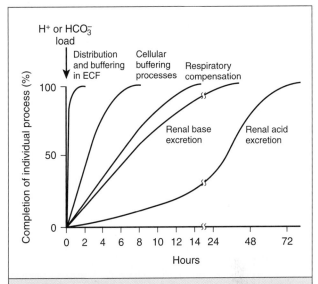

Figure 5-2. Time course of acid-base compensatory mechanisms. In response to a metabolic acid or alkaline load, individual approaches to completion of distribution and extracellular buffering mechanisms, cellular buffering events, and respiratory and renal regulatory processes are presented as a function of time. ECF, extracellular fluid. (From Brenner BM: Brenner and Rector's The Kidney, 7th ed. Philadelphia, WB Saunders, 2004.)

SUMMARY BOX: RESPIRATORY ALKALOSIS

- A respiratory alkalosis is either due to primary hyperventilation (pain, anxiety, central nervous system disease) or induced by hypoxemia (various forms of lung disease), or both (acute asthma attack).

- Maximal compensation by the kidneys takes a couple of days.

- It is "easier" for the kidneys to excrete bicarbonate than to retain it when a respiratory acid-base disturbance exists, resulting in greater compensation for respiratory alkaloses than for respiratory acidoses.

CASE 5-3

A 41-year-old woman comes in for a pre-employment physical examination and is found to have mild to moderate hypertension, with the following laboratory values:
pH: 7.55
$[HCO_3^-]$: 35 mEq/L
P_{CO_2}: 19 mm Hg

1. **What is the primary acid-base disorder?**
   Following the algorithm given earlier, we see that the primary disorder is consistent with a metabolic alkalosis.

2. **What is the differential diagnosis in this patient?**
   Loss of gastric secretions (i.e., vomiting), diuretics, volume depletion, hypokalemia, mineralocorticoid excess, Cushing disease, excessive licorice consumption, and some rare diseases including Bartter, Gitelman, and Liddle syndromes and 11β-hydroxysteroid dehydrogenase (11β-HSD) deficiency. Patients who are in the ICU and who have a chronic respiratory acidosis corrected too quickly can also develop a similar picture, because their kidneys, which have become used to excreting a large acid load to compensate, will take several days to readjust.

3. **What is the pathophysiology of each of the conditions in the differential diagnosis?**
   - Volume depletion ("contraction alkalosis"):
     - Sodium and bicarbonate reabsorption are directly linked in the proximal tubule. Volume depletion results in an attempt to retain Na^+ and thereby leads to increased bicarbonate reabsorption.
     - Volume depletion stimulates the renin-angiotensin system. The increased aldosterone promotes Na^+ reabsorption in exchange for K^+ and H^+ in the distal tubule.
   - Hypokalemia:
     - K^+ and H^+ compete for secretion in the distal tubule; hypokalemia stimulates K^+ retention, resulting in increased H^+ secretion.
     - Hypokalemia results in transcellular shift of K^+ out of cells, which is electrically balanced (in part) by a shift of H^+ into cells, directly lowing serum H^+.
     - The transcellular shift of H^+ also results in intracellular acidification, which, at the proximal tubule (where the nephron's "pH sensor" is located), stimulates increased ammonia production, ultimately resulting in increased excretion of H^+ in the form of NH_4^+.
   - Loss of gastric secretions:
     - Loss of H^+ will directly cause a decrease in HCO_3^- and an increase in pH.
     - Loss of chloride ions will inhibit HCO_3^- secretion in the distal tubule and collecting duct (because of decreased Cl^-/HCO_3^- exchange by intercalated cells).
     - See mechanisms involved in volume depletion, as described earlier in list.
     - No wonder vomiting and nasogastric tube (NGT) suctioning are such powerful producers of metabolic alkalosis!
   - Diuretics (loop diuretics and thiazides only!) Remember that acetazolamide and, to a lesser extent, K^+-sparing diuretics tend to cause an acidosis:
     - Volume depletion
     - Hypokalemia
   - Mineralocorticoid excess: The action of aldosterone in the distal tubule results in an increase in H^+ (and K^+) secretion in exchange for Na^+.
   - Cushing disease: An excess of corticosteroids will activate the mineralocorticoid receptor.
   - Bartter syndrome: Defective $Na^+/K^+/Cl^-$ transporter in the loop of Henle mimics the effect of a loop diuretic!
   - Gitelman syndrome: Defective Na^+/Cl^- transporter mimics the effect of a thiazide diuretic!

- Liddle syndrome: A defect in the Na^+ channel in the distal tubule that is normally stimulated by aldosterone results in the channel being permanently activated (mimics mineralocorticoid excess; in this setting spironolactone will not work, so one must use triamterene or amiloride instead).
- 11β-HSD deficiency: Defect of the enzyme that normally breaks down cortisol into cortisone within aldosterone-responsive cells causes cortisol to build up and activate the mineralocorticoid receptor.
- Licorice: "Real" licorice (black licorice, not Twizzler's red candy) contains a substance that inhibits 11β-HSD.

4. **Is there appropriate compensation or is there a mixed disorder?**
No, there is not appropriate compensation. The expected compensation for a metabolic alkalosis would be an increase in P_{CO_2} of $0.7 \times \Delta HCO_3^- = 0.7 \times 10 = 7$ mm Hg. Therefore, a mixed disorder is present.

CASE 5-3 continued:

When the patient is further questioned at the follow-up appointment, she also admits to having polyuria, polydipsia, muscle weakness, and headaches. She has the following laboratory values:
[K^+]: 3.1 mEq/L
[Na^+]: 149 mEq/L
Aldosterone/renin ratio: >20

5. **What is the most likely diagnosis?**
The presentation and laboratory values are classic for primary hyperaldosteronism (Conn syndrome). Conn syndrome should be suspected in any patient with hypertension and hypokalemia.
This patient's hypokalemia and hypernatremia and, to a lesser extent, her signs and symptoms can be seen in all syndromes of high aldosterone activity, including secondary hyperaldosteronism (renin-secreting tumor, CHF, renovascular disease) and "nonaldosterone mineralocorticoid excess" (Cushing syndrome, Liddle syndrome, 11β-HSD deficiency, licorice ingestion, exogenous mineralocorticoids). However, it is only in primary hyperaldosteronism that the aldosterone-renin ratio is > 20. For secondary hyperaldosteronism both renin and aldosterone are increased, but in "nonaldosterone mineralocorticoid excess" they are both decreased.

6. **Would administration of saline be helpful in this patient?**
No, it would not. The causes of metabolic alkalosis can be divided into saline-responsive and saline-resistant categories (Fig. 5-3). Even without knowing the diagnosis, it is possible to figure out if a saline infusion will help by looking at the urine chloride level (U_{Cl}). A $U_{Cl} < 10$ mEq/L indicates saline infusion *would not* be helpful, whereas a $U_{Cl} > 20$ mEq/L indicates saline infusion *would* be helpful. The range of U_{Cl} 10 to 20 mEq/L is a grayer area but most often indicates a saline-resistant process.
This patient needs an adrenal computed tomography (CT) scan or magnetic resonance imaging (MRI) to determine if the primary hyperaldosteronism is due to adrenal hyperplasia or to an adenoma or carcinoma. Spironolactone is the treatment for hyperplasia, whereas surgery is the treatment for adenoma or carcinoma.
Do not worry about getting too caught up in the details of this question. This topic is beyond the scope of Step 1 and is simply included to expand your knowledge in preparation for your clinical years.

SUMMARY BOX: METABOLIC ALKALOSIS

- The most common causes of metabolic alkalosis are loss of gastric secretions (vomiting or nasogastric suctioning), diuretics (loops and thiazides), volume depletion, and mineralocorticoid excess.

■ Loss of gastric contents is a very powerful stimulant of metabolic alkalosis because it works through three separate but additive mechanisms: direct loss of H^+, loss of Cl^-, and volume depletion.

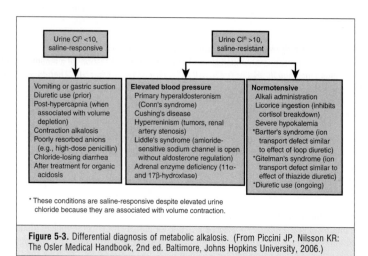

* These conditions are saline-responsive despite elevated urine chloride because they are associated with volume contraction.

Figure 5-3. Differential diagnosis of metabolic alkalosis. (From Piccini JP, Nilsson KR: The Osler Medical Handbook, 2nd ed. Baltimore, Johns Hopkins University, 2006.)

CASE 5-4

An 18-year-old man presents with 2 days of fatigue, abdominal pain, and vomiting. Examination shows tachycardia with pulse rate of 120 beats/min.

pH: 7.15
$[Na^+]$: 140 mEq/L
$[Cl^-]$: 90 mEq/L
$[HCO_3^-]$: 22 mEq/L
P_{CO_2}: 36 mm Hg
[K]: 5.2 mEq/L
BUN: 52 mg/dL

1. **What is the primary acid-base disorder?**
   This looks like a primary metabolic acidosis (pH is less than 7.4 and bicarbonate is less than 25).

2. **Is there appropriate compensation or is this a mixed disorder?**
   The P_{CO_2} is decreased by 4, which is consistent with appropriate respiratory compensation $(1.2 \times \Delta HCO_3^- = 1.2 \times 3 = 3.6)$.

3. **What is the next step in diagnosis of this disorder?**
   Calculate the anion gap! It is critical to distinguish between AG acidosis and non-AG acidosis because the differentials for each are drastically different.
   Remember, $AG = Na - (Cl^- + HCO_3^-)$. In this patient, $AG = 140 - (90 + 22) = 28$ mEq/L.

STEP 1 SECRET ✔

You will be expected (but not necessarily instructed) to calculate anion gap on Step 1 if the diagnosis involves metabolic acidosis. Be on the lookout for this type of question!

4. **How can there be such a large anion gap with such an *extremely* low pH when the disturbance in HCO_3^- is so minimal?**
   This effect is caused by a superimposed metabolic alkalosis! For every 1 mEq of anion contributing to the changing AG, $[HCO_3^-]$ should fall by 1 mEq from its normal value. Therefore, the change in AG should equal the change in bicarbonate concentration if the AG acidosis is the only metabolic disturbance present. However, if a discrepancy exists, more than one metabolic process is present: the AG acidosis and either a second, a hyperchloremic, metabolic acidosis or a metabolic alkalosis.

   This idea can be summarized through the concept of the "delta-delta." The "delta-delta" simply represents the comparison of the ΔAG and the ΔHCO_3^-. It should be interpreted as follows (Fig. 5-4):
   - If $\Delta AG = \Delta HCO_3^-$ the high AG acidosis is the sole metabolic acid-base disorder.
   - If $\Delta AG < \Delta HCO_3^-$ there is a hyperchloremic metabolic acidosis in addition to the high AG acidosis (since the *change* in bicarbonate is *greater* than expected).
   - If $\Delta AG > \Delta HCO_3^-$ there is a metabolic alkalosis in addition to the high AG acidosis (since the *change* in bicarbonate is *smaller* than expected).
   - In this case, the $\Delta AG = 28 - 12 = 16$ mEq/L. The ΔHCO_3^- is $24 - 12 = 2$ mEq/L. Thus, $\Delta AG > \Delta HCO_3^-$, indicating a "hidden" metabolic alkalosis as we suspected.

CASE 5-4 continued:

The history reveals that the patient has polyuria, polydipsia, and an odor of acetone on his breath.

5. **What is the most likely diagnosis in this patient?**
   This patient most likely has diabetic ketoacidosis (DKA)! DKA is a board favorite, so you need to understand it well. This condition occurs mainly in type 1 diabetics (although rarely it can occur in type 2 diabetics as well). It is not uncommon for an 18-year-old man to present in DKA without having previously been diagnosed with type 1 diabetes; in fact, about 20% of patients present with no previous history of diabetes. The clinical manifestations consist of polyuria and polydipsia (result of hyperglycemia-induced osmotic diuresis); nausea, vomiting, abdominal pain, and ileus (due to effects of hyperglycemia and electrolyte disturbance on the gastrointestinal [GI] tract); Kussmaul's (deep) respirations (to compensate for the metabolic acidosis); odor of alcohol on the breath (acetone, a volatile ketone body, being expired in the lungs); signs of volume depletion, such as tachycardia and hypotension (result of diuresis and vomiting); and changes in mental status (from acidosis and electrolyte disturbances).

   The laboratory findings in a typical case include AG acidosis (from the ketoacids, such as β-hydroxybutyrate [β-HB], pseudohyponatremia (due to hyperglycemia), increased blood urea nitrogen (volume depletion), increased serum glucose, serum and urine ketones (measured as serum β-HB or on urine dip), and leukocytosis (which sometimes reflects an infection that triggered the episode).

   Total body potassium is usually reduced (as a result of the osmotic diuresis and volume depletion). However, serum K^+ levels are usually normal or even elevated at presentation due to transcellular shift of K^+ out of cells (caused by both the lack of insulin and the acidosis). Serum K^+ must be followed closely because it can drop precipitously once treatment (with intravenous fluids and insulin) is initiated.

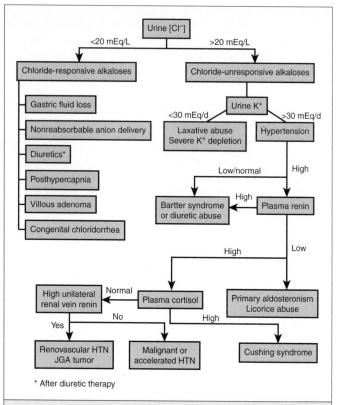

Figure 5-4. Diagnostic algorithm for metabolic alkalosis. The algorithm is based on the urine chloride concentration. HTN, hypertension; JGA, juxtaglomerular apparatus. (From Brenner BM: Brenner and Rector's The Kidney, 7th ed. Philadelphia, WB Saunders, 2004.)

In this case, the superimposed metabolic alkalosis is due to the vomiting and volume contraction. Remember that vomiting rids the body of gastric acid, thus increasing pH. Metabolic alkalosis can be especially dangerous because the body's compensatory response involves respiratory acidosis, which potentially results in hypoxemia (recall that increased P_{CO_2} results in an obligatory decrease in P_{O_2}).

Although DKA often occurs when a type 1 diabetic fails to take insulin, it is also quite often precipitated by a triggering illness. Infections, such as pneumonia, urinary tract infections (UTIs), and skin or soft tissue infections, are particularly common. Other serious illnesses, such as myocardial infarction (MI) or pancreatitis, can serve as triggers as well.

The hyperglycemia seen in DKA is due to increased gluconeogenesis and increased glycogenolysis by the liver in the setting of decreased consumption of glucose by the peripheral tissues, all a result of insufficient insulin relative to glucagon and the other counterregulatory hormones. The ketosis also arises from the inability of the peripheral tissues to utilize glucose. The lack of available glucose stimulates the release of free fatty acids by peripheral adipose tissues into the bloodstream. The fatty acids are then converted in the liver to the ketones β-HB and acetoacetate so that they can used by vital organs (such as the CNS and heart), which normally depend on glucose for energy.

6. **What is on the differential diagnosis for large anion gap metabolic acidosis?**
   The classic mnemonic is MUDPILES: **M**ethanol and **M**etformin, **U**remia (renal failure) **D**iabetic and other ketoacidoses, **P**henformin and **P**araldehyde (rarely seen anymore), **I**soniazid and **I**ron supplements, **L**actic acidosis, **E**thylene glycol and **E**thanol, **S**alicylates.

   In each case, an unmeasured organic acid or anion accumulates to produce the AG. Methanol and ethylene glycol are metabolized to formic and oxalic acid, respectively. The AG seen in renal failure results from the accumulation of phosphates, sulfates, and other organic anions normally excreted by healthy kidneys. Salicylates include aspirin and other derivates of salicylic acid. The antituberculosis drug isoniazid is also a derivative of an organic acid (isonicotinic acid).

   It is important to remember there are many causes of lactic acidosis. Sepsis, seizures (with increased muscle activity or impaired breathing), ischemia of limbs or organs (especially small bowel ischemia), cyanide or carbon monoxide poisoning, and circulatory or respiratory failure can all cause lactic acidosis. Liver failure results in impaired clearance of lactic acid.

   In addition, recall that ketosis can also result from starvation and chronic alcoholism, albeit much less commonly and usually with a much less severe acidosis. In chronic alcoholics this is most often seen a few days after heavy binge drinking in the setting of poor food intake; there are numerous mechanisms involved, including depletion of NAD^+ by hepatic oxidation of alcohol, reduced nutrient intake, and dehydration (which decreases urinary ketone excretion).

STEP 1 SECRET

The **MUDPILES** mnemonic is a must-know for Step 1. Among these common causes of metabolic acidosis, diabetic ketoacidosis and lactic acidosis (caused by ischemia, diabetic drugs, etc.) are USMLE favorites.

---

7. **What is the correct treatment?**
   Insulin, aggressive rehydration starting with normal saline, potassium repletion (once the K^+ drops down to high-normal levels), and treatment of possible precipitants such as infections. Treatment of the acidosis with bicarbonate is controversial (as there is no documented improvement in outcome) and is generally done only in severe cases with a $pH < 7.0$.

CASE 5–5

A 38-year-old homeless man suffering from chronic alcoholism comes into the emergency department with nausea, vomiting, and blurry vision. Interestingly, he denies any recent ingestion of alcohol, saying that he "ran out of booze." His blood alcohol level is undetectable. His laboratory values are as follows:
   pH: 7.29
   $[Na^+]$: 135 mEq/L
   $[Cl^-]$: 100 mEq/L
   $[HCO_3^-]$: 14 mEq/L
   [Glucose]: 90 mg/dL

1. **What is the most likely diagnosis?**
   This man has methanol intoxication. The AG is 21 mEq/L. Visual impairment in the setting of an AG acidosis is highly suggestive of methanol poisoning (see **MUDPILES** mnemonic). Methanol is found in windshield washer fluid and is therefore an easily accessible alcohol. It is also found in shellac and varnish. Methanol, like ethanol, is metabolized by the enzyme alcohol dehydrogenase. The formic acid that results is a mitochondrial toxin that acts by inhibiting cytochrome oxidase of oxidative phosphorylation. The retina, optic nerve, and basal ganglia are especially vulnerable. A component of lactic acidosis often contributes to the AG due to the impairment of oxidative

phosphorylation (similar to cyanide poisoning) and due to the overconversion of nicotinamide adenine dinucleotide (NAD) to its reduced form, NADH, in the liver (similar to ethanol poisoning). In the first 6 hours of ingestion, the signs and symptoms of methanol intoxication resemble those of ethanol intoxication. Following this period, visual disturbances and depressed consciousness then become prominent. Examination might reveal papilledema. Blurry vision (in the setting of elevated AG acidosis) is the buzz word to recognize on the boards.

CASE 5-5 continued:

Now assume that this homeless man comes into the emergency department merely 6 weeks later with apparent inebriation and signs of pulmonary edema and cardiovascular collapse on examination. Again he denies alcohol consumption! In addition, he is found to have calcium oxalate stones on urine microscopy. His urine also fluoresces when under a Wood's lamp.

2. **Now what is the most likely diagnosis?**
   Now this man has ethylene glycol intoxication. Ethylene glycol can be found in antifreeze and de-icing solutions. Antifreeze in the United States commonly has an additive that produces the Wood's lamp fluorescence. Alcohol dehydrogenase is again the metabolizing enzyme, producing oxalic acid. Oxalic acid can combine with calcium to produce crystals in the urine seen on microscopic examination; if extensive crystal precipitation occurs within the kidneys, acute renal failure could result. Again, a component of lactic acidosis can result from the overconversion of NAD^+ to NADH, resulting from oxidation of the alcohol. In severe cases, renal failure occurs, along with depressed consciousness, coma, and cardiopulmonary collapse.

3. **What is the treatment for the man in questions 1 and 2?**
   Fomepizole inhibits alcohol dehydrogenase and is therefore very effective in both methanol and ethylene glycol intoxication because it can prevent the buildup of the toxic metabolites formic and oxalic acids, respectively. Intravenous ethanol has also been used effectively in the past, as high ethanol levels can competitively inhibit the metabolism of methanol or ethylene glycol by alcohol dehydrogenase, but fomepizole does not have the side effects of ethanol (and its use in clinical practice is much less controversial). In severe cases, such as those resulting in severe acidemia, severe end-organ damage, or visual disturbances (from methanol ingestion), hemodialysis is indicated, as it effectively removes methanol, ethylene glycol, and their acid metabolites.

STEP 1 SECRET

As mentioned throughout this book, drug side effects and toxicities are extremely high yield for Step 1. Knowing antidotes to common drug overdoses (e.g., fomepizole for methanol, ethanol, and ethylene glycol poisoning) is an easy way to earn points on the USMLE.

CASE 5-6

A patient with a history of depression is brought into the emergency department with nausea, vomiting, and tinnitus. Her laboratory values are as follows:
  $[Na^+]$: 140 mEq/L
  $[K^+]$: 3.5 mEq/L
  $[Cl^-]$: 104 mEq/L
  $[HCO_3^-]$: 16 mEq/L
  [glucose]: 100 mg/dL
  pH: 7.50

Pco₂: 20 mm Hg
Po₂: 125 mm Hg

1. **What is the most likely diagnosis?**
   This patient has a mixed disorder consisting of a respiratory alkalosis, a large AG acidosis, and a near-normal pH. The AG in this case is 20 mEq/L. Remember that an elevated AG, even in the setting of a normal pH or an alkalemia, *always* reflects a metabolic acidosis. For that reason, it is often worth while to calculate the AG in acid-base problems regardless of the pH (particularly if the question makes little sense otherwise!).

   The prototypical mixed disorder that appears on the boards is aspirin intoxication. In this case, the patient's history of depression suggests a risk of suicidal ingestion, while the tinnitus in particular is a major clue for salicylate poisoning. However, on the boards you should also consider aspirin ingestion in a patient with the combination of an AG acidosis and respiratory alkalosis (**Note:** Initial aspirin overdose directly activates the respiratory center in the medulla, resulting in hyperventilation and a respiratory alkalosis.)

   Although aspirin is itself an acid, most of the AG produced in aspirin poisoning occurs from lactic acid buildup that results from aspirin's ability at toxic levels to interfere with cellular metabolism.

   Side effects of aspirin can be recalled using the mnemonic **ASPIRIN: A**sthma, **S**alicylism, **P**eptic ulcers, **I**ntestinal Bleeding, **R**eye syndrome, **I**diosyncratic reactions, and **N**oise (tinnitus).

SUMMARY BOX: ANION GAP METABOLIC ACIDOSIS

- For causes of anion gap (AG) acidosis, remember **MUDPILES: M**ethanol, **M**etformin, **U**remia (renal failure), **D**iabetic and other ketoacidoses, **P**araldehyde, **P**henformin, **I**soniazid, **I**ron supplements, **L**actic acidosis, **E**thylene glycol, **E**thanol, **S**alicylates.

- If $\Delta AG = \Delta HCO_3^-$ the high AG acidosis is the sole metabolic acid-base disorder.

- If $\Delta AG < \Delta HCO_3^-$ there is a hyperchloremic metabolic acidosis in addition to the high AG acidosis (because the *change* in bicarbonate is *greater* than expected).

- If $\Delta AG > \Delta HCO_3^-$ there is a metabolic alkalosis acidosis in addition to the high AG acidosis (because the *change* in bicarbonate is *smaller* than expected).

- Diabetic ketoacidosis (DKA) could be the presentation for previously undiagnosed type 1 diabetes (know the presentation of DKA well !).

- AG acidosis + blurry vision: Think methanol ingestion.

- AG acidosis + urine with oxalate crystals and/or Wood's lamp fluorescence: Think ethylene glycol ingestion.

- AG acidosis + respiratory alkalosis ± tinnitus: Think aspirin intoxication.

- Remember all the causes of lactic acidosis: sepsis, circulatory or respiratory failure, limb or organ (especially small bowel) ischemia, cyanide or carbon monoxide, hepatic failure.

CASE 5-7

The emergency department admits a CHF patient presenting in severe respiratory distress. His laboratory values are as follows:
pH: 7.0
Pco₂: 60 mm Hg
[HCO₃⁻]: 28 mEq/L

1. **What is the primary acid-base disorder?**
   Respiratory acidosis ($P_{CO_2} > 40$) is the disorder.

2. **What is the differential diagnosis in this patient?**
   The differential diagnosis of CO_2 retention is vast and includes not only lung disease but central hypoventilation from any cause (sedatives, CNS trauma, pickwickian syndrome), neuromuscular disorders (e.g., myasthenia gravis, Guillain-Barré syndrome, amyotrophic lateral sclerosis [ALS], muscular dystrophy, poliomyelitis), upper airway obstruction (acute airway obstruction, laryngospasm, obstructive sleep apnea), and thoracic cage abnormalities (pneumothorax, flail chest, scoliosis).
   Note: Lung disease generally impairs gas exchange through dead space (lung that is ventilated but not perfused) or shunting (lung that is perfused but not ventilated) or, most commonly, a combination of both (i.e., ventilation-perfusion mismatch). Disorders with prominent dead space ventilation (such as emphysema) tend to cause prominent and early CO_2 retention. Disorders with prominent intrapulmonary shunting (such as asthma, pulmonary edema, pneumonia, atelectasis, or PE) tend to cause prominent hypoxia but can result hypercapnia later as well.

3. **What is the most likely diagnosis in this patient?**
   From the limited amount of information we are given, acute pulmonary edema due to CHF is the most likely explanation. An intrapulmonary shunt is created when alveoli are filled with fluid, such as in pneumonia, pulmonary edema (from ARDS or CHF), or atelectasis. Intrapulmonary shunts generally lead to hypoxemia, which often in turn stimulates hyperventilation and a *decreased* (or normal) P_{CO_2}. However, when the shunt fraction is very large or when the increased hyperventilation and increased work of breathing lead to muscle fatigue, respiratory acidosis is the result.

4. **Is there appropriate compensation or is this a mixed disorder?**
   The increase in HCO_3^- is $28 - 25 = 3$ mEq/L. An acute respiratory acidosis would be expected to raise bicarbonate by $0.1 \times \Delta P_{CO_2} = 0.1 \times 20 = 2$ mEq/L (see Table 5-3). There is, therefore, appropriate compensation. Recall that maximal compensation by the kidney in the setting of a respiratory acidosis takes about 3 days (see Fig. 5-2).

CASE 5-7 continued:

The patient was intubated and admitted to the ICU; he steadily improved over the next couple of days and then suddenly developed a respiratory acidosis again.

5. **How can you determine if this exacerbation is due to central hypoventilation from sedation or due to a ventilation-perfusion ($\dot{V}/\dot{Q}$) mismatch, such as worsening of his pulmonary edema or development of a ventilator-associated pneumonia?**
   Often the history will reveal an obvious cause of a respiratory acidosis. However, it can get very tricky when there are multiple possible causes that fit with the patient's history. To determine if the patient's hypercapnia is a result of sedation or of a lung process, you can check the patient's A-a gradient (alveolar-arterial O_2 gradient). A normal/unchanged A-a gradient indicates that the lungs are exchanging gases normally but that the impairment is from a separate process, such as central hypoventilation from oversedation (or neuromuscular disease, etc.). Lung disease resulting in $\dot{V}/\dot{Q}$ mismatch will reveal an increased A-a gradient.
   If neuromuscular disease were included in the differential diagnosis in this patient, it could be distinguished from central hypoventilation by measuring inspiratory pressures. Neuromuscular disorders will have a normal A-a gradient but low peak inspiratory pressures, whereas both the A-a gradient and inspiratory pressures would be normal in central hypoventilation.

SUMMARY BOX: RESPIRATORY ACIDOSIS

- The differential diagnosis includes lung disease (usually via ventilation/perfusion mismatch) as well as central hypoventilation, neuromuscular disorders, upper airway obstructions, and thoracic cage abnormalities.

- Maximal compensation (i.e., bicarbonate retention) by the kidney in the setting of a respiratory acidosis takes about 3 days.

- Dead space ventilation (such as in emphysema) results in hypercarbia early, but in disorders involving intrapulmonary shunts (such as asthma, pulmonary edema, pneumonia, atelectasis, or pulmonary embolism [PE]) hypercarbia does not occur until there is a large shunt or respiratory muscle fatigue develops.

- An increased alveolar-arterial (A-a) gradient suggests a $\dot{V}/\dot{Q}$ abnormality and a lung defect.

- A normal/unchanged A-a gradient suggests central hypoventilation or a neuromuscular disorder as the cause.

- Neuromuscular disorders will reveal low peak inspiratory pressures, which will be normal in central hypoventilation.

CHAPTER 6

GASTROENTEROLOGY

Thomas A. Brown, MD, and Sonali J. Shah

INSIDER'S GUIDE TO GASTROENTEROLOGY FOR THE USMLE STEP 1

Gastroenterology is a comprehensive subject on boards that tends to integrate a number of fields into its questions. You will, for example, see gastrointestinal (GI) questions related to physiology, pathology, and microbiology. And although GI pharmacology is indeed fair game for the test, it is not as high yield as the aforementioned topics. You may have also noticed that the GI section in First Aid includes an extensive anatomy section—there is a reason for this! Some of the highest-yield anatomy points come from this section, and it is therefore important that you know the branches of the celiac trunk, the relationship of the pancreatic head to the common bile duct, the locations of various types of hernias, etc. It is also advisable that you spend time learning the roles of the various GI hormones. GI pathology on the boards covers an extensive number of topics, but do not panic. Several USMLE favorites are described throughout the cases in this chapter, and you should read them carefully to discern the subtle differences between the various diseases. GI pathology is not an intrinsically difficult subject, but disease presentations can blend together if you do not classify them well as you are attempting to learn them.

BASIC CONCEPTS

1. **What is the major stimulus for gastrin secretion? What are the physiologic actions of gastrin in the stomach?**
   Protein in the stomach is the primary stimulus for the secretion of gastrin by G cells in the antrum of the stomach (other stimuli include stomach distention, stomach alkalinization, and vagal stimulation). The secreted gastrin stimulates the secretion of hydrochloric acid and intrinsic factor (IF) by the gastric parietal cells and stimulates secretion of pepsinogen by the chief cells. Notice that all these secretions are important in protein/meat digestion, because the acid environment created helps hydrolyze proteins and creates an optimal pH in which pepsin works ($\sim$pH 2). Additionally, the secreted IF binds and protects the vitamin B_{12} that is present in meat. A major inhibitor of gastrin secretion is decreased gastric pH, which stimulates somatostatin secretion from D cells in the pancreas and gastrointestinal mucosa. Somatostatin and decreased pH are both negative feedback mechanisms to keep the stomach from becoming too acidic.

2. **What are the main pancreatic enzymes and what are their functions?**
   Pancreatic enzymes are all involved in digestion (degradation) of food macromolecules. Pancreatic amylase degrades starch/complex carbohydrate, trypsin and chymotrypsin degrade proteins, and lipase hydrolyzes triglycerides; there are also DNase and RNase enzymes in pancreatic secretions. The pancreas also secretes bicarbonate, which neutralizes acidic chyme entering the duodenum and creates the pH necessary for pancreatic enzymes to work.

Pancreatic enzymes are secreted as zymogens (inactive precursor molecules), which are cleaved into their active form within the intestinal lumen. This prevents autodigestion of the pancreatic tissue by the active enzyme forms. Trypsinogen is cleaved into trypsin by enterokinase within the intestinal mucosa. Trypsin then activates more trypsinogen as well as other pancreatic enzymes.

Note: The pancreatic acinar cells are rich in secretory granules full of enzymes, and the pancreatic ductal cells are principally responsible for bicarbonate and fluid secretion.

3. **What are the primary hormonal stimuli for the pancreatic exocrine secretions and how do these secretions differ in content?**
   Cholecystokinin (CKK) primarily stimulates the secretion of enzymes (e.g., proteases such as trypsinogen) from the pancreatic acinar cells, whereas secretin primarily stimulates the secretion of a bicarbonate-rich fluid from pancreatic ductal cells.

4. **What are the primary stimuli for the secretion of cholecystokinin and secretin and from where are these hormones secreted?**
   CCK is secreted primarily in response to fatty acids entering the duodenum, whereas secretin is released primarily in response to acidification of the duodenum. Both are secreted from the duodenum.

5. **What other digestive processes does cholecystokinin stimulate?**
   CCK also stimulates contraction of the gallbladder and relaxation of the sphincter of Oddi (where the common bile duct enters the duodenum), thereby promoting bile entry into the duodenum. By stimulating pancreatic secretion of lipolytic enzymes as well as the delivery of bile to the small intestine, this hormone creates the appropriate milieu for the digestion of fats.

   Note: CCK also delays gastric emptying. This explains why the sensation of fullness lasts longer after a fatty meal.

6. **What is the function of the bile salts? How are they formed?**
   The bile salts solubilize fats in meals, creating a bigger surface area on which pancreatic lipase can work. They additionally form micelles that facilitate the delivery of fatty acids to the intestinal enterocytes for absorption. Bile salts are formed from the degradation of cholesterol in the liver via the enzyme 7α-hydroxylase. As a point of interest, this is the primary method the body has for eliminating cholesterol.

7. **What is the enterohepatic circulation and why is it important in the digestion of fats?**
   Enterohepatic circulation occurs when substances are secreted by the liver, reabsorbed by the intestine, and returned to the liver. The majority of the bile salts that are delivered to the intestine during digestion are from intestinal reabsorption of secreted bile salts. In diseases that decrease bile salt reabsorption (e.g., Crohn's disease), the enterohepatic circulation and secretion of bile salts from the liver are impaired, resulting in impaired fat digestion.

8. **What defines the foregut, midgut, and hindgut anatomically? Which main arteries provide the blood supply to each segment? What nerves supply these regions?**
   The foregut comprises the upper gastrointestinal (GI) tract down to a site just distal to the ampulla of Vater (where the common bile duct empties into the secondary part of the duodenum). Its main vascular supply comes from the celiac artery. The midgut extends from the second part of the duodenum down to the splenic flexure of the colon and is served by the superior mesenteric artery. The hindgut extends from the splenic flexure of the colon to the anus and is supplied by the inferior mesenteric artery. The foregut and midgut are innervated by the vagus nerve, and the hindgut is innervated by the pelvic nerve.

Note: The pancreas and liver are embryologic outgrowths of the foregut and share the vascular supply of the foregut (i.e., celiac artery). Although the spleen is not an embryologic derivative of the foregut (it is mesodermal in origin), it is supplied by the celiac artery as well.

9. **What are the anatomic layers of the gut wall?**
From the lumen out, the layers of the GI tract are as follows: (1) mucosa, comprising the mucosal epithelium, lamina propria, and muscularis mucosae; (2) submucosa, which contains the submucosal (Meissner's) nerve plexus; (3) muscularis propria, comprising an inner circular smooth muscle layer, myenteric plexus, and outer longitudinal smooth muscle layer; and (4) serosa (adventitia), which is the fibrous outer covering (Fig. 6-1).
Note: The taeniae coli are band-like muscles composing the outer longitudinal smooth muscle layer of the large intestine, except in the appendix and the rectum.

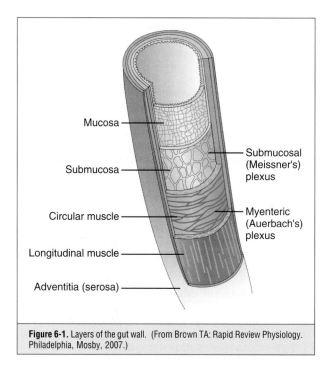

Figure 6-1. Layers of the gut wall. (From Brown TA: Rapid Review Physiology. Philadelphia, Mosby, 2007.)

CASE 6-1

A 45-year-old obese man presents with a 2-year history of chest discomfort following heavy meals. He describes the discomfort as a substernal burning sensation that radiates to his neck. The discomfort worsens when he is lying down in bed at night. He mentions that he also has a chronic cough and hoarse voice in the morning.

1. **What is the differential diagnosis?**
The differential diagnosis includes gastroesophageal reflux disease (GERD), esophageal spasm, and myocardial ischemia. Note that myocardial infarction and angina should be part of

the differential diagnosis in any case in which there is chest discomfort/pain, especially considering that this patient is a middle-aged, obese male, all of which are risk factors for heart disease. GERD characteristically presents with heartburn, which can mimic myocardial ischemia, and regurgitation of sour material into the mouth. The heartburn from GERD is typically exacerbated by both eating large meals and bending over or being recumbent in bed. In addition to heartburn, patients with GERD can also present with chronic cough from gastric acid irritation of the tracheobronchial tree and a hoarse voice in the morning from the gastric acid irritation of the vocal cords at night.

CASE 6-1 continued:

Physical examination is significant for obesity. There is no chest wall tenderness. Cardiac examination is unremarkable, except for auscultating bowel sounds in the patient's chest. A cardiac stress test is negative for inducible ischemia. A barium swallow is shown in Figure 6-2.

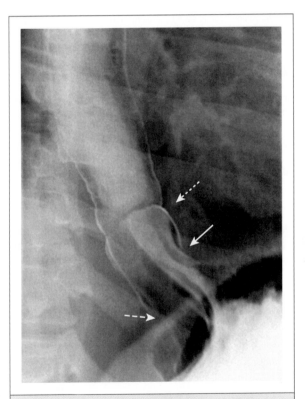

Figure 6-2. Sliding hiatal hernia. A bulbous collection of contrast representing the stomach herniated is evident above the diaphragm. Gastric folds are present in the hernia, identifying it as part of the stomach (*solid white arrow*). Notice the esophagus does not narrow as it normally does when passing through the esophageal hiatus (*dashed white arrow*). Just above the hernia is a thin, weblike filling defect characteristic of a **Schatzki's ring** (*dotted white arrow*). The Schatzki's ring marks the level of the esophagogastric junction. (From Herring W: Learning Radiology: Recognizing the Basics, 2nd ed. Philadelphia, Saunders, 2012.)

2. **Based on the findings in Figure 6-2, what is the patient's likely diagnosis?**
   The patient has a sliding hiatal hernia. In a sliding hiatal hernia, the gastroesophageal junction herniates upward through the esophageal hiatus in the diaphragm. The additional sphincteric pressure that is provided by the diaphragm is then lost, allowing reflux of gastric contents to occur more easily. This contrasts with a paraesophageal hiatal hernia, in which a portion of the gastric fundus "rolls" into and herniates through the diaphragm but the gastroesophageal junction remains in place. Although paraesophageal hiatal hernias usually do not cause reflux, they are more serious because they can become incarcerated (strangulated) and ischemic.

3. **Discuss the pathophysiology of gastroesophageal reflux disease.**
   GERD is caused by the reflux of acidic or bilious gastric contents into the esophagus, which irritates the esophageal mucosa and causes pain. Many factors can predispose to this reflux. One of the most important factors is abnormal transient relaxation of the lower esophageal sphincter (LES) unrelated to swallowing. A continually relaxed (atonic) LES will also allow reflux. Increased intra-abdominal pressure (due to obesity, pregnancy, Valsalva maneuver, etc.), increased gastric volume (due to eating a large meal or gastroparesis), and decreasing distance of gastric contents from the gastroesophageal junction (occurring when lying down or with hiatal hernia) may exacerbate reflux of gastric contents into the esophagus.

CASE 6-1 continued:

The patient is started on a 1-week therapeutic trial of omeprazole, which provides substantial relief. He is therefore started on a long-term course of omeprazole.

4. **Cover the far left column of Table 6-1 and attempt to name the drugs used in the treatment of GERD based on the class of drug, the mechanism of action, and the primary side effects listed in the table.**

TABLE 6-1. DRUGS USED FOR TREATMENT OF GASTROESOPHAGEAL REFLUX DISEASE

Drug	Class	Mechanism of Action	Primary Side Effect
Cimetidine Ranitidine Nizatidine Famotidine	Histamine H_2 receptor antagonists	Inhibits histamine-stimulated release of hydrochloric acid by blocking H_2 receptors on parietal cells	Cimetidine inhibits hepatic cytochrome P-450 enzymes and causes gynecomastia
Metoclopramide	Antiemetic Prokinetic	Prokinetic drug (increases gastric emptying and LES tone) via cholinergic side effects	Parkinsonian symptoms, seizures
Omeprazole Lansoprazole Rabeprazole	Proton pump inhibitors	Irreversibly inhibits the parietal cell H^+/K^+-ATPase "pump"	Hypergastrinemia

GI, gastrointestinal; LES, lower esophageal sphincter.

5. **Which of the drugs in Table 6-1 are contraindicated in a patient in whom bowel obstruction is suspected and why?**
Prokinetic drugs should be avoided whenever bowel obstruction is suspected, as they can exacerbate the obstruction and potentially cause perforation.

6. **Why may the omeprazole this patient was given cause him to develop hypergastrinemia?**
Proton pump inhibitors such as omeprazole inhibit gastric hydrochloric acid (HCl) secretion by irreversibly inhibiting the H^+/K^+-ATPase pump on gastric parietal cells. This raises gastric pH, which disinhibits gastric secretion by the G cells, resulting in hypergastrinemia.

CASE 6-1 continued:

Unfortunately, the patient initially is lost to follow-up, but he shows up at his physician's office 3 years later complaining of 6 months of progressively worsening dysphagia to solids and unintentional weight loss. He says he tried to be diligent about taking his omeprazole for the first month, but soon stopped taking his pills and learned to tolerate the discomfort.

7. **Which complications of gastroesophageal reflux disease could be responsible for the patient's difficulty swallowing?**
Esophageal stricture results from fibrosing and scarring of the esophageal mucosa from chronic irritation by gastric acid. This scarring narrows the lumen, which prevents a food bolus from passing through, causing food to get stuck. Another complication of GERD is Barrett's esophagus, which is columnar metaplasia of stratified squamous esophageal epithelium that can lead to esophageal adenocarcinoma. Esophageal carcinoma usually presents with rapidly progressive dysphagia and weight loss.

8. **Differentiate between the two types of esophageal cancers—adenocarcinoma and squamous cell carcinoma—in terms of risk factors and location.**
Adenocarcinoma typically occurs in the lower one third of the esophagus. Barrett's esophagus and chronic irritation of esophageal epithelium from untreated GERD are risk factors for this type of cancer. Squamous cell carcinoma usually occurs in the upper two thirds of the esophagus. Smoking and alcohol, especially together (synergistic effect), increase the risk for this type of cancer. Both of these esophageal cancers can cause dysphagia to solids.

9. **Why would a patient with Sjögren's syndrome be more susceptible to esophageal pathology in gastroesophageal reflux disease?**
Sjögren's syndrome is an autoimmune disease characterized by lymphocytic infiltration of the lacrimal and salivary glands, causing dry eyes and dry mouth due to deficient secretions. Because saliva is rich in bicarbonate, it functions to neutralize acid in the esophagus. The absence of this protective function predisposes patients with this condition to esophageal damage with even minimal gastroesophageal reflux.

SUMMARY BOX: GASTROESOPHAGEAL REFLUX DISEASE, HIATAL HERNIAS, AND ESOPHAGEAL CARCINOMAS

- Gastroesophageal reflux disease (GERD) classically presents with regurgitation of "sour" contents into the esophagus or oropharynx and substernal chest discomfort that worsens after large meals and when in a recumbent position.

- The pathogenesis of GERD involves *inappropriate* relaxation of the lower esophageal sphincter (LES).

- Sliding hiatal hernias can predispose to GERD. Paraesophageal "rolling" hiatal hernias are subject to incarceration.

- GERD is typically treated with proton pump inhibitors, H_2 receptor antagonists, or surgery (Nissen fundoplication in refractory cases).

- Long-term complications of GERD include Barrett's esophagus, adenocarcinoma, esophageal stricture, and esophageal ulceration.

STEP 1 SECRET

Gastroesophageal reflux disease (GERD) is a board favorite. Be able to recognize the symptoms of chest pain following meals (may be described as a burning sensation in the chest), sour taste in the mouth, and nocturnal cough as a classic presentation for this condition. You should also know how to recognize complications of GERD (e.g., Barrett's esophagus, strictures, adenocarcinoma) by both medical history and histologic appearance (refer to Chapter 27, Pathology, for images).

CASE 6-2

A 50-year-old woman complains of recent dysphagia to solids and liquids.

1. **In pathophysiologic terms, how do you approach dysphagia?**
   Dysphagia can be approached in terms of oropharyngeal or esophageal etiology.
   Oropharyngeal dysphagia is caused by difficulty initiating a swallow reflex, due to either neurologic or muscular problems. Typical causes include stroke, amyotrophic lateral sclerosis (Lou Gehrig's disease), and myasthenia gravis. Patients usually have coughing or choking with dysphagia of oropharyngeal etiology.
   Esophageal dysphagia is caused by food getting "stuck" in the esophagus after being swallowed. This is due to either mechanical obstruction or esophageal dysmotility. History can often distinguish between an obstructive etiology or a motility disorder. If the patient has problems with only solid foods initially, then this suggests mechanical obstruction. This can progress to advanced obstruction, such as from esophageal adenocarcinoma, causing dysphagia to both solids and liquids. If the patient has dysphagia to both solids and liquids from the beginning, this suggests a dysmotility disorder, such as achalasia, scleroderma-like esophagus, or diffuse esophageal spasm.

CASE 6-2 continued:

The patient also notes occasional chest pain with eating, nocturnal cough, and an unintentional 15-lb weight loss in the last 2 months. She was recently admitted to the hospital for treatment of pneumonia. Esophageal manometry shows increased LES pressure with incomplete LES relaxation and a complete absence of peristalsis in the lower esophagus. A barium swallow is shown in Figure 6-3.

2. **What is the likely diagnosis in this woman? Describe the pathophysiology of this disease.**

The initial dysphagia to solids and liquids, barium swallow showing the classic "bird's beak" appearance, and esophageal manometry findings of aperistalsis and increased LES pressure are classic for achalasia.

The LES is normally tonically constricted, generating enough intraluminal pressure to prevent the reflux of gastric contents into the esophagus. During the esophageal phase of swallowing, the LES relaxes in response to a food bolus descending through the esophagus, a phenomenon referred to as *receptive relaxation*. In achalasia, there is destruction of the myenteric plexus, which mediates receptive relaxation and also mediates esophageal peristalsis (hence the aperistalsis). Although the exact mechanism of increased LES tone in patients with achalasia is not known, research suggests that these patients have loss of nitric oxide–secreting neurons, a key factor in LES relaxation. The failure of the LES to relax together with the failure of the distal esophagus to undergo peristalsis allows food to accumulate and dilate the lower esophagus, creating the "bird's beak" appearance on barium swallow (Fig. 6-3).

Note: The myenteric (Auerbach's) plexus is located between the inner circular and the outer longitudinal smooth muscle layers (muscularis propria) of the esophagus.

3. **Chagas' disease is also known to be a cause of achalasia. What is the pathologic mechanism and what organism is the primary culprit?**

Chagas' disease (American trypanosomiasis) can cause destruction of the myenteric plexus in the esophagus. This disease is caused by the protozoal parasite *Trypanosoma cruzi* and is particularly common in South America. In addition to achalasia, Chagas' disease can also cause megacolon by destroying the myenteric plexus of the colon.

4. **What was the likely cause of this woman's previous episode of pneumonia?**

The pneumonia was probably caused by aspiration of esophageal contents, especially while sleeping, due to the presence of undigested material in the esophagus.

5. **In addition to pneumatic dilatation of the lower esophageal sphincter and surgical myotomy, injection of botulinum toxin into the lower esophageal sphincter is a treatment option for this woman. What is this drug's mechanism of action in this context?**

Much of the tonic constriction of the LES is due to vagal cholinergic innervation. Because botulinum toxin exerts its effects by inhibiting the release of acetylcholine from nerve endings, it reduces this input to LES tone.

SUMMARY BOX: ACHALASIA

- Because it is a motility disorder, patients with achalasia typically present with dysphagia to both solids and liquids.

- Achalasia is caused by destruction of the myenteric (Auerbach's) plexus. In Chagas' disease, this destruction is mediated by the protozoan *Trypanosoma cruzi*.

- Esophageal manometry will classically show distal aperistalsis and increased LES tone.

- Barium swallow will show a "bird's beak" appearance.

- Treatment options include LES dilatation, LES myotomy, and injection of botulinum toxin into the LES.

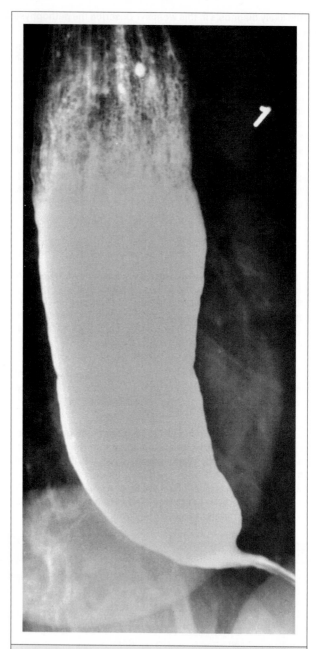

Figure 6-3. Barium swallow of patient in case 6-2. (From Cummings CW, Flint PW, Haughey BH, et al: Otolaryngology: Head and Neck Surgery, 4th ed. Philadelphia, Mosby, 2005.)

STEP 1 SECRET

Whenever you see a clinical vignette that mentions progressive dysphagia to solids and liquids, consider achalasia, scleroderma, and esophageal cancer in your differential diagnosis. Consider an oropharyngeal etiology (e.g., stroke) if associated with a history of choking or cough.

CASE 6-3

A 33-year-old man presents to his primary care physician complaining of a 2-month history of gnawing epigastric pain that develops a couple of hours after meals. The pain is particularly bothersome at night and often awakens him from sleep.

1. **What is the differential diagnosis?**
    The differential diagnosis of postprandial epigastric pain includes biliary colic, GERD, irritable bowel syndrome (IBS), and peptic ulcer disease (PUD). Biliary colic is severe, right upper quadrant pain caused by gallstones and usually precipitated by fatty meals. It has a higher frequency in women but is still common in men. GERD may cause epigastric or substernal discomfort that worsens with large meals, bending over, or lying flat. IBS can produce abdominal pain and bloating that is worsened by stress or food but relieved by defecation. Patients typically have altered bowel habits (e.g., diarrhea or constipation), which this patient's history does not mention. PUD encompasses both gastric and duodenal ulcers. Duodenal ulcers typically cause most pain 1 to 3 hours after a meal, when the acidic chyme enters the small bowel. Pain also occurs at night, due to circadian rhythm–induced acid secretion. Food or antacids can relieve the epigastric pain. Gastric ulcers have a more variable presentation, but epigastric pain is typically precipitated by food and therefore patients may experience weight loss due to food avoidance. Based on the patient's history, duodenal ulcer is the most likely diagnosis.

CASE 6-3 continued:

After a brief history and physical examination the physician prescribes some antacids and schedules a follow-up visit in 2 weeks to see if this treatment provides relief.

2. **If you were this man's physician, what would you have done differently in the treatment of this patient?**
    The patient with epigastric pain warrants a thorough history and physical examination, looking for any "red-flag" symptoms, such as GI bleeding, anemia, dysphagia, persistent vomiting, or unintentional weight loss, as these problems could point toward more serious pathologic process, such as malignancy. The two usual culprits for PUD are nonsteroidal anti-inflammatory drugs (NSAIDs) and *Helicobacter pylori*. A more thorough history could have discovered if the patient was taking NSAIDs, which you would have recommended that he stop taking. Testing for *H. pylori* would also be necessary to prevent recurrence.
    In the absence of red-flag symptoms in a young adult with suspected PUD, visualization of the ulcer by upper endoscopy or barium swallow is not necessary, and the patient can be empirically treated with H_2 receptor antagonists (e.g., ranitidine) or proton pump inhibitors.

3. **How are nonsteroidal anti-inflammatory drugs thought to predispose to the formation of gastric ulcers? What alternatives exist to lessen gastrointestinal side effects?**

NSAIDs inhibit the production of prostaglandins in the gastric mucosa. These prostaglandins normally function to protect the gastric mucosa by increasing mucus and bicarbonate secretion and by stimulating local vasodilation, which maintains mucosal perfusion and prevents ischemic injury.

Two options exist to circumvent this problem: taking misoprostol with NSAIDs (rarely done) or using cyclooxygenase (COX)-2 inhibitors. Misoprostol is a prostaglandin E_1 analog that decreases gastric acid secretion and increases mucus and bicarbonate secretion, thereby decreasing the deleterious effects of NSAIDs. As the name indicates, COX-2 inhibitors selectively inhibit COX-2 and do not affect COX-1 activity. The constitutively expressed form, COX-1, is present in multiple tissues and is responsible for the production of protective prostaglandins in the stomach. The inducible form, COX-2, is present *primarily* in inflammatory cells and is responsible for producing proinflammatory substances. By potently inhibiting COX-2 and minimally inhibiting COX-1, COX-2 inhibitors cause fewer GI side effects. Unfortunately, COX-2 inhibitors can be prothrombotic and exacerbate hypertension, increasing the risk of myocardial infarction and stroke. This major side effect led to rofecoxib (Vioxx) being pulled from the U.S. market in recent years.

CASE 6–3 continued:

The patient misses his 2-week appointment and returns 7 months later looking pale and tired. The antacids initially provided some relief, but now the pain is back and is worse than before. In addition, the patient has noticed he has dark, tarry stools and feels tired all the time.

4. **Based on the appearance of the stool, is this more likely a lower gastrointestinal bleed or an upper gastrointestinal bleed?**

Our patient presents with melena, paleness, and fatigue, the latter two of which are suggestive of anemia. The melena indicates an upper GI bleed (UGIB), likely caused by a bleeding duodenal ulcer. UGIB is anatomically distinguished from a lower GI bleed (LGIB) in that it occurs proximal to the ligament of Treitz. UGIB presents with either hematemesis or melena. Melena occurs because the hemoglobin has time to be broken down by bacteria in the gut to give dark, tarry stools. Hematochezia (bright red rectal bleeding) is *typically* indicative of LGIB, in which bacteria do not have the time to break down hemoglobin. However, brisk UGIBs such as bleeding esophageal varices can present with hematochezia because blood stimulates GI motility and decreases transit time.

5. **What are the major complications of peptic ulcer disease?**

Hemorrhage is the most common complication and can present as hematemesis or melena. Potential sources of hemorrhage include a posterior penetrating duodenal ulcer (gastroduodenal artery) or penetrating gastric ulcer on the lesser curvature (gastric artery). Perforation into the abdominal cavity usually presents as sudden onset of pain with peritonitis. A chest or kidney, ureter, and bladder (KUB) x-ray study will usually demonstrate free air under the diaphragm. Gastric outlet obstruction can rarely result from chronic ulcers and typically presents with persistent vomiting and weight loss. Gastric carcinoma can ulcerate and cause pain just like PUD. Therefore, gastric ulcers should typically be biopsied during upper endoscopy to rule out gastric carcinoma. Chronic gastritis and *H. pylori* predispose to development of gastric carcinoma. Gastric carcinoma is associated with metastases to the left supraclavicular node (Virchow's node) and bilateral metastases to the ovaries (Krukenberg tumors), which have "signet ring" cells as a pathologic finding.

Note: Pancreatic adenocarcinoma also metastasizes to Virchow's node.

CASE 6-3 continued:

Laboratory evaluation reveals a hemoglobin level of 10 g/dL. The patient is referred to a gastroenterologist, who performs an upper endoscopy that reveals a well-demarcated, clean-based ulcer in the proximal duodenum, as shown in Figure 6-4.

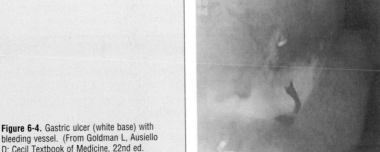

Figure 6-4. Gastric ulcer (white base) with bleeding vessel. (From Goldman L, Ausiello D: Cecil Textbook of Medicine, 22nd ed. Philadelphia, WB Saunders, 2004.)

6. **What enzyme does *Helicobacter pylori* produce that can be tested for?**
   H. pylori produces the enzyme urease, which breaks down urea to liberate ammonia and carbon dioxide. Consequently, *H. pylori* can be detected by having a patient ingest [13]C- or ^{14}C-labeled urea and then determining if the patient's breath contains radiolabeled CO_2. Interestingly, the liberation of ammonia by *H. pylori* neutralizes gastric acid and facilitates the survival of this organism in the stomach. *H. pylori* infection can also be detected by serum antibodies to this organism, but this test does not discriminate between current and previous infection unless IgM is specifically requested.

7. **During endoscopy, if multiple duodenal ulcers had been found in our patient, what disease would we suspect and how would we test for it?**
   Whenever peptic ulcers are refractory to aggressive therapy, there are multiple ulcers, or the ulcers are located in abnormal positions such as the jejunum, Zollinger-Ellison syndrome (ZES) (due to a gastrin-secreting tumor or gastrinoma) should be suspected. The increased gastrin secretion by these tumors causes excessive secretion of acid. A markedly elevated gastrin level, usually with levels >1000 pg/mL (fasting levels <150 pg/mL), is indicative of ZES. The secretin test will also show a paradoxical increase in gastrin.
   Note: Recall that patients on PPIs may also have substantially elevated gastrin levels, so it may be difficult to immediately differentiate between a patient on PPIs and one with ZES.

CASE 6-3 continued:

The patient's urea breath test is positive and he is therefore prescribed "triple therapy."

8. **Why was our patient prescribed triple therapy?**
   The patient has an *H. pylori* infection that needs to be eradicated to reduce the rate of recurrence of peptic ulcer and the risk of developing gastric adenocarcinoma.
   Note: Triple therapy typically includes two antibiotics and an H_2 blocker or a proton pump inhibitor.

CASE 6-3 continued:

At his 4-week follow-up, the patient denies any abdominal symptoms but does note that he has noticed fatty enlargement of his breasts.

9. **What was the most likely cause of his gynecomastia?**
    One of the distinctive side effects of cimetidine is gynecomastia. Another noteworthy fact about cimetidine is that it is the only H_2 receptor antagonist that inhibits one of the hepatic cytochrome P-450 enzymes, which makes it particularly dangerous when given with warfarin, as warfarin is metabolized through this pathway.

STEP 1 SECRET

Know which drugs upregulate and downregulate the hepatic cytochrome P-450 enzymes. These drugs have been known to show up on many USMLE forms:

Inhibitors	Inducers
Cimetidine	Barbiturates
Macrolides	Quinidine
Azole antifungals	Rifampin
Isoniazid	Phenytoin
Sulfonamides	Griseofulvin
Grapefruit juice	Carbamazepine
Protease inhibitors	St. John's wort
Ciprofloxacin	Chronic alcohol use

10. **What alternative pharmacologic treatment strategies exist for this patient with peptic ulcer disease?**
    1. Proton pump inhibitors, such as omeprazole, lansoprazole, and pantoprazole
    2. Other H_2 receptor antagonists, such as ranitidine
    3. Anticholinergics, such as atropine
    4. Mucosal protective agents, such as misoprostol, and sucralfate
    5. Antacids, such as calcium carbonate, magnesium hydroxide, and aluminum hydroxide
        Note: Magnesium causes diarrhea, whereas aluminum causes constipation, so these two compounds are often mixed together in antacid formulations to balance these effects.

SUMMARY BOX: PEPTIC ULCER DISEASE

- Classically, pain with gastric ulcers occurs with meals, while pain with duodenal ulcers occurs 1 to 3 hours after meals, but there is substantial overlap.

- Two major causes of peptic ulcer disease (PUD) are *Helicobacter pylori* and nonsteroidal anti-inflammatory drugs (NSAIDs).

- Misoprostol with NSAIDS or cyclooxygenase (COX)-2 inhibitors decrease gastrointestinal (GI) side effects.

- Melena usually indicates an upper GI bleed. Hematochezia indicates a lower GI bleed or a brisk upper GI bleed.

- Hemorrhage and perforation are major complications of PUD.

- Always biopsy gastric ulcers to rule out gastric carcinoma.

- Think Zollinger-Ellison syndrome with refractory PUD, multiple ulcers or ulcers in unusual locations, and a markedly elevated gastrin level.

- Use urea breath test (more accurate) and IgM serum antibody test to diagnose current *H. pylori* infection.

- Cimetidine inhibits P-450 (contraindicated with warfarin) and causes gynecomastia.

CASE 6-4

A 42-year-old obese woman presents with a history of epigastric pain that has worsened in the past week and is exacerbated by food. She has lost 20 lb over the past 2 months and has felt a little feverish in the past week. She has also been bothered by nausea and vomiting.

1. **What is the differential diagnosis for postprandial epigastric pain?**
   The differential diagnosis for postprandial epigastric pain in the presence of nausea and vomiting includes gallstone disease, GERD, PUD, pancreatitis, and acute gastritis. Gallstone disease, such as biliary colic and acute cholecystitis, is the leading diagnosis because the patient has several risk factors—obesity, middle-aged, female, and recent weight loss (which may have been lost due to fasting, which is another risk factor)—that predispose her to gallstone formation. Also, pain associated with biliary colic is exacerbated by eating (classically associated with fatty foods). GERD, PUD (particularly gastric ulcers), and acute gastritis are also all typically exacerbated by food.

CASE 6-4 continued:

Upon further questioning, the patient attributes the weight loss to not eating because it exacerbates the pain. She also admits to drinking six alcoholic drinks a day and taking ibuprofen regularly for lower back pain.

2. **How does this information alter the differential diagnosis?**
   Now, gastric ulcers, acute gastritis, and acute pancreatitis are the most likely diagnoses. Gastric ulcers are related to NSAID use and are associated with weight loss, but alcohol does not usually play a role in their onset. NSAIDs and alcohol are major risk factors for acute gastritis and the pain from food usually leads to anorexia and weight loss. Acute pancreatitis due to alcohol or a gallstone is another concern.

CASE 6-4 continued:

Physical examination reveals mild epigastric tenderness. Serum amylase and lipase are within normal limits. A urease breath test is negative. Endoscopy is positive for punctate erosions in the antrum (Fig 6-5), and a tissue biopsy reveals diffuse inflammation of the gastric mucosa with no evidence of malignancy.

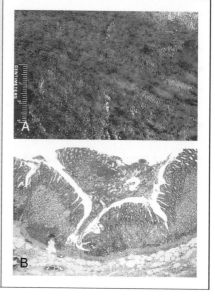

Figure 6-5. Acute gastritis. **A,** Gross view showing punctate erosions in an otherwise unremarkable mucosa; adherent blood is dark because of exposure to gastric acid. **B,** Low-power microscopic view of focal mucosal disruption with hemorrhage; the adjacent mucosa is normal. (From Kumar V, Abbas AK, Fausto N: Robbins and Cotran Pathologic Basis of Disease, 7th ed. Philadelphia, WB Saunders, 2005.)

3. **Based on these findings, the diagnosis of acute gastritis is confirmed. What are the two primary classifications of this disease?**
Acute gastritis can be divided into infectious and noninfectious gastritis. Noninfectious gastritis (as in this case) is caused by exposure to toxins and drugs (ethanol, NSAIDs) and severe physical stress (burns, head trauma, surgery), and infectious gastritis is typically caused by *H. pylori*.

CASE 6-4 continued:

You counsel the patient about cutting back on alcohol and stopping the NSAIDs, which the patient does, and her symptoms resolve within weeks. Years later, the patient brings her 68-year-old mother to you because she thinks you are "the greatest doctor in the world" after solving her "belly" problem. The patient's mother has been experiencing fatigue, memory difficulties, and numbness and tingling in her feet for the past 6 months.

4. **What is the differential diagnosis for the mother's symptoms?**
The differential diagnosis is broad but includes depression, dementia, vitamin B_{12} (cobalamin) deficiency, diabetic peripheral neuropathy, and alcoholic peripheral neuropathy. The depression could explain the memory difficulties, especially in the elderly (pseudodementia), and the fatigue. Dementia is consistent with memory difficulties, which should be a consideration in any elderly patient with memory complaints. Vitamin B_{12} deficiency can cause memory difficulties and paresthesias, as this patient describes, and the anemia associated with vitamin B_{12} deficiency can explain the fatigue. Diabetic and alcoholic peripheral neuropathies can cause paresthesias in the extremities.

CASE 6-4 continued:

Physical examination is significant for epigastric tenderness and impaired vibratory sense and proprioception in the lower extremities. Her hemoglobin is 9.5 g/dL and

mean corpuscular volume (MCV) is 105 fL. A peripheral blood smear is shown in
Figure 6-6.

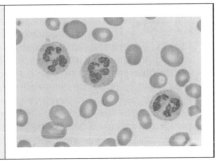

Figure 6-6. Peripheral blood smear for patient in Case 6-4. (From Hoffman R, Benz EJ Jr, Shattil SJ, et al: Hematology: Basic Principles and Practice, 4th ed. Philadelphia, Churchill Livingstone, 2005.)

5. **What most likely explains the macrocytic anemia and peripheral blood smear as shown in Figure 6-6?**
   This woman has a megaloblastic anemia secondary to vitamin B_{12} or folate deficiency. The peripheral blood smear shows hypersegmented (generally >5 lobes) neutrophils, which confirms the diagnosis of megaloblastic anemia. Vitamin B_{12} is required for DNA synthesis in rapidly proliferating erythrocyte progenitor cells. A deficiency of vitamin B_{12} therefore may result in a macrocytic anemia. Given her other symptoms, vitamin B_{12} deficiency is almost certainly the diagnosis.

STEP 1 SECRET

Figure 6-6 is a high-yield image for Step 1. Immediately associate hypersegmented neutrophils with folate and vitamin B_{12} deficiency. If neurologic changes are mentioned in the clinical vignette, vitamin B_{12} deficiency is likely.

CASE 6-4 continued:

A serum vitamin B_{12} (cobalamin) level is 120 pg/mL (normal ≥ 300 pg/mL).

6. **What are the various causes of vitamin B_{12} deficiency?**
   A vitamin B_{12} deficiency is caused by either a nutritional deficiency or various malabsorption syndromes. Dietary sources of vitamin B_{12} include red meat, fortified cereals, and dairy products. Reserves of vitamin B_{12} are long-lasting (2-7 years) even with severe malabsorption. At-risk groups for this type of deficiency are elderly with "tea and toast" diets and chronic alcoholics (secondary to nutritional deficiency). Malabsorption syndromes that cause vitamin B_{12} deficiency include pernicious anemia, celiac disease, bacterial overgrowth, *Diphyllobothrium latum* infection, Crohn's disease, and pancreatic insufficiency. Parietal cells produce intrinsic factor (IF), which is needed for proper absorption of vitamin B_{12} in the terminal ileum. Pernicious anemia or type A chronic gastritis is caused by autoimmune destruction of parietal cells in the fundus and body of the stomach, which will decrease the amount of IF (and hydrochloric acid) produced. Through various mechanisms, celiac disease, bacterial overgrowth, and Crohn's disease

may affect absorption at the terminal ileum. Pancreatic insufficiency results in a deficiency in pancreatic enzymes that usually separate vitamin B_{12} from other factors that allow IF to bind to it.

7. **What test can help with diagnosing the cause of vitamin B_{12} deficiency?**
The Schilling test can help determine the cause of malabsorption in patients with vitamin B_{12} deficiency. The first stage of the Schilling test is to saturate all the blood and tissue vitamin B_{12}–binding sites with an intramuscular injection of vitamin B_{12}. Radiolabeled vitamin B_{12} is then given orally. In the absence of vitamin B_{12} malabsorption, the vitamin B_{12}/IF complex would normally be absorbed in the terminal ileum and excreted in the urine because all tissue and blood vitamin B_{12} binding sites are saturated. If the level of urine radioactivity is low (suggesting that malabsorption is indeed present), then the second stage of the test is repeated with oral vitamin B_{12} plus intrinsic factor (IF), which specifically determines whether the patient has pernicious anemia (recall that since the parietal cells produce intrinsic factor, supplementation with IF should increase B_{12} absorption in patients with pernicious anemia). If the urine radioactivity is still low after the second stage, then a third stage uses oral vitamin B_{12} plus either antibiotics or pancreatic enzymes to test for bacterial overgrowth or pancreatic insufficiency, respectively.

Note: Even though the Schilling test is now rarely used, you are still expected to understand the principles behind it for boards.

CASE 6-4 continued:

The patient's Schilling test shows normal vitamin B_{12} absorption with the addition of IF, and the diagnosis of pernicious anemia is therefore made.

8. **What are the two primary classifications of chronic gastritis?**
Chronic gastritis is also subdivided into two types: type A (noninfectious) and type B (infectious). Type A chronic gastritis is caused by autoimmune destruction of parietal cells in the fundus and body of the stomach. Type B chronic gastritis is associated with *H. pylori* colonization of the gastric antrum. Type B chronic gastritis is more common than type A, accounting for approximately 80% of the cases of chronic gastritis. Type A causes pernicious anemia (as described previously) and achlorhydia (deficiency of hydrochloric acid), which can result in G cell hyperplasia from elevated gastrin levels and predispose to enteric infections, especially salmonella. Both types of chronic gastritis are risk factors for the development of gastric carcinoma.

SUMMARY BOX: ACUTE/CHRONIC GASTRITIS

- Possible causes of acute gastritis: (1) *Helicobacter pylori*, (2) nonsteroidal anti-inflammatory drugs (NSAIDs) or alcohol, and (3) stress-induced.

- Two types of chronic gastritis: type A (autoimmune) and type B (*H. pylori*).

- Autoimmune gastritis affects parietal cells, inhibiting production of intrinsic factor (pernicious anemia) and hydrochloric acid (achlorhydria).

- Polysegmented neutrophils = megaloblastic anemia = vitamin B_{12} or folate deficiency until proven otherwise.

- The Schilling test can help distinguish between the various malabsorption syndromes causing vitamin B_{12} deficiency.

CASE 6-5

A 38-year-old alcoholic man presents to the emergency room with sudden-onset, severe epigastric pain that radiates to his back. He also complains of nausea and vomiting.

1. **What is the differential diagnosis for abdominal pain radiating to the back?**
The differential diagnosis includes acute pancreatitis, ruptured abdominal aortic aneurysm, perforated duodenal ulcer, biliary colic, and renal colic. In a middle-aged man with heavy alcohol use, acute pancreatitis seems likely.

CASE 6-5 continued:

Physical examination is significant for fever (101° F), tachycardia, blood pressure (BP) of 98/60 mm Hg, epigastric tenderness, and absent bowel sounds. Laboratory tests reveal elevated serum amylase and lipase, hypocalcemia, and a leukocytosis.

2. **What is the diagnosis? What are the causes of this disease?**
Acute pancreatitis characteristically has epigastric pain radiating to the back, elevated amylase and lipase, leukocytosis, and a low-grade fever. Although uncommon, you should also know that acute pancreatitis may also be associated with hypocalcemia (due to fatty acid saponification of calcium salts). The most common causes are alcohol abuse and gallstones. Other less common but well-established causes of acute pancreatitis include severe hypertriglyceridemia (typically >2000 mg/dL), marked hypercalcemia, trauma, medications, iatrogenic causes (e.g., following endoscopic retrograde cholangiopancreatography [ERCP]), annular pancreas, and scorpion bite.

3. **How can gallstones cause pancreatitis?**
Gallstones can pass into the lower common bile duct and obstruct the egress of bile into the intestine. The bile can then back up into the pancreatic duct, irritating and inflaming the pancreatic tissue. The pancreatic duct also cannot empty, so pancreatic secretions may build up and contribute to the inflammatory process.
   Note: Patients with cystic fibrosis often develop chronic pancreatitis because thick pancreatic secretions can block the pancreatic duct.

CASE 6-5 continued:

The patient spends 4 days in the hospital and is discharged home feeling well. However, he continues to drink alcohol, and several years later, he is evaluated for a 2-month history of abdominal pain, diarrhea, and weight loss. An abdominal x-ray study is shown in Figure 6-7.

4. **What is the likely diagnosis in this case and what is the most common cause of this disease?**
The combination of chronic alcohol use, abdominal pain, diarrhea, weight loss, and pancreatic calcifications on an abdominal x-ray film is classic for chronic pancreatitis. Alcohol is the most common cause of chronic pancreatitis (gallstones are *not* a major cause).

5. **What are the primary complications of chronic pancreatitis?**
The sequelae of chronic pancreatitis include fat malabsorption, fat-soluble vitamin deficiency (vitamins A, D, E, K), persistent diarrhea, and insulin-dependent diabetes mellitus. A lack of various pancreatic enzymes that help in the digestion of fat in the small intestine results in fat malabsorption and fat-soluble vitamin (A, D, E, and K) deficiency. These and other poorly absorbed nutrients are then available to be catabolized/fermented by the bacterial flora in the large intestine. The final products of this catabolism are typically osmotically active, and draw water into the lumen of the intestine, leading to an osmotic diarrhea. Diabetes mellitus results from chronic inflammation, eventually destroying the beta cells of the islets of Langerhans.

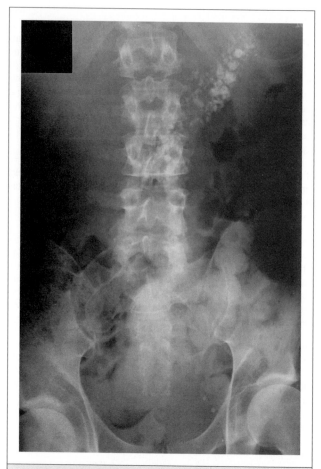

Figure 6-7. Calcification in pancreas. (From Noble J: Textbook of Primary Care Medicine, 3 rd ed. St. Louis, Mosby, 2001.)

SUMMARY BOX: ACUTE/CHRONIC PANCREATITIS

- Acute pancreatitis is classically characterized by epigastric pain radiating to the back, elevated amylase and lipase levels, leukocytosis, and low-grade fever.

- The most common cause of chronic pancreatitis is heavy consumption of alcohol and gallstones.

- Chronic pancreatitis can lead to persistent diarrhea, diabetes mellitus, fat malabsorption, and vitamin A, D, E, and K deficiencies.

CASE 6-6

A 2-week-old boy is brought to the emergency department with nonbilious, projectile vomiting that began earlier in the day.

1. **What is the differential diagnosis for projectile vomiting in a newborn?**
The differential diagnosis includes infantile hypertrophic pyloric stenosis, tracheoesophageal fistula, esophageal atresia, duodenal atresia, annular pancreas, and gastroenteritis. The most likely diagnosis in this case is infantile hypertrophic pyloric stenosis, which usually presents with nonbilious, projectile vomiting around 3 to 4 weeks of life. Tracheoesophageal fistula is an abnormal communication between the trachea and esophagus that usually presents with coughing and cyanosis during the first feeding. The fistulas typically occur at the midlevel of the esophagus, which is where the lungs bud off from the foregut during embryologic development. Esophageal atresia is another embryologic esophageal disorder in which the esophagus ends in a blind pouch, resulting in food accumulation and reflux into the airway, also causing coughing and cyanosis during the first feedings. Duodenal atresia typically presents with vomiting within the first day of life, and the vomitus tends to be bilious if the atresia occurs below where the common bile duct enters the second part of the duodenum. Finally, annular pancreas is caused by the ventral and dorsal pancreatic bud's being abnormally fused around the second part of the duodenum, which can result in duodenal obstruction and projectile vomiting within the first few days of life.

2. **What acid-base and electrolyte disorder can be caused by prolonged vomiting in this baby and how does it develop?**
Hypochloremic metabolic alkalosis. Because gastric parietal cells secrete hydrochloric acid into the lumen of the stomach, prolonged vomiting can deplete the body of both hydrogen and chloride ions. The alkalosis that develops is caused by the loss of hydrochloric acid and the simultaneous retention of the bicarbonate that is generated when the parietal cells make hydrochloric acid.

CASE 6-6 continued:

Physical examination reveals a firm, palpable olive-like mass in the epigastric region, and ultrasound reveals a thickened and elongated pylorus muscle (Fig 6-8).

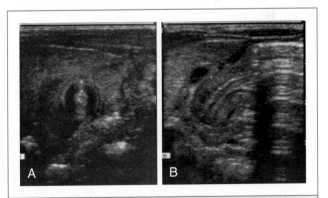

Figure 6-8. A, Transverse sonogram demonstrating a pyloric muscle wall thickness of greater than 4 mm (*distance between crosses*). **B,** Horizontal image demonstrating a pyloric channel length greater than 14 mm (*wall thickness outlined between crosses*). (From Kliegman RM, Behrman RE, Jenson HB, et al: Nelson Textbook of Pediatrics, 18th ed. Philadelphia, WB Saunders, 2007.)

3. **What is the most likely diagnosis?**

Projectile vomiting in a 2-week-old infant and the findings on physical examination and ultrasound point to the diagnosis of infantile hypertrophic pyloric stenosis.

STEP 1 SECRET

"Palpable olive-like mass" in the epigastric region is a popular buzzword for pyloric stenosis. The mass is the result of muscular hypertrophy of the pyloric sphincter.

CASE 6-6 continued:

The infant undergoes surgical pyloromyotomy. One week later, the mother returns to the physician because the infant is experiencing severe diarrhea after being breast-fed.

4. **What is the cause of the diarrhea?**

Dumping syndrome is caused by the delivery of excessive amounts of hyperosmotic chyme from the stomach to the small intestine, which may occur with a dysfunctional pyloric sphincter. The intestine is unable to "process" such a large quantity of chyme, resulting in an osmotic diarrhea, which may cause dizziness, weakness, and tachycardia following meals.

   Note: Dumping syndrome may also result following gastric bypass surgery. Because the meal is delivered to the small intestine more quickly than usual, the increased tonicity of the small intestine causes a large fluid shift into the gut lumen. This increases the motility of the small intestine and results in diarrhea. In severe cases, the luminal shift of fluid stimulates blood flow to the intestine, which decreases total blood volume. Hypotension and reflex tachycardia can result.

SUMMARY BOX: HYPERTROPHIC PYLORIC STENOSIS

- Infantile hypertrophic pyloric stenosis typically presents in 2- to 3-week-old infants with nonbilious, projectile vomiting.

- Dumping syndrome can result from a dysfunctional pyloric sphincter caused, for example, by surgical pyloromyotomy.

- Prolonged vomiting may result in a hypochloremic metabolic acidosis.

- Tracheoesophageal fistula presents with coughing and cyanosis with the first feeding.

- Duodenal atresia presents in the first day of life, demonstrates a "double-bubble" sign on radiographs, and can cause bilious vomiting. It is associated with Down syndrome.

CASE 6-7

A 33-year-old woman complains of a long history of diarrhea, flatus, and abdominal pain. More recently, she has experienced unintentional weight loss despite a preserved appetite. She has never left the United States.

1. **What is the differential diagnosis?**

The differential diagnosis includes inflammatory bowel disease (IBD), celiac disease, giardiasis, IBS, Whipple's disease, tropical sprue, disaccharidase (lactase) deficiency, and abetalipoproteinemia. From the history, IBD, giardiasis, and celiac disease are the most likely possibilities because of the chronic diarrhea, weight loss, and abdominal pain. Weight loss does not usually occur in IBS and lactose intolerance. Whipple's disease is unlikely because it typically occurs in men over the age of 40. Tropical sprue is unlikely because the patient has not traveled outside of the United States. Abetalipoproteinemia normally presents within the first few months of life; therefore, this condition is unlikely in this patient.

CASE 6-7 continued:

Physical examination is unremarkable. Stool examination for ova and parasites is negative. A complete blood count (CBC) reveals microcytic anemia. A pathology report from a small intestinal biopsy (Fig 6-9A) describes an intestinal mucosa significant for "villous atrophy, lymphocytic infiltration of the lamina propria, and hyperplastic crypts." The woman is told she has a malabsorption syndrome and is put on a special diet devoid of wheat, barley, and rice. Weeks later, a repeat biopsy shows complete resolution of mucosal damage to the small intestines (Fig. 6-9B), and she is encouraged to stay on her diet.

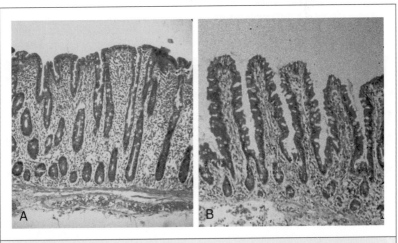

Figure 6-9. A, Duodenal biopsy specimen from patient in Case 6-7. **B,** Repeat duodenal biopsy from patient in Case 6-7 after implementation of strict gluten-free diet. (From Feldman M, Friedman LS, Brandt LJ: Sleisenger and Fordtran's Gastrointestinal and Liver Disease, 8th ed. Philadelphia, WB Saunders, 2006.)

2. **What is the likely diagnosis in this case?**

The diagnosis of celiac disease (celiac sprue or nontropical sprue) is established by resolution of mucosal damage following a gluten-free diet. Celiac disease is caused by hypersensitivity to the gliadin in gluten, which is present in wheat, barley, rice, and a multitude of processed foods. Through an unknown molecular mechanism the exposure to gliadin in a hypersensitive person causes damage to the intestinal mucosa.

3. **How is celiac disease associated with microcytic anemia in this patient?**
   Celiac disease typically affects the proximal small bowel (duodenum and jejunum), where iron and folate are absorbed. This can result in iron-deficiency (microcytic) anemia and a folate-deficiency (macrocytic) anemia. In this case, the iron malabsorption is greater than the folate, as is typically seen. Vitamin B_{12} malabsorption, which can also cause macrocytic anemia and neurologic symptoms, can occur with more severe celiac disease that affects the terminal ileum (although this is rare).

4. **How do the signs, symptoms, and intestinal biopsy findings in Whipple's disease differ from celiac disease?**
   Whipple's disease is due to infection with *Torphyrema whipelli*. It typically occurs in men over the age of 40. The signs and symptoms are fairly similar, but intestinal biopsy shows "lipid vacuolation with infiltration of PAS (periodic acid–Schiff)-positive macrophages with small bacilli" in Whipple's disease.

5. **How does celiac disease differ from tropical sprue?**
   Both these diseases have the same symptoms, but tropical sprue does not respond to a gluten-free diet. Intestinal biopsy findings are similar in both diseases, although tropical sprue affects the entire small intestine, and celiac disease mostly concentrates in the proximal small bowel. In addition, tropical sprue is most commonly found, as its name implies, in the tropics (e.g., Southeast Asia, Central and South America, Caribbean). Although an infectious organism is suspected, the precise etiology of tropical sprue remains unknown. Broad-spectrum antibiotics remain the treatment of choice for tropical sprue.

SUMMARY BOX: CELIAC DISEASE/DIARRHEA

- Celiac disease has a pseudo-autoimmune cause, but tropical sprue is infectious in origin.

- Celiac disease improves with a gluten-free diet, whereas tropical sprue does not.

- Celiac disease often causes an iron-deficiency anemia although rarely can cause folate- or B_{12}-deficient anemia.

- Whipple's disease has a similar presentation to celiac disease, although it typically occurs in men older than 40, and intestinal biopsy shows characteristic intestinal mucosa infiltrated with PAS (periodic acid–Schiff)-positive macrophages.

CASE 6–8

A 32-year-old woman, of Ashkenazi Jewish descent, complains of a long history of abdominal pain and diarrhea. On a typical day, she usually passes 15 to 20 loose stools. In the last few weeks, she has lost 15 lb and has experienced several episodes of bloody diarrhea. She denies any pain with bowel movements (tenesmus) but does complain of abdominal pain following meals.

1. **What is the differential diagnosis?**
   The differential diagnosis includes IBD (Crohn's disease and ulcerative colitis), infectious colitis (*Clostridium difficile*, *Shigella*, *Campylobacter*, *Escherichia coli*), and mesenteric ischemia. Crohn's disease and ulcerative colitis are both characterized by abdominal pain, frequent loose stools, bloody diarrhea, and weight loss. The diarrhea tends to be nonbloody in Crohn's disease if

the colon is not involved. Infectious colitis is likely if the patient has significant travel history (*Shigella, Campylobacter, E. coli*) or taken antibiotics recently (*C. difficile*). Mesenteric ischemia is more common in adults >50 years old with atherosclerotic disease. Pain is acute and usually occurs following a meal.

CASE 6-8 continued:

Physical examination is significant for mild fever as well as abdominal tenderness in the right lower quadrant (RLQ). Laboratory studies show an elevated erythrocyte sedimentation rate (ESR) as well as decreased plasma levels of vitamin B_{12}, vitamin D, and vitamin K. Lower endoscopy reveals a "cobblestone" appearance and the presence of lesions in the terminal ileum and proximal colon. Biopsy of the terminal ileum reveals granulomas and transmural chronic inflammation.

2. **What is the diagnosis?**
   The diagnosis of Crohn's disease can be made based on the patient's history of bloody diarrhea and presence of classic pathologic features of the disease, such as "cobblestone" appearance of the bowel, absence of continuous lesions along the bowel (so called "skip" lesions), granulomas, and transmural inflammation.

3. **Compare and contrast the characteristics of Crohn's disease and ulcerative colitis. Try testing yourself by covering the entries in the appropriate columns of Table 6-2 for each respective characteristic.**

TABLE 6-2. CHARACTERISTICS OF CROHN'S DISEASE AND ULCERATIVE COLITIS		
Feature	**Crohn's Disease**	**Ulcerative Colitis**
Associations	↑ Prevalence in Ashkenazi Jews (though most cases occur in non-Jews)	Patient who recently quit smoking
Location in gastrointestinal tract	Anywhere (mostly terminal ileum), spares rectum, "skip" lesions	Limited to colon, contiguous inflammation from the rectum
Wall thickness involved	Transmural inflammation, "cobblestone" appearance of mucosa	Mucosal inflammation only
Complications	Strictures, fistulas, abscess, malabsorption, ↑ risk of colon cancer	Toxic megacolon, hemorrhage, primary sclerosing cholangitis, ↑↑ risk of colon cancer
Dermatologic manifestations	Erythema nodosum	Pyoderma gangrenosum
Other non-intestinal manifestations	Arthritis, aphthous ulcers, uveitis, perianal fistulas, cholelithiasis	Uveitis

STEP 1 SECRET

Learn the information listed in Table 6-2 thoroughly. The USMLE commonly asks students to differentiate between Crohn's disease and ulcerative colitis.

4. **In what special situation does transmural inflammation of the colon occur in ulcerative colitis?**
   Transmural inflammation of the colon occurs in toxic megacolon, which is a medical emergency. Surgery (usually a colectomy with ileoanal pull-through) is required to prevent peritonitis and sepsis and restore some semblance of normal bowel activity.

5. **What congenital disorder results in constipation and a severely dilated colon (similar to toxic megacolon)? What is this disease caused by?**
   Hirschsprung's disease, also known as congenital megacolon or aganglionic megacolon, is caused by neural crest cells that form the myenteric plexus failing to migrate to the colon. The rectum is always involved because neural crest cells migrate caudally along the intestine. Rectal examination yields an absence of stool on the finger (can also be a finding with cystic fibrosis). Hirschsprung's disease is also associated with Down syndrome. Treatment of this disease involves surgical resection of the aganglionic segment.

6. **How can Crohn's disease cause deficiencies of the fat-soluble vitamins?**
   Crohn's disease commonly involves the terminal ileum, where vitamin B_{12} is absorbed. The terminal ileum is also where bile salts are reabsorbed, and because most of the bile salts secreted into the intestine are from the enterohepatic circulation, a deficiency of bile salt secretion develops. This can impair the absorption of fats and fat-soluble vitamins (A, B_{12}, D, E, and K). Surgical resection of the ileum can also cause these vitamin deficiencies.

7. **Why might cholestyramine help with this patient's diarrhea?**
   Cholestyramine is a bile acid sequestrant that binds bile salts, which are poorly absorbed in Crohn's disease and might otherwise cause colonic irritations and diarrhea upon entering the colon.

CASE 6-8 continued:

The patient is started on sulfasalazine for treatment of her active Crohn's disease.

8. **What pharmacokinetic properties of sulfasalazine make it particularly suited to treating inflammatory bowel disease?**
   Sulfasalazine is a precursor of the active compound 5-aminosalicylic acid, a nonsteroidal anti-inflammatory agent that can reduce inflammation in the bowel. However, if 5-aminosalicylic acid itself is given orally in sufficient quantities to reduce inflammation in the large bowel, significant gastric irritation will develop. Sulfasalazine avoids this problem because it is not broken down into 5-aminosalicylic acid until it reaches the distal ileum and colon. Sulfasalazine is also poorly absorbed from the GI tract, thus increasing the concentration of active drug that reaches the large bowel.

9. **What extraintestinal complication of ulcerative colitis should be suspected in a patient who presents with signs of obstructive jaundice?**
   Primary sclerosing cholangitis, which is caused by fibrosis of the large bile ducts, is a rare complication associated with both ulcerative colitis and Crohn's disease. For boards, associate primary sclerosing cholangitis with ulcerative colitis.

CASE 6-8 continued:

Several years later, the patient is seen by her physician for progressively worsening lower back pain. X-ray films of the pelvis and lumbar spine are shown in Figure 6-10.

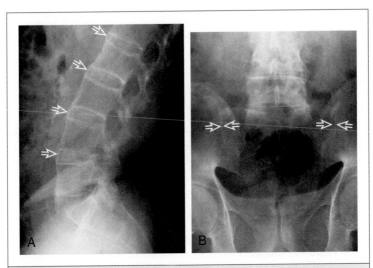

Figure 6-10. Ankylosing spondylitis. **A,** A lateral view of the lumbar spine demonstrates calcific bridging across the disk spaces (*arrows*), causing the typical "bamboo spine" appearance. **B,** Anteroposterior view of the pelvis shows that the region of the sacroiliac joints (*arrows*) is not easily visualized owing to fusion of both sacroiliac joints. (From Mettler FA: Essentials of Radiology, 2nd ed. Philadelphia, WB Saunders, 2005.)

10. **What extraintestinal complication of inflammatory bowel disease should be suspected?**
    Ankylosing spondylitis, with the characteristic "bamboo spine" appearance and bilateral sacroiliitis, is more commonly associated with Crohn's disease than with ulcerative colitis.

11. **Will a complete colectomy alleviate the extraintestinal complications of inflammatory bowel disease?**
    No. The extraintestinal manifestations (i.e., arthritis, sclerosing cholangitis) often persist.

SUMMARY BOX: INFLAMMATORY BOWEL DISEASE

- Abdominal pain, bloody (or mucous) diarrhea, and unintentional weight loss are characteristic of inflammatory bowel disease (IBD) (Crohn's disease and ulcerative colitis).

- Crohn's disease has a higher prevalence among Ashkenazi Jews.

- Ulcerative colitis might occur after a person *stops* smoking.

- Crohn's disease most commonly involves the terminal ileum but can affect any part of the gastrointestinal tract. It is associated with "skip" lesions, transmural inflammation, and cobblestone appearance.

- Ulcerative colitis causes a continuous lesion that occurs only in the colon and affects the mucosa and submucosa (is not transmural). It is associated with diffuse ascending inflammation from the rectum and pseudopolyp formation.

- Generally, sulfasalazine is used for initial treatment for IBD.

- Bile salts can cause diarrhea in two ways: (1) secondary to their secretory effect on the colon or (2) malabsorption caused by their depletion from the enterohepatic circulation.

CASE 6-9

A 13-year-old girl with a history of ovarian cysts is brought to the emergency department because of severe abdominal pain. She was awakened from sleep several hours earlier with pain that she now complains is in the right lower abdomen. She also complains of nausea and loss of appetite.

1. **What is the differential diagnosis?**
   The differential diagnosis includes acute appendicitis, ovarian torsion, ruptured ovarian cyst, ectopic pregnancy, pelvic inflammatory disease (PID), *Yersinia enterocolitis*, acute onset of IBD, Meckel's diverticulitis, and right-sided diverticulitis. In this girl, with a history of ovarian cysts, ruptured ovarian cysts or ovarian torsion are on the top of the differential list. Acute appendicitis should also be considered in any person with RLQ abdominal pain. Ectopic pregnancy would also warrant investigation with a pregnancy test. Right-sided diverticulitis would be unlikely in a girl this young.

CASE 6-9 continued:

Examination is significant for a temperature of 100.2° F, and the patient's abdomen is tender at McBurney's point. Laboratory workup reveals a mild leukocytosis and a negative β-hCG (human chorionic gonadotropin). A pelvic ultrasound reveals a small ovarian cyst on the left ovary but adequate blood flow to both ovaries. A computed tomography (CT) scan reveals a thickened and inflamed appendix (Fig. 6-11).

2. **What is the diagnosis?**
   Although the patient's initial presentation may be suggestive of ovarian torsion or a ruptured ovarian cyst, the physical examination findings and the CT scan confirmed the diagnosis of acute appendicitis.

3. **What is the most common cause of appendicitis?**
   Appendicitis is most often caused by obstruction of the lumen of the appendix, most commonly by a fecalith, but obstruction can also be due to lymphoid hyperplasia, tumors, or an intestinal stricture. Obstruction of the appendix lumen leads to bacterial overgrowth and acute inflammation. Polymorphonuclear cells (PMNs) are seen in the wall of the appendix.

4. **Note that Meckel's diverticulitis can present similarly to appendicitis. What is its pathophysiology?**
   Most Meckel's diverticula are an asymptomatic, embryologic remnant that connected the lumen of the developing gut to the yolk sac in the developing embryo. About 50% of these diverticula are lined with heterotopic gastric or pancreatic tissue. The gastric mucosa can secrete acid, eventually creating adjacent intestinal ulcerations that can bleed and cause pain that mimics acute appendicitis. Alternatively, diverticula can lead to intussusception, incarceration, or perforation.

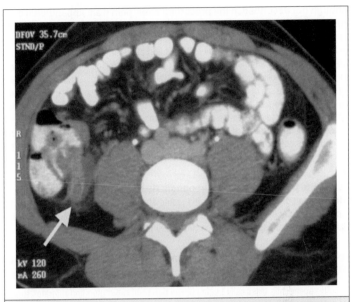

Figure 6-11. Computed tomographic scan showing acute appendicitis. The appendix is edematous, and there is surrounding stranding of the mesenteric fat (*arrow*). (From Goldman L, Ausiello D: Cecil Textbook of Medicine, 22nd ed. Philadelphia, WB Saunders, 2004.)

Note: Recall the law of the "three 2s" pertaining to Meckel's diverticulum: it affects about 2% of the population, is about 2 inches long, and is located about 2 feet from the ileocecal valve.

CASE 6-9 continued:

The patient is taken to the operating room for a laparoscopic appendectomy and returns home the same day.

5. What type of cancer of the appendix is occasionally seen as an incidental finding during an appendectomy? What substance do these tumors secrete and what syndrome can it cause?
    Carcinoid tumors secrete large quantities of serotonin, resulting in elevated levels of 5-hydroxyindoleacetic acid (5-HIAA), which can be easily detected. Intestinal carcinoid tumors that metastasize to the liver can cause a carcinoid syndrome, which is a constellation of symptoms including episodic flushing, diarrhea, wheezing, and right-sided heart valve lesions (serotonin is degraded by monoamine oxidase [MAO] in the lungs, so it is unable to reach the left side of the heart). Hepatic metastases are necessary for this syndrome to occur with intestinal carcinoid tumors because the liver would otherwise metabolize serotonin and other biogenic amines as they pass through the liver from the intestines.
    Note: The appendix is the most common site of gut carcinoid tumor.

STEP 1 SECRET

Carcinoid syndrome is a favorite on boards. It refers to a tumor of neuroendocrine cells and is associated with the symptoms of wheezing, diarrhea, flushing, and right-sided heart murmurs that increase on inspiration.

6. **Although not described in the preceding case, pain from appendicitis classically begins around the umbilicus and migrates to the right lower quadrant. What is the neuroanatomic basis for this pattern?**
The initial pain from appendicitis is due to activation of visceral pain receptors in the inflamed appendix and *visceral peritoneum*. The sensory nerves that carry this information synapse on spinal neurons that also receive sensory signals from the anterior abdominal wall in the periumbilical area. Because the origin of the signal cannot be discerned, the brain misinterprets the visceral pain as a poorly localized pain arising from the periumbilical area (T10 dermatome). Later, when the *parietal peritoneum* adjacent to the appendix becomes inflamed, the pain becomes sharper and is more accurately localized to the RLQ by somatic pain fibers. This exact position is referred to as McBurney's point, which is located two thirds of the distance between the umbilicus and the iliac crest. You should know this reference point for boards *and* for your clinical years.

7. **What is the principal danger if appendicitis remains untreated?**
Perforation can occur, causing peritonitis (acute abdomen) and possibly abdominal abscess formation. Perforation may be detected by the presence of free air on an abdominal x-ray study or as air under the hemidiaphragm on a chest x-ray film.

SUMMARY BOX: APPENDICITIS

- Pain from appendicitis classically begins in the periumbilical region and migrates to the right lower quadrant (RLQ). Patients are typically anorexic and may have nausea, vomiting, and a low-grade fever.

- Remember that many different diseases can present similarly to acute appendicitis (see previous text discussion of differential diagnosis).

- Gastric mucosa can be present in Meckel's diverticulum as heterotopic gastric tissue and cause symptoms similar to those of acute appendicitis.

- Know the "three 2s" for Meckel's diverticulum: 2% of population, 2 inches long, and 2 feet from ileocecal valve.

- Carcinoid syndrome causes flushing, diarrhea, bronchospasm, and right-sided heart lesions.

CASE 6-10

A 50-year-old man visits the doctor with a history of severe colicky abdominal pain, vomiting, and constipation. Past medical history is unremarkable with the exception of appendectomy 6 years prior.

1. **What is the differential diagnosis for this patient's condition?**
This presentation is classic for small bowel obstruction. General causes of bowel obstruction include surgical adhesions, hernia, tumor, volvulus, intussusception, Crohn's disease, gallstone ileus, stricture, congenital malformation, and enteritis.

2. **What is the cause of this patient's condition?**
Given this patient's past surgical history of appendectomy and otherwise unremarkable medical history, a surgical adhesion is the most likely diagnosis. Adhesions are fibrous bands that form after injury during surgery. They connect organs and tissues that are otherwise not normally

connected. Abdominal adhesions can result in small bowel obstruction if they tug on or kink the bowel and prevent the passage of bowel contents.

3. **What would be expected on abdominal auscultation in this patient?**
   High-pitched, tinkling bowel sounds are generally heard with a small bowel obstruction.

STEP 1 SECRET

You may be given a multimedia question with a finding of tinkling bowel sounds on abdominal examination. Associate this with small bowel obstruction and use the medical history to prioritize your differential diagnosis.

SUMMARY BOX: SURGICAL ADHESIONS AND SMALL BOWEL OBSTRUCTION

- Surgical adhesions are a common cause of small bowel obstruction. Adhesions are fibrous bands that form after surgical injury and join two organs or tissues that are not normally connected.

- Symptoms of small bowel obstruction include colicky abdominal pain, abdominal distention, vomiting, constipation, and an inability to pass gas with severe obstruction.

- Physical examination of a patient who presents with small bowel obstruction may reveal a high-pitched tinkling sound on auscultation of the abdomen.

CHAPTER 7

HEPATOLOGY

Eric B. Roth, Thomas A. Brown, MD, and Sonali J. Shah

INSIDER'S GUIDE TO HEPATOLOGY FOR THE USMLE STEP 1

Many medical students struggle with hepatology on the USMLE Step 1, and understandably so. Although a fair number of questions will be straightforward, certain hepatology-related topics on boards will demand that you make fine distinctions between various clinical findings and laboratory results to arrive at the correct diagnosis. Some of these high-yield details are covered but not explained well in First Aid. Not surprisingly, the students who do best on hepatology are the ones who know how to analyze (and not just memorize) these details. Therefore, it is our goal to teach you how to approach confusing hepatology-related topics within this chapter. For those of you looking to turn hepatology into a strength on test day, we suggest the following approach: Read through the First Aid section and then study this chapter carefully. You should then go back and thoroughly study First Aid again, but this time, you should annotate your copy of First Aid with notes from this chapter. Be sure to include detailed information from the subjects we have laid out in boxes within this chapter. This will prepare you to tackle hepatology on Step 1.

BASIC CONCEPTS

1. **Review the anatomy of the hepatic lobule and portal triad. In what manner do blood and bile flow through a lobule?**

   A central hepatic vein is located at the center of each hepatic lobule. Multiple portal triads (hepatic artery, portal venule, bile duct) surround this central vein. Hepatocytes are arranged in sheets of single-cell thickness and are surrounded by blood-filled sinusoids. Blood flows from the hepatic artery and portal vein toward the central vein through the sinusoids. Bile is formed by the hepatocytes and emptied into bile canuliculi in the lateral wall of the hepatocyte. The bile flows from here toward the bile ducts (Fig. 7-1).

   Blood flows from the portal triad toward the central vein, and bile flows from the hepatocytes toward the portal triads.

   Knowing the structure of the hepatic lobule is clinically relevant. The hepatocytes located near the portal triad (zone 1) are closest to the oxygenated blood supply and are thus the first cells affected by toxins that reach the liver via the bloodstream. On the other hand, hepatocytes closest to the central vein (zone 3) are the furthest from the oxygenated blood supply of the lobule and are thus the first cells affected by ischemia.

2. **What is the chemical difference between conjugated and unconjugated bilirubin and how are these substances formed?**

   Bilirubin is a breakdown product of the heme moiety found in red blood cells (RBCs), bone marrow, liver, and mitochondrial cytochrome enzymes. Unconjugated bilirubin is the breakdown

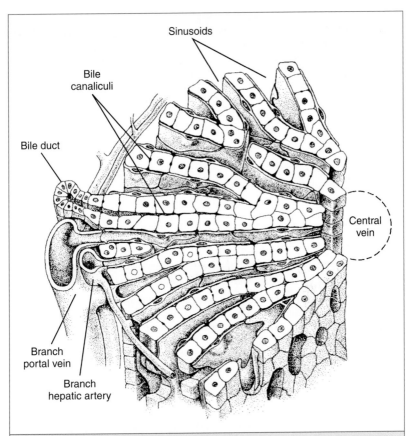

Figure 7-1. Diagrammatic representation of a hepatic lobule. A central vein is located in the center of the lobule, with plates of hepatocytes disposed radially. Branches of the portal vein and hepatic artery are located on the periphery of the lobule, and blood from both perfuses the sinusoids. Peripherally located bile ducts drain the bile canaliculi that run between the hepatocytes. (From Bloom W, Fawcett DW: A Textbook of Histology, 10th ed. Philadelphia, 1975, WB Saunders.)

product formed in the peripheral tissues. Conjugated bilirubin then is formed in the liver by *conjugating* glucuronic acid to bilirubin to make it more soluble.

Note: Jaundice is a yellowish discoloration of the skin, mucus membranes, and sclera due to elevated levels of either conjugated (direct) or unconjugated (indirect) bilirubin.

3. **Why is unconjugated bilirubin not normally excreted in the urine?**
   Unconjugated bilirubin is hydrophobic and circulates bound to albumin. Albumin, a negatively charged protein, cannot cross a healthy glomerular basement membrane because the glycosaminoglycans that form this membrane are negatively charged and repel the albumin.

4. **What are the main causes of jaundice and how does each affect the type of hyperbilirubinemia observed?**
   See Table 7-1 for the causes of jaundice and the characteristics of each.

TABLE 7-1. CAUSES OF JAUNDICE

Jaundice Type	Hyperbilirubinemia	Urine Bilirubin Levels	Urobilinogen Formation	Urine and Stool Color
Hemolytic	Unconjugated (<20% conjugated bilirubin)	↓↓	↑	Normal
Hepatocellular	Conjugated/unconjugated (20-50% conjugated bilirubin)	↑	↓	Normal
Obstructive	Conjugated	↑	↓	Normal urine, clay-colored feces

STEP 1 SECRET

You should be able to differentiate between the causes and presentations of conjugated and unconjugated hyperbilirubinemias shown in Table 7-1. This is a commonly tested principle on boards. For those of you who do not fully understand the details of Table 7-1, we have provided our handy approach to reasoning through the causes of jaundice.

Secret to Diagnosing Common Causes of Jaundice

For those of you who still struggle with this concept, we will attempt to explain our easy method for approaching evaluation of jaundice. In order to understand jaundice, you must first understand the pathway of bilirubin formation and excretion. Red blood cell (RBC) breakdown leads to the formation of unconjugated bilirubin, which is bound to albumin in the bloodstream. This unconjugated bilirubin is referred to as indirect bilirubin and is water-insoluble (therefore, it cannot be excreted into urine). The indirect bilirubin is then taken up by the liver and conjugated to glucuronic acid by the enzyme uridine diphosphate (UDP) glucuronyltransferase. This forms a water-soluble product called direct bilirubin. Direct bilirubin is then excreted into the bile that is formed in the liver. Bile itself is composed of bile salts, bilirubin, phospholipids, cholesterol, electrolytes, and water. It is stored in the gallbladder, where it is concentrated. When bile is secreted into the gut lumen, the conjugated bilirubin is deconjugated by bacterial flora into urobilinogen. Urobilinogen has three possible fates: (1) it is excreted into feces, where it gives the characteristic brown color of stool; (2) it returns to the liver via the enterohepatic circulation; or (3) it is reabsorbed via the systemic circulation and excreted by the kidney, giving the characteristic color of urine.

Now that you have the background on bilirubin formation and excretion, we can begin to explore the causes of jaundice. Jaundice may be the result of any abnormality along the aforementioned pathway. It can therefore occur as a result of (1) excessive bilirubin production, (2) decreased hepatic uptake or conjugation of indirect bilirubin, (3) decreased hepatocellular secretion of bilirubin into bile, or (4) impaired or obstructed bile flow. If this makes sense to you, it becomes very formulaic to tease apart the various causes of jaundice. All you have to do is match the various causes of jaundice listed in Table 7-1 to these basic mechanisms.

Let's start with increased bilirubin production (item 1 in our preceding list). The most notable cause of increased bilirubin production is hemolytic jaundice, which leads to an unconjugated hyperbilirubinemia. Why does this occur? Hemolysis refers to accelerated breakdown of RBCs, which rapidly increases indirect bilirubin levels in the bloodstream. The liver, which must uptake and conjugate all of this bilirubin, has trouble keeping up with the rapid rate of bilirubin production.

As a result, indirect bilirubin levels increase in the bloodstream. Do not confuse this with hepatocellular jaundice. The liver, in this case, is perfectly functional! It can uptake and conjugate bilirubin, but it cannot do so at the required pace. In fact, absolute amounts of conjugated bilirubin and urobilinogen increase above normal because of the increased production and conjugation of indirect bilirubin. The bilirubin that is conjugated is responsible for maintaining urobilinogen concentrations in urine and feces. Thus, both are normally colored.

Decreased hepatic uptake and conjugation of bilirubin (items 2 and 3 in our list) are additional causes of jaundice. Consider a scenario in which the liver does not function normally, such as viral hepatitis. This leads to hepatocellular jaundice because the "sick" liver is unable to perform its normal task of conjugating bilirubin. Some bilirubin will be conjugated (thus maintaining the normal color of urine and feces), but indirect bilirubin levels will also increase above normal. Note that conjugated bilirubin in the liver also leaks out into the bloodstream through the damaged hepatic tissue. It is *never* normal to see bilirubin (whether indirect or direct) in the bloodstream. If this finding appears on laboratory tests, it is a red flag for disease.

The final cause of jaundice mentioned in Table 7-1 is obstructive jaundice. Obstructive jaundice results when conjugated bilirubin is unable to be excreted into the gut either due to impaired liver secretion of bile (see item 3) or impaired bile flow (see item 4). The most common cause of obstructive jaundice is bile duct obstruction (e.g., gallstones, pancreatic tumor). Although conjugated bilirubin is produced and secreted into bile, the bile is unable to be secreted into the gut lumen due to an obstruction in the bile duct system. Bile backs up into the liver, causing engorgement and rupture of intrahepatic ducts. This leads to spillage of conjugated bilirubin into sinusoidal blood and, ultimately, the systemic circulation. Thus, conjugated bilirubin levels become elevated while urobilinogen levels decrease due to inadequate concentrations of conjugated bilirubin in the gut lumen. Urine color remains normal (conjugated bilirubin in the systemic circulation is water soluble and can be excreted by the kidneys), but stool becomes clay-colored due to lack of urobilinogen excretion into feces.

Now that you have a better understanding of the causes of jaundice, revisit Table 7-1 and attempt to fill it in on your own.

5. **Which veins feed into the portal vein?**

   Venous return from the foregut, midgut, and hindgut feeds into the portal vein from the gastric veins, splenic vein, and superior and inferior mesenteric veins. Consequently, portal hypertension can cause venous congestion in any and all of these vascular beds (e.g., congestive splenomegaly from splenic vein, esophageal varices from gastric veins).

6. **What are the symptoms of portal hypertension?**

   Portal hypertension leads to increased resistance to flow in the systemic venous system. As a result, blood cannot pass freely from the portal system to the systemic system and backs up into the portacaval anastomoses, which causes them to become engorged, dilated, or varicose. The location of these anastomoses determines the specific symptoms that result from portal hypertension. These symptoms and signs are listed in Table 7-2. General symptoms of portal hypertension include ascites (secondary to increased hydrostatic pressure), spontaneous bacterial peritonitis (note that ascitic fluid is a wonderful culture medium for bacteria), hepatorenal syndrome, and splenomegaly due to decreased drainage of venous blood from the spleen. Splenomegaly can result in anemia, thrombocytopenia, or pancytopenia due to cellular sequestration within the engorged spleen.

   Note: Portal hypertension results from prehepatic, intrahepatic, and posthepatic causes. Cirrhosis is a common cause of intrahepatic portal hypertension, while portal vein thrombosis is a prehepatic cause. Right-sided heart failure and Budd-Chiari syndrome (see next question) are common precursors to posthepatic portal hypertension.

TABLE 7-2.   PORTAL HYPERTENSION: ANASTOMOSES AND RELATED SIGNS

Portacaval Anastomosis	Clinical Sign
Left gastric vein with esophageal vein (branch of azygos vein)	Esophageal varices (leading to heavy bleeding/hematemesis)
Paraumbilical vein with epigastric vessels	Caput medusae
Superior rectal vein with middle and inferior rectal veins	Internal hemorrhoids (unlike external hemorrhoids, these are not painful because the visceral nerves that are above the dentate line sense pressure and not pain)

STEP 1 SECRET

You should memorize each portacaval anastomosis and the symptoms that result from portal hypertension.

7. **How can Budd-Chiari syndrome arise and what can it lead to?**
   Budd-Chiari syndrome occurs when the hepatic venous outflow becomes obstructed, usually because of thrombosis. Polycythemia vera, pregnancy, and clotting disorders predispose to thrombus formation and can lead to hepatic venous outflow obstruction. The obstruction may result in portal hypertension with a classic presentation of abdominal pain, ascites, and hepatomegaly. Although this may be confused with right-sided heart failure, Budd-Chiari syndrome does *not* cause jugular venous distention because it affects only the inferior vena cava.

8. **What are the common liver biochemical tests and what do they indicate?**
   The most common laboratory tests ordered are the aminotransferases (alanine transaminase [ALT], aspartate transaminase [AST]), alkaline phosphatase (ALP), γ-glutamyl transpeptidase (GGTP), bilirubin, prothrombin time (PT), and albumin. Serum protein concentration and PT tests evaluate synthetic function of the liver because albumin (the predominant serum protein) and clotting factors are manufactured by hepatocytes. PT, in particular, is not generally elevated until severe liver disease has occurred. Serum bilirubin concentration is used to evaluate functional clearance by the liver. ALT, AST, ALP, and GGTP more accurately reflect liver injury. Serum elevations in ALT and AST result from leakage of these enzymes from damage to hepatocytes. ALT is generally elevated more than AST with viral infection, but AST is elevated more than ALT with alcohol abuse. Serum elevations in ALP and GGTP are seen when increased production of these enzymes are induced by bile duct damage. ALP is less specific for bile duct/liver damage than GGTP, as it is often elevated during bone remodeling. Both ALP and GGTP levels should be obtained if bile duct damage is suspected. GGTP levels are also elevated with alcohol abuse because it is a marker of mitochondrial damage. As a general rule of thumb, ALT and AST show greater elevation in hepatitis, and ALP and GGTP show greater elevation in cholestatic disease.

STEP 1 SECRET

It is expected that you know the significance of abnormal liver function test (LFT) results for boards and for your clinical years. A silly trick for remembering that alanine transaminase (ALT) is elevated with viral hepatitis is to picture the **ALT** key on the keyboard of a **VIRALLY** infected computer.

CASE 7-1

You are working in the emergency department when a man presents at 5 AM vomiting blood (hematemesis). At first glance, you can see that his mental status is impaired, his skin is jaundiced, and he has scleral icterus. Because you recognize him as the man you frequently see drinking from a brown paper bag in the park, you think you know why he is here.

1. **What is the most common cause of upper gastrointestinal bleeding?**
   The most common causes of upper gastrointestinal (GI) bleeding are ulcers or erosions. These can occur in the esophagus, stomach, or duodenum and develop when acid secretion overruns protective factors (mucus and bicarbonate secretion). Infection with *Helicobacter pylori*, nonsteroidal anti-inflammatory drug (NSAID) use, and cigarette smoking all disrupt the protective factors. In other cases, there is hypersecretion of gastric acid, such as seen in Zollinger-Ellison syndrome (gastrinoma). Other causes of upper GI bleeding include Mallory-Weiss tear and ruptured esophageal or gastric varices.

2. **Why should a Mallory-Weiss tear be included in the differential diagnosis?**
   Mallory-Weiss tears are seen most commonly in alcoholics, and are due to excessive vomiting that causes mucosal lacerations that extend through the gastroesophageal junction. It is another common cause of hematemesis in alcoholics or people with conditions causing excessive vomiting (e.g., bulimia). However, Mallory-Weiss tears do not typically cause massive hematemesis like that seen with ruptured esophageal varices.

3. **What is scleral icterus?**
   Scleral icterus is yellow discoloration (icterus) seen in the "whites of the eye" (sclerae). It is an indication of increased unconjugated bilirubin in the serum, and is often the first place you will see jaundice on physical examination. Jaundice usually indicates hepatic or cholestatic pathology but may indicate bleeding or hemolysis.
   Note: Vitamin A toxicity can cause yellow discoloration of the skin, which is distinct from the scleral icterus observed with jaundice.

4. **To confirm your suspicion about severe liver disease in this patient, what physical examination findings might you expect and why?**
   Gynecomastia and testicular atrophy can be present, resulting from impaired ability of the damaged liver to metabolize estrogen. Estrogen also weakens vascular walls, leading to spider angiomata with increased estrogen levels. Hemorrhoids may result from a portacaval anastomosis between the superior rectal vein and the inferior rectal vein, and a caput medusae (engorged veins radiating from the umbilicus) can result from blood being diverted from the portal vein into the periumbilical veins that run along the round ligament of the liver to the anterior abdominal wall (see Table 7-2). An enlarged liver may be palpated with alcoholic hepatitis, but once cirrhosis develops, the liver will become firm and shrunken. A spleen tip may be palpable, as congestive splenomegaly may occur with portal hypertension because the splenic vein drains into the portal vein.

CASE 7-1 continued:

On examination you do indeed find spider angiomata on his face and thorax, gynecomastia, and a periumbilical caput medusae. His abdomen is distended, his spleen is enlarged, he has pedal and periorbital edema, and his breath has a sweet, ammoniacal odor (fetor hepaticus).

5. **What is the pathophysiology of his ascites, pedal edema, and periorbital edema?**
   In severe liver disease there is inadequate production of serum albumin, the major determinant of plasma oncotic pressure. Consequently, fluid reabsorption from the interstitium back into the capillary beds is reduced. This explains his pedal and periorbital edema. In addition to the reduced capillary oncotic pressure, the increased venous pressure in the portal system from

portal hypertension causes greater intracapillary hydrostatic pressure, which opposes movement of fluid from the interstitium into the capillaries and results in ascites.

6. **What is the pathogenesis of the suspected cause of hematemesis in this patient?**
    He most likely has ruptured esophageal varices (see Table 7-2). This patient has portal hypertension secondary to alcohol-induced cirrhosis. This creates portacaval anastomoses, in which the pressure in the portal venous system diverts blood from the portal system into the systemic circulation at sites where there are anastomoses. In this patient's case, blood from the gastric veins backed up into his esophageal tributaries, which became distended and eventually ruptured (Fig. 7-2).
    Note: The round ligament of the liver (ligamentum teres hepatica) is an embryologic remnant of the umbilical vein. The major morphologic characteristics of cirrhosis are extensive fibrosis with nodules of regenerating hepatocytes.

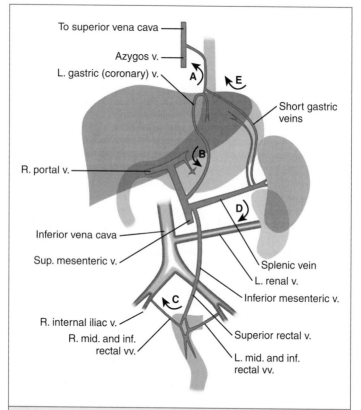

Figure 7-2. Diagram of the portal circulation. The most important sites for the potential development of portosystemic collaterals are shown. **A,** Esophageal submucosal veins, which are supplied by the left gastric vein and drain into the superior vena cava via the azygous vein. **B,** Paraumbilical veins, which are supplied by the umbilical portion of the left portal vein and drain into abdominal wall veins near the umbilicus. These veins may form a caput medusae at the umbilicus. **C,** Rectal submucosal veins, which are supplied by the inferior mesenteric vein through the superior rectal vein and drain into the internal iliac veins through the middle (*mid.*) and inferior (*inf.*) rectal veins. **D,** Splenorenal shunts, which are created spontaneously or surgically. **E,** Short gastric veins, which are supplied by the esophageal submucosal veins and drain into the splenic vein. (From Feldman M, Friedman LS, Brandt LJ: Sleisenger & Fordtran's Gastrointestinal and Liver Disease, 8th ed. Philadelphia, WB Saunders, 2006.)

CASE 7-1 continued:

When an intravenous (IV) line is started to administer fluids, a fairly large hematoma develops at the IV site. Laboratory tests reveal an elevated direct bilirubin, indirect bilirubin, and PT; low blood urea nitrogen (BUN); and a normal creatinine level. Serologic tests for hepatitis B and C, as well as antimitochondrial antibodies, are negative. Serum iron, transferrin, iron saturation (%), ferritin, and ceruloplasmin are all within normal limits.

7. **What is the value of the following tests: hepatitis serology, serum iron, ceruloplasmin, and antimitochondrial antibodies?**
   These tests all identify different causes of liver cirrhosis. Hepatitis B and C both can cause liver cirrhosis, as can hemochromatosis (too much iron), Wilson's disease (too much copper), and primary biliary cirrhosis (antimitochondrial antibodies).
   Note: All of the above-listed causes of liver cirrhosis increase the risk for hepatocellular carcinoma (HCC), as do α_1-antitrypsin deficiency and aflatoxin exposure.

8. **Assuming he is not taking any anticoagulants, what is the most likely reason this patient developed a large hematoma at the intravenous site?**
   The liver is where most of the clotting factors are produced, and some (factors I, II, VII, IX, X) are modified post-translationally. Severe liver disease impairs their production and processing, producing a coagulopathy. Notice that his PT was elevated because of this.

9. **List all the laboratory findings you would expect in a patient with liver failure.**
   See Table 7-3 for the laboratory findings in liver failure and their underlying mechanisms.

TABLE 7-3.	COMMON FINDINGS IN PATIENTS WITH LIVER FAILURE
Laboratory Value	**Mechanism**
Elevated or normal LFT values	Liver enzymes may be elevated during initial damage, but if cirrhosis is present or the liver shrinks over time, liver enzyme levels may appear normal in the context of decreased hepatic tissue.
Elevated PT	The liver is the site of coagulation factor production. With severe liver damage, PT becomes elevated.
Elevated serum bilirubin concentration	The liver is responsible for bilirubin uptake. Liver failure causes a spike in serum bilirubin concentration due to decreased hepatic uptake.
Hypoalbuminemia	The liver is the predominant site of albumin production. Decreased serum protein concentration may clinically manifest as ascites.
Fasting hypoglycemia	Impaired gluconeogenesis and glycogenolysis during fasting.
Elevated estrogen levels	The liver is the site of estrogen breakdown. Liver damage elevates estrogen levels, which can lead to testicular atrophy and formation of spider angiomata.

Continued

TABLE 7-3. COMMON FINDINGS IN PATIENTS WITH LIVER FAILURE—continued

Laboratory Value	Mechanism
Elevated ammonia levels with decreased BUN	The liver produces the enzymes involved in the urea cycle, which converts ammonia to urea. Elevated ammonia levels can result in hepatic encephalopathy, marked by confusion, loss of consciousness, asterixis, irritability, tremor, and coma. Increased ammonia also can result in fetor hepaticus ("breath of the dead"), which is characteristic of liver disease.

ADH, antidiuretic hormone; BUN, blood urea nitrogen; LFT, liver function test; PT, prothrombin time.

10. **Would you expect the ascitic fluid to be a transudate or an exudate?**
A transudate develops as a result of fluid moving across a membrane as a result of hemodynamic forces. Because there is no alteration in the permeability of the membranes that the fluid is moving across, the fluid that accumulates has low protein content. In contrast, exudates are fluid collections that develop because of alterations in membrane/vessel permeability, so proteins and cells accumulate in these fluid collections. Because this ascites is caused by lowered oncotic pressure (secondary to hypoalbuminemia) and portal hypertension, both of which alter hemodynamic forces but not vessel permeability, the result is a transudate. Table 7-4 lists the differences between transudates and exudates.

STEP 1 SECRET

Transudates and exudates can both result in edema. You should know the difference between transudates and exudates and the causes of each. These comparisons are listed for you in Table 7-4.

11. **How does liver cirrhosis cause the following abnormalities?**
A. Unconjugated and conjugated hyperbilirubinemia
Because there are fewer functional hepatocytes there is a reduced ability to take up and conjugate bilirubin, which results in an unconjugated hyperbilirubinemia. Additionally, bilirubin that is conjugated may leak back into the bloodstream due to hepatocyte damage. This concept is explained in further detail later in the chapter.
B. Reduced blood urea nitrogen, fetor hepaticus, and mental status abnormalities
The liver is a major site of amino acid metabolism and is the site of the urea cycle. Reduced output of the urea cycle because of hepatocyte destruction results in a lower BUN. Because the urea cycle is also the major site of ammonia detoxification, elevated blood ammonia levels become detectable as a sweet odor in the breath (fetor hepaticus). The elevated blood ammonia, which can enter the brain, can alter cerebral metabolism and contribute to confusion (hepatic encephalopathy) (see Table 7-3).

TABLE 7-4. TRANSUDATES VERSUS EXUDATES

Fluid Type	Mechanism	Common Causes	Characteristics
Transudate	Disturbances of hydrostatic or oncotic pressures	Nephrotic syndrome Liver failure CHF	Clear fluid, protein-poor, specific gravity <1.012, fluid [LDH]/plasma [LDH] ratio <0.6, often results in pitting edema
Exudate	Increased vessel permeability; often mediated by acute-phase cytokines	Inflammation Septic shock	Cloudy fluid, protein-rich, specific gravity >1.020, fluid [LDH]/plasma [LDH] ratio >0.6

CHF, congestive heart failure; LDH, lactate dehydrogenase.

12. **How can an acute alcohol binge cause a fatty liver to develop?**
This is also called hepatic steatosis and results from the shunting of substrates to lipid biosynthesis, impaired secretion of lipoproteins from the liver, and increased peripheral catabolism of fat. It is reversible.

13. **How does chronic alcohol consumption lead to a more rapid catabolism of ingested alcohol?**
Alcohol can be degraded by two separate metabolic pathways, as shown in Figure 7-3.
    The pathway that begins with alcohol dehydrogenase (ADH), in the cytosol of most tissues, is constitutively active and can only metabolize a fixed amount of alcohol. Individuals who do not abuse alcohol rely principally on this pathway for metabolism. In contrast, the microsomal ethanol-oxidizing system (MEOS) pathway begins in liver microsomes with enzymes that are

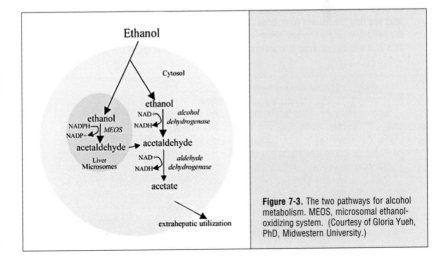

Figure 7-3. The two pathways for alcohol metabolism. MEOS, microsomal ethanol-oxidizing system. (Courtesy of Gloria Yueh, PhD, Midwestern University.)

induced by alcohol and other drugs. Such induction enhances the capacity to metabolize ethanol. In alcoholics, the MEOS pathway is substantially upregulated.

14. **Why are ethanol and fomepizole used to treat methanol poisoning and ethylene glycol poisoning?**
Methanol and ethylene glycol are metabolized through the same pathway as ethanol, and the intermediate substances that are formed in this process (formaldehyde from methanol and oxalic acid from ethylene glycol) are very toxic. Alcohol competes with both methanol and ethylene glycol for metabolism by ADH, thereby reducing the rate of formation of the toxic metabolites. Fomepizole further inhibits conversion of methanol or ethylene glycol to their toxic intermediates by directly inhibiting ADH.

SUMMARY BOX: ALCOHOLIC HEPATITIS AND RUPTURED ESOPHAGEAL VARICES

- The pathogenesis of hepatic damage in chronic alcohol abuse is poorly understood, but the result is often hepatic cirrhosis and portal hypertension.

- Alcoholic steatohepatitis (fatty liver) is initially reversible but can progress to cirrhosis with continued alcohol abuse. Cirrhosis is irreversible.

- Ruptured esophageal varices and Mallory-Weiss tears are uncommon in the general population but are often associated with alcoholic liver disease.

- Ascitic fluid resulting from portal hypertension is a transudate. It has a low protein concentration and results from alterations in hemodynamic forces. Exudates have higher protein content and result from alterations in vessel permeability, and most commonly result from infection.

- Hepatic encephalopathy is in part caused by increased levels of plasma ammonia. Because dietary protein increases production of ammonia, patients with cirrhosis may be placed on a low-protein diet to minimize the risk of hepatic encephalopathy.

CASE 7-2

The third-year medical student that you are supervising in your primary care clinic does the initial history and annual physical examination on an 18-year-old man. The student tells you that the patient complains only of malaise and anorexia. On physical examination, the patient is jaundiced and has golden brown rings at the limbus of the cornea (Fig. 7-4). This reminds the student of a disease for which she cannot recall the name.

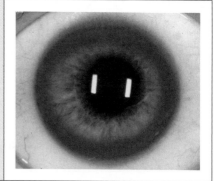

Figure 7-4. Ocular examination of patient in Case 7-2. (From Goldman L, Ausiello D: Cecil Textbook of Medicine, 22nd ed. Philadelphia, WB Saunders, 2004.)

1. **To what disease is the student referring?**
In Wilson's disease (hepatolenticular degeneration) the golden brown corneal deposits (typically seen through slit-lamp examination of the eyes) are termed Kayser-Fleischer rings and result from copper deposition in the corneal limbus.

2. **What laboratory tests and further physical examination components would you like to do to strengthen your suspicion for this disease?**
In addition to hepatic enzymes, you will want to order a serum ceruloplasmin, total serum copper, free copper, and urine copper. A slit-lamp examination would help confirm the suspected eye abnormality.

CASE 7–2 continued:

Laboratory workup reveals reduced total serum copper but an increased level of free copper. Increased urinary copper excretion is also demonstrated. Slit-lamp examination confirms the presence of Kayser-Fleischer rings. Your suspicion for Wilson's disease is now quite high.

3. **How is the diagnosis of Wilson's disease made definitively?**
A liver biopsy showing an elevated free copper concentration is required. Histologic staining for copper can also be done, but this test is not as sensitive, and a negative result does not exclude the diagnosis because copper can be deposited heterogeneously. The biopsy will also show piecemeal necrosis and lymphocytosis, which can evolve to cirrhosis.
Note: Total serum copper levels are *decreased* secondary to decreased ceruloplasmin levels. Elevated free copper levels are toxic and thus responsible for the symptoms observed in Wilson's disease.

4. **What is the pathogenesis of Wilson's disease?**
As mentioned previously, deficiency in ceruloplasmin, which normally functions to bind plasma copper, results in low total plasma copper but elevated free plasma copper. It is this elevated free plasma copper that causes the disease, resulting in deposition of copper in the lenticular nuclei (neurologic symptoms), cornea (Kayser-Fleischer rings), liver (cirrhosis, HCC), and other organs throughout the body.
Note: There are over 200 mutations of the *ATP7B* gene known to cause Wilson's disease, which is inherited in an recessive manner and usually manifests at a young age (between 6 and 20 years); prenatal genetic screening is available within an affected family if the responsible mutation has been identified.

5. **If this patient remains untreated, what neurologic manifestations may develop?**
Because of the degeneration of the lenticular nuclei (putamen and globus pallidus) in the basal ganglia, a Parkinson-like syndrome, characterized by tremors, dysarthria, bradykinesia, and spasticity, can develop.

6. **What is the treatment for Wilson's disease and how does it work?**
Copper chelation therapy with lifelong use of ᴅ-penicillamine or trientine hydrochloride, which are drugs that help remove copper from tissue. Taking extra zinc, which competes with copper for intestinal absorption, is commonly used in combination with copper chelation therapy.

SUMMARY BOX: WILSON'S DISEASE

- Wilson's disease is caused by deficient production of the copper-carrying protein ceruloplasmin. It is inherited in an autosomal recessive manner.

- Golden brown rings around the limbus of the cornea (Kayser-Fleischer rings resulting from copper deposition) are an important diagnostic clue.

- Laboratory tests typically show low serum ceruloplasmin and total copper but increased free copper. Urinary copper excretion is also typically increased.

- A liver biopsy showing increased copper concentration is the diagnostic gold standard.

- Neurologic manifestations in later stages of the disease include a Parkinson-like syndrome.

- Treatment is copper chelation therapy. If left untreated, Wilson's disease is fatal.

CASE 7-3

A 32-year-old man develops fever, nausea, vomiting, malaise, anorexia, and abdominal pain within a few weeks of returning to the United States from vacationing in a Third-World country. He also mentions that his urine is dark.

1. **In terms of infections, what do you include in the differential diagnosis for a patient who has recently traveled out of the country?**
   You must broaden your differential diagnosis to include diseases endemic to that area, such as schistosomiasis in sub-Saharan Africa; infections potentially obtained from local food, such as *Vibrio cholerae* infection from drinking contaminated water in South America; diseases associated with wildlife, such as plague in countries with infected rodents; and infection from insects, such as malaria transmitted by *Anopheles* mosquitoes in tropical and subtropical countries. Sexually transmitted diseases, such as human immunodeficiency virus/acquired immunodeficiency syndrome (HIV/AIDS), can be more abundant in other countries. It is estimated that up to 80% of sex workers in some parts of Africa are infected with HIV/AIDS. These are just a few examples, but it is important to remember to consider such possibilities in travelers.

CASE 7-3 continued:

The patient states that he ate some shellfish that were harvested from a bay in which sewage enters. He was bitten by several mosquitoes and thinks he may have been infected with malaria. He had not received any immunizations before leaving for his vacation. On physical examination, he is jaundiced and has tender hepatomegaly. Laboratory studies reveal a peripheral smear negative for malaria, marked elevations of AST and ALT, mildly elevated ALP, and elevated direct and indirect bilirubin. A hepatitis profile reveals + anti-HAV IgM (hepatitis A virus immunoglobulin M), − anti-HAV IgG (hepatitis A virus immunoglobulin G), and − HBsAg (hepatitis B surface antigen).

2. **What is the diagnosis?**
   Acute hepatitis A infection is most likely. Hepatitis A is an enterically transmitted virus that is highly endemic in parts of the developing world where sanitation is poor. It is usually transmitted from an infected food handler who does not thoroughly wash hands before handling food others will consume.

3. **Why is there an elevation of both direct and indirect bilirubin?**
   In viral hepatitis, the indirect hyperbilirubinemia is caused by reduced ability of the infected hepatocytes to take up unconjugated bilirubin. The direct hyperbilirubinemia is caused by leakage of conjugated bilirubin from infected hepatocytes into the systemic circulation.

4. **Explain how the results of the hepatitis profile facilitate the diagnosis of an acute infection rather than a chronic one.**

    IgM is the first antibody isotype produced in response to a new infectious agent and remains in the circulation for about 12 weeks in hepatitis A infection. A previous infection would have been negative for anti-HAV IgM and positive for anti-HAV IgG, because the IgG isotype is produced later in the infection, and memory B cells do not make IgM but generally make IgG.

5. **Should he be concerned about developing a chronic infection or hepatic cirrhosis?**

    No, because in the vast majority of cases, hepatitis A does not develop into a chronic infection or lead to cirrhosis. However, hepatitis B and C viruses can cause both chronic infection and cirrhosis.

6. **How would you expect liver "function" test patterns to differ between parenchymal liver disease and cholestatic (biliary) disease?**

    Generally, in diseases that primarily affect the liver parenchyma, both AST and ALT are elevated to a greater extent than ALP and γ-glutamyltransferase (GGT). In biliary (cholestatic) diseases, the converse is generally the case, with ALP and GGT being elevated to a greater extent than AST and ALT.

7. **Now let's review some characteristic features of the different hepatitis viruses.**

    See Table 7-5.

STEP 1 SECRET

Hepatitis is very commonly tested on boards. You must know all the characteristics of the different hepatitis viruses. The one that confuses students most is hepatitis B because it is associated with a variety of antigens and antibodies that are either positive or negative depending on the stage of the disease. Do not worry! We will discuss hepatitis B in extensive detail later in this chapter.

8. **Can hepatitis A be prevented?**

    A live inactivated vaccine for hepatitis A is now available. It has been added to the vaccine recommendations of the Centers for Disease Control and Prevention (CDC) for all children over 1 year of age.

SUMMARY BOX: ACUTE HEPATITIS A

- Hepatitis A is contracted from the fecal-oral route and is often associated with foods that are processed in an unsanitary way, including inadequate handwashing by infected food handlers.

- Hepatitis A and E generally do not result in chronic hepatitis. Hepatitis B and C both have potential for chronic disease.

- The pattern of liver enzyme abnormalities varies depending on the cause of liver disease. Viral hepatitis typically causes a marked transaminitis. Alcoholic liver disease classically causes an AST elevation that is $\geq 2 \times$ ALT. Cholestatic liver disease typically causes greater elevations in ALP and GGT than AST and ALT.

TABLE 7-5. CHARACTERISTICS OF HEPATITIS VIRUSES

Hepatitis Virus	Type of Virus	Transmission	Chronicity	Cirrhosis	Hepatocellular Carcinoma Risk	Comments
A	ssRNA	Fecal-oral	No	No	No	
B	dsDNA	Parenteral	Yes	Yes	Yes	
C	ssRNA	Parenteral	Yes	Yes	Yes	Most common cause of posttransfusion hepatitis
D	ssRNA		No	No	No	Requires hepatitis B virus to replicate
E	ssRNA	Fecal-oral	No	No	No	20% mortality rate in pregnant women

dsDNA, double-stranded DNA; ssRNA, single-stranded RNA.

- Anti-HAV IgM is present for roughly 12 weeks after acquiring hepatitis A infection. Anti-HAV IgG becomes present shortly after IgM and persists for several years, indicating past infection and providing protective immunity.

- A vaccine to prevent hepatitis A is now available. There is also a vaccine for hepatitis B. No vaccines are currently available for hepatitis C, D, or E.

CASE 7-4

A 3-day-old, full-term baby presents with jaundice that started on his face and spread to his body. On close inspection, there are no hematomas present. Laboratory tests show elevated indirect bilirubin, a negative direct Coombs' test, normal reticulocyte count (for his age), and normal complete blood count (CBC). Enzyme assays for glucuronyltransferase activity are within normal limits.

1. **What is the most likely diagnosis?**
   Physiologic jaundice of the newborn is most likely. The unconjugated hyperbilirubinemia suggests hemolysis or a liver that cannot adequately process the bilirubin load. The negative direct Coombs' test helps exclude more serious hemolytic diseases of newborns in which the body produces autoantibodies against the newborn's native RBCs. Hemolytic diseases of newborns also cause CBC abnormalities, including anemia from extensive hemolysis and neutropenia and thrombocytopenia from suppression of myelopoiesis and platelet production in favor of erythropoiesis. Normal glucuronyltransferase activity excludes congenital enzyme deficiencies.

2. **Why does physiologic jaundice develop?**
   In the process of converting from RBCs with fetal hemoglobin to RBCs with adult hemoglobin, there is an approximate sixfold increase in the amount of unconjugated bilirubin presented to the liver. The neonatal liver often does not have the capacity to completely take up and conjugate this amount of bilirubin due to immature uridine diphosphate (UDP) glucuronyltransferase, resulting in a transient "physiologic" jaundice with unconjugated hyperbilirubinemia and possible kernicterus. Treatment involves phototherapy, which converts the unconjugated bilirubin into a water-soluble form that can be excreted in the urine.
   Note: This condition is more common among breastfed babies because breast milk contains deconjugating enzymes. No treatment is required.

3. **Why did the physician check for hematomas on physical examination?**
   Breakdown of RBCs in hematomas and the attendant bilirubin formation can be a cause of jaundice.

4. **Why are a normal reticulocyte count and a normal complete blood count important in the diagnostic workup for this neonate?**
   A hemolytic anemia can cause jaundice and will generally show an elevated reticulocyte count.

5. **What is the most serious complication of neonatal jaundice and how does it develop?**
   Kernicterus, which is deposition of insoluble unconjugated bilirubin in the brain, can result when the bilirubin concentration is especially high. Kernicterus is dangerous because it can lead to brain damage.

CASE 7-4 continued:

The mother and baby return to your office when the child is 1 week old for a scheduled follow-up visit with a lactation consultant. The jaundice has resolved, but the anxious first-time mother is concerned about long-term consequences for the baby.

6. **Are there long-term risks associated with physiologic jaundice of the newborn?**
    No. Most newborns will appear somewhat jaundiced in the first few days of life and this does not predispose them to any future disorders, hepatic or otherwise. The mother should be reassured. However, had the jaundice been severe and the bilirubin concentration greater than 20 mg/dL, there would be an increased risk for kernicterus.

7. **Would you expect physiologic jaundice to be exacerbated or attenuated by Gilbert's syndrome?**
    Gilbert's syndrome is characterized by mildly decreased UDP glucuronyltransferase activity, resulting in increased unconjugated bilirubin levels, so this disease would exacerbate physiologic jaundice.

8. **What is the hereditary syndrome with a more serious deficiency of uridine diphosphate glucuronyltransferase than in Gilbert's syndrome?**
    Crigler-Najjar syndrome, which also causes an unconjugated hyperbilirubinemia. Two forms of Crigler-Najjar syndrome have been described. Type 1 is characterized by high levels of unconjugated hyperbilirubinemia and kernicterus. Type 2 demonstrates a lower degree of hyperbilirubinemia and carries a much smaller risk of kernicterus.
    Note: Phenobarbital can be used to treat type 2 Crigler-Najjar syndrome, as it upregulates UDP glucuronyltransferase activity, thereby increasing the capacity of the liver to conjugate bilirubin.

9. **What are the hereditary forms of conjugated hyperbilirubinemia and what is the major histologic difference between them?**
    Dubin-Johnson and Rotor's syndromes. Dubin-Johnson syndrome is characterized by black, coarse pigmentation of centrilobular hepatocytes. Table 7-6 outlines the differences between the hereditary forms of bilirubin metabolism and transport.

SUMMARY BOX: PHYSIOLOGIC JAUNDICE OF THE NEWBORN

-   Many newborns develop jaundice shortly after birth; the vast majority of these cases are physiologic.

-   Pathologic causes of neonatal jaundice include hemolysis, hematoma formation, polycythemia, vertical transmission of hepatitis B, and hereditary hyperbilirubinemias.

-   A high bilirubin concentration (>20 mg/dL) in a newborn can result in kernicterus. For unclear reasons, extreme hyperbilirubinemia does not cause kernicterus in adults.

-   A hereditary deficiency of uridine diphosphate (UDP) glucuronyltransferase activity, as occurs in Gilbert's and Crigler-Najjar syndromes, may result in an unconjugated hyperbilirubinemia.

-   Dubin-Johnson syndrome and Rotor's syndrome are the two hereditary forms of conjugated hyperbilirubinemia, resulting from an inability to transfer conjugated bilirubin from the liver to the gastrointestinal (GI) system.

TABLE 7-6. HEREDITARY DISORDERS OF HEPATIC BILIRUBIN METABOLISM AND TRANSPORT

Feature	Gilbert's Syndrome	Crigler-Najjar Type I Syndrome	Crigler-Najjar Type II Syndrome	Dubin-Johnson Syndrome	Rotor's Syndrome
Incidence	6-12%	Very rare	Uncommon	Uncommon	Rare
Gene affected	*UGT1A1*	*UGT1A1*	*UGT1A1*	*MRP2*	Unknown
Metabolic defect	↓ Bilirubin conjugation	No bilirubin conjugation	↓↓ Bilirubin conjugation	Impaired canalicular export of conjugated bilirubin	Impaired canalicular export of conjugated bilirubin
Plasma bilirubin (mg/dL)	≤3 in absence of fasting or hemolysis, nearly all unconjugated	Usually >20 (range, 17–50), all unconjugated	Usually <20 (range, 6–45), nearly all unconjugated	Usually <7, about one half conjugated	Usually <7, about one half conjugated
Liver histologic appearance	Usually normal, occasional ↑ lipofuscin	Normal	Normal	Coarse pigment in centrilobular hepatocytes, leading to a grossly black liver	Normal
Other features	↓ Bilirubin concentration with phenobarbital	No response to phenobarbital	↓ Bilirubin concentration with phenobarbital	↑ Bilirubin concentration with estrogens, ↑↑ urinary coproporphyrin I/III ratio, slow BSP elimination kinetics with secondary rise	Mild ↑ urinary coproporphyrin I/III ratio, very slow BSP elimination kinetics without secondary rise

Continued

TABLE 7-6. HEREDITARY DISORDERS OF HEPATIC BILIRUBIN METABOLISM AND TRANSPORT—continued

Feature	Gilbert's Syndrome	Crigler-Najjar Type I Syndrome	Crigler-Najjar Type II Syndrome	Dubin-Johnson Syndrome	Rotor's Syndrome
Prognosis	Normal Jaundice may be evident only with fasting and stress	Death in infancy if untreated	Usually normal	Normal	Normal
Treatment	None	Phototherapy as a bridge to liver transplantation	Phenobarbital for ↑↑ bilirubin concentration	Avoid estrogens	None available

BSP, sulfobromophthalein; *MRP2*, multidrug resistance–associated protein-2 gene; *UGT1A1*, bilirubin UDP-glucuronyltransferase gene.
From Feldman M, Friedman LS, Brandt LJ: Sleisenger and Fordtran's Gastrointestinal and Liver Disease, 8th ed, Philadelphia, WB Saunders, 2006.

CASE 7-5

A 60-year-old male smoker who was infected with hepatitis B in his late 20s presents to your clinic. He had been feeling well until recently and has avoided seeing a doctor for the past 10 years.

1. **To what ailments are persons infected with hepatitis B susceptible?**
   The ones that should come immediately to mind are liver disease and HCC. Others include glomerulonephritis (from antibody-antigen [Ab-Ag] deposition in the glomerulus which elicits an inflammatory cascade) and polyarteritis nodosa (PAN) (from immune complex deposition in the blood vessels).
   Note: Hepatitis D virus is also parenterally and sexually transmitted, and infection can occur only with concominant hepatitis B infection.

CASE 7-5 continued:

He decides to see his gastroenterologist because over the last 2 months he has noticed a dull epigastric pain that is now nearly constant and he is feeling increasingly fatigued. He notes an unintentional 30-lb weight loss in recent months and a yellow discoloration of his skin. He asks the physician if "maybe that old virus is up to something."

2. **How does the preceding additional information change the differential diagnosis? What specific laboratory tests might you want to order to further investigate?**
   Fatigue and unintentional weight loss should always make you consider malignancy in your differential diagnosis, especially in older patients. In a patient with a history of hepatitis B infection we need to consider HCC, which can present with jaundice, right upper quadrant (RUQ) pain, ascites, and nausea. α-fetoprotein (AFP) is a nonspecific serum marker for HCC.

CASE 7-5 continued:

In addition to the usual liver enzyme blood tests, a test for AFP and ultrasound are ordered. The AFP is markedly elevated at 1200 ng/mL (normal <10 ng/mL), and a hyperechoic pattern is appreciated on ultrasound (Fig. 7-5).

3. **What is the likely diagnosis and how can it be confirmed?**
   HCC is most likely. HCC is the most common primary hepatic malignancy; it is the fifth most common cancer in men and the eighth most common in women. Histologic diagnosis is definitive, and samples can be obtained by fine needle aspiration (FNA) or percutaneous biopsy.

4. **What other type of malignancy will produce a markedly elevated α-fetoprotein?**
   Nonseminomatous germ cell tumors (think yolk sac tumor) and HCC are the only primary malignancies that will yield a value greater than 500 ng/mL; liver metastases can also yield a value this high. AFP is also used in prenatal screening for Down syndrome (decreased levels) and neural tube defects (increased levels).

5. **What are some risk factors for hepatocellular carcinoma?**
   The four major risk factors that have been identified are chronic hepatitis B infection, chronic hepatitis C infection, cirrhosis, and dietary exposure to aflatoxin B_1. Aflatoxin B_1 is derived from *Aspergillus* species that can contaminate foodstuffs in tropical and subtropical regions of Africa

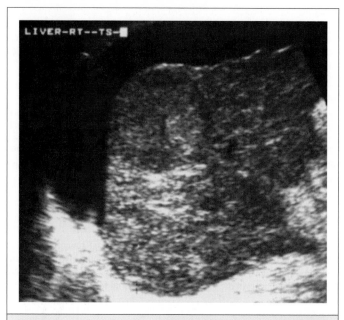

Figure 7-5. Liver ultrasound of patient in Case 7-5. (From Grainger RG, Allison D: Grainger & Allison's Diagnostic Radiology: A Textbook of Medical Imaging, 4th ed. London, Churchill Livingstone, 2001.)

and Asia. There are several minor risk factors, including cigarette smoking, oral contraceptive steroids, Wilson's disease, α_1-antitrypsin deficiency, and hereditary hemochromatosis.

6. **Where are likely sites for metastatic hepatocellular carcinoma?**
The most common sites of metastases are the lung, regional lymph nodes, and adrenal glands. The liver is the most common site for metastases of other malignancies because of the high degree of blood supply to the liver from the portal venous system. In addition to malignancies in organs whose blood supply feeds into the portal system, lung and breast cancers often metastasize to the liver.
   You can generally differentiate primary cancer from metastatic cancer with imaging techniques by the presence of single versus multiple tumors within the organ of interest, respectively.

7. **What paraneoplastic syndromes are associated with hepatocellular carcinoma?**
HCC is associated with the production of insulin-like factor, erythropoietin, and parathyroid hormone-related peptide (PTHrP). Clinical findings may include polycythemia and constitutive hypoglycemia. Note that the latter contrasts with liver failure secondary to noncancerous causes, which leads to fasting hypoglycemia only.

8. **In a woman who takes oral contraceptives and has a single hepatic nodule detected on ultrasound and a normal α-fetoprotein, what kind of neoplasm might you suspect?**
Hepatocellular adenomas are benign neoplasms that were very rare before oral contraceptives became widely used. Steroid use is also associated with hepatocellular adenoma risk. Hepatic angiography can be useful in making the diagnosis because many hepatocellular adenomas are

avascular. Surgical resection is recommended because of the risk of rupture and, in a very small percentage of cases, transformation to HCC.

9. **What are the treatment options for hepatocellular carcinoma and what factors guide decision making?**
No one of these options has been proved to be better than any other in terms of survival (Table 7-7).

STEP 1 SECRET

The information in Table 7-7 is beyond what is expected for Step 1, but may be useful to you in your clinical years.

SUMMARY BOX: HEPATOCELLULAR CARCINOMA

- Hepatocellular carcinoma (HCC) is the most common primary hepatic malignancy; it is the fifth most common cancer in men and eighth most common in women worldwide.

- α-Fetoprotein (AFP) is a serum marker for HCC as well as nonseminomatous germ cell tumors.

- The prognosis for HCC is grim. Those whose cancer is too advanced for treatment can expect a median survival of 3 to 6 months.

- HCC commonly metastasizes to the lungs, regional lymph nodes, and adrenal glands.

- Hepatitis B has been associated with glomerulonephritis, polyarteritis nodosa, fulminant hepatic failure, and HCC.

- Infection with hepatitis D occurs only in a patient already infected with hepatitis B because it requires hepatitis B viral particles to replicate and infect other hepatocytes.

TABLE 7-7. TREATMENT OPTIONS FOR HEPATOCELLULAR CARCINOMA

Treatment Modality	Indications/Comments
Arterial embolization or chemoembolization	Multiple small tumors or those that are inaccessible Embolization also can be used to decrease the size of larger tumors, to allow for resection
Chemotherapy	Response rates are less than 20%, multiple agents are almost always required, and multidrug resistance is a major problem
Liver transplantation	Unresectable tumors or highly cirrhotic or dysfunctional liver Recurrence rates are high, and lifelong immunosuppression is required after transplantation
Surgical resection	Tumor confined to one lobe of the liver and accessible, ideally without significant cirrhosis Only 15% of symptomatic patients are surgical candidates

CASE 7-6

Your first clinic patient of the day is a 15-year-old boy who moved to the United States from Indonesia at the age of 5. He is home schooled by his mother, who reports that he has been less active than normal and has lost his appetite. He points to the RUQ of his abdomen and tells you that he has been having a stomach ache in that area. Laboratory workup reveals an elevated ALT and AST. Other laboratory tests are unrevealing.

1. **What structures are located in the right upper quadrant?**
   The RUQ contains the liver, the gallbladder and biliary tree, the first, second, and third parts of the duodenum, the head of the pancreas and pancreatic duct, the hepatic flexure of the colon, and the right hemidiaphragm.

2. **What is the differential diagnosis considering the relevant anatomy?**
   Hepatitis (viral being most common), biliary colic, cholelithiasis, cholecystitis, cholangitis, peptic ulcer, pancreatitis, mesenteric ischemia, perforated bowel, peritoneal abscess, and malignancy should be considered.
   Note: Using anatomic cues is important for building a differential diagnosis, but abdominal pain does not always follow anatomic division. Pathology in other anatomic locations can present as RUQ pain, such as a dissecting abdominal aortic aneurysm, a right lower lobe pneumonia, or an atypical appendicitis, to name a few.

CASE 7-6 continued:

A hepatitis profile reveals the following:
- − Anti-HAV IgM
- − Anti-HAV IgG
- + HBsAg
- − Anti HBsAg
- + Anti-HBcAg (IgG)
- − Anti-HBcAg (IgM)
- − Anti-HCV

3. **What is the diagnosis?**
   Chronic active hepatitis B virus (HBV) infection is indicated. The hepatitis profile indicates a chronic hepatitis B infection; review Table 7-5. The symptoms of fatigue, poor appetite, and low-grade RUQ pain as well as elevated aminotransferases (ALT>AST) suggest active infection. Patients with chronic inactive hepatitis B are often asymptomatic with normal aminotransferases.
   Diagnosing hepatitis B infection based on laboratory values is important for Step 1. For those of you who struggle with this concept or simply wish for additional clarification, you will find it helpful to study Figure 7-6 and the description in the Secrets box (Secrets for Scrutinizing Hepatitis B Infection).

SECRETS FOR DIAGNOSING STAGES OF HEPATITIS B INFECTION

The easiest way to think about hepatitis B is to first group the three types of antigens associated with this infection. These are surface antigen (HBsAg), core antigen (HBcAg), and an antigen that circulates in the blood during viral replication called hepatitis B e antigen (HBeAg). HBcAg is not clinically useful because it is not detectable in serum, so don't even worry about that one. HBsAg is the most important of the three. It is the first antigen to appear and last antigen to disappear, and if you have it, you *are infected* with hepatitis B virus (although you cannot tell from

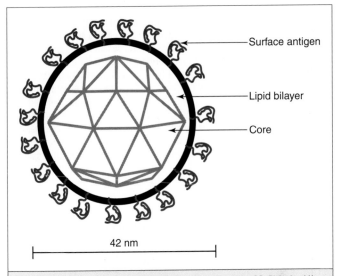

Surface antigen

Lipid bilayer

Core

42 nm

Figure 7-6. Schematic diagram of hepatitis B virus. (From Long SS, Pickering LK, Prober CG: Principles and Practice of Pediatric Infectious Diseases, 2nd ed. Philadelphia, Churchill Livingstone, 2003.)

this quite yet whether it is an acute, chronic, or carrier state infection). HBeAg is your infectivity marker. This is especially important in pregnant women. The presence of HBeAg indicates a high infectivity rate, period. Approximately 90% of neonates will acquire hepatitis B infection from mom if she is HBeAg-positive.

Let's say someone is acutely infected with hepatitis B virus (HBV). Right off the bat, serum HBsAg will become positive (core antigen will also be positive, but remember that we do not see this). HBeAg becomes positive soon after, and anti-HBcAg is then produced. This antibody is hugely important for two reasons—one we will mention now and the other we will mention later. First, think of anti-HBcAg as your chronicity marker (remember "C" for chronicity). If a patient is positive for anti-HBcAg of the IgM isotype, it indicates acute/recent infection. If the isotype is IgG, the patient has chronic disease (>6 months of infection) or has recovered from disease.

As many of you probably know, most people with HBV do not develop chronic hepatitis because their immune system will eventually fix the problem that it caused in the first place. The immune system will start to make antibodies to HBsAg and HBeAg. In this case, the antibody isotype really isn't important. What is important is that when this starts to happen, the patient will enter the *window period*. The best way for understanding the window period is to picture the following scenario: Let's say you have concentration X of HBsAg in your serum. As the body produces antibodies to this antigen, the antigen precipitates out of serum through immune complex formation. When the concentration of antibody matches concentration X of antigen, all of the antigen precipitates out, and HBsAg becomes undetectable in serum. This also applies to HBeAg and its antibody.

To summarize, the window period marks the time when the patient produces surface and "e" antibodies in equal concentrations to their antigens such that neither antibody nor antigen is detectable in serum.

This is where anti-HBcAg again becomes important. The *only* marker that is positive during the window period is anti-HBcAg, and it can thus be used to test for infection during the window period if you suspect it. *Remember that someone who has been vaccinated against HBV will be positive only for anti-HBsAg and not anti-HBcAg.*

Once the window period has ended, levels of anti-HBsAg and anti-HBeAg rise over the levels of antigen, and these antibodies will become detectable in the serum. If a patient has detectable levels of anti-HBsAg, HE IS CURED, no matter what. How do you distinguish between a cured patient versus an immunized patient? Easy! Look for anti-HBcAg (IgG).

The only other thing that you need to know is what a carrier will look like. These are people who are positive for surface antigen but do not have antibodies to surface antigen, although they are otherwise asymptomatic. In this case it is helpful to think of immunocompromised patients, because these are people whose CD8+ T cells will not attack the viral antigens on hepatocytes and mount symptoms of the disease. Carriers can, however, pass the disease onto others but will not be symptomatic for hepatitis themselves.

We hope this makes more sense to you now and recommend rereading this section while studying Figure 7-6 to test yourself.

4. What is the most likely mode of transmission in this case?

Vertical transmission to neonates from HBV carrier mothers is the most common mode of transmission in endemic regions of the world, such as Southeast Asia, China, and Africa. In the United States, sexual contact is the most common mode of transmission. Most neonatal infections become chronic, whereas only a small percentage of infections acquired in adulthood do. HBV is thought to be 10 times more infectious than hepatitis C virus (HCV) and 100 times more infectious than HIV.

5. What is the significance of hepatitis B e antigen?

Hepatitis B e antigen (HBeAg) is present in the serum early in acute infection. Persistence in the serum for longer than 3 months indicates higher infectivity and a greater likelihood of transition to chronic HBV. Mothers who are HBeAg-positive have the highest risk of perinatal transmission to their children.

6. If a patient with hepatitis B infection also presented with arthralgias, mononeuritis, fever, abdominal pain, renal disease, and hypertension, what disease might you suspect?

Polyarteritis nodosa (PAN) is often associated with HBV. Although only a small percentage of HBV patients will develop PAN, almost one third of patients with PAN have acute or, more commonly, chronic HBV. Membranous glomerulonephritis and membranoproliferative glomerulonephritis are also sometimes associated with HBV.

STEP 1 SECRET

If symptoms of polyarteritis nodosa are suggested in a clinical vignette on boards, the question stem will most likely mention hepatitis B association.

7. When is the hepatitis B virus vaccine typically given?

Universal vaccination of all children in the United States is recommended. The first of three doses is usually given at birth, the second at 1 to 2 months, and the third at 6 to 18 months. Children born to HBsAg+ mothers should also be given hepatitis B immunoglobulin within 12 hours of birth to achieve passive immunity. Members of other high-risk groups, including health care workers (YOU!!), should also be vaccinated if they previously were not.

8. **What are the two most common treatment options for hepatitis B virus?**
The primary goal of treatment is long-term suppression of the virus. INF-α and nucleoside analogs are both used to achieve this. Interferon is less expensive and only needs to be taken for a limited time (4-12 months), but it has many side effects. Nucleoside analogs have fewer side effects but need to be taken long term. In some cases, combination treatment is optimal.

9. **What are some other infectious causes of hepatitis?**
Less common causes of hepatitis are given in Table 7-8.

TABLE 7-8.	LESS COMMON CAUSES OF HEPATITIS
Pathogenic Category	**Potential Etiologic Disorder(s)**
Amebic	*Entamoeba histolytica* abscess
Bacterial	Pyogenic hepatic abscess—may be caused by gram-positive aerobic cocci in neonates and gram-negative rods in adults
Parasitic	Leptospirosis, schistosomiasis, liver flukes (trematodes), toxoplasmosis
Viral	Cytomegalovirus (CMV), Epstein-Barr virus (EBV), herpes simplex virus (HSV), varicella-zoster virus (VZV) infections

SUMMARY BOX: HEPATITIS B VIRUS

- Hepatitis B is a hepadnavirus that can be transmitted by bodily fluids or perinatally.

- Hepatitis B and C viruses are capable of producing chronic infection.

- Hepatitis D infection can occur only along with hepatitis B infection.

- Presence of hepatitis B e antigen (HBeAg) indicates higher viral titers and higher infectivity.

- The goal of treatment is long-term suppression of the virus; interferon-α and nucleoside analogs are currently the main approved therapies.

CASE 7-7

A 19-year-old college student presents with nausea, vomiting, and abdominal pain. Initially, she is slightly confused and withdrawn, making it difficult to collect a good history, but she does tell you that she was at a fraternity party 2 nights ago and got "pretty drunk." She denies using any other drugs at the party. You do a pelvic examination and a rectal examination to assess for occult blood and order stat laboratory tests including a CBC, basic metabolic panel, liver enzymes, urinalysis, urine pregnancy test, and lipase. You also prepare to do an abdominal ultrasound.

1. **What are the some of the common causes of acute abdominal pain with nausea and vomiting?**
   See Table 7-9.

TABLE 7-9. COMMON CAUSES OF ACUTE ABDOMINAL PAIN	
Causative Condition	**Nature of Pain/Associated Findings**
Acute appendicitis	Pain may be located in the periumbilical area or in the RLQ; anorexia is common.
Acute cholecystitis	Pain is located in the RUQ, and ultrasound imaging may show gallstones.
Acute gastroenteritis	Diarrhea often is a prominent component, and its characteristics, along with characterization of its onset with regard to meals, can help to determine the underlying disorder.
Acute pancreatitis	Epigastric pain radiates to the back, associated with anorexia, nausea, and vomiting; plasma amylase and lipase (a more specific marker) levels may be elevated (although often not in chronic pancreatitis).
Acute salpingitis	Bilateral adnexal pain is common, with cervical motion tenderness on bimanual examination.
Biliary colic	RUQ pain is intermittent; ultrasound imaging may show gallstones.
Ectopic pregnancy	Nausea and vomiting often are absent, and a urine pregnancy test is positive; pelvic ultrasound imaging is used to rule out an intrauterine pregnancy and will sometimes reveal an adnexal mass or blood.
Intestinal obstruction	Pain often is diffuse and crampy in nature.
Perforated duodenal ulcer	Pain usually is epigastric; dark, tarry blood may be found in the stool.
Renal colic	Flank and costovertebral angle pain are severe; hematuria is common.

RLQ, right lower quadrant; RUQ, right upper quadrant.

CASE 7-7 continued:

Pelvic and rectal examinations are unrevealing with stool negative for blood. Laboratory tests reveal a mild anemia and thrombocytopenia as well as significantly elevated transaminases. The urine pregnancy test is negative, and other laboratory tests are normal. Abdominal ultrasound is unremarkable. You present these findings to the patient, telling her that it appears that her liver seems to have been damaged. Somewhere along the way, you garnered her trust and she now tells you more about the party. She saw her boyfriend kissing one of her sorority sisters, and after chugging three more beers, she went back to her dorm and took a bunch of Tylenol before passing out to avoid a hangover in the morning. After learning this, you order laboratory tests for total bilirubin and PT, which are elevated and prolonged, respectively.

2. **What is the diagnosis and suspected etiology?**
She has fulminant hepatic failure (FHF) resulting from acetaminophen toxicity. FHF is defined as the rapid development of hepatocellular dysfunction and mental status changes in a patient without previously known liver disease.
   Note: FHF often manifests as a coagulopathy or encephalopathy. Coagulopathy occurs because the liver is not able to adequately produce clotting factors, and there can be platelet destruction. Cerebral edema may lead to encephalopathy of varying severity. Indeed, the duration of time before encephalopathy begins is sometimes used to characterize the severity of FHF. Hypoglycemia, infections, and renal failure are other complications that can arise from FHF.

3. **What is the mechanism of hepatic damage in acetaminophen toxicity?**
Acetaminophen is oxidized by the cytochrome P-450 system into *N*-acetyl-*p*-benzoquinoneimine (NAPQI). NAPQI is toxic to liver cells, but normally it is detoxified in a phase II reaction by glutathione. If a toxic dose of acetaminophen is ingested, the glutathione supply is depleted, leaving NAPQI to cause liver damage.

4. **What is the antidote for acetaminophen toxicity?**
In addition to supportive treatment, acetaminophen toxicity should be treated with N-acetylcysteine (Mucomyst)—the sooner the better. Treatment within 8 hours of ingestion is nearly 100% hepatoprotective. Acetylcysteine substitutes for glutathione and detoxifies NAPQI. Activated charcoal should be given if the patient presents shortly after ingestion. The charcoal absorbs toxins such as acetominophen in the stomach. The effectiveness of activated charcoal drops sharply if more than 1 hour has passed from time of toxin ingestion.

5. **What is the maximum daily dosage of acetaminophen for adults?**
The maximum dose for adults is 4 g/day. The maximum dose for children is variable by age. Acetaminophen is an ingredient in many medications, such as Vicodin, Percocet, and cold and flu formulations. Patients often do not realize this and can accidentally overdose when using multiple medications.

STEP 1 SECRET

You do NOT need to know brand names or medication dosages for the USMLE.

6. **Why should alcoholics avoid acetaminophen?**
Alcohol consumption increases the activity of the enzyme that metabolizes acetominophen into NAPQI, which, as you know, is hepatotoxic. Chronic alcohol use can also deplete glutathione stores in the liver thus reducing its protection against damage caused by reactive oxygen species.

7. **What other potentially hepatotoxic drugs should you know for the boards?**
There are far too many potentially hepatotoxic drugs to mention here, but some of the more commonly used ones include the following: amiodarone, amoxicillin, chlorpromazine, ciprofloxacin, erythromycin, fluconazole, isoniazid, methotrexate, methyldopa, statins, niacin,

rifampin, salicylates, and valproic acid, as well as several antiretrovirals and anticancer drugs. It is also worth reminding you that many drugs undergo hepatic metabolism and their dosages should be adjusted in patients with liver disease.

SUMMARY BOX: ACETAMINOPHEN-INDUCED FULMINANT LIVER FAILURE

- Fulminant hepatic failure (FHF) is the rapid onset of hepatocellular dysfunction and mental status changes in a patient without previous liver disease.

- Encephalopathy and coagulopathy are common manifestations of FHF; other complications include hypoglycemia, infection, and renal failure.

- Hyperbilirubinemia, elevated transaminases, and prolonged prothrombin time can be expected in FHF.

- Many drugs are hepatotoxic, but acetaminophen toxicity is the most common cause of FHF in the United States.

- *N*-acetyl-*p*-benzoquinoneimine (NAPQI), a metabolite of acetaminophen, is responsible for hepatic damage in acetaminophen toxicity.

- Activated charcoal and acetylcysteine (Mucomyst) are used to treat acetaminophen toxicity.

- The maximum daily dose of acetaminophen is 4 g for adults. The maximum dose in patients with liver disease is lower, typically 2 g/day.

CASE 7-8

A 41-year-old obese mother of four complains of nausea, vomiting, fever, and right-sided upper abdominal pain after eating fatty meals. On examination, she is not jaundiced, has a temperature of 100.5° F, and experiences sharp pain on inspiration when pressure is provided to the lower edge of her right costal cartilage (Murphy's sign). Laboratory tests show a leukocytosis with a left shift.

1. **What diagnosis do you suspect?**
   Cholecystitis (inflammation of the gallbladder), which is usually due to obstruction of the gallbladder neck or cystic duct by a gallstone, is likely. However, other diagnoses such as ascending cholangitis should be considered.

2. **What risk factors for gallstones does the patient exhibit?**
   This classic presentation includes the risk factors that can be remembered as the four F's: female, fat (although not politically correct, this is a useful mnemonic), fertile, forties (age).

3. **Why do patients with gallstones experience pain, particularly after eating a high-fat meal?**
   Entry of fatty acids into the duodenum stimulates the release of cholecystokinin (CCK), which causes gallbladder contraction. This creates pain by increasing biliary pressure.

CASE 7-8 continued:

Ultrasound of the RUQ reveals a distended gallbladder containing gallstones and demonstrates a sonographic Murphy's sign. She is admitted to the hospital and placed on antibiotics, and a surgery consult is obtained.

4. **What is a sonographic Murphy's sign?**
   Tenderness with pressure from the ultrasound probe directly over where the gallbladder is visualized. This response can be negative in greater than 50% of cases of acute cholecystitis. In contrast, Murphy's sign on physical examination refers to a maneuver in which the physician places the hands below the costal margin at the right midclavicular line (immediately below the level of the gallbladder) after instructing the patient to exhale. The patient is asked to breathe in, and the diaphragm and abdominal contents are shifted downward as the lungs expand. The gallbladder now makes contact with the examiner's hands, which causes the patient to wince in pain if gallbladder disease (e.g., inflammation, gallstones) is present. This is considered a Murphy's sign. Murphy's sign is not generally positive with cholangitis.

   Note: Ultrasound is the imaging of choice to evaluate for gallstones and cholecystitis. It is quick and noninvasive and can be done at the bedside.

CASE 7-8 continued:

A laparoscopic cholecystectomy is scheduled and carried out without complication during the same hospitalization.

5. **What are the most common types of gallstones?**
   Cholesterol monohydrate (80%) or calcium bilirubinate (20%) are most common.

6. **Why does an obstructing stone in the common bile duct predispose to jaundice, whereas a stone in the cystic duct generally does not?**
   A stone in the common bile duct (choledocholithiasis) can completely prevent the flow of bile to the intestines (cholestasis), causing biliary backpressure that damages the liver and results in hyperbilirubinemia and jaundice. However, a stone in the cystic duct will only prevent bile from flowing into or out of the gallbladder, leaving bile flow from the liver to the intestines unimpeded.

7. **What is cholangitis?**
   Cholangitis is an infection of the biliary tree, usually occurring as a result of a stone in the common bile duct. It requires aggressive treatment.

8. **What is Charcot's triad for cholangitis?**
   Charcot's triad consists of (1) fever, (2) RUQ pain, and (3) jaundice and is present in approximately 50% of patients with cholangitis. The fever is due to the response to infection, the jaundice is due to obstruction of the common bile duct (or other bile ducts), and the cause of RUQ pain is obvious. RUQ pain secondary to ascending cholangitis can radiate to the shoulder or tip of the scapula.

9. **Where in the pancreas would a neoplasm causing obstructive jaundice most likely be located and why?**
   It would be in the head of the pancreas. The common bile duct runs through the head of the pancreas on its way to the second part of the duodenum and can get obstructed along the way. The USMLE loves this anatomic relationship between the pancreas and the common bile duct. Note that the classic presentation is one of "painless jaundice" in a patient with malaise and unintentional weight loss.

10. **How can cholestasis cause pale stools?**
Conjugated bilirubin is normally metabolized to urobilinogen (clear color) by colonic bacteria and ultimately to stercobilin (brown color) via auto-oxidation, which causes the normal stool color. Neither of these processes occurs if bile does not reach the intestines.

11. **Define steatorrhea and explain why it can develop from complete obstruction of the common bile duct.**
Steatorrhea, typically characterized by foul-smelling stools, refers to the presence of significant amounts of fat in stool. Bile acids emulsify fats so that they can be digested by pancreatic lipases, then form micelles of the digested fatty acids and deliver them to the intestinal mucosa for absorption. Consequently, impaired delivery of bile to the intestines interferes with all these processes and causes steatorrhea.

12. **What prevents the formation of cholesterol stones in the normal physiologic setting?**
Bile salts and phospholipids solubilize cholesterol and prevent it from precipitating out of solution. In fact, for patients with small stones who are poor surgical candidates, oral bile acids are given to facilitate dissolution of the stone. Decreased bile salt and phospholipid concentrations or increased cholesterol concentrations can all lead to stone formation.

13. **Why are people with Crohn's disease predisposed to the development of cholesterol stones?**
Crohn's disease often involves the terminal ileum, where bile salts are reabsorbed. Because these salts are important in the solubilization of cholesterol, reduced reabsorption facilitates stone formation.

14. **Which cholesterol-lowering drugs bind bile acids in the intestine? Explain how these drugs lower serum cholesterol.**
Cholestyramine and colestipol, which are nonabsorbable ionic resins, bind bile acids in the intestine and are eliminated in the feces, promoting the excretion of bile salts. As a result, more bile acids need to be produced de novo. Because serum cholesterol is used as a substrate for bile acids, bile acid synthesis results in reduced plasma cholesterol. Recall that the formation of bile salts is the only method available to the body to eliminate cholesterol.

15. **How can infection with *Clonorchis sinensis* also lead to obstructive jaundice?**
This trematode infects the hepatobiliary tree. Chronic inflammation from this infection can cause fibrotic strictures within the bile ducts that impede the egress of bile.

SUMMARY BOX: BILIARY DISEASE

- Cholelithiasis is the presence of stones in the gallbladder or cystic duct. Cholecystitis is inflammation of the gallbladder. Choledocholithiasis is the presence of stones in the common bile duct. Cholangitis is inflammation of the biliary tree.

- Most gallstones are cholesterol stones. Calcium bilirubinate stones are the next most common type.

- Ultrasound is the initial imaging of choice for suspected biliary disease.

- Release of cholecystokinin (CCK) results in gallbladder contraction, which occurs following fatty meals and thereby exacerbates RUQ pain.

- Charcot's triad is fever, right upper quadrant pain, and jaundice; it is associated with acute cholangitis but is present in only ~50% of patients.

CASE 7-9

A mother brings her 4-year-old child into your office and complains that he has been lethargic, sleepy, irritable, and quiet for the past few days. He has also displayed heavy vomiting that has not been relieved by meals. You ask if the child has been feverish at all. "Not anymore," his mother answers. "He just got over the chickenpox a few days ago and had several high fevers during that time, but we gave him aspirin around the clock and they eventually resolved."

1. **What is the most likely diagnosis?**
   This is a classic presentation of Reye syndrome, which is a rare but serious childhood hepatoencephalopathy. It is associated with salicylate administration in children, especially following viral infection. For this reason, aspirin use is almost never recommended for children. However, a notable exception to this guideline is to decrease risk of coronary artery aneurysm in children with Kawasaki disease.

2. **What is the pathophysiology of Reye syndrome?**
   Aspirin metabolites can reversibly inhibit a mitochondrial enzyme involved in β-oxidation of fatty acids, leading to buildup of fatty acids and microvesicular fatty change in the liver. This may induce hepatic damage and disrupt other processes that occur in the liver such as gluconeogenesis, glycogenolysis, and the urea cycle. Clinical manifestations of these disruptions include hypoglycemia and encephalopathy or coma with increased ammonia levels in the blood.

3. **List the components of the postinfectious triad associated with Reye syndrome.**
   Encephalopathy, fatty liver degeneration, and transaminase elevation occur.

SUMMARY BOX: REYE SYNDROME

- Reye syndrome occurs in children secondary to salicylate administration. In general, children should not be given aspirin except to prevent coronary artery aneurysm with Kawasaki disease.

- Reye syndrome leads to microvesicular fatty change in the liver. Damage is reversible.

- Clinical symptoms of Reye syndrome include lethargy, irritability, somnolence, heavy vomiting, and coma.

CHAPTER 8

ENDOCRINOLOGY

Sonali J. Shah, Thomas A. Brown, MD, Anna Radwan,
and Henry L. Nguyen

INSIDER'S GUIDE TO ENDOCRINOLOGY FOR THE USMLE STEP 1

Endocrinology on the USMLE tests your ability to reason through complex-appearing problems and is therefore a favorite subject among examiners. Luckily, these problems become quite straightforward with a bit of practice. This chapter is aimed at giving you this practice. The most important secret to doing well on Step 1 endocrinology questions is to understand hormonal pathways and the concept of negative feedback. This information alone will help you answer a large number of endocrinology questions on board examinations. Study the cases in this chapter and test yourself by drawing out hormonal feedback loops whenever possible.

BASIC CONCEPTS

1. **What is the cellular mechanism of action of the steroid hormones?**
   Steroid hormones are lipophilic. Therefore, they diffuse across the plasma membrane and form complexes with cytosolic or nuclear receptors; the bound complexes then activate transcription of various genes. Because steroid hormones rely on the intermediary process of gene expression and protein translation, it can take hours to days for their effects to manifest. Examples of steroid hormones are testosterone, estrogen, progesterone, cortisol, and aldosterone. Cholesterol is the precursor to all steroid hormones. Although thyroid hormone is not a steroid hormone, it uses the same cellular mechanism as the steroids (Fig. 8-1).

2. **What is the cellular mechanism of action of the peptide hormones and the catecholamines?**
   The peptide hormones and catecholamines are not highly lipid-diffusible and thus cannot cross the plasma membrane. They bind to cell surface receptors (see Fig. 8-1), which initiate a variety of biochemical events, including activation or inhibition of enzymes, alteration of membrane proteins, and mediation of cellular trafficking. These processes can occur within seconds to minutes. Nevertheless, the peptide hormones can stimulate gene expression as well, and this effect is delayed as it is with the steroid hormones. Examples of peptide hormones are insulin, parathyroid hormone (PTH), vasopressin (antidiuretic hormone), and oxytocin. Table 8-1 shows a comparison of polypeptide and steroid hormones.

3. **Why is the total serum hormone level not an accurate reflection of hormone activity?**
   Many of the hormones in the serum are inactive because they are attached to serum binding proteins. It is only the *free* hormone that is biologically active. Another important factor that

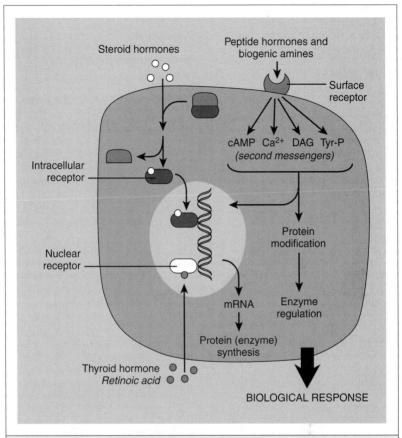

Figure 8-1. Mechanisms by which peptide and steroid hormones signal. Ca²⁺, calcium; cAMP, cyclic adenosine monophosphate; DAG, diacylglycerol; mRNA, messenger RNA; Tyr-P, phosphorylated tyrosine residue. (From Goldman L, Ausiello D: Cecil Textbook of Medicine, 22nd ed. Philadelphia, WB Saunders, 2004.)

TABLE 8-1. COMPARISON OF THE DIFFERENT TYPES OF HORMONES

Feature	Polypeptides	Modified Amino Acids	Steroids
Size	Medium-large	Very small	Small
Ability to cross cell membrane	No	Yes	Yes
Receptor type	Cell surface	Cell surface or intracellular	Intracellular
Solubility	Water	Water	Fat
Action	Protein activation	Protein activation or synthesis	Protein synthesis
Transport in the blood	Dissolved in the plasma	Dissolved in the plasma or bound to plasma proteins	Bound to plasma proteins

From Meszaros JG, Olson ER, Naugle JE, et al: Crash Course: Endocrine and Reproductive Systems. Philadelphia, Mosby, 2006.

affects hormone activity is the concentration of cellular hormone receptors available for binding a specific hormone and mediating its action.

Note: Free hormone is in equilibrium with bound hormone:

$$[\text{Free hormone}] + [\text{Binding protein}] \leftrightarrow [\text{Hormone} - \text{binding protein complex}]$$

4. **How does a hormone's binding to the same type of receptor have different effects in different cell types?**
   Different tissues are different because they express different genes (i.e., *differential transcription*). Therefore, although different target tissues may express the same hormone receptor, they may also express entirely different downstream protein targets. For example, by binding the same β_2-adrenergic receptors, epinephrine is able to elicit a host of different physiologic responses depending on the tissue location of that receptor (e.g., glycogenolysis in the liver, lipolysis in adipose tissue).

5. **What are the four primary classes of membrane-spanning receptors to which peptide hormones bind?**
   The four primary classes of membrane-spanning receptors to which peptide hormones bind are (1) tyrosine and serine kinase receptors, (2) receptor-linked kinases, (3) G protein–coupled receptors, and (4) ligand-gated ion channels (Fig. 8-2 and Table 8-2). As a gross simplification, the "prototypical" agonists for these receptor types can be considered to be growth *factors*, growth *hormones* (GHs), peptide hormones, and neurotransmitters, respectively.

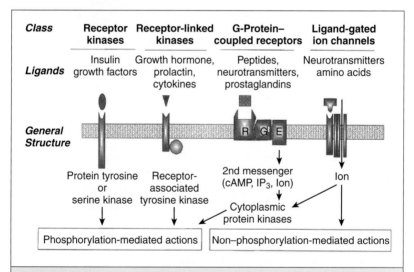

Figure 8-2. The four major classes of membrane receptors for hormones and neurotransmitters. cAMP, cyclic adenosine monophosphate; E, effector enzyme; G, G protein; IP₃, inositol triphosphate; R, receptor. (From Brown TA, Brown D: USMLE Step 1 Secrets. Philadelphia, Hanley & Belfus, 2004.)

STEP 1 SECRET

Classes of receptors used by various hormones are commonly tested on Step 1. You should memorize the information listed in Table 8-2.

TABLE 8-2. CLASSES OF RECEPTORS USED BY VARIOUS HORMONES

Receptor Class	Hormones and Related Substances
cAMP	LH, FSH, ACTH, TSH, PTH, hCG, CRH, glucagon
cGMP	NO, ANP
IP$_3$	GnRH, GHRH, oxytocin, TRH
Steroid receptor	Estrogen, testosterone, glucocorticoids, vitamin D, aldosterone, progesterone, T$_3$/T$_4$
Tyrosine kinase	Insulin, growth factors (e.g., IGF, PDGF), GH, prolactin

ACTH, adrenocorticotropic hormone; ANP, atrial natriuretic peptide; cAMP, cyclic adenosine monophosphate; cGMP, cyclic guanosine monophosphate; CRH, corticotropin-releasing hormone; FSH, follicle-stimulating hormone; GH, growth hormone; GHRH, growth hormone–releasing hormone; GnRH, gonadotropin-releasing hormone; hCG, human chorionic gonadotropin; IGF, insulin-like growth factor; IP$_3$, inositol triphosphate; NO, nitric oxide; PDGF, platelet-derived growth factor; PTH, parathyroid hormone; T$_3$, triiodothyronine; T$_4$, thyroxine; TRH, thyrotropin-releasing hormone; TSH, thyroid-stimulating hormone.

6. **How do the tyrosine kinase receptors transduce their messages?**
As depicted in Figure 8-3, binding of peptide hormone to the extracellular domain of the receptor initiates a signal transduction cascade by promoting autophosphorylation of the kinase receptor and subsequent phosphorylation of downstream target proteins, thereby activating or inhibiting these proteins.

7. **How do the ligand-gated ion channels work?**
Activation of ligand-gated ion channels results in an influx (or efflux) of ions into (or out of) the cell. The nicotinic receptor on skeletal muscle is an example of such a receptor. Binding of acetylcholine to this receptor results in an influx of principally sodium ions into the cell.

8. **How do the G proteins transduce their signals?**
Binding of hormone/agonist to G protein–coupled receptors causes an $\alpha\beta\gamma$ subunit complex to exchange guanosine diphosphate (GDP) for guanosine triphosphate (GTP). Once GTP is bound to the subunit complex, it dissociates into the α subunit and a separate $\beta\gamma$ subunit. These dissociated subunits then activate or inhibit enzymes (adenylate cyclase, phospholipase) and ion channels (Ca^{2+} channels) (Fig. 8-4).
Note: Adenylate cyclase synthesizes cyclic adenosine monophosphate (cAMP) from adenosine triphosphate (ATP), and the cAMP activates various target proteins. G$_s$ receptors stimulate adenylate cyclase, whereas G$_i$ receptors inhibit adenylate cyclase.

STEP 1 SECRET

G proteins are a five-star topic on boards. Study the pathways for G$_s$, G$_i$, and G$_q$ signaling depicted in Figure 8-4. You should know the details of these pathways, including the predominant cellular changes that occur with activation of each protein (e.g., cyclic adenosine monophosphate [cAMP] increase with G$_s$ activation, intracellular [Ca^{2+}] increase with G$_q$ activation).

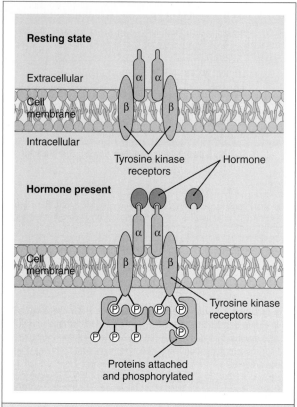

Figure 8-3. Mechanism of activation of a tyrosine kinase receptor. (From Meszaros JG, Olson ER, Naugle JE, et al: Crash Course: Endocrine and Reproductive Systems. Philadelphia, Mosby, 2006.)

9. **How do endocrine, paracrine, and autocrine mechanisms of cell communication differ?**

   Endocrine secretions (i.e., hormones) affect their target organs at considerable distance from their site of secretion, so they must be carried by the bloodstream. Paracrine secretions act locally on adjacent cells and tissues. Paracrine communication seems particularly important in endocrine tissues, such as the pancreatic islets, where constant communication between adjacent cells (e.g., α and δ cells) is critical for optimal functioning. Autocrine secretions are secretions from a cell that bind to receptors on that same cell and exert regulatory actions on that cell. Neuroendocrine secretions involve the secretion of peptides into the blood from specialized neurons (hence the term *neuroendocrine*). Hypothalamic peptides released into the blood from the terminal boutons of axons located in the posterior pituitary are one example of this mechanism of regulation (Fig. 8-5).

10. **Describe the concept of negative feedback. What is a feedback loop?**

    Hormone synthesis and release are governed at multiple levels. Hormone synthesis/release from an organ of interest typically involves regulation by a pituitary hormone, which itself is regulated by a hypothalamic hormone. This general pathway structure is commonly referred to as a hypothalamic-pituitary-(organ) axis (e.g., HPO axis refers to the ovary, HPA axis refers to the adrenal gland). Negative feedback occurs when a product downstream of an axis inhibits

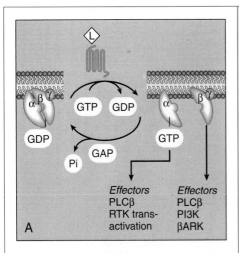

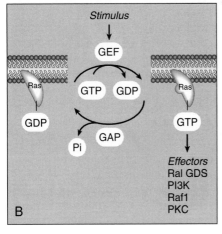

Figure 8-4. Signal transduction by G proteins. βARK, β-adrenergic receptor kinase; GAP, GTPase-activating protein; GDP, guanosine diphosphate; GEF, guanine nucleotide exchange factor; GTP, guanosine triphosphate; Pi, inorganic phosphate, PI3K, phosphatidylinositol 3-kinase; PKC, protein kinase C; PLCβ, phospholipase Cβ; Raf1, effector protein; Ral GDS, Ras-related GTPase guanine nucleotide dissociation stimulator; RTK, receptor tyrosine kinase. (From Mann DL: Heart Failure: A Companion to Braunwald's Heart Disease. Philadelphia, WB Saunders, 2004.)

production of a reactant by which it is regulated; for example, thyroid hormone inhibition of thyroid-stimulating hormone (TSH). These relationships are often depicted using feedback loops. An example of the thyroid hormone feedback loop is depicted in Figure 8-6.

CASE 8-1

A 38-year-old woman developed a massive postpartum hemorrhage, for which she was eventually stabilized with multiple blood transfusions. A few weeks later she complains that she has not been able to lactate since delivering her baby. She also feels lethargic and weak, and often gets dizzy upon standing. Physical examination is unremarkable except for sparse axillary and pubic hair, and her pulse rate increases by 20 beats/min upon standing from a supine position. Injection of corticotropin-releasing hormone (CRH) causes only a blunted elevation of serum adrenocorticotropic hormone (ACTH) level. Similarly, injection of a gonadotropin-releasing hormone (GnRH) analog causes only a blunted elevation of follicle-stimulating hormone (FSH) and luteinizing hormone (LH). Serum prolactin concentration is abnormally low.

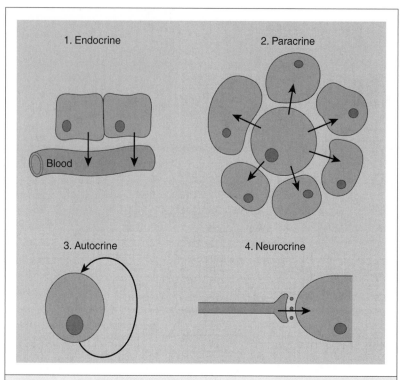

Figure 8-5. The routes by which chemical signals are delivered to cells. (From Meszaros JG, Olson ER, Naugle JE, et al: Crash Course: Endocrine and Reproductive Systems. Philadelphia, Mosby, 2006.)

1. **What is the diagnosis?**
   She has Sheehan's syndrome (or postpartum necrosis), which is an infarction of the anterior pituitary.

2. **Why is the pituitary more susceptible to infarction in postpartum hemorrhage than in hemorrhagic shock unrelated to pregnancy?**
   During pregnancy, there is hyperplasia of the lactotrophs (prolactin-secreting cells) in the anterior pituitary (adenohypophysis) without proportional increase in blood supply, which increases this tissue's minimal perfusion needs. During postpartum hemorrhage, blood supply to the anterior pituitary can become sufficiently inadequate to meet this increased need, causing infarction.

3. **Why is the posterior pituitary typically spared in Sheehan's syndrome?**
   The posterior pituitary (neurohypophysis) differs in embryologic origin from the anterior pituitary and therefore has a different blood supply. Remember, the embryologic origin of the anterior pituitary is Rathke's pouch (an endodermal evagination from the roof of the mouth), whereas the posterior pituitary is derived from a ventral outgrowth from the primitive hypothalamus. Table 8-3 shows a review of the functions of the posterior pituitary hormones.

4. **Secretion of which pituitary hormones may be affected in this woman?**
   The hormones secreted by the anterior pituitary include FSH, LH, ACTH, TSH, prolactin, and GH. FLAT P(i)G is a useful mnemonic to remember these hormones.

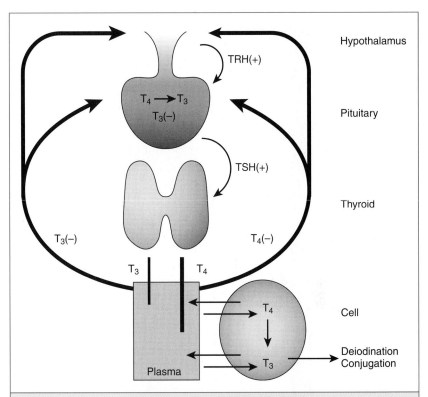

Figure 8-6. Thyroid hormone physiology. Under normal conditions, thyrotropin-releasing hormone (TRH) is released from the hypothalamus, which causes the release of thyroid-stimulating hormone (TSH) from the anterior pituitary. TSH then causes the release of triiodothyronine (T_3) and thyroxine (T_4) by the thyroid gland, which act on various peripheral organs. T_3 and T_4 also regulate TRH and TSH secretion through negative feedback mechanisms. In primary hypothyroidism (due to thyroid dysfunction), T_3 and T_4 are low despite high TSH levels. In secondary hypothyroidism (due to pituitary or hypothalamic dysfunction), the levels of TSH, T_3, and T_4 are all low. (From Goldman L, Ausiello D: Cecil Textbook of Medicine, 22nd ed. Philadelphia, WB Saunders, 2004.)

Depending on the extent of the infarction, all the anterior pituitary hormones may be affected (Fig. 8-7). This patient is unable to lactate, which is consistent with decreased prolactin secretion. (Whenever you see a patient who is unable to lactate shortly after delivery, consider Sheehan's syndrome!) Note that her axillary and pubic hair is sparse, which is consistent with decreased gonadotropin (FSH, LH) secretion. The patient is also weak and lethargic, which is consistent with hypocortisolism due to decreased ACTH secretion.

5. **Why may hypothalamic releasing hormone secretion increase because of an infarction of the anterior pituitary?**
   The loss of pituitary hormone secretion will decrease negative feedback on the hypothalamic hormones both from low pituitary hormone levels and from low target organ hormone production. Table 8-4 reviews the hypothalamic releasing hormones.

TABLE 8-3.   HORMONES SECRETED BY THE POSTERIOR PITUITARY AND THEIR EFFECTS

Hormone	Synthesized by	Stimulated by	Inhibited by	Target Organ	Effect
Antidiuretic hormone (ADH)	Supraoptic vasopressinergic neurons	Raised osmolarity; low blood volume	Lower osmolarity	Kidney	Increases permeability of the collecting duct to reabsorb water
Oxytocin	Paraventricular oxytocinergic neurons	Stretch receptors in the nipple and cervix, estrogen	Stress	Uterus and mammary glands	Smooth muscle contraction leading to birth or milk ejection

From Meszaros JG, Olson ER, Naugle JE, et al: Crash Course: Endocrine and Reproductive Systems. Philadelphia, Mosby, 2006.

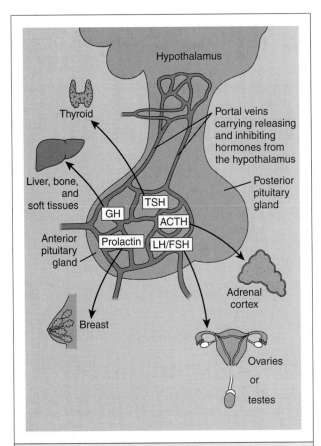

Figure 8-7. Hormones of the anterior pituitary gland and their respective target organs. ACTH, adrenocorticotropic hormone; FSH, follicle-stimulating hormone; GH, growth hormone; LH, luteinizing hormone; TSH, thyroid-stimulating hormone. (From Meszaros JG, Olson ER, Naugle JE, et al: Crash Course: Endocrine and Reproductive Systems. Philadelphia, Mosby, 2006.)

6. **Why wouldn't hypothalamic dopamine secretion be elevated from an anterior pituitary infarction?**
   In contrast with the other hypothalamic hormones, dopamine is inhibitory in nature and reduces the secretion of prolactin by the lactotrophs. Because serum prolactin normally stimulates dopamine secretion from the hypothalamus, in a setting of *hypo*prolactinemia secondary to pituitary infarction, we would expect decreased secretion of hypothalamic dopamine.

SUMMARY BOX: SHEEHAN'S SYNDROME

- Postpartum necrosis of the anterior pituitary is termed Sheehan's syndrome.

- Anterior pituitary hormones include follicle-stimulating hormone (FSH), luteinizing hormone (LH), adrenocorticotropic hormone (ACTH), thyroid-stimulating hormone (TSH), growth hormone (GH), and prolactin. (Remember FLAT P(i)G and disregard the i.)

TABLE 8-4. HORMONES SYNTHESIZED AND SECRETED BY THE ANTERIOR PITUITARY AND THEIR EFFECTS

Hormone	Synthesized by	Stimulated by	Inhibited by	Target organ	Effect
GH	Somatotrophs	GHRH	GHIH and IGF-1	Liver	Stimulates IGF-1 production and opposes insulin
TSH	Thyrotrophs	TRH	T_3	Thyroid gland	Stimulates thyroxine release
ACTH	Corticotrophs	CRH	Glucocorticoids	Adrenal cortex	Stimulates glucocorticoid and androgen release
LH + FSH	Gonadotrophs	GnRH, sex steroids	Prolactin, sex steroids	Reproductive organs	Release of sex steroids
Prolactin	Lactotrophs	PRH and TRH	Dopamine	Mammary glands and reproductive organs	Promotes growth of these organs and initiates lactation
MSH	Corticotrophs	—	—	Melanocytes in skin	Stimulates melanin synthesis
Beta-endorphin	Corticotrophs	—	—	Unknown	May be involved in pain control

ACTH, adrenocorticotropic hormone; CRH, corticotropin-releasing hormone; FSH, follicle-stimulating hormone; GH, growth hormone; GHIH, growth hormone–inhibiting hormone; GHRH, growth hormone–releasing hormone; IGF, insulin-like growth factor; LH, luteinizing hormone; MSH, melanocyte-stimulating hormone; PRH, prolactin-releasing hormone; T_3, triiodothyronine; TRH, thyrotropin-releasing hormone; TSH, thyroid-stimulating hormone.
From Meszaros JG, Olson ER, Naugle JE, et al: Crash Course: Endocrine and Reproductive Systems. Philadelphia, Mosby, 2006.

- The posterior pituitary secretes vasopressin (antidiuretic hormone [ADH]) and oxytocin.

- The embryologic origin of the anterior pituitary is Rathke's pouch.

- The posterior pituitary is derived from a ventral outgrowth of the primitive hypothalamus.

CASE 8-2

A 32-year-old woman complains of recent visual problems and slight breast discharge (galactorrhea). She has not had her period for the past 6 months (secondary amenorrhea) and is upset that she has been unable to become pregnant, despite trying for the past year with her husband. She denies any history of schizophrenia or of being treated with neuroleptics (antipsychotics). Laboratory workup reveals a negative pregnancy test result, normal TSH level, and significantly elevated levels of prolactin. Magnetic resonance imaging (MRI) of the head shows enlargement of the structure located in the sella turcica.

1. **What is the diagnosis?**
   Prolactinoma is a pituitary adenoma caused by abnormal proliferation of lactotrophs; it is the most common type of hypersecreting pituitary adenoma. Note that the pituitary is situated in the sella turcica. Table 8-5 reviews pituitary adenomas.

2. **What are the normal physiologic functions of prolactin preceding, during, and following pregnancy?**
   - *Preceding pregnancy:* Prolactin levels are normal due to tonic hypothalamic inhibition via dopamine and to the absence of stimulatory factors such as suckling or high estrogen. It has numerous physiologic functions in countless organ systems in the nonpregnant woman, none of which are high yield for boards.
   - *During pregnancy:* Prolactin levels are high secondary to high estrogen levels (secreted by the placenta), which stimulate breast maturation and lactogenesis. However, actual lactation is prevented by high estrogen and progesterone (which antagonize actions of prolactin on the breast).
   - *Following pregnancy:* Estrogen levels drop, and prolactin levels also will drop *unless* stimulation by suckling occurs; levels increase and lactation occurs with suckling stimulation. It is important for you to know that prolactin will also inhibit GnRH secretion, often (but not always!) resulting in anovulatory infertility while nursing.
   Figure 8-8 outlines the other physiologic functions of prolactin.

3. **Why does this patient have galactorrhea, whereas pregnant women with similar levels of serum prolactin generally do not have this problem?**
   Although prolactin stimulates milk production, the high concentrations of estrogen and progesterone that are present during pregnancy inhibit lactation, and therefore, galactorrhea. In contrast, this patient has hyperprolactinemia in the absence of elevated levels of estrogen and progesterone, which is causing her galactorrhea.
   Note: Milk letdown occurs after childbirth because, during pregnancy, the placenta makes most of the estrogen and progesterone. Levels of both hormones decrease after this structure is expelled in delivery. Additionally, oxytocin is secreted in response to suckling, and this hormone stimulates contraction of myoepithelial cells around the glandular tissue of the breast, causing milk ejection.

4. **Hyperprolactinemia can also occur in men. What symptoms might be expected in men?**
   In men, inhibition of GnRH secretion by prolactin decreases gonadotropin-mediated testosterone, production and low testosterone may lead to erectile dysfunction (impotence) and the loss of sex drive (libido). Galactorrhea can also rarely occur in men in response to certain stimuli such as

TABLE 8-5.   DISORDERS CAUSED BY THE DEFICIENCY OR EXCESS OF ANTERIOR PITUITARY HORMONES

Hormone(s)	Deficiency	Excess
GH	Dwarfism in children or adults GH deficiency syndrome	Gigantism in children, acromegaly in adults
LH and FSH	Gonadal insufficiency (decreased sex steroids)	Extremely rare but causes infertility
ACTH	Adrenocortical insufficiency (decreased cortisol and adrenal androgens)	Cushing disease (increased cortisol and adrenal androgens)
TSH	Hypothyroidism (decreased thyroid hormones)	Extremely rare but causes hyperthyroidism (increased thyroid hormones)
Prolactin	Hypoprolactinemia (failure in postpartum lactation)	Hyperprolactinemia (impotence in males, amenorrhea in females, and decreased libido)

ACTH, adrenocorticotropic hormone; FSH, follicle-stimulating hormone; GH, growth hormone; LH, luteinizing hormone; TSH, thyroid-stimulating hormone.
From Meszaros JG, Olson ER, Naugle JE, et al: Crash Course: Endocrine and Reproductive Systems. Philadelphia, Mosby, 2006.

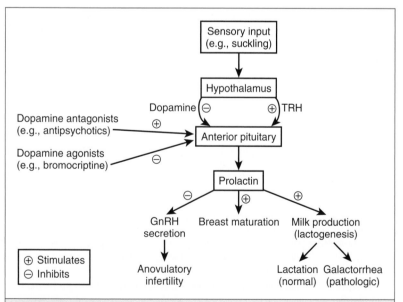

Figure 8-8. Physiologic actions of prolactin. TRH, thyrotropin-releasing hormone. (From Brown TA: Rapid Review Physiology. Philadelphia, Mosby, 2007.)

severe stress and prolonged starvation. Of note, be suspicious of hyperprolactinemia in men presenting with malaise and depression. This correlation is a board favorite.

5. **How does elevated prolactin prevent pregnancy (i.e., what is the mechanism of infertility and amenorrhea in this patient)?**
Prolactin inhibits the hypothalamic release of GnRH, which is a stimulus for FSH and LH secretion. The consequent reduction of FSH and LH eliminates the ovulatory cycle, resulting in infertility and amenorrhea. Note that hyperprolactinemia in men can cause impotence and infertility through a similar mechanism, except in this case testosterone is lowered as a result of the decreased LH.

6. **Why is asking about a history of schizophrenia and use of antipsychotic medications a relevant question in the diagnostic workup of this patient?**
Several antipsychotics (particularly the typical antipsychotics) can cause hyperprolactinemia. This is not a fact you have to memorize if you simply recall that antipsychotics are dopamine antagonists, and that hypothalamic dopamine is the major inhibitor of pituitary prolactin secretion. The USMLE loves these types of correlations!

7. **What is the mechanistic basis for using bromocriptine (used to treat Parkinson's disease) in the treatment of a prolactinoma?**
Bromocriptine is a dopamine agonist (recall that Parkinson's disease is caused by a lack of dopamine) that inhibits prolactin secretion by the anterior pituitary.

8. **How can head trauma with a severed pituitary stalk cause a similar increase in prolactin (assuming the anterior pituitary itself was not damaged)?**
This increase is due to disruption of the tuberoinfundibular tract, which runs from the hypothalamus through the pituitary stalk and is the source of dopamine, which inhibits prolactin release.
   Note: Plasma levels of all other anterior pituitary hormones (e.g., TSH, ACTH) will decrease with a severed pituitary stalk.

STEP 1 SECRET

Be sure to understand the concept of tuberoinfundibilar tract disruption. It is especially important for you to know that all pituitary hormones decrease except for prolactin, which increases owing to decreased levels of dopamine.

9. **Why does hypothyroidism need to be considered in the evaluation of hyperprolactinemia?**
Hypothalamic thyrotropin-releasing hormone (TRH) stimulates the secretion of both TSH and prolactin by the anterior pituitary. Because hypothyroidism causes elevated levels of TRH, it should be ruled out as a potential cause of hyperprolactinemia.

SUMMARY BOX: PROLACTINOMA AND HYPERPROLACTINEMIA

- The pituitary is located in the sella turcica.
- Prolactinoma is the most common type of hypersecreting pituitary adenoma.

- Hyperprolactinemia can be caused by a prolactinoma, antipsychotics (via inhibition of hypothalamic dopamine secretion), hypothyroidism (via increased thyrotropin-releasing hormone [TRH]), and breast feeding or excessive nipple stimulation.

- The increase in prolactin secretion that occurs with suckling is important in allowing for lactation. It can also inhibit gonadotropin-releasing hormone (GnRH) secretion and cause an anovulatory infertility, explaining why nursing women may have difficulty becoming pregnant.

- In women, in addition to causing infertility, hyperprolactinemia can cause galactorrhea. It can also cause malaise and depression.

- In men, hyperprolactinemia can cause impotence and lack of libido but only rarely will cause galactorrhea.

- Treatment for prolactinoma includes the use of dopamine agonists (for small adenomas) or, less commonly, surgical resection (for larger adenomas).

CASE 8-3

A 38-year-old man presents complaining of gradually enlarging hands and feet over the past several years. In comparison with a photo from 15 years ago, his facial features have become obviously coarsened. Laboratory evaluation shows mildly elevated plasma glucose, and MRI of the brain reveals an enlarged mass in the sella turcica. Given the suspected diagnosis, specialized testing is performed in which GH levels are measured following administration of an oral glucose load; no measurable decrease is seen.

1. **What is the diagnosis?**
   Acromegaly (from the Greek roots *akros* [extremities] and *megalos* [large]: *large extremities*) is caused by a GH-secreting tumor of the anterior pituitary. It most commonly affects middle-aged adults.
   Note: One good way to diagnose this disorder is to look at an old picture of the patient and compare it with the patient's current appearance. Because the physical changes take place over decades, family members and friends often do not recognize them.

2. **Why is hyperglycemia commonly associated with this disease?**
   GH increases serum glucose levels, and its release in response to decreasing glucose concentration is one of the body's mechanisms for preventing serious hypoglycemia. The elevation of blood glucose can be significant enough in acromegaly that many of these patients will have frank diabetes. In normal individuals, a glucose load will cause almost complete suppression of GH secretion, but it will not suppress GH secretion as much or at all by an independently functioning pituitary adenoma that is secreting GH.

3. **What are the normal physiologic functions of growth hormone and how is its secretion regulated?**
   GH secretion occurs primarily at night and in response to various stressors such as starvation and hypoglycemia. When released during a good night of sleep, its anabolic actions on muscle and bone are of primary importance. When released in response to physiologic stressors such as starvation and hypoglycemia, its metabolic actions to conserve carbohydrate fuels (for use by the central nervous system [CNS] and other glucose-dependent tissues) and maintain protein stores (to preserve muscle strength needed for mobility) take center stage.

   GH secretion is inhibited by elevated somatostatin, glucose levels, emotional stress, illness, malnutrition, obesity, glucocorticoids, and decreased thyroid hormone. Triiodothyronine (T_3) is required for normal function of GH.

4. **Given the normal physiology of growth hormone, how can we explain this patient's presentation?**
    The enlarged mass in the sella turcica is explained by a pituitary adenoma composed of proliferating somatotrophs. The enlarged hands and feet result from the anabolic effects of GH and insulin-like growth factor-1 (IGF-1) on the bones. As discussed previously, failure of GH suppression by a glucose load is typically seen in acromegaly. We were not told that this patient had hyperglycemia, but one would expect it in acromegaly because of the insulin-antagonizing ("diabetogenic") actions of GH on the liver and skeletal muscle, as well as stimulation of lipolysis in adipose tissue.
    Note: Most of the metabolic effects of GH are mediated through IGF-1, which is secreted by the liver. IGF-1 acts on bone to stimulate linear and lateral bone growth. IGF-1 also promotes the growth of cartilage and other soft tissues (Fig. 8-9).

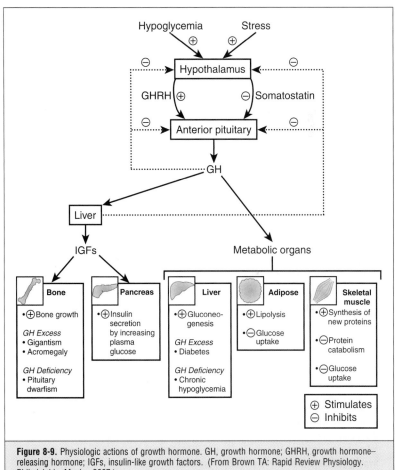

Figure 8-9. Physiologic actions of growth hormone. GH, growth hormone; GHRH, growth hormone–releasing hormone; IGFs, insulin-like growth factors. (From Brown TA: Rapid Review Physiology. Philadelphia, Mosby, 2007.)

5. **Why is octreotide, a somatostatin analog, useful in the treatment of acromegaly?**
    Somatostatin is a peptide hormone secreted by the hypothalamus. It inhibits GH secretion by the anterior pituitary. Its analog octreotide is also effective in inhibiting GH secretion.

Note: Somatostatin is also synthesized by pancreatic islets and gastric mucosa and inhibits intestinal activity and gastrointestinal motility.

6. **If this patient developed a growth hormone–secreting tumor in his early teens, how might the clinical manifestations differ?**
   GH stimulates bone growth, and if the epiphyseal plates have not yet closed, excess GH can cause patients to attain extremes of body height. When this occurs, the disease is called gigantism. "André the Giant," a professional wrestler and actor, suffered from this disease.

7. **What growth abnormality results from deficient secretion of growth hormone during the growing years?**
   Pituitary dwarfism is the most common result of this deficiency.
   Note: The dwarfism caused by deficient GH secretion is proportional (i.e., the limbs and trunk are of normal relative proportions), as opposed to the comparatively shorter limbs characteristic of dwarfism caused by achondroplasia. Of note, achondroplasia is caused by mutations of the fibroblast growth factor receptor gene 3 (*FGFR3*), which inhibit bone growth.

SUMMARY BOX: ACROMEGALY AND PHYSIOLOGY OF GROWTH HORMONE

- A growth hormone (GH)-hypersecreting pituitary adenoma can result in gigantism and acromegaly depending on the age at onset (i.e., whether the epiphyseal plates have fused).

- GH promotes anabolic actions on skeletal muscle and bone, stimulates lipolysis in adipose tissue, and stimulates hepatic gluconeogenesis. It generally antagonizes the actions of insulin.

- The metabolic actions of GH are largely mediated by insulin-like growth factor-1 (IGF-1).

- GH secretion is stimulated by hypoglycemia, stress, and sleep. It is inhibited by somatostatin, glucose, and IGF-1. Glucose administration does *not* inhibit GH secretion in acromegaly.

- Patients with acromegaly may present with prominent jaw (macrognathia), coarsening of facial features, hyperglycemia or frank diabetes, and organomegaly.

CASE 8-4

A 35-year-old woman presents for evaluation of a 6-month history of fatigue, weakness, and hip pain. She has also not had her period for the past 6 months and notes that her voice seems deeper than usual. The patient appears moderately obese (with primarily a central distribution) and has a jovial rounded face. No facial hair can be appreciated, but she does admit to shaving on a regular basis. Physical examination is significant for a myriad of additional findings, including a pronounced dorsocervical fat pad, acanthosis nigricans, purple abdominal striae, and proximal muscle weakness. Laboratory tests show hyperglycemia and an elevated random cortisol.

1. **What are the general causes of the hormonal abnormality most likely present in this woman?**
   This woman has hypercortisolism (Cushing syndrome), as indicated by her symptoms (muscle weakness, amenorrhea, deepening voice), classic examination findings (central obesity,

abdominal striae, dorsocervical fat pad or "buffalo hump," acanthosis nigricans), and laboratory findings (hyperglycemia, elevated random cortisol).

Perhaps the most common cause of Cushing syndrome is the iatrogenic prescription of glucocorticoids for inflammatory conditions. Other causes include a cortisol-hypersecreting adrenal adenoma (common) or carcinoma (rare), ACTH-secreting pituitary adenoma (Cushing disease), and ectopic (paraneoplastic) secretion (think small cell carcinoma of the lung for boards).

The hirsutism and deepening voice in this patient are suggestive of an ACTH-dependent cause of Cushing syndrome, in which shunting of glucocorticoid precursors into the androgenic pathway occurs, but further workup is clearly needed.

CASE 8-4 continued:

Further workup shows elevated 11 PM salivary cortisol and plasma ACTH levels, both of which suppress moderately in response to the administration of high-dose dexamethasone.

2. **What is the cause of the hypercortisolism in this patient?**
Cushing *disease* is due to the elevated cortisol *and* ACTH. One would expect suppressed ACTH levels if the adrenal glands were hypersecreting cortisol. Paraneoplastic ACTH secretion (e.g., small cell carcinoma) is suggested by the increased ACTH level, but ectopic ACTH secretion occurs independently of the HPA (hypothalamic-pituitary-adrenal) axis and does *not* normally suppress in response to glucocorticoids such as dexamethasone. In contrast, pituitary adenomas, which are well differentiated, typically retain *some* feedback responsiveness to glucocorticoids; thus, ACTH secretion may not suppress with low-dose dexamethasone but typically will with high-dose dexamethasone (Table 8-6).

TABLE 8-6. FEATURES OF CUSHING SYNDROME			
Cause of Cushing Syndrome	**ACTH**	**Cortisol**	**Results of Dexamethasone Suppression Test on Plasma Cortisol**
Cushing disease	High	High	High dose lowers cortisol
Ectopic ACTH production	High	High	No effect
Adrenal adenoma/ carcinoma	Low	High	No effect
Iatrogenic	Low	High	No effect
ACTH, adrenocorticotropic hormone.			

3. **Why are the results of a dexamethasone suppression test read at a specific time of day?**
Cortisol secretion has a wide circadian rhythm, with plasma levels varying several-fold throughout a 24-hour period (normal range 5-20 µg/dL) and peaking in the morning hours. The morning upsurge is necessarily preceded by an upsurge in ACTH, so ACTH levels should also be measured at a specific time (usually 5 AM).

4. **Why has hirsutism developed in this woman?**
Hirsutism is the presence of excess facial and body hair in women, especially in a male pattern, and typically reflects elevated androgens. Elevated androgens in this woman are due to increased

levels of ACTH, which in addition to stimulating cortisol synthesis by the adrenals also promotes "shunting" of the glucocorticoid precursors to the androgen pathway,.

5. **Why isn't hyperaldosteronism typically seen in Cushing disease?**
Although aldosterone is secreted by the adrenal cortex, its synthesis and secretion are influenced only minimally by ACTH levels. Rather, the principal regulators of aldosterone secretion are angiotensin II and serum potassium.

6. **What morphologic feature of the adrenal glands would you expect to see in this woman?**
Bilateral adrenal *hyperplasia* (with widening of the zona fasciculata and reticularis, specifically) is typically seen because ACTH is trophic for the adrenal glands. This feature is also present in ectopic production of ACTH.

7. **How is hypercortisolism contributing to hyperglycemia in this patient?**
Cortisol promotes hyperglycemia by stimulating hepatic gluconeogenesis and inhibiting the peripheral utilization of glucose (similar to GH). The increase in gluconeogenesis is due to stimulation of the synthesis of gluconeogenic enzymes by cortisol and also to greater mobilization of amino acids from skeletal muscle to participate in gluconeogenesis (hence the muscle wasting) (Fig. 8-10).

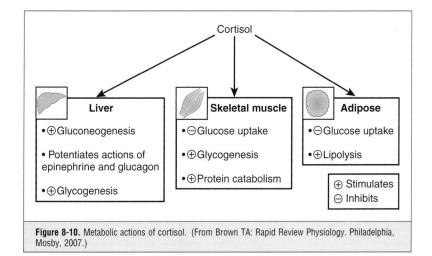

Figure 8-10. Metabolic actions of cortisol. (From Brown TA: Rapid Review Physiology. Philadelphia, Mosby, 2007.)

8. **How is hypercortisolism contributing to hypertension and hypokalemia in this patient?**
At higher plasma levels, cortisol exerts mineralocorticoid effects similar to those of aldosterone. This causes sodium retention and an ensuing plasma volume expansion that contributes to hypertension. The sodium is retained in exchange for secreting more potassium, which explains this patient's hypokalemia. Another contributing factor to this patient's hypertension is that cortisol stimulates the expression of adrenergic receptors in vascular smooth muscle.

9. **Why doesn't cortisol have mineralocorticoid actions in the normal physiologic setting?**
Cortisol can bind mineralocorticoid receptors with an affinity similar to that of aldosterone, but cells in mineralocorticoid-sensitive tissues (kidneys, colon, salivary glands) produce 11β-hydroxysteroid

dehydrogenase (11β-HSD), which breaks down cortisol into cortisone. Cortisone cannot bind to the aldosterone receptor. When the plasma cortisol is significantly elevated, 11β-HSD becomes saturated, thereby allowing intracellular cortisol to exert its mineralocorticoid effects in these tissues. This explains the plasma volume expansion and hypertension discussed previously.

Note: Licorice candy (if it contains licorice root from the licorice plant) also increases plasma cortisol levels by decreasing the activity of 11β-HSD, thereby potentially causing hypertension.

10. **What would an x-ray study of her bones likely reveal?**
An x-ray study of her bones would likely show a loss of bone density due to osteoporosis. Cortisol inhibits osteoblasts and stimulates osteoclasts, a double whammy. As a result, this promotes bone resorption, leading to osteoporosis. Osteoporosis is an especially significant side effect in patients taking steroids chronically.

11. **What are the three layers of the adrenal cortex, and which one is responsible for the excess production of cortisol in this patient?**
Just think of glomerular filtration rate (GFR) for the three layers—zona *g*lomerulosa, *f*asciculata, and *r*eticularis—which secrete mineralocorticoids (e.g., aldosterone), glucocorticoids (e.g., cortisol), and androgens (e.g., dehydroepiandrosterone [DHEA]), respectively (Fig. 8-11).

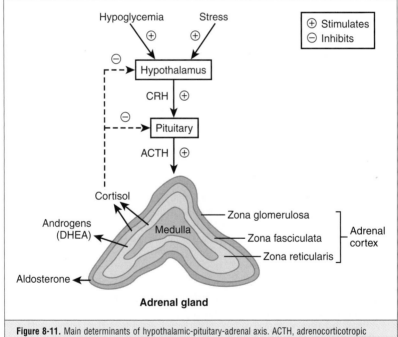

Figure 8-11. Main determinants of hypothalamic-pituitary-adrenal axis. ACTH, adrenocorticotropic hormone; CRH, corticotropin-releasing hormone; DHEA, dehydroepiandrosterone. (From Brown TA: Rapid Review Physiology. Philadelphia, Mosby, 2007.)

12. **One treatment for Cushing disease is to remove both adrenal glands (bilateral adrenalectomy). What might happen to the pituitary gland following such a surgery?**
The removal of both adrenal glands will stop the production of cortisol. Lacking the negative feedback of cortisol, the pituitary will synthesize ACTH and melanocyte-stimulating hormone

(MSH) unchecked, leading to enlargement of the preexisting pituitary adenoma with resulting headache and diffuse hyperpigmentation. This is known as *Nelson's syndrome*.

Note: MSH production is elevated when ACTH production is increased because both are produced from the same precursor polypeptide (pro-opiomelanocortin [POMC]).

SUMMARY BOX: HYPERCORTISOLISM

- Hypercortisolism regardless of cause is termed Cushing syndrome. The most common cause of Cushing syndrome is the iatrogenic administration of steroids.

- Hypercortisolism from a hypersecreting pituitary adenoma is termed Cushing disease.

- Classic signs and symptoms of Cushing syndrome include:

  - Central obesity: Cortisol stimulates protein breakdown in the extremities, but the hyperinsulinemia from the cortisol-induced hyperglycemia promotes fat deposition.

  - Purple abdominal striae are the result of weight gain and capillary fragility or rupture from the effects of hypercortisolism.

  - Hypertension is due to mineralocorticoid actions of cortisol at the kidney.

  - Hirsutism is due to adrenocorticotropic hormone (ACTH)–induced shunting of glucocorticoid precursors to the androgenic pathway.

  - Osteoporosis is due to cortisol-induced bone breakdown.

- Bilateral adrenalectomy for Cushing disease (rarely done!) can cause Nelson's syndrome, which is characterized by diffuse hyperpigmentation as a result of increased melanocyte-stimulating hormone (MSH) production.

CASE 8-5

An 18-year-old man presents for evaluation of a 6-month history of fatigue and weakness. He also complains of anorexia, nausea, and an unintentional 10-lb weight loss. On physical examination, his blood pressure is 90/55 mm Hg, and his skin appears tan despite its being midwinter. Laboratory workup is significant for low sodium, high potassium, and low glucose levels.

1. **What do you suspect at this point?**
   Vague symptoms (fatigue, weakness), hypotension, and the metabolic disturbances in this case are all concerning for adrenal insufficiency.

   Recall that aldosterone (and cortisol at high levels) stimulates sodium retention and potassium excretion from the kidneys. Recall also that cortisol and epinephrine antagonize the actions of insulin. Given these physiologic functions, one can see how a lack of mineralocorticoid, glucocorticoid, and catecholamines can result in hypotension, hyponatremia (see following note), and hyperkalemia.

   There are many causes of adrenal insufficiency but the hyperpigmentation observed in this patient suggests elevated ACTH levels (recall that MSH is a byproduct of ACTH synthesis). We can deduce from this that the "problem" exists at the level of the adrenals (low cortisol levels decrease negative feedback on the pituitary, leading to elevated ACTH levels).

2. **What are some general causes of primary adrenal insufficiency (Addison's disease)?**

Autoimmune destruction is perhaps the most common cause of Addison's disease. Tubercular invasion of the adrenals in miliary (disseminated) tuberculosis is a common cause of Addison's disease in developing countries. Metastatic invasion of the adrenals, which occurs frequently with lung cancer, is another cause. Other rarer causes include disseminated fungal infections (e.g., histoplasmosis) and drugs such as ketoconazole and metyrapone, which selectively inhibit the steroidogenesis pathway.

CASE 8–5 continued:

Further workup reveals elevated AM plasma ACTH and low plasma cortisol. Injection of ACTH (cosyntropin) elicits only a blunted increase in plasma cortisol. He is started on routine hydrocortisol and fludrocortisone.

3. **What was the cause of adrenal insufficiency in this patient?**

All we can say with the given information is that this young man has primary adrenal insufficiency due to the elevated ACTH and lack of response to cosyntropin. Because there are no clues to suggest malignancy or infection, and we are not told that he is taking any medications, the likely cause is autoimmune destruction of the adrenals.

RELATED QUESTIONS

4. **What adrenal disease should be suspected in a young patient with bacterial meningitis due to *Neisseria meningitidis* who also becomes acutely hypotensive?**

Waterhouse-Friderichsen syndrome typically causes bilateral adrenal hemorrhage, which can be rapidly fatal. The responsible bacterium is *Neisseria meningitidis*. This is a board favorite.

STEP 1 SECRET

Waterhouse-Friderichsen syndrome is a high-yield diagnosis for clinical vignettes on boards. Be on the lookout for symptoms of septicemia, disseminated intravascular coagulation (DIC), adrenal hemorrhage, and petechial rash.

5. **How would we expect plasma aldosterone levels to be affected in a patient with secondary (pituitary) adrenal insufficiency?**

Aldosterone secretion is primarily stimulated by angiotensin II and serum potassium levels. ACTH has little influence on aldosterone secretion, so this hormone will continue to be secreted at normal levels.

SUMMARY BOX: ADRENAL INSUFFICIENCY

- Primary adrenal insufficiency (Addison's disease) can present with vague symptoms such as weakness and malaise as well as with specific metabolic abnormalities such as hyponatremia, hyperkalemia, and hypoglycemia. Hypotension due to vascular collapse is also common.

- Causes of Addison's disease include autoimmune destruction, tubercular and metastatic invasion, fungal infections such as disseminated histoplasmosis, and drugs such as ketoconazole and metyrapone, which selectively inhibit the glucocorticoid pathway.

- The most common cause of adrenal insufficiency is the iatrogenic administration of steroids for inflammatory conditions.

- An elevated adrenocorticotropic hormone (ACTH) level suggests primary adrenal insufficiency, whereas a low ACTH level suggests pituitary, or rarely, a hypothalamic etiology.

- Another adrenal disease that should be considered in the appropriate clinical scenario is Waterhouse-Friderichsen syndrome. This disease is caused by *Neisseria meningitidis* and results in bilateral adrenal hemorrhage. It can be rapidly fatal.

CASE 8-6

A 38-year-old man with a history of generalized anxiety disorder complains of intermittent episodes of headache, palpitations, profuse sweating, and fear of "impending death." He was recently started on a beta blocker for mild hypertension, but surprisingly, his hypertension has worsened. He denies any history of cocaine or amphetamine abuse.

1. **What do you suspect at this point?**
    Intermittent episodes of headache, palpitations, profuse sweating, and fear of "impending death" are classic for pheochromocytoma. The worsening of his hypertension with initiation of beta blockers also points toward pheochromocytoma. However, other diagnoses to consider include panic attack (disorder), hypoglycemia, mastocytosis, and carcinoid syndrome.

2. **Why does hypertension often worsen after starting a beta blocker in patients with pheochromocytoma?**
    Plasma epinephrine, which is elevated in pheochromocytoma, has vasodilatory and vasoconstrictor effects depending on which adrenergic receptor (β or α) it binds. In the presence of a beta blocker, epinephrine will primarily bind α-adrenergic receptors, resulting in *unopposed α-receptor–mediated vasoconstriction*, thereby raising the blood pressure.

CASE 8-6 continued:

A 24-hour urine collection reveals elevated levels of catecholamine metabolites, and a positron emission tomography (PET) scan shows what appears to be a highly vascular mass above the left kidney. The administration of clonidine does not suppress plasma catecholamine levels.

3. **What is the likely diagnosis?**
    Pheochromocytoma, a tumor that episodically releases large amounts of catecholamines and results in symptomatic episodes of hypertension, tachycardia, palpitations, sweating, and headache, is most likely. Pheochromocytomas generally arise from neural crest–derived chromaffin cells of the adrenal medulla. Tumors arising in paraganglia are termed paragangliomas or extra-adrenal pheochromocytomas.

STEP 1 SECRET ✓

You should know all of the derivatives of neural crest cells. Believe it or not, this is a commonly tested boards topic. They include chromaffin cells, parafollicular cells of the thyroid, Schwann cells, autonomic nervous system (ANS), dorsal root and celiac ganglia, melanocytes, cranial nerves, pia and arachnoid, odontoblasts, skull bones, and the aorticopulmonary septum.

Knowing the embryologic derivatives of other tissue types is fair game for boards but not nearly as high yield as neural crest derivatives.

4. **How can the administration of clonidine be used to differentiate pheochromocytoma from a "high-stress state"?**
Clonidine is a centrally acting α_2-agonist that inhibits sympathetic outflow from the CNS. Its administration should reduce catecholamine production by the CNS and adrenal medulla but does not reduce catecholamine production by an autonomously functioning pheochromocytoma.

5. **What is the "rule of 10s" for pheochromocytomas?**
   - 10% are familial (see following note)
   - 10% are extra-adrenal in location
   - 10% are malignant
   - 10% occur in children
   - 10% are calcified
   - 10% affect the adrenals bilaterally

   Note: Most pheochromocytomas arise sporadically, but approximately 10% are associated with hereditary disorders such as multiple endocrine neoplasia (MEN) IIA or MEN IIB, von Hippel-Lindau (VHL) disease, or neurofibromatosis.

6. **What malignant tumor that most often occurs in children under 5 years of age also shows increased urinary levels of catecholamine metabolites?**
Neuroblastoma is a neuroendocrine tumor arising from neural crest cells. Children with neuroblastoma may manifest with hypertension and a palpable abdominal mass. Approximately 50% of cases are also associated with opsoclonus-myoclonus syndrome, in which patients exhibit chaotic eye movements. Neuroblastoma commonly metastasizes to skin, bone, and the posterior mediastinum. The tumor itself is associated with *N-myc* oncogene overexpression and Homer-Wright rosettes (neuroblasts surrounding spaces filled with eosinophilic neuropil). You should be aware of these associations for boards.

CASE 8-6 continued:

The patient is prescribed antihypertensive therapy that includes prazosin and propranolol and is informed that surgical correction can offer a cure.

7. **What type of receptors do norepinephrine and epinephrine bind to on the heart to increase the rate and force of cardiac contraction?**
They bind to β_1-adrenergic receptors on nodal cells (positive chronotropic effect) and cardiac myocytes (positive inotropic effect). This is why a beta blocker, like propranolol, is used as part of the management of hypertension in patients with pheochromocytoma *as long as an α-blocker is started first.*

8. **Why was this patient given propranolol, a nonselective beta blocker, if it can cause a hypertensive crisis?**
You'll notice he was also given prazosin, which is an α_1-receptor antagonist and can prevent this problem. In fact, it is important to achieve α-blockade first with a drug like prazosin before beta blockers are even started in order to avoid such a hypertensive crisis.
The "-osins," which include doxazosin, terazosin, and prazosin, are α_1-receptor antagonists. These receptors are located predominantly on vascular smooth muscle.

9. **On a related note, what class of antihypertensive agent, if given prior to epinephrine, would make it so that epinephrine actually lowered the blood pressure?**
In this case, the initial administration of α_1-blockers (e.g., prazosin) will "block" all of the α_1-receptors, leaving only β_2-adrenergic receptors available for binding to subsequently administered epinephrine. Stimulation of β_2-adrenergic receptors results in vasodilation, which lowers peripheral vascular resistance and causes a drop in blood pressure.

STEP 1 SECRET

Questions like these are board favorites because they stress a broad conceptual understanding of physiology and pharmacology. Automatic nervous system (ANS) drugs are a five-star boards topic.

CASE 8–6 continued:

Prior to surgery, blood pressure was normalized with phenoxybenzamine. Surgical resection of the affected adrenal gland is performed without complications.

10. **Why was phenoxybenzamine given prior to surgery?**
Phenoxybenzamine is an irreversible noncompetitive antagonist of α_1-adrenergic receptors. Because of its irreversible binding of α_1-adrenergic receptors, it is preferred over other α_1-blockers in preoperative preparation. It minimizes the hypertensive effects of catecholamines released during the surgery.

SUMMARY BOX: PHEOCHROMOCYTOMA

- Intermittent episodes of headache, palpitations, profuse sweating, and fear of "impending death" are classic for pheochromocytoma. Worsening of hypertension with initiation of beta blockers is also suggestive of pheochromocytoma.

- Remember the "rule of 10s" for pheochromocytoma: 10% are familial, 10% are extra-adrenal in location, 10% are malignant, 10% occur in children, 10% are calcified, and 10% affect the adrenal glands bilaterally.

- Clonidine is used to differentiate pheochromocytoma from increased sympathoadrenal outflow due to stress or pain.

- In pheochromocytoma, an α-blocker should be given *before* beta blockade to prevent unopposed α-blocker–mediated vasoconstriction. Phenoxybenzamine is an irreversible α_1-blocker that is preferred over other α_1-blockers in preoperative preparation because it minimizes the hypertensive effects of catecholamines released during the surgery.

- Neuroblastoma is a malignant tumor that typically manifests in young children and also shows increased urinary levels of catecholamine metabolites.

CASE 8-7

A 40-year-old woman complains of easy fatigability, heat intolerance, excessive sweating, and palpitations. She also notes an unintentional 20-lb weight loss despite an excellent appetite, as well as occasional diarrhea.

1. **What do you suspect at this point?**
   There are only a few conditions associated with unintentional weight loss despite normal food intake. These possibilities include diabetes mellitus, malabsorption syndromes such as sprue, cancer, and hyperthyroidism. Both hyperthyroidism and malabsorption can cause diarrhea, but given this patient's heat intolerance and palpitations, hyperthyroidism seems likely.

CASE 8-7 continued:

Physical examination is significant for a blood pressure of 165/75 mm Hg, a systolic ejection murmur, and tachycardia, as well as diffuse nontender enlargement of the thyroid, slight resting tremor, fine hair, separation of the fingernail plate from the nail bed (onycholysis), and brisk reflexes. Laboratory tests reveal elevated free plasma thyroxine (T_4) and reduced TSH.

2. **What is the diagnosis?**
   Hyperthyroidism, the most common cause of which is Graves' disease. Other causes of hyperthyroidism are listed in Table 8-7.

TABLE 8-7. FEATURES OF HYPERTHYROIDISM

Cause	Pathophysiology	Pattern of Radioiodine Uptake	Classic Presentation
Permanent Causes			
Graves' disease (diffuse toxic goiter)	Activating antibodies to TSH receptor	Diffuse uptake throughout gland	Goiter, ophthalmopathy, dermopathy
Toxic multinodular goiter	Multiple hyperactive nodules, may have mutations in genes encoding TSH receptor or G proteins	Uptake in one or a few overly active "hot" nodules Uptake in remainder of thyroid is suppressed	History of nontoxic multinodular goiter in older adult May include cardiac complications such as atrial fibrillation or heart failure
Toxic adenoma (Plummer's disease)	Hyperactive adenoma(s); may have mutations in genes encoding TSH receptor or G proteins	Uptake in one or a few "hot" nodules Uptake in remainder of thyroid is suppressed	History of a slowly growing "lump" in the neck in a younger adult

Continued

TABLE 8-7. FEATURES OF HYPERTHYROIDISM—continued

Cause	Pathophysiology	Pattern of Radioiodine Uptake	Classic Presentation
Pituitary adenoma	Hypersecretion of TSH	Diffuse uptake throughout thyroid	May include additional symptoms (e.g., headaches, bitemporal hemianopia, nausea and vomiting)
Transient Causes			
Autoimmune thyroiditis (e.g., Hashimoto's disease)	Autoimmune destruction of thyroid	Suppressed uptake throughout thyroid	Hyperthyroidism initially, followed by hypothyroidism
Subacute thyroiditis (de Quervain's thyroiditis)	Probably secondary to viral infection of thyroid Follows upper respiratory tract infection	Suppressed uptake throughout thyroid	Thyroid exquisitely painful to palpation
Iodine-induced (Jod-Basedow effect)	Iodine overload may stimulate autonomous nodules, which function independently of TSH stimulation, to hypersecrete thyroid hormone	Suppressed uptake throughout thyroid	Thyrotoxicosis in a patient with toxic multinodular goiter after administration of iodine-rich radiographic contrast media and iodinated drugs such as amiodarone
Thyrotoxicosis factitia	Inadvertent or intentional ingestion of large amounts of thyroid hormone	Suppressed uptake throughout thyroid	Ingestion of thyroid hormone to lose weight, typically by medical personnel
Struma ovarii	Thyroid tissue forms part of ovarian germ cell tumor (teratoma) and secretes excessive thyroid hormone	Suppressed uptake throughout thyroid	Hyperthyroidism in female

Continued

TABLE 8-7. FEATURES OF HYPERTHYROIDISM—continued

Cause	Pathophysiology	Pattern of Radioiodine Uptake	Classic Presentation
Trophoblastic tumors	Malignant trophoblastic tissue secretes human chorionic gonadotropin (hCG), which stimulates the TSH receptor	Diffuse uptake throughout thyroid	Hydatidiform moles, choriocarcinoma, metastatic embryonal carcinoma of the testis

TSH, thyroid-stimulating hormone.

3. **Why has this woman experienced weight loss?**
   The thyroid hormones increase the basal metabolic rate (BMR), principally through increasing the production and insertion of the Na^+/K^+-ATPase pumps in various cell types. Thyroid hormones also increase the BMR via production of glycolytic enzymes. The increased metabolic rate results in weight loss and contributes to heat intolerance (Table 8-8).

TABLE 8-8. INTRACELLULAR AND PHYSIOLOGIC ACTIONS OF TRIIODOTHYRONINE (T_3)

Site of Action	Intracellular Effects	Physiologic Results
Cell membrane	Stimulates the Na^+/K^+-ATPase pump	Increased demand for metabolites, e.g., glucose
Mitochondria	Stimulates growth, replication, and activity; basal metabolic rate is raised	Increased heat production, oxygen demand, heart rate, and stroke volume
Nucleus	Increases expression of enzymes necessary for energy production	Lipolysis, glycolysis, and gluconeogenesis increased to raise blood metabolite levels and cellular metabolite use
Neonatal cells	Essential for cell division and maturation	Essential for normal development of central nervous system and skeleton

From Meszaros JG, Olson ER, Naugle JE, et al: Crash Course: Endocrine and Reproductive Systems. Philadelphia, Mosby, 2006.

4. **What are the two thyroid hormones and which is more potent?**

T_4 and T_3 are the hormones. T_3 is much more potent than T_4 ($\sim$5 times more so) and is primarily produced by the peripheral conversion of T_4 to T_3 (which is catalyzed by the intracellular enzyme 5'-deiodinase), although as much as 20% of T_3 can be secreted from the thyroid gland. Some authors prefer to call T_4 a "prohormone," because its activity is largely dependent on conversion to the more active T_3 (Table 8-9).

TABLE 8-9. COMPARISON OF T_3 AND T_4

Feature	T_3	T_4
Proportion of secreted thyroid hormone	10%	90%
Percentage free in plasma	1%	0.1%
Relative activity	10	1
Half-life (days)	1	7

T_3, triiodothyronine; T_4, thyroxine. (From Meszaros JG, Olson ER, Naugle JE, et al: Crash Course: Endocrine and Reproductive Systems. Philadelphia, Mosby, 2006.)

5. **How are the thyroid hormones synthesized?**

Ultimately, four iodine residues have to be attached to two tyrosine residues to form T_4, or three iodine residues are attached to form T_3. The first step in the synthesis is the uptake of iodide ion (I^-) from plasma into follicular cells and eventually the follicular lumen via the iodide "pump." Within the lumen, the enzyme *thyroid peroxidase* then catalyzes the next two steps, in which iodide is oxidized to iodine (I_2) and iodine molecules are attached to tyrosine residues on thyroglobulin (*organification step*). Iodinated tyrosine residues are then coupled together to form either T_4 or T_3. Endocytosis of this modified thyroglobulin protein into the follicular cells and its subsequent hydrolysis yield T_4 and T_3, which diffuse across the plasma membrane into the circulation (Fig. 8-12).

6. **Assuming the plasma levels of catecholamines are normal in this patient, what explains the tachycardia, tremors, palpitations, and increased pulse pressure?**

Thyroid hormones increase the expression of adrenergic receptors in target tissues, resulting in increased sensitivity to circulating catecholamines. Thyroid hormone also increases β-adrenergic receptor synthesis in the heart and has a direct stimulating effect (both inotropic and chronotropic) on the heart, independent of the sympathetic nervous system.

As stroke volume increases and the diastolic pressure is reduced due to widespread vasodilation that is caused by the thyroid hormone–dependent tissue metabolism needs, the resulting effect is an increase in pulse pressure. Figure 8-13 shows other potential pathologic manifestations of Graves' disease.

Note: Beta blockers are often given to alleviate the sympathomimetic effects (palpitations, tremor) of hyperthyroidism. Of note, untreated hyperthyroidism can predispose to osteoporosis and atrial fibrillation.

7. **What is the difference between primary, secondary, and tertiary hyperthyroidism and which does this patient have?**

Primary hyperthyroidism results from excessive production of thyroid hormones by the thyroid gland, which in turn suppresses pituitary TSH production. In contrast, secondary hyperthyroidism results from excessive pituitary secretion of TSH. Tertiary hyperthyroidism is caused by increased hypothalamic secretion of TRH. This patient most likely has Graves' disease due to elevated thyroid hormone levels in the face of decreased TSH levels (Table 8-10).

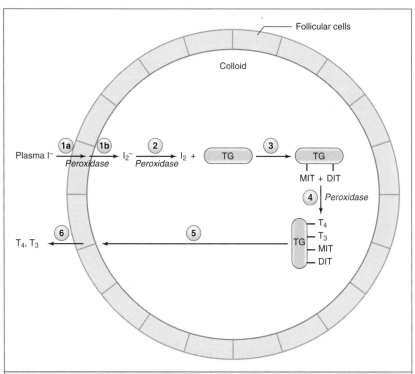

Figure 8-12. Thyroid hormone synthesis in the thyroid follicle. DIT, diiodotyrosine; I, iodide ion; I_2, iodine; MIT, monoiodotyrosine; T_3, triiodothyronine; T_4, thyroxine; TG, thyroglobulin. (From Brown TA: Rapid Review Physiology. Philadelphia, Mosby, 2007.)

8. **Based on your suspected diagnosis, what additional laboratory and physical findings might you expect?**
   Graves' disease is the most common cause of hyperthyroidism and is additionally characterized by exophthalmos, pretibial myxedema, and antibodies (IgG) to the TSH receptor in the thyroid. The antibodies presumably stimulate the thyroid in the same way as TSH does. Notice that this woman had a diffusely enlarged thyroid, which is consistent with TSH receptor stimulation causing diffuse thyroid enlargement.

CASE 8-7 continued:

On further examination, you note the appearance of the skin of the lower extremities, as shown in Figure 8-14.

9. **What is the pathophysiology of this complication of Graves' disease?**
   Pretibial myxedema is a *nonpitting* edema caused by accumulation of interstitial glycosaminoglycans (GAGs) within the dermis. Paradoxically, pretibial myxedema can also be seen in severe hypothyroidism.

10. **What would a thyroid iodide-131 uptake scan likely reveal in this patient?**
    Because iodide is used to synthesize thyroid hormone, Graves' disease would show an increased diffuse uptake, corresponding to an increased synthesis of T_4. When the gland is inactive owing to exogenous hormone therapy or because of the inflammation of the gland (e.g., thyroiditis), uptake would be low. See Figures 8-15 and 8-16 for comparison.

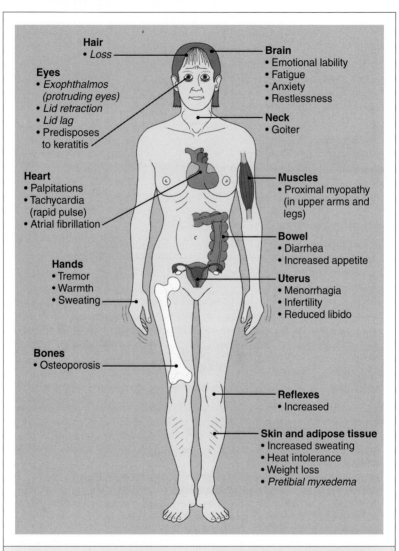

Figure 8-13. Symptoms and signs of thyrotoxicosis (hyperthyroidism). The features in *italics* are found only in Graves' disease. (From Meszaros JG, Olson ER, Naugle JE, et al: Crash Course: Endocrine and Reproductive Systems. Philadelphia, Mosby, 2006.)

TABLE 8-10. LABORATORY VALUES ASSOCIATED WITH HYPERTHYROIDISM

Type	Example	TRH	TSH	T₄
Primary hyperthyroidism	Graves' disease	↓	↓	↑
Secondary hyperthyroidism	Pituitary adenoma	↓	↑	↑
Tertiary hyperthyroidism	Hypothalamic tumor	↑	↑	↑

T_4, thyroxine; TRH, thyrotropin-releasing hormone; TSH, thyroid-stimulating hormone.

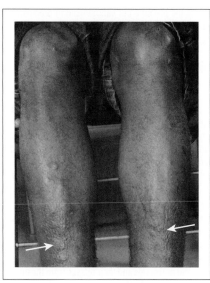

Figure 8-14. Appearance of lower extremities in patient in case 8-7. (From Noble J: Textbook of Primary Care Medicine, 3rd ed. St. Louis, Mosby, 2001.)

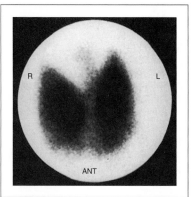

Figure 8-15. Graves' disease, showing diffusely increased radiolabeled iodine uptake. (From Mettler FA Jr: Essentials of Radiology, 2nd ed. Philadelphia, WB Saunders, 2005.)

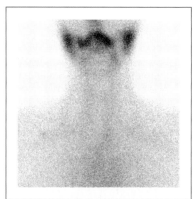

Figure 8-16. Thyroiditis, showing near absence of radiolabeled iodine uptake. (From Rakel RE: Conn's Current Therapy 2007, 59th ed. Philadelphia, WB Saunders, 2007.)

11. **What therapeutic options are available to this patient?**
   She has the options of medications (thionamides, beta blockers), surgery, radioactive[131]I ablation, and watchful waiting.

12. **Why might a physician prescribe propylthiouracil or methimazole for this woman? How do these drugs work?**
   Both propylthiouracil (PTU) and methimazole are largely concentrated in the thyroid and inhibit thyroid hormone synthesis. To a small extent, PTU also acts by preventing the peripheral deiodination of T_4 to T_3.

Note: PTU and methimazole both freely cross the placenta but can be used in pregnancy (though there are some risks, particularly with methimazole), whereas radioactive iodide is clearly contraindicated in pregnancy because it permanently destroys thyroid function.

13. **What is thyroid storm? Why is propylthiouracil used for this condition instead of methimazole?**
Thyroid storm results from excessive levels of thyroid hormone, causing a substantial elevation in the BMR and extreme fever in which patients can seem to "burn up right in front of you." It is potentially fatal. Both PTU and methimazole inhibit thyroid hormone synthesis, but because the thyroid has an abundant store of thyroid hormone it may take weeks for this effect to manifest. However, because at higher doses PTU also inhibits the conversion of T_4 to T_3 in the peripheral tissues, and T_3 is the more active form of thyroid hormone, PTU can have a fairly rapid effect.
Note: Both of these drugs can cause a fatal agranulocytosis, often preceded by a sore throat, so periodic monitoring is therefore required.

14. **Why is iodide therapy generally initiated 2 weeks prior to thyroidectomy in hyperthyroid patients?**
By an unknown mechanism, administration of a large amount of iodide decreases the vascularity of the thyroid gland, which reduces bleeding complications during surgery. Excess iodide also appears to inhibit the synthesis of thyroid hormones and their release from the thyroid gland (the so-called *Wolff-Chaikoff* effect), which may be an intrinsic mechanism to protect against hyperthyroidism in a setting of iodine excess.

SOME DIFFERENTIAL DIAGNOSIS AND PHYSIOLOGY CONCEPTS

15. **How would a patient with hyperthyroidism secondary to de Quervain's thyroiditis (subacute granulomatous thyroiditis) typically present clinically?**
Patients with this disease have an exquisitely tender thyroid gland and generally have signs of infection (e.g., fever).

16. **How can a teratoma produce hyperthyroidism?**
A rare form of female teratoma called *struma ovarii* is made up exclusively of functional thyroid tissue, which can produce enough thyroid hormone to cause clinical hyperthyroidism.

SUMMARY BOX: HYPERTHYROIDISM AND GRAVES' DISEASE

- Hyperthyroidism classically presents with some combination of the following: heat intolerance, weight loss despite an excellent appetite, tremor, palpitations, anxiety, diarrhea, osteoporosis, hypercalcemia, atrial fibrillation, and high-output heart failure.

- Graves' disease is the most common cause of hyperthyroidism and may be additionally characterized by exophthalmos, pretibial myxedema, and antibodies (IgG) to the thyroid-stimulating hormone (TSH) receptor in the thyroid. Toxic multinodular goiter is the second most common cause of hyperthyroidism disease.

- Radiolabeled iodide uptake is diffusely increased in Graves' disease but decreased in hyperthyroidism caused by exogenous thyroid hormone administration or in transient cases of hyperthyroidism due to thyroiditis.

- Thyroid hormones increase the basal metabolic rate (BMR) principally through increasing the production and insertion of the Na^+/K^+-ATPase pumps in various cell types, as well as by stimulating the production of glycolytic enzymes.

- Thyroxine (T_4) is a prohormone whose activity is largely dependent on conversion to the more active triiodothyronine (T_3).

- Thyroid hormone synthesis: (1) uptake of iodide ion (I^-) from plasma into follicular cells and the follicular lumen; (2) oxidation of iodide ion (I^-) to iodine (I_2) and attachment of iodine to tyrosine on thyroglobulin, both catalyzed by thyroid peroxidase; (3) coupling of iodinated tyrosine molecules to form T_4 or T_3; and (4) endocytosis of modified thyroglobulin into follicular cells and hydrolysis to T_4 and T_3, which then diffuse across the plasma membrane and enter the circulation.

- Thyroid hormones increase the sensitivity to circulating catecholamines, contributing to tachycardia, tremor, and palpitations.

- Pretibial myxedema is a *nonpitting* edema caused by accumulation of interstitial glycosaminoglycans (GAGs) within the dermis.

- Treatment options for Graves' disease include thionamides, surgery, radioactive iodine-131 ablation, beta blockers, and watchful waiting.

- The thionamides propylthiouracil (PTU) and methimazole are largely concentrated in the thyroid and inhibit thyroid hormone synthesis.

- Iodide therapy before surgery reduces the vascularity of the thyroid and therefore the bleeding complications of the surgery. Via the *Wolff-Chaikoff* effect, excess iodide also inhibits thyroid hormone synthesis, which may be an intrinsic mechanism to protect against hyperthyroidism in settings of iodine excess.

CASE 8-8

A 42-year-old woman complains of recent weight gain, fatigue, and heavy periods (menorrhagia). On physical examination she appears pale, speaks slowly, and has a diffusely enlarged nontender thyroid gland and a yellowish tinge to her skin.

1. **What do you suspect at this point?**
   Weight gain, fatigue, and menorrhagia, as well as constipation and cold intolerance (which this patient does not have), are all classic symptoms of hypothyroidism. The pallor and psychomotor retardation also point toward hypothyroidism. However, other conditions such as depression and anemia need to be considered.

CASE 8-8 continued:

She denies any history of bipolar disorder or treatment with lithium.

2. **Why was asking about lithium use relevant in the diagnostic workup of this patient?**
   Lithium inhibits the uptake and organification of iodine by the thyroid gland and also inhibits the peripheral conversion of T_4 to T_3 by 5'-monodeiodinase, thereby causing hypothyroidism. Amiodarone, an antiarrhythmic agent, is also known to cause hypothyroidism.

CASE 8-8 continued:

Workup reveals elevated TSH and reduced T$_4$.

3. **What is the diagnosis?**
   She has hypothyroidism, the most common cause of which is Hashimoto's (autoimmune) thyroiditis. Other causes of hypothyroidism include subacute granulomatous thyroiditis (de Quervain's thyroiditis), Reidel's thyroiditis, iatrogenic causes (e.g., thyroidectomy, thyroid radiotherapy), cretinism, endemic goiter, and medications such as lithium and amiodarone.
   For boards, you should recognize the following associations with regard to hypothyroidism:
   - Hashimoto's thyroiditis is caused by autoimmune destruction of the thyroid gland.
   - De Quervain's thyroiditis typically develops after a viral upper respiratory tract infection.
   - Reidel's thyroiditis is caused by fibrosis of the thyroid gland such that the thyroid gland may have a "woody" consistency on examination.
   - Cretinism results in short stature, protruding umbilicus, pot belly, and coarse facial features, including a protuberant tongue. Mental retardation occurs secondary to iodine deficiency at early developmental stages, and endemic goiter results from dietary iodide insufficiency in adulthood.

4. **Does this patient have primary, secondary, or tertiary hypothyroidism?**
   This woman has primary hypothyroidism. Reduced hormone production by the thyroid gland disinhibits the hypothalamic-pituitary axis, resulting in increased TRH and TSH. Secondary and tertiary hypothyroidism is caused by pituitary and hypothalamic dysfunction, respectively (Table 8-11). TSH levels would not be elevated in either of these cases.

TABLE 8-11. FORMS OF HYPOTHYROIDISM			
Clinical Form	**T$_4$/T$_3$**	**TSH**	**TRH**
Primary hypothyroidism	Low	High	High
Secondary hypothyroidism	Low	Low	High
Tertiary hypothyroidism	Low	Low	Low
Subclinical hypothyroidism	Normal	High	Normal

T$_3$, triiodothyronine; T$_4$, thyroxine; TRH, thyrotropin-releasing hormone; TSH, thyroid-stimulating hormone.

5. **What diagnosis should you suspect in a hospitalized patient with abnormal thyroid hormone levels?**
   Sick euthyroid syndrome refers to abnormalities in thyroid function that occur in ill patients without underlying thyroid or pituitary disease. Sick euthyroid syndrome may in part be caused by reduced peripheral conversion of T$_4$ to T$_3$, and commonly occurs following illness, nutritional deficiencies and glucocorticoid administration. The exact cause of sick euthyroid syndrome is not known, but it is thought to be the body's attempt to conserve calories during states of caloric deficit or increased caloric need. Because of the prevalence of sick euthyroid syndrome and the difficulty in interpreting thyroid studies in sick patients, most endocrinologists do not recommend testing thyroid function in hospitalized patients.

CASE 8-8 continued:

Further workup reveals the presence of plasma antimicrosomal (antiperoxidase) antibodies, and a thyroid biopsy shows a diffuse lymphocytic infiltrate.

6. **What is the diagnosis? Why might you also want to check serum vitamin B$_{12}$ levels in this patient?**

Plasma antimicrosomal (antiperoxidase) antibodies and biopsy showing lymphocytic infiltration of the thyroid gland is typical of Hashimoto's thyroiditis. This disease is frequently associated with autoimmune conditions such as pernicious anemia, which is characterized by impaired absorption of vitamin B$_{12}$ (Table 8-12). Therefore, checking a vitamin B$_{12}$ level would not be unreasonable.

TABLE 8-12. AUTOIMMUNE CONDITIONS

Disease	Autoantibody
Hashimoto's thyroiditis	Antimicrosomal, antithyroglobulin
SLE	Antinuclear antibody (most sensitive, nonspecific)
	Anti-dsDNA (present with lupus-associated renal disease; indicates poor prognosis)
	Anti-Smith (very specific)
Drug-induced lupus	Antihistone
Scleroderma	Anticentromere (CREST)
	Anti-Scl-70/anti-topoisomerase (diffuse)
Graves' disease	Anti-TSH
Myasthenia gravis	Anti-AChR
Pernicious anemia	Anti-intrinsic factor, anti-parietal cell
Rheumatoid arthritis	Rheumatoid factor (anti-IgG)
Primary biliary cirrhosis	Antimitochondrial
Sjögren's syndrome	Anti-Ro, anti-La
Celiac disease	Antigliadin, antiendomysial
Autoimmune hepatitis	Anti-smooth muscle
Goodpasture disease	Anti-basement membrane
Wegener's granulomatosis	c-ANCA (cytoplasmic)
Microscopic polyangiitis	p-ANCA (peripheral)
Pauci-immune crescentic glomerulonephritis	MPO-ANCA
Polymyositis Dermatomyositis	Anti-Jo-1
Diabetes type 1	Anti-glutamic acid decarboxylase

AChR, acetylcholine receptor antibody; ANCA, antineutrophil cytoplasmic antibodies; CREST, *c*alcinosis, *R*aynaud syndrome, *e*sophageal dysmotility, *s*clerodactyly, *t*elangiectasia; dsDNA, double-stranded DNA; IgG, immunoglobulin G; MPO, myeloperoxidase; SLE, systemic lupus erythematosus; TSH, thyroid-stimulating hormone.

STEP 1 SECRET

Autoimmune conditions are most widely seen in young to middle-aged females. You are expected to know the antibodies associated with common autoimmune conditions, and are likely to be asked at least one question from Table 8-12.

7. **Why does this patient have the weight gain and yellow skin?**
This patient's weight gain is due to her low metabolic state (i.e., low BMR) along with retention of salt and water. The retention of salt and water will put her at risk for congestive cardiomyopathy. The yellowing of her skin is due to the impaired conversion of β-carotenes into retinoic acid, which is normally driven by thyroid hormone.

8. **Given her history of menorrhagia, what hematologic disorder should we be worried about?**
Iron deficiency anemia is a concern. Because she is having heavy periods, she is losing blood and iron. The combination of pallor and fatigue also points to this condition.

CASE 8-8 continued:

The patient returns 10 years later for evaluation of profound fatigue. Examination is significant for periorbital edema, blunted deep tendon reflexes, and sinus bradycardia. Laboratory workup shows sodium level of 126 mEq/dL (normal range is 135–145 mEq/dL).

9. **What is the diagnosis?**
Myxedema coma, which can manifest as profound lethargy or coma, weakness, hypothermia, hypoventilation, hypoglycemia, and hyponatremia, is the diagnosis.

SOME DIFFERENTIAL DIAGNOSIS CONCEPTS

10. **If this woman's history was significant for a recent upper respiratory infection and her thyroid was tender to palpation, what would be the probable diagnosis?**
Those findings would suggest subacute thyroiditis (de Quervain's thyroiditis). This disease starts out as *hyperthyroidism*, due to inflammation causing release of stored thyroid hormones, but then progresses to hypothyroidism. It is thought to involve viral infection of the thyroid gland and classically occurs following an upper respiratory infection. It usually resolves on its own.

11. **How can a thyroidectomy cause muscle cramps and paresthesias?**
Accidental removal of the parathyroid glands may occur with thyroidectomy. This can lead to hypocalcemia, which manifests with these symptoms.

12. **What is the treatment option for hypothyroidism?**
Thyroid hormone replacement (levothyroxine) is needed, with a goal of normalizing TSH and relieving symptoms of hypothyroidism.

RELATED QUESTIONS

13. **How is it possible for a thyroid gland to develop at the back of the tongue?**
The thyroid begins its development at the back of the tongue and then migrates to its position below the thyroid cartilage in the neck. Failure to migrate along the thyroglossal duct may therefore result in a thyroid gland at the back of the tongue. This is an important embryologic correlation to make for Step 1.
   Note: Persistence of the thyroglossal duct that facilitates the migration of the thyroid can cause a thyroglossal duct cyst.

14. **Why are thyroid hormone levels routinely evaluated in newborns?**
Hypothyroidism is one of the preventable causes of mental retardation.

15. Cover the two columns on the right side of Table 8-13 and list the manifestations of hypothyroidism and hyperthyroidism for each feature in column 1.

TABLE 8-13. MANIFESTATIONS OF HYPOTHYROIDISM AND HYPERTHYROIDISM		
Feature	Hypothyroidism	Hyperthyroidism
Metabolic rate	Decreased	Increased
Body weight	Gain	Loss
Intestinal activity	Constipation	Diarrhea
Mental status	Memory loss/dementia	Psychosis, agitation
Body temperature	Cold intolerance	Heat intolerance
Deep tendon reflexes	Hypoactive	Hyperactive
Most severe complication	Myxedema coma	Thyroid storm

SUMMARY BOX: HYPOTHYROIDISM

- Hypothyroidism classically presents with some combination of the following: weight gain, fatigue, cold intolerance, constipation, menorrhagia, and depression.

- The most common cause of hypothyroidism is Hashimoto's thyroiditis, which is caused by autoimmune destruction of the thyroid gland. Hashimoto's thyroiditis is often associated with other autoimmune conditions such as pernicious anemia.

- Other causes of hypothyroidism include subacute granulomatous thyroiditis (de Quervain's thyroiditis), Reidel's thyroiditis, iatrogenic thyroiditis (e.g., caused by thyroidectomy or thyroid radiotherapy), cretinism, endemic goiter, and medications such as lithium and amiodarone.

- Sick euthyroid syndrome refers to abnormalities in thyroid function that occur in ill patients without obvious thyroid or pituitary disease. It is very common in hospitalized patients and may be related to reduced peripheral conversion of thyroxine (T_4) to triiodothyronine (T_3).

- Treatment for hypothyroidism is replacement therapy with thyroid hormone, with a goal of normalizing thyroid-stimulating hormone (TSH) and relieving symptoms.

- Typically in the presence of a stressor such as infection, untreated hypothyroidism can occasionally progress to myxedema coma, which can manifest as profound lethargy or coma, weakness, hypothermia, hypoventilation, hypoglycemia, and hyponatremia.

- Hypothyroidism is one of the preventable causes of mental retardation.

CASE 8-9

A previously healthy 12-year-old boy presents complaining of fatigue and excessive thirst (polydipsia). His mother mentions that he uses the bathroom quite frequently (polyuria), and his friends at school always tease him about this. His mother is also concerned because he has lost 10 lb despite eating "everything in sight." A random (nonfasting) plasma glucose level is 220 mg/dL.

1. **What is the likely diagnosis?**
   He most likely has diabetes mellitus, probably type 1 given his young age, but it could just as easily be early-onset type 2 associated with sedentary lifestyle and obesity.

2. **Differentiate among type 1, type 2, and maturity-onset diabetes of youth.**
   Type 1 diabetes is caused by autoimmune destruction of the beta cells. It classically occurs in children and adolescents. Patients are typically thin, and their initial presentation may be one of diabetic ketoacidosis (DKA).

   Type 2 diabetes is caused by a combination of insulin resistance and beta cell dysfunction. It classically occurs in sedentary and overweight adults. Type 2 diabetics are prone to hyperosmolar nonketotic syndrome and may occasionally experience DKA.

   Maturity-onset diabetes of youth (MODY) is a group of dominantly inherited disorders caused by impaired insulin secretion. MODY mimics type 1 diabetes because of the impaired insulin secretion. There are currently six known types of MODY, with MODY2 and MODY3 being the most common. Patients with MODY typically do not experience DKA because they produce enough insulin for fatty acid uptake (Fig. 8-17).

   ## CASE 8-9 continued:

   An oral glucose tolerance test (OGTT) shows plasma glucose level of 225 mg/dL 2 hours after the administration of a 75-g glucose load. Further workup reveals low levels of plasma insulin and C-peptide.

3. **Which type of diabetes does this boy have?**
   Type 1 diabetes mellitus is associated with low levels of insulin and C-peptide due to autoimmune destruction of the beta cells, as discussed previously. Recall that C-peptide is cosecreted (in equimolar amounts) with insulin.

4. **How can measurements of plasma C-peptide be used to differentiate between factitious hypoglycemia and an insulinoma?**
   Because plasma C-peptide is cosecreted with endogenous insulin, they will both be high in an insulinoma but very low in factitious hypoglycemia, in which only recombinant insulin is injected.

5. **Explain the mechanism by which the major metabolic pathways behave as though the body is in the fasting state during insulin deficiency (i.e., why has this patient lost weight)?**
   After consumption of a meal, insulin secretion is stimulated, which in turn activates glycolysis, glycogenesis, fatty acid synthesis, and protein synthesis. In the setting of insulin deficiency, all these pathways become less active and the opposing pathways (gluconeogenesis, glycogenolysis, and fatty acid catabolism) are stimulated; in essence, insulin deficiency causes a "hypercatabolic state."

6. **What is the biochemical mechanism by which diabetic ketoacidosis develops in the setting of insulin deficiency?**
   Ordinarily, insulin stimulates fatty acid uptake by adipocytes via stimulating lipoprotein lipase. In the absence of insulin (or significant insulin deficiency) fewer fatty acids are taken up by the adipocytes, and these fatty acids are then delivered to the liver, where they are metabolized, and ketoacids are a byproduct. Further exacerbating this problem, because insulin normally inhibits fatty acid catabolism by the liver, in the absence of insulin this pathway is even more active and more ketone bodies are produced. Finally, the acidosis is exacerbated because the corresponding hyperglycemia causes dehydration, making it more difficult for the kidneys to excrete acid.

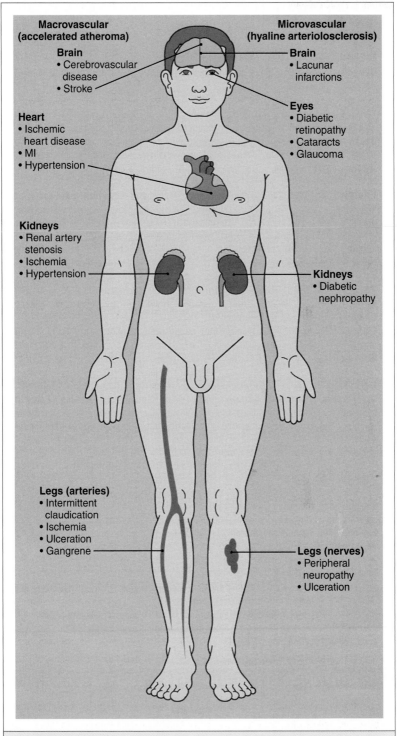

Figure 8-17. Chronic complications of diabetes mellitus. MI, myocardial infarction. (From Meszaros JG, Olson ER, Naugle JE, et al: Crash Course: Endocrine and Reproductive Systems. Philadelphia, Mosby, 2006.)

7. **What is the short-term value of controlling the blood sugar in this boy?**
   This will prevent the symptoms of hyperglycemia, such as polyuria, polydipsia, and polyphagia, as well as preventing weight loss. Additionally, in type 1 diabetes, the correction of insulin deficiency will prevent DKA.

8. **What is the long-term value of glycemic control in this boy?**
   Tight glycemic control has been proved to reduce the incidence of microvascular complications, including retinopathy, neuropathy, and nephropathy. However, it has not yet been shown to reduce macrovascular events such as heart attack and stroke, although future long-term studies may show such an effect.

9. **What is the value of measuring the hemoglobin A_{1c} level routinely in this patient?**
   The hemoglobin A_{1c} (HbA_{1c}) represents glycosylated hemoglobin, and the levels of HbA_{1c} are directly associated with levels of plasma glucose. It is an effective measure of long-term diabetes control because the life span of hemoglobin-laden red blood cells (RBCs) is approximately 120 days in the circulation. Moreover, reduced HbA_{1c} levels have been shown to correlate with better clinical outcomes.

10. **Why should blood pressure be closely scrutinized in this boy as he ages and high blood pressure be treated aggressively with angiotensin-converting enzyme inhibitors if it develops?**
    Blood pressure reduction substantially reduces the incidence of nephropathy and myocardial infarction. The angiotensin-converting enzyme (ACE) inhibitors are most effective at preventing nephropathy.

11. **For boards, why are beta blockers relatively contraindicated in diabetics?**
    Beta blockers may mask the warning signs of hypoglycemia, such as tremors, shakes, and tachycardia. Additionally, by antagonizing hepatic β-receptors, these drugs make it more difficult for the liver to respond to epinephrine, a counterregulatory hormone that elevates the blood glucose by stimulating glycogenolysis and gluconeogenesis. In type 1 diabetes, hypoglycemia is predominantly due to insulin overdosing.

CASE 8-9 continued:

The patient is diagnosed with type 1 diabetes mellitus and started on insulin therapy. One night he inadvertently takes his nighttime insulin dose twice. He notices no ill effects that night, but the following morning his prebreakfast glucose value is substantially higher than normal.

12. **What has happened?**
    Insulin-induced hypoglycemia during the night triggers release of "stress" hormones (e.g., cortisol, GH, glucagon, catecholamines), which cause a compensatory increase in plasma glucose. If the patient is not educated about this, he may inappropriately increase the nighttime dose of insulin to reduce the morning blood sugar levels and potentially precipitate hypoglycemic coma or even death during the night.

SUMMARY BOX: TYPE 1 DIABETES MELLITUS

- Type 1 diabetes usually occurs in children and adolescents. Newly diagnosed patients are often thin and may present initially in diabetic ketoacidosis (DKA).

- The pathophysiology of type 1 diabetes is related to inadequate insulin secretion. The body therefore behaves as if it is in the fasting state, and the processes of gluconeogenesis, glycogenolysis, and fatty acid catabolism are all stimulated. Treatment for type 1 diabetes is the administration of insulin.

- DKA occurs because in the absence of insulin, rather than being taken up by adipocytes, fatty acids are delivered to the liver and metabolized to ketone bodies. The hyperglycemia also causes an osmotic diuresis, which causes dehydration and exacerbates the metabolic derangements.

- Maturity-onset diabetes of the young (MODY) is an autosomal dominant inheritance disorder in which people present with mild hyperglycemia due to impaired glucose-induced release of insulin.

- Long-term tight glycemic control will retard the development of the microvascular (retinopathy, neuropathy, nephropathy) and macrovascular (myocardial infarction, peripheral vascular disease) complications of diabetes.

- The hemoglobin A_{1c} (HbA$_{1c}$) reflects the percent glycosylated hemoglobin at any time. It is an effective measure of long-term diabetes control because the life span of hemoglobin-laden red blood cells (RBCs) is approximately 120 days. Reduced HbA$_{1c}$ levels have been shown to correlate with better clinical outcomes.

- Beta blockers may mask the warning signs of hypoglycemia, such as tremors, shakes, and tachycardia.

- Taking too much nighttime insulin may result in an elevated morning plasma glucose level due to the pronounced sympathetic response to hypoglycemia.

CASE 8-10

A middle-aged obese man evaluated for a pre-employment physical examination complains of increased thirst and frequent urination. His nonfasting (random) plasma glucose level is 275 mg/dL. Both of his parents were overweight, had "sugar problems," and died of cardiovascular complications.

1. **Does this patient more likely have type 1 or type 2 diabetes mellitus?**
   Type 2 diabetes mellitus is most commonly seen in overweight sedentary middle-aged adults with a strong family history of diabetes. Many of these patients are diagnosed after complaining of increased thirst (polydipsia) and increased urinary frequency (polyuria), although more cases are now diagnosed from routine screening in asymptomatic patients.

2. **What is the pathogenesis of type 2 diabetes mellitus?**
   The early stage is characterized by insulin resistance and hyperinsulinemia but a *relative* insulin deficiency (due to insulin resistance). The later stages are characterized by beta cell dysfunction ("burnout"), which may result in insulin deficiency.
   Whether due to insulin resistance or insulin deficiency, hyperglycemia uniformly occurs in type 2 diabetes. Hyperglycemia results from increased lipolysis in adipose tissues (with the glycerol acting as a gluconeogenic substrate in the liver) as well as reduced glucose uptake by skeletal muscle and adipose tissue.
   Note: The increased atherogenesis that occurs in diabetes may be explained *in part* by the increased plasma levels of free fatty acids.

3. **How does binding of insulin to the insulin receptor result in glucose uptake into cells?**
It causes GLUT4 (insulin-dependent glucose transporter) to be incorporated into the plasma membrane of cells in skeletal muscle and adipose tissue. Glucose is then cotransported with potassium into the cell.

4. **What is the primary metabolic fuel in the fasting (between-meals) state?**
Fatty acids are the primary fuel. A notable exception to this is the CNS, which relies exclusively on serum glucose in both the fed and fasting states, except in periods of prolonged starvation, in which case the CNS will metabolize ketone bodies as well.

CASE 8-10 continued:

You take time to educate him about diabetes and plan a follow-up visit for 2 weeks, when fasting laboratory tests show plasma glucose of 180 mg/dL, total cholesterol of 250 mg/dL, low-density lipoprotein cholesterol of 175 mg/dL, and high-density lipoprotein cholesterol of 30 mg/dL, and a urinalysis reveals microalbuminuria. He is told he has diabetes and is educated about the importance of diet and exercise. Pharmacotherapy is started with metformin. He returns to the clinic 3 months later and his HbA$_{1c}$ has decreased from 8.5% to 7.5%.

5. **Why might therapy with a biguanide such as metformin make sense in this patient?**
This patient has type 2 diabetes mellitus, is obese, and has dyslipidemia, all of which can be improved by metformin therapy.
  Metformin (Glucophage) is a wonder drug for the management of type 2 diabetes mellitus. It normalizes plasma glucose primarily by inhibiting hepatic glucose production and by stimulating peripheral uptake of glucose by adipose and skeletal muscle. Furthermore, it has a beneficial effect on the lipid profile. In addition, it is very cheap. Finally, and perhaps most important to some patients, it has an anorexic effect and may result in modest weight loss.
  Note: Metformin can very rarely cause a life-threatening lactic acidosis. For this reason, it should be avoided in patients with congestive heart failure (CHF), liver disease, or renal disease. In terms of cardiac risk stratification, diabetes is considered a coronary heart disease (CHD) risk equivalent, and low-density lipoprotein (LDL) target goals are therefore <100 mg/dL in diabetics. Most diabetics should be on a statin, ACE inhibitor, and daily aspirin.

6. **What other classes of oral hypoglycemic agents are available to treat type 2 diabetes mellitus?**
Sulfonylureas such as tolbutamide, α-glucosidase inhibitors such as acarbose, and peroxisome proliferator-activated receptor (PPAR)-γ agonists (glitazones) such as pioglitazone.

7. **Why do the α-glucosidase inhibitors cause frequent gastrointestinal symptoms and annoying flatulence?**
This class of drugs, which includes *acarbose* and *miglitol,* work by inhibiting intestinal α-glucosidases (e.g., sucrase, maltase, isomaltase) that break down disaccharides into monosaccharides that can be absorbed by the intestines. The undigested sugars are metabolized by colonic bacteria to generate large volumes of gas.
  Note: These drugs do not cause hypoglycemia, but in the event that hypoglycemia occurs from a different oral hypoglycemic agent while the patient is taking one of these drugs, oral glucose should be given because its intestinal absorption will not be impeded. Clearly, intravenous glucose would be given in a hospital setting.

8. **What is the mechanism of action of the sulfonylureas?**
Sulfonylureas such as tolbutamide (first-generation agent) and glyburide (second-generation agent) act by stimulating insulin secretion. They do this by closing membrane-spanning K$^+$

channels on pancreatic beta cells. This results in depolarization of the cell, which triggers opening of voltage-gated calcium channels on the plasma membrane. The resultant influx of extracellular calcium stimulates insulin secretion, which lowers plasma glucose.

9. **What are some side effects of sulfonylureas?**
Improved glycemic control via increased insulin secretion may result in weight gain, because insulin stimulates fat synthesis. However, the more serious side effect of sulfonylureas is their propensity to cause hypoglycemia by causing excessive insulin secretion, particularly if a meal is skipped.
   First-generation sulfonylureas can cause a disulfiram-like reaction and are now rarely used.

10. **Why should this patient be educated about the importance of examining his feet periodically?**
Long-standing hyperglycemia in diabetes is associated with microvascular disease, as well as diabetic neuropathy. The microvascular disease may cause poor perfusion of the feet (macrovascular disease can do this, too), such that foot ulcers do not heal well. In addition, diabetic neuropathy allows ulcers to fester without causing any noticeable pain.
   Note: Diabetic neuropathy is typically in a "stocking-glove" distribution, with the distal feet affected before the more distal hands. This "stocking-glove" distribution is seen in other metabolic neuropathies as well, as the longer axons are more susceptible to a metabolic abnormality.

CASE 8-10 continued:

The patient's creatinine gradually increased from 0.7 to 3.2 mg/dL over 2 years. A renal biopsy is as shown in Figure 8-18.

11. **What renal pathology should you suspect?**
Diabetics are susceptible to nodular glomerulosclerosis and the so-called Kimmelstein-Wilson lesion. The image in Figure 8-18 shows nodular glomerulosclerosis with expansion of the mesangium by intensely PAS (periodic acid–Schiff)-positive material but without appreciable thickening of the glomerular capillary walls.

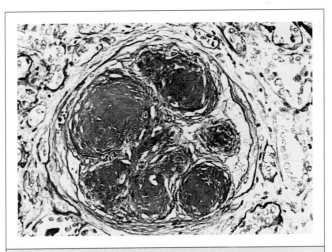

Figure 8-18. Light chain deposition disease. (From Brenner BM: Brenner and Rector's The Kidney, 7th ed. Philadelphia, WB Saunders, 2004.)

12. How can poor glycemic control cause this man to go into coma?

If he overdoses on sulfonylureas, he can go into a hypoglycemic coma. On the other hand, if his blood sugar runs too high, he can develop hyperosmolar nonketotic coma. Finally, although type 2 diabetics rarely go into DKA because of the presence of some insulin, if he becomes ill, DKA is another possibility.

SUMMARY BOX: TYPE 2 DIABETES MELLITUS

- Type 2 diabetes mellitus accounts for approximately 90% of cases of diabetes. Most people with type 2 diabetes are sedentary and overweight.

- The initial stage of type 2 diabetes is caused by insulin resistance and hyperinsulinemia. The later stage is caused by beta cell dysfunction and impaired insulin secretion.

- Clinical findings in type 2 diabetes include polyuria, polydipsia, recurrent blurry vision, and recurrent infections.

- Treatment for type 2 diabetes is exercise, weight loss, and oral hypoglycemic agents. Some type 2 diabetics require insulin.

CASE 8-11

A 33-year-old pregnant woman with an unremarkable medical history is admitted to the hospital for her 24-week gestational screening. One hour after the administration of a 50-g glucose load, her plasma glucose is 166 mg/dL. She has no history of diabetes, and none of her family members have diabetes. She is asked to return 1 week later, and a 3-hour glucose tolerance test (100-g glucose drink) is administered. Her results are shown in Table 8-14.

TABLE 8-14.	RESULTS OF GLUCOSE TOLERANCE TEST IN CASE 8-11	
Time	Serum Glucose Level	Normal Range
Fasting	95 mg/dL	95 mg/dL or below
At 1 hour	200 mg/dL	180 mg/dL or below
At 2 hours	181 mg/dL	155 mg/dL or below
At 3 hours	160 mg/dL	140 mg/dL or below

1. What is the diagnosis?

This woman has gestational diabetes. Gestational diabetes is defined as diabetes diagnosed for the first time during pregnancy and resolving 6 weeks or more after the pregnancy ends. It portends an increased risk for developing type 2 diabetes later in life.

All pregnant women should be screened when they are between 24 and 28 weeks' gestation. In a 50-g glucose challenge test (GCT), a 1-hour postglucose challenge plasma glucose level of >140 mg/dL is a positive finding. Confirmation of gestational diabetes is done using a 3-hour oral glucose tolerance test with a positive result having two or more values above the threshold value.

2. What is the cause of the relative maternal insulin resistance that develops during pregnancy and how is this valuable to the fetus?

Maternal insulin resistance during pregnancy is thought to result from the placental secretion of human placental lactogen (hPL), a glycoprotein that antagonizes the actions of maternal insulin. Because glucose moves across the placenta by passive diffusion, this physiologic alteration may facilitate delivery of glucose to the fetus.

3. **What is the most common undesired effect of maternal diabetes on fetal size and why does this happen?**
Fetal macrosomia (large fetus) is a complication of maternal diabetes and is a problem because of the increased risk of birth injury when an oversized fetus passes through the birth canal. Fetal size is increased because the maternal hyperglycemia stimulates increased fetal insulin secretion, which in turn stimulates fetal growth.

4. **Should hypoglycemia or hyperglycemia be expected in a baby born to a poorly controlled diabetic mother immediately following delivery? Explain.**
Hypoglycemia is expected. During in utero life, elevated fetal glucose levels (secondary to high maternal glucose levels) cause chronic fetal hyperinsulinemia. Just after delivery, when the fetus is no longer exposed to the elevated maternal glucose, the residual hyperinsulinemia can cause hypoglycemia. The treatment for this is to give the baby glucose after birth.

5. **What respiratory syndrome is the fetus at risk for at birth if the gestational diabetes is not corrected in the mother?**
Respiratory distress syndrome is due to the lack of surfactant synthesized by type II pneumocytes. Surfactant synthesis is *decreased* by insulin and increased by cortisol and T_4. Because mothers with gestational diabetes have higher-than-normal levels of insulin, this risk to the newborn should be noted.

SUMMARY BOX: GESTATIONAL DIABETES

- Gestational diabetes is defined as diabetes detected for the first time during pregnancy and resolving 6 weeks or more after the pregnancy ends. It is due to the insulin resistance associated with pregnancy.

- All pregnant women should be screened with a glucose challenge test between 24 and 28 weeks' gestation. A 1-hour after the challenge test a glucose level of >140 mg/dL is a positive screen. This then needs to be confirmed with a 3-hour glucose tolerance test.

- Gestational diabetes portends an increased risk for diabetes later in life. It also predisposes newborns to macrosomia, hypoglycemia, and respiratory distress syndrome.

CASE 8-12

A 42-year-old registered nurse complains of episodes of tremor, diaphoresis, and palpitations several hours after eating. She also notes similar symptoms when first waking in the morning. Symptoms are alleviated by eating. Her plasma glucose is low during symptomatic episodes, ranging from 30 to 60 mg/dL (she has access to a glucometer because her husband is diabetic). Review of systems is significant only for a 15-lb weight gain in recent months. Physical examination is unrevealing.

1. **What is the differential diagnosis for hypoglycemia in this woman?**
Hypoglycemia can be "reactive" or can be due to insulin excess. Reactive or postprandial hypoglycemia can occur in various situations (more on this later). Excess insulin can be due to either an endogenous source (insulinoma, nesidioblastosis) or an exogeneous source (factitious hypoglycemia).

For boards, realize that a patient with a significant psychiatric history or with access to prescription drugs (e.g., nurses, doctors) is suspect for exogenous insulin administration (factitious hypoglycemia).

2. **What is reactive (postprandial) hypoglycemia?**
Reactive hypoglycemia can be categorized as functional or alimentary or representing early (occult) diabetes.

Functional hypoglycemia is the most common type. It occurs following meals and is associated with high-energy, type A personalities. The mechanism of the hypoglycemia is unclear but is thought not to be related to excessive insulin secretion.

Alimentary hypoglycemia occurs in response to rapid glucose absorption. This is typically seen following gastric resections, in which gastric contents are delivered to the small bowel at a rapid rate, resulting in a surge of insulin secretion and hypoglycemia. Symptoms will often respond to reduced carbohydrate intake as well as smaller, more frequent meals.

Early or occult diabetes mellitus can also cause hypoglycemia. The mechanism is felt to be related to a delay in early insulin release from beta cells, resulting in hyperglycemia. An exaggerated late-phase insulin secretion then occurs in response to the hyperglycemia.

3. **How can the C-peptide level help differentiate factitious from true hypoglycemia?**
C-peptide is cosecreted with insulin in equivalent amounts. Exogenous insulin preparations do not contain C-peptide. Therefore, patients self-administering insulin should be expected to have low levels of C-peptide, whereas patients with endogenous hyperinsulinism (e.g., insulinoma) should have high levels of C-peptide. It is important to recognize that sulfonylureas are an exception to this rule. Sulfonylureas increase insulin and C-peptide secretion by beta cells such that a patient ingesting sulfonylureas will have elevated levels of insulin and C-peptide. Sulfonylurea ingestion can be very difficult to differentiate from insulinoma; therefore, obtaining a plasma sulfonylurea level can be helpful.

CASE 8-12 continued:

The patient returns the next day to the clinic, and blood work is performed. Fasting plasma glucose is low at 35 mg/dL, and simultaneous plasma insulin is markedly elevated. The patient is moderately symptomatic from her hypoglycemia. She is given some crackers and soda and her symptoms resolve.

4. **Has Whipple's triad been satisfied by this patient?**
Yes. The constellation of documented hypoglycemia, symptoms that can be reasonably attributed to hypoglycemia (e.g., confusion), and the resolution of these symptoms with eating (or the administration of glucose) is known as Whipple's triad. Whipple's triad is suggestive of, but not specific for, an insulinoma.

CASE 8-12 continued:

The patient is admitted for an observed 48-hour fast. A plasma sulfonylurea screen is negative. After 28 hours of observed fasting, the patient becomes confused and diaphoretic, and simultaneous measurements of glucose and insulin are again low and high, respectively. An MRI of the abdomen shows a small mass in the tail of the pancreas.

5. **What is the diagnosis?**
Short of a definitive pathologic diagnosis, we can be fairly certain that this patient has an insulinoma. Her insulin levels are inappropriately high in the presence of hypoglycemia. Furthermore, she does not appear to be abusing sulfonylureas, and the abdominal MRI is suggestive of a pancreatic insulinoma. The next step for this patient would be surgery.

SUMMARY BOX: HYPOGLYCEMIA AND INSULINOMA

- Hypoglycemia can manifest clinically as lethargy, tremor, and palpitations, which are due to stimulation of the sympathetic and parasympathetic (sweating) arms of the autonomic nervous system.

- Hypoglycemia can be factitious in origin (as in a health care worker with access to insulin) "reactive" following meals, or secondary to endogenous hyperinsulinism, the most common cause of which is an insulinoma.

- The diagnosis of an insulinoma requires demonstration of Whipple's triad—hypoglycemia, hypoglycemic symptoms, and resolution of symptoms with glucose.

- Proinsulin, when cleaved, produces two products: C-peptide and insulin.

- Another cause of hypoglycemia can be nesidioblastosis, or beta islet cell hyperplasia. This is a rare hyperplasia disorder of the beta islet cells that results in excess insulin secretion, leading to a hypoglycemic state.

- For boards, treatment of an insulinoma is surgical resection.

CASE 8–13

A 49-year-old man with a history of recurrent calcium oxalate kidney stones and peptic ulcer disease, which has been refractory to therapy with proton pump inhibitors, is evaluated for new-onset visual deficits. MRI of the head reveals an enlarged structure located in the sella turcica.

1. **What do you suspect?**
Recurrent calcium oxalate kidney stones are suggestive of hyperparathyroidism, refractory peptic ulcer disease is suggestive of the Zollinger-Ellison syndrome, and visual deficits and the MRI finding are suggestive of a pituitary adenoma. The constellation of a pituitary adenoma, pancreatic neuroendocrine tumor, and hyperparathyroidism should make one think of multiple endocrine neoplasia type I (MEN I). However, more information is needed.

CASE 8–13 continued:

Laboratory workup reveals elevated levels of gastrin, prolactin, and PTH.

2. **What is the diagnosis?**
Hyperparathyroidism, hyperprolactinemia, presumably from a pituitary adenoma, and hypergastrinemia confirm the diagnosis of MEN I. Hyperparathyroidism is the most common abnormality in MEN I, present in more than 90% of patients. It occurs 10 to 20 years earlier than the sporadic form of hyperparathyroidism and is much more aggressive. It typically involves all four parathyroid glands, and subtotal parathyroidectomy is therefore rarely curative. MEN I is caused by mutations in the menin gene, a presumptive tumor suppressor gene.

3. **What is the danger of missing a diagnosis of multiple endocrine neoplasia type IIA?**
MEN IIA is associated with medullary thyroid carcinoma, pheochromocytoma, and primary hyperparathyroidism. Cutaneous lichen amyloidosis has also been recently added. Medullary

thyroid carcinoma, which can be life-threatening, has a frequency of greater than 90% in MEN IIA patients. Therefore, making the diagnosis and initiating early genetic screening are critical. MEN IIA is caused by mutations in the *RET* proto-oncogene.

4. **What is multiple endocrine neoplasia type IIB?**

   MEN IIB is very rare and is associated with medullary thyroid carcinoma, pheochromocytoma, mucosal neuromas, intestinal ganglioneuromas, and occasionally a marfanoid habitus. As with MEN IIA, medullary thyroid carcinoma is the most common component. However, unlike in MEN I and MEN IIA, primary hyperparathyroidism is not present. MEN IIB is also caused by mutations in the *RET* proto-oncogene.

5. **What is Zollinger-Ellison syndrome and how is it related to multiple endocrine neoplasia type I?**

   Zollinger-Ellison syndrome is a disorder in which the hormone gastrin is produced in excess, directly causing the stomach to produce excessive hydrochloric acid. This tumor can arise in the duodenum or pancreas. In this patient, a tumor of the pancreatic islet cell (gastrinoma) is causing the continuous excretion of gastrin. Thirty percent of patients with gastrinoma of the pancreatic islet cell also have tumors of the parathyroid glands and the pituitary. These collective tumors are known as MEN I.

   Note: Other causes of hypergastrinemia include G cell hyperplasia, pernicious anemia, gastric outlet obstruction, renal failure, and proton pump inhibitors.

STEP 1 SECRET

Multiple endocrine neoplasia (MEN) syndromes are a boards favorite! You should know the tumors associated with all three MEN syndromes and the constellation of symptoms that result from them. Boards questions on MEN syndromes are often straightforward but will most likely require you to recognize the diagnosis, which can be tricky for some students. The best way to get good at this is to do USMLE practice questions.

SUMMARY BOX: MULTIPLE ENDOCRINE NEOPLASIA

- The constellation of a pituitary adenoma, pancreatic neuroendocrine tumor, and hyperparathyroidism should make one think of multiple endocrine neoplasia (MEN) type I. Hyperparathyroidism is the most common abnormality in MEN I, present in more than 90% of patients. It occurs 10 to 20 years earlier than the sporadic form of hyperparathyroidism and is much more aggressive. It typically involves all four parathyroid glands, and subtotal parathyroidectomy is therefore rarely curative. MEN I is caused by mutations in the menin gene, a presumptive tumor suppressor gene.

- MEN IIA is associated with medullary thyroid carcinoma, pheochromocytoma, and primary hyperparathyroidism. Cutaneous lichen amyloidosis has also been recently added.

- Medullary thyroid carcinoma, which can be life-threatening, has a frequency of greater than 90% in MEN IIA patients. Therefore, making the diagnosis and initiating early genetic screening are critical. MEN IIA is caused by mutations in the *RET* proto-oncogene.

- MEN IIB is rare and is associated with medullary thyroid carcinoma, pheochromocytoma, mucosal neuromas, intestinal ganglioneuromas, and occasionally a marfanoid habitus.

- As with MEN IIA, medullary thyroid carcinoma is the most common component. However, unlike in MEN I and MEN IIA, primary hyperparathyroidism is not present. MEN IIB is also caused by mutations in the *RET* proto-oncogene.

- Zollinger-Ellison syndrome is caused by a tumor in the duodenum or pancreas that hypersecretes the hormone gastrin. Approximately 30% of patients with a gastrinoma of the pancreatic islet cells have MEN I.

CASE 8-14

A 41-year-old woman with an unremarkable past medical history is noted to have asymptomatic hypercalcemia on routine screening. She takes no medications. Physical examination is unremarkable.

1. **What are some causes of hypercalcemia?**
   In healthy "outpatients," primary hyperparathyroidism is the most common cause of hypercalcemia. In hospitalized patients, hypercalcemia of malignancy is the most common cause of hypercalcemia. Together these two are responsible for approximately 90% of cases of hypercalcemia. However, there are many other causes of hypercalcemia to be considered. Primary hyperparathyroidism associated with other endocrine disorders or with a family history of endocrine disorders evokes the possibility of the MEN syndromes. Frequent use of calcium-containing antacids evokes milk-alkali syndrome. Other medications such as thiazide diuretics and lithium can also cause hypercalcemia. Endocrinopathies resulting in excessive bone breakdown such as hyperthyroidism and Cushing syndrome can cause hypercalcemia. Paraneoplastic syndromes associated with production of parathyroid hormone–related peptide (PTHrP) can cause hypercalcemia. A genetic disorder of the calcium-sensing receptor in familial hypocalciuric hypercalcemia (FHH) is another cause of hypercalcemia. Finally, excessive vitamin D (which may occur with toxic ingestion, lymphomas, or granulomatous diseases such as sarcoidosis) can cause hypercalcemia.

CASE 8-14 continued:

A review of her medical records shows that she has had mild hypercalcemia since the age of 21. Upon questioning, it is discovered that her mother and an aunt both have mild hypercalcemia.

2. **How does this information suggest the likely cause of her hypercalcemia?**
   Given the strong family history, she likely has primary hyperparathyroidism associated with a MEN syndrome or she has FHH. It would be nice to know whether she has ever had kidney stones before.

CASE 8-14 continued:

She denies a personal or family history of kidney stones. A 24-hour urine collection reveals low amounts of urinary calcium excretion. Polymerase chain reaction (PCR) testing shows a mutation of her calcium-sensing receptor (*CASR*) gene.

3. **What is the diagnosis?**
She has FHH. As its name implies, FHH is associated with hypercalcemia resulting in part from deficient renal calcium excretion. It is inherited in an autosomal dominant manner. In contrast with primary hyperparathyroidism, which is often associated with markedly elevated PTH, hypercalciuria causing calcium oxalate kidney stones, and osteoporosis, FHH patients typically have a modest elevation in PTH and rarely get kidney stones. Nonetheless, FHH is often confused with mild cases of primary hyperparathyroidism. The danger in misdiagnosing FHH for primary hyperparathyroidism is that these patients may unnecessarily undergo a parathyroidectomy, with all its attendant risks.

4. **How does an inactivated calcium-sensing receptor gene in familial hypocalciuric hypercalcemia cause hypercalcemia?**
The *CASR* gene in the parathyroid glands mediates feedback inhibition of PTH secretion in response to rising serum calcium. An inactivated CASR therefore disinhibits PTH secretion in response to hypercalcemia. The result is that a higher-than-normal serum calcium level is required to inhibit PTH secretion, resulting in a mild hypercalcemia and modest elevation in PTH. The degree of hypercalcemia depends on how severely the *CASR* gene is inactivated.

5. **What is the treatment for familial hypocalciuric hypercalcemia?**
FHH usually does not require treatment, and most affected persons are asymptomatic. However, for those who are symptomatic, thiazide diuretics can be given.

RELATED QUESTIONS

6. **What are the three hormones that regulate calcium levels in the blood and tissues and their origin of secretion?**
   1. PTH is secreted from the chief cells in the parathyroid glands. PTH is released in response to low serum calcium, and its purpose is to raise the serum calcium level.
   2. Vitamin D is produced from the diet as well as from synthesis through cholesterol with the help of ultraviolet (UV) light. Its purpose is to raise the serum calcium level.
   3. Calcitonin comes from parafollicular cells in the thyroid gland. Calcitonin is secreted in response to high serum calcium and will lower the serum calcium level.

7. **How does inactive vitamin D get converted to the active form?**
See Figure 8-19.

SUMMARY BOX: FAMILIAL HYPOCALCIURIC HYPERCALCEMIA

- Familial hypocalciuric hypercalcemia is caused by autosomal dominant loss-of-function mutations in the calcium-sensing receptor (*CASR*) gene. Familial hypocalciuric hypercalcemia (FHH) patients are typically asymptomatic and present with hypercalcemia, hypocalciuria, and normal or modestly elevated parathyroid hormone (PTH) levels.

- FHH can be diagnosed with genetic testing for mutation in *CASR*, checking family history for hypercalcemia, and measuring 24-hour urine calcium excretion.

- Treatment for asymptomatic FHH patients is simply observation. If the patient is symptomatic from the hypercalcemia, a thiazide diuretic is often enough.

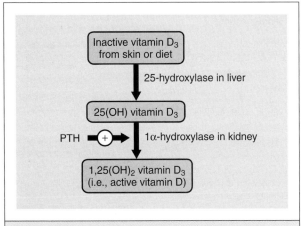

Figure 8-19. Activation of vitamin D. PTH, parathyroid hormone.(From Meszaros JG, Olson ER, Naugle JE, et al: Crash Course: Endocrine and Reproductive Systems. Philadelphia, Mosby, 2006.)

CASE 8-15

A newborn baby presents with ambiguous external genitalia. The child seems to have an enlarged clitoris rather than a penis, but there is a scrotum-like structure that appears to be the result of labial fusion. Physical examination also reveals tachycardia, hypotension, irritability, and hyperpigmentation seen most readily in the areolae and genitalia. Laboratory tests show hypoglycemia, hyponatremia, and hyperkalemia. An ultrasound reveals normally developed ovaries. Upon testing, the child's karyotype is found to be 46,XX.

1. **What is the most likely diagnosis?**
    The baby girl most likely has congenital adrenal hyperplasia (CAH), which is most commonly due to 21α-hydroxylase deficiency. All forms of CAH are characterized by deficient cortisol production, but depending on the specific enzymatic defect, levels of other adrenal steroids can be increased or decreased. Deficiency of 21α-hydroxylase accounts for about 90% of CAH cases, while 11β-hydroxylase deficiency accounts for most of the remaining 10%.

2. **How does 21α-hydroxylase deficiency cause virilization of females?**
    The adrenal steroid biosynthetic pathways produce three major hormones: mineralocorticoids (such as aldosterone), glucocorticoids (such as cortisol), and sex hormones (androgens or estrogens). In CAH, 21α-hydroxylase is usually partially deficient such that the production of aldosterone and cortisol decrease owing to the metabolic block (Fig. 8-20). This leads to an overproduction of steroid precursors (such as 17-hydroxyprogesterone). These precursors are shunted into the pathway of sex hormone biosynthesis, leading to excessive accumulation of adrenal androgens, which causes in utero masculinization of the external genitalia in developing females.

    Male pseudohermaphroditism occurs when an individual is a genetic and gonadal male with a 46,XY karyotype and (undescended) testes but has female genitalia. The most common disorder of male pseudohermaphroditism is testicular feminization syndrome (also known as androgen insensitivity) caused by a defective androgen receptor. Female pseudohermaphrodites are genetic and gonadal females with a 46,XX karyotype and ovaries but have male external genitalia and secondary sex characteristics. Female pseudohermaphrodites are usually the result of CAH. Unlike true hermaphrodites, pseudohermaphrodites have gonadal tissue of only one sex.

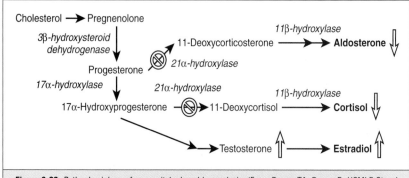

Figure 8-20. Pathophysiology of congenital adrenal hyperplasia (From Brown TA, Brown D: USMLE Step 1 Secrets. Philadelphia, Hanley & Belfus, 2004.)

3. **Why did this patient exhibit hyperkalemia, hyponatremia, tachycardia, hypotension, and hypoglycemia?**

Aldosterone is normally responsible for the maintenance of plasma volume and potassium concentration by promoting the reabsorption of sodium in exchange for potassium in the early distal tubule of the nephron. Aldosterone deficiency leads to hypovolemia, hyperkalemia, and in the case of severe deficiency, hyponatremia from salt wasting. Recall that sodium loss usually does not cause hyponatremia, but severe hypovolemia from sodium wasting will eventually stimulate ADH release, which in turn causes hyponatremia in an attempt to maintain volume.

Hypoglycemia is due to decreased activity of the counterregulatory (i.e., insulin-opposing) hormone cortisol.

Note: Cortisol deficiency is also a major contributor (if not the primary contributor) to hypotension in the setting of adrenal insufficiency. Cortisol plays a major role in the maintenance of "cardiovascular tone" and blood pressure that, although relatively poorly understood, is clinically very important. Acute cortisol deficiency can lead to severe hypotension that will be refractory to fluid resuscitation in the absence of glucocorticoid replacement. This is a common phenomenon in adult intensive care unit (ICU) patients, who often fail to adequately increase their cortisol secretion in response to the stress of critical illness (so-called relative adrenal insufficiency).

It is these electrolyte and hemodynamic consequences of cortisol deficiency that make CAH or other forms of acute adrenal insufficiency rapidly fatal if left untreated. Once the condition is diagnosed, treatment is fairly straightforward with replacement of cortisol. Often a synthetic mineralocorticoid (i.e., fludrocortisone) is given as well. (Because cortisol has some mineralocorticoid activity, some patients do well with cortisol alone.)

4. **Why are there bilateral adrenal hyperplasia and hyperpigmentation?**

The low cortisol level reduces negative feedback on pituitary ACTH production such that ACTH levels dramatically increase and stimulate glandular hyperplasia. Recall that ACTH also stimulates adrenal androgen synthesis, which further contributes to the virilization of females with CAH.

The hyperpigmentation is an indirect consequence of increased ACTH production. ACTH is synthesized from a POMC that is cleaved into ACTH, endorphins (i.e., endogenous opioids), and MSH. Thus, any increase in ACTH release is obligatorily accompanied by increases in MSH and endorphin release. As its name suggests, a rise in MSH levels results in stimulation of melanin production by melanocytes, producing the hyperpigmentation.

Note: Except for the virilization, many of the disease manifestations of CAH are identical to those seen in adults with disorders of primary adrenal insufficiency such as autoimmune adrenalitis (i.e., Addison's disease). These features include hypotension, salt wasting with hypovolemia and hyponatremia, hyperkalemia, hypoglycemia, and hyperpigmentation.

RELATED QUESTIONS

5. **Why does 11β-hydroxylase deficiency exhibit virilizing manifestations similar to those in 21α-hydroxylase deficiency but not the same salt-wasting manifestations?**
   When 11β-hydroxylase is deficient, aldosterone and cortisol synthesis are decreased as in 21α-hydroxylase deficiency. Again, steroid precursors accumulate and are shunted into androgen production, and low cortisol results in increased ACTH levels, which further stimulate androgen production.
   However, in contrast with classical CAH, 11β-hydroxylase deficiency results in the accumulation of 11-deoxycorticosterone (11-DOC), which is a weak mineralocorticoid. The levels of 11-DOC are high enough to cause fluid retention and hypertension despite the deficiency of aldosterone.

6. **Why are patients with 17α-hydroxylase deficiency phenotypically female?**
   With regard to external genitalia, all fetuses are female by default; it is only the production of androgens that masculinizes the external genitalia in normal males. However, with low levels of 17α-hydroxylase, insufficient levels of these androgens are produced in fetuses that are genetically male, resulting in male pseudohermaphrodism (genetic and gonadal males with 46,XY karyotypes and undescended testes, but female external genitalia).
   Note: Because estrogens are invariably synthesized from androgens (via aromatization of androgens) there is also low estrogen production in patients with 17α-hydroxylase deficiency. Thus, females with this rare form of CAH will usually present for investigation of failure to undergo pubertal development or menarche.

7. **Why are patients with 17α-hydroxylase deficiency often hypertensive?**
   The block in the pathway to make androgens or cortisol increases flux of substrate through the aldosterone synthesis pathway. The resulting increased aldosterone levels cause increased salt and water retention, resulting in hypervolemia and hypertension.

8. **Quick review: Cover the columns on the right side of Table 8-15 and list the signs and symptoms for the major congenital metabolic disorders within each metabolic pathway and their clinical manifestations.**

TABLE 8-15. MAJOR CONGENITAL METABOLIC DISORDERS			
Metabolic Pathway	**Genetic Diseases**	**Primary Cause of Clinical Symptoms**	**Major Signs/ Symptoms**
Glycogenolysis	Glucose-6-phosphatase deficiency (von Gierke disease)	Hypoglycemia	Hypoglycemic episodes, massive hepatomegaly
	Muscle glycogen phosphorylase deficiency (McArdle disease)	Inability of muscle to utilize glucose stored as glycogen	Muscle pain, exercise intolerance

Continued

TABLE 8-15. MAJOR CONGENITAL METABOLIC DISORDERS—continued

Metabolic Pathway	Genetic Diseases	Primary Cause of Clinical Symptoms	Major Signs/ Symptoms
Hexose monophosphate shunt (i.e., pentose phosphate pathway)	Glucose-6-phosphate dehydrogenase (G6PD) deficiency	RBC susceptibility to oxidative stress (e.g., sulfa or antimalarial drugs, infection)	Hemolytic anemia
Fatty acid oxidation	Medium-chain fatty acid decarboxylase (MCAD) deficiency	Hypoglycemia	Hypoketotic hypoglycemia, hyperammonemia
Urea cycle	Various enzymes deficiencies	Hyperammonemia	Encephalopathy
Amino acid metabolism	Phenylketonuria (PKU)	Toxic accumulation of phenylalanine and phenylketone derivatives; lack of tyrosine	Mental retardation, light pigmentation, eczema, "mousy" odor
	Maple syrup urine disease	Toxic accumulation of branched-chain amino acids (especially leucine) and their ketoacid derivatives	Poor feeding, psychomotor retardation, maple syrup odor to urine
Heme synthesis	Acute intermittent porphyria (AIP) and other acute porphyrias	Accumulation of porphyrin intermediates toxic to neurons	Neurovisceral symptoms (neuropathy, episodic abdominal pain)
	Porphyria cutanea tarda and other cutaneous porphyrias	Accumulation of photoreactive porphyrins within skin and/or RBCs	Photosensitive chronic blistering
	Hemolytic porphyrias		Hemolytic anemia
Adrenal corticosteroid synthesis	Congenital adrenal hyperplasia	Deficiency of cortisol and deficiency and/ or excess of mineralocorticoids and sex steroids	*All forms*: adrenal insufficiency with glandular hyperplasia and hyperpigmentation

Continued

TABLE 8-15. MAJOR CONGENITAL METABOLIC DISORDERS—continued

Metabolic Pathway	Genetic Diseases	Primary Cause of Clinical Symptoms	Major Signs/ Symptoms
	21α-Hydroxylase deficiency	Low cortisol and mineralocorticoids; excess androgens	Virilization in females; salt wasting with hypotension, hyponatremia, hyperkalemia
	11β-Hydroxylase deficiency	Low cortisol, excess mineralocorticoids (11-DOC) and androgens	Virilization in females; hypertension and fluid overload

11-DOC, 11-deoxycorticosterone; RBCs, red blood cells.

SUMMARY BOX: CONGENITAL ADRENAL HYPERPLASIA

- Congenital adrenal hyperplasia (CAH) is due to defects in glucocorticoid (i.e., cortisol) synthesis, with resulting hypoadrenalism and, depending on the specific enzyme involved, either increased or decreased levels of mineralocorticoids or sex steroids.

- The 21α-hydroxylase deficiency accounts for 90% of CAH. It results in deficiency of cortisol and aldosterone but excess adrenal androgens, resulting in ambiguous external genitalia in females; salt wasting with hypotension, tachycardia, hyponatremia, and hyperkalemia; hypoglycemia; and hyperpigmentation (due to increased adrenocorticotropic hormone [ACTH] and melanocyte-stimulating hormone [MSH] synthesis).

- Other forms of CAH, such as 11β-hydroxylase deficiency, can lead to virilization and fluid retention and hypertension due to excess mineralocorticoid production. Others, such as the rare 17α-hydroxylase deficiency, can lead to androgen and estrogen deficiency.

CHAPTER 9

MALE AND FEMALE REPRODUCTIVE SYSTEMS

David Austin Schirmer, III, MD, Thomas A. Brown, MD, and Sonali J. Shah

INSIDER'S GUIDE TO MALE AND FEMALE REPRODUCTIVE SYSTEMS FOR THE USMLE STEP 1

Students tend to brush off reproductive physiology and pathology during their boards studying, but in our opinion, this is a huge mistake. This subject is incredibly straightforward (and bound to give you a lot of free points!) if you work hard at it. Reproductive physiology is tremendously important. You should have a thorough understanding of the menstrual cycle, hormonal regulation, and the factors controlling male and female sexual differentiation. This will be of enormous help when it comes to understanding pathology and pathophysiology. We have done our best to offer the most boards-relevant case presentations in this chapter. Whenever relevant, you should pay close attention to the laboratory findings associated with these diseases as they relate to disorders of the hypothalamic-pituitary-gonadal axis.

BASIC CONCEPTS

1. **What is the normal duration of the menstrual cycle? What are the two ovarian phases, and which occurs first?**
    Normal cycle time is approximately 28 days, and the ovarian phases consist of the follicular and luteal phases, with the follicular phase occurring first. The first day of the menstrual cycle (and follicular phase) is defined as the day on which menstruation begins (Fig. 9-1).

2. **Which phase of the ovarian cycle is generally responsible for the cycle being longer or shorter?**
    The luteal phase is fixed at 14 days in a majority of women, so the differences in the length of the follicular phase account for cycle length differences. For boards, you should simply assume that the luteal phase accounts for 14 days of the menstrual cycle.

3. **During the follicular phase, what hormonal changes occur in the pituitary and the ovary?:**
    A. Pituitary
       Because the corpus luteum has involuted prior to the beginning of the follicular phase, and because this structure is the principal source of estrogen during the preceding luteal phase, plasma estrogen levels at the beginning of the follicular phase are low. This reduces estrogen's negative feedback effect on pituitary production of follicle-stimulating hormone (FSH), so FSH secretion begins to rise. Note that the corpus luteum is also the major source of progesterone during the luteal phase, so progesterone levels are low during the follicular phase.

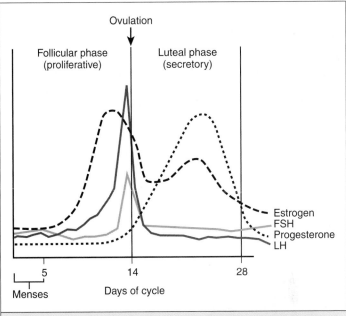

Figure 9-1. Menstrual cycle. FSH, follicle-stimulating hormone; LH, luteinizing hormone. (From Brown TA: Rapid Review Physiology. Philadelphia, Mosby, 2007.)

B. Ovary

During the follicular phase, the rising FSH stimulates the development of several ovarian follicles, eventually causing the emergence of a dominant follicle, which becomes a site of estrogen synthesis. The growing follicle secretes increasing amounts of estrogen, which has the effect of inhibiting pituitary FSH production, thereby gradually reducing serum FSH levels in the later part of the follicular phase. However, the dominant follicle becomes increasingly sensitive to circulating FSH, so plasma estrogen levels still continue to rise throughout the follicular phase.

Note: Inhibin is also secreted by the ovaries and selectively inhibits FSH secretion with no effect on luteinizing hormone (LH) secretion.

4. **What occurs in the uterus during the follicular phase?**
The estrogen secreted by the ovaries stimulates proliferation of the endometrial lining of the uterus throughout the follicular phase.

5. **What happens to cause ovulation at the end of the follicular phase?**
When plasma estrogen reaches a critical level, it switches from causing negative feedback on the pituitary to causing positive feedback by sensitizing gonadotropes to gonadotropin-releasing hormone (GnRH). This stimulates the pituitary to release a surge of LH and FSH. The surge of these hormones causes rupture of the follicle and release of the ovum. This is an elegant design feature, because high estrogen levels indicate to the pituitary that the ovarian follicle is sufficiently "mature" to be released.

6. **What happens in the ovary and endometrium during the luteal phase?**

   After ovulation, the cells that lined the follicle (granulosa cells and theca interna cells) form the corpus luteum ("yellow body") under the influence of LH. The corpus luteum synthesizes both estrogen and a large amount of progesterone. The progesterone stimulates the endometrium to become more secretory and glandular in preparation for implantation. It also stimulates the spiral arteries to develop. These arteries empty into the intervillous space so that chorionic villi from the cytotrophoblast can extract oxygen if fertilization occurs. If fertilization does not occur, the corpus luteum degenerates, the levels of estrogen and progesterone fall, and the endometrium sloughs off as the menstrual flow.

   You are expected to be able to differentiate between the histologic appearances of the endometrial lining during the follicular and luteal phases (Fig. 9-2). Notice the glandular hypertrophy, irregular shape of glands, and well-developed spiral arteries in the luteal (secretory) phase. In contrast, the glands in the follicular phase are smaller and straighter, and there is less vascularity in the stroma.

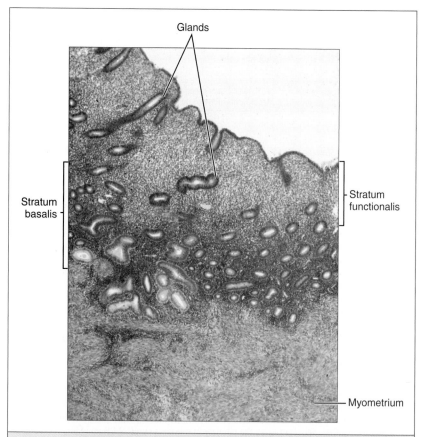

Figure 9-2. Low-magnification view of the uterine endometrium during the proliferative (estrogenic) phase of the reproductive cycle. Growing endometrial glands have straight profiles. (From Telser A, Young J, Baldwin K: Elsevier's Integrated Histology. Philadelphia, Mosby, 2008.)

7. **In women with amenorrhea (absence of menses), why does bleeding after the cessation of a brief course of progesterone indicate that the cause of amenorrhea is due to the lack of ovulation?**
In order to answer this question, one has to have a thorough comprehension of the normal physiology of the menstrual cycle; hence, this is a good board-style question.
   If the administration and withdrawal of progesterone cause menses, this indicates that the endometrium has been sufficiently primed by estrogen and requires only a course of progesterone to have menses. However, the only source of endogenous progesterone is the corpus luteum, which forms only after ovulation. If there is no ovulation, there is no progesterone secretion, and there will not be menses.
   The most common causes of anovulation are obesity, polycystic ovary syndrome, eating disorders (can result in decreased GnRH levels), premature ovarian failure, hyperprolactinemia (prolactin inhibits GnRH release), thyroid disorders (increased thyrotropin-releasing hormone [TRH] levels can stimulate prolactin release), adrenal insufficiency, and Asherman's syndrome.

8. **How does fertilization prevent degeneration of the corpus luteum?**
If the ovum is fertilized, the developing embryo will synthesize human chorionic gonadotropin (hCG), which acts similarly to LH and maintains the corpus luteum.

9. **How does the corpus luteum function in the maintenance of pregnancy?**
During the first 6 weeks of pregnancy the corpus luteum is the primary producer of estrogen and progesterone, hormones required for the continuation of pregnancy. After the sixth week of pregnancy, the placenta begins to take over as the principal site of steroidogenesis. After delivery and removal of the placenta, both estrogen and progesterone levels fall markedly.

10. **Describe the hormones associated with normal testicular descent.**
Normal testicular descent involves a transabdominal phase, which is mediated by müllerian-inhibiting factor (MIF) (a product of Sertoli cells), and a scrotal phase, which is mediated by androgens and β-hCG. Cryptorchidism refers to incomplete descent of the testes into the scrotal sac. The most common location of undescended testes is in the inguinal canal. Generally, the condition is unilateral and resolves spontaneously by 3 months. If uncorrected, cryptorchidism can result in infertility secondary to arrested germ cell maturation (sperm prefer the cooler temperature of the scrotal sac), increased risk of seminoma, and testicular infarction secondary to torsion of the undescended testes.

11. **What is the function of the *SRY* gene?**
The *SRY* gene is located on the Y chromosome and is responsible for testicular development (mediated by testis-determining factor). Testes contain Leydig and Sertoli cells. Leydig cells secrete testosterone, which stimulates the development of the mesonephric ducts. The mesonephric ducts develop into all of the male internal genitalia except for the prostate (epididymis, seminal vesicles, ejaculatory duct, and ductus deferens). Testosterone can also be converted into dihydrotestosterone (DHT), which stimulates the development of the male external genitalia and prostate. Sertoli cells produce MIF, which permits the degeneration of the paramesonephric duct. If degeneration does not occur, the paramesonephric duct develops by default into the female internal genitalia (uterus, fallopian tubes, and upper third of the vagina).

12. **What is hermaphroditism?**
A true hermaphrodite is a person who has both male and female internal genitalia (ovotestes). This condition is very rare. Pseudohermaphroditism is more common; the term describes any person in whom there is discordance between the sex of the internal and external genitalia. Because female pseudohermaphrodites lack a Y chromosome, they do not have an *SRY* gene and thus do not develop testes. Lack of MIF production results in development of female internal genitalia from the paramesonephric duct. Exposure to excessive androgen concentrations during

the early gestational period (either by exogenous intake during pregnancy or through congenital adrenal hyperplasia) stimulates production of virilized external genitalia. Male pseudohermaphrodites, on the other hand, do contain a Y chromosome and thus develop testes. Because their testes produce MIF, they do not develop female internal genitalia. However, their external genitalia are feminized. This is most often due to androgen insensitivity syndrome, in which there is a defect in the androgen receptor. As a result, genotypic males are unable to develop male external genitalia but have high concentrations of testosterone and estrogen because there is no negative feedback from the pituitary due to lack of receptor stimulation.

13. **What is 5α-reductase deficiency?**
The enzyme 5α-reductase is responsible for converting testosterone into DHT. Because DHT stimulates the production of male external genitalia and the prostate, lack of DHT at birth leads to ambiguous external genitalia in these males. Internal genitalia are unaffected, because testicular development is governed exclusively by the presence of the Y chromosome. At puberty, increased concentrations of testosterone are adequate to stimulate development of the male external genitalia (Table 9-1). Patients with this autosomal recessive condition are thus said to develop a "penis at 12."

TABLE 9-1.   CONDITIONS AFFECTING DEVELOPMENT OF THE GENITALIA

Condition	Testosterone	LH	Explanation
Exogenous steroid use	↑	↓	The body perceives that there is too much testosterone, so it reduces production of LH and intratesticular testosterone, leading to testicular atrophy.
Androgen insensitivity syndrome	↑	↑	Although testosterone concentration is much higher than normal, LH production is not inhibited, because the testosterone receptors on the pituitary that mediate feedback also are dysfunctional.
Primary hypogonadism	↓	↑	Problem with testosterone production; originates at the level of the testes.
Hypogonadotropic hypogonadism	↓	↓	Problem with production of GnRH or LH leads to decreased production of testosterone.

GnRH, gonadotropin-releasing hormone; LH, luteinizing hormone.

STEP 1 SECRET

Disorders that influence the development of male and female genitalia are high-yield for Step 1. Do not be surprised if you receive a question on your test that asks you to identify whether various hormone levels are increased/decreased/normal in a patient with a genital development disorder. Use Table 9-1 as a guide.

CASE 9-1

A 29-year-old G2P2 (gravida 2 para 2) woman who just delivered her second baby wants to start birth control pills for contraception. She plans on breastfeeding her newborn.

1. **What important information should you find out before prescribing hormonal contraceptives?**

   It would be important to ask about tobacco use, breastfeeding, risk for sexually transmitted diseases (STDs), past medical history, and current medications because these factors may influence decisions about which type of contraceptive to prescribe.

CASE 9-1 continued:

You find out she has smoked one pack per day for the past 10 years. Her past medical history is significant for hypertension, for which she takes a beta blocker. She has no personal history of breast or endometrial cancer, but her mother did have endometrial cancer.

2. **What are you concerned about in this woman's history in regard to hormonal contraception?**

   Estrogen-containing hormonal contraceptives alone increase the risk for various thrombotic and thromboembolic phenomena, including stroke, myocardial infarction, deep venous thrombosis, and pulmonary embolism (PE). In women who smoke, such contraceptives increase this risk substantially (as does this woman's hypertension) and should therefore be used with caution. If this woman were over 35 as well as a smoker, estrogen-containing contraceptives would be contraindicated.

3. **What are the absolute contraindications to using estrogen-containing contraceptives?**

   Smoker older than 35, history of thromboembolic phenomena (PE, stroke), coronary artery disease, hepatic tumors (estrogens can make hepatic tumors grow and rupture), and personal history of estrogen-dependent cancers such as endometrial carcinoma or breast carcinoma, unexplained vaginal bleeding, and impaired liver function.

4. **What do oral contraceptives typically consist of and what is their mechanism of action?**

   The two general types of oral contraceptive are the combination pills (estrogen and progesterone) and the progesterone-only pills. In the combination pills, the *constant* level of estrogen supplied continuously suppresses pituitary gonadotropin secretion, thereby removing the stimulus for ovulation. The progesterone in the combination pills serves two functions: first, it thickens the cervical mucus secretions, essentially making the vaginal/uterine environment less "receptive" to sperm, and second, it opposes the proliferative effects of estrogen, causing thinning of the uterine lining (which is important in reducing the risk of endometrial cancer from unopposed estrogen). The progesterone-only pills are only about 50% effective at inhibiting ovulation, but as mentioned, they also work by thickening the cervical mucus and altering the motility and secretions of the fallopian tubes, as well as thinning the endometrium.

   Important in this woman's history is that she wishes to breastfeed her baby. Combination hormonal contraceptives post partum can interfere with milk production, so prescribing a progesterone-only contraceptive would be recommended.

   Other methods of hormonal contraception:

   - Transdermal patch and the vaginal ring are other forms of the estrogen and progesterone therapy.
   - Injectable progesterone is an intramuscular form of progesterone injected every 3 months.

Other types of contraception include the intrauterine device (IUD) with or without hormones; barrier methods (condoms, diaphragm, cervical cap); or tubal ligation/vasectomy.

5. **How can menstrual cycles be made regular by hormonal contraceptives?**
In order for menstruation to occur, there must first be estrogenic stimulation of endometrial proliferation; then progesterone must induce maturation and stimulate secretion by the endometrial glands. Menses begin following the decline in progesterone and estrogen levels near the end of the menstrual cycle. In many women, these hormonal events do not occur in such a well-orchestrated manner. Consequently, the estrogen and progesterone stimulation of the uterus can be provided artificially, which can mimic the natural menstrual period. Typically, to achieve this type of control, estrogens are given with progesterones for 21 days, and then placebo pills are given for 7 days to allow for menstruation.

6. **Your patient asks if taking hormonal contraceptives will increase her risk for endometrial cancer. How does taking oral contraceptives affect the risk of endometrial, ovarian, and breast cancer? What is supposed to explain this effect?**
Hormonal contraceptives (combined) actually decrease the risk of ovarian as well as endometrial cancer. The proposed explanation for decreasing risk of ovarian cancer is that by inhibiting ovulation, oral contraceptives reduce the inflammatory response and cell proliferation that usually occurs on the ovarian surface after each follicle ruptures through the ovarian surface, which is what predisposes ovarian surface epithelium to malignancy. The proposed explanation for decreasing the risk of endometrial cancer is the effect progesterone has on thinning the uterine lining and preventing unopposed growth by estrogen.
The risk of breast cancer is controversial: Studies show either no effect or a slight increase in risk.

7. **How do ovarian cysts form and how do oral contraceptives reduce their occurrence?**
The most common ovarian cysts are "functional cysts" that form when the normal follicular maturation and the corpus luteum formation process becomes somewhat aberrant. These are the follicular cysts and corpus lutein cysts, respectively. Follicular cysts develop after failure of a mature ovarian follicle to rupture and be ovulated. Corpus lutein cysts are formed during the luteal phase and occur when the corpus luteum becomes abnormally large or hemorrhagic (corpus hemorrhagicum). Clearly, the inhibition of follicular maturation and ovulation by oral contraceptives should reduce the chance that these cysts will develop.

8. **Why may the drugs phenytoin, phenobarbital, and rifampin make oral contraceptives less effective at preventing pregnancy?**
These drugs all induce hepatic cytochrome P-450 enzymes, which can accelerate the rate of hepatic catabolism of estrogen and progesterone compounds.

SUMMARY BOX: ORAL CONTRACEPTIVES

- Hormonal contraceptives increase the risk for thromboembolic events. They are contraindicated for smokers over age 35.

- Hormonal contraceptives can be progesterone-only or a combination of estrogen and progesterone.

- It is principally the withdrawal of progesterone (not estrogen) that causes normal menses.

- Hormonal contraceptives decrease risk of ovarian and endometrial cancer. How they affect the risk of breast cancer is unclear.

CASE 9-2

A 26-year-old woman has not had a period for approximately 2 months, whereas she was previously regular. She has also had several episodes of nausea and vomiting but has not otherwise felt ill.

1. **What is the differential diagnosis for secondary amenorrhea?**
   The differential diagnosis for secondary amenorrhea includes pregnancy (which is most common), tumor of ovary or adrenals, anatomic abnormalities (such as Asherman's syndrome, in which intrauterine adhesions may occur following uterine surgery), ovarian failure or polycystic ovary syndrome (PCOS), hypothyroidism, hyperprolactinemia, and central nervous system (CNS) or hypothalamic disorder.

CASE 9-2 continued:

She is absolutely and positively emphatic that she cannot be pregnant. Physical examination does not reveal any palpable abdominal or pelvic masses or tenderness.

2. **What laboratory tests should you order?**
   Even though the woman is emphatic that she cannot be pregnant, a serum β-hCG should always be done first to rule out pregnancy. If the β-HCG test is negative, one then can then proceed with further testing: thyroid-stimulating hormone (TSH), prolactin level, a progesterone-only challenge test, estrogen and progesterone challenge, FSH level, and LH level.
   If withdrawal bleeding is present with the progesterone-only challenge test, then the amenorrhea is secondary to anovulation (see question 7 under Basic Concepts section for further discussion). If withdrawal bleeding is absent with progesterone alone, but present with estrogen and progesterone, then suspect inadequate endogenous estrogen and evaluation of FSH and LH levels might help distinguish between a hypothalamic/pituitary process and ovarian failure. If withdrawal bleeding is completely absent, an anatomic disorder such as Asherman's syndrome might be present. Asherman's syndrome refers to the removal of the stratum basalis owing to repeated curettage. Because the stratum basalis serves as the stem cell layer of the endometrium, destruction of this layer prevents regeneration of the functional endometrial tissue. Instead, endometrial fibrosis persists.

CASE 9-2 continued:

A serum β-hCG is done and is positive.

3. **Does an elevated β-human chorionic gonadotropin level always indicate a developing embryo/fetus?**
   It does not necessarily mean she is pregnant, because gestational trophoblastic tumors (hydatiform moles/invasive moles/choriocarcinoma) as well as several germ cell tumors of the ovary also elaborate β-hCG. Note, however, that these are all rare entities. You should confirm the presence of a developing embryo within the uterus by ultrasound.

4. **What is β-human chorionic gonadotropin and what is its normal function, aside from serving as a marker for pregnancy?**
   The hormone β-hCG is similar in structure and activity to LH. It is secreted early in pregnancy by the placenta (specifically, the syncytiotrophoblast cells) and functions to maintain the corpus luteum, which is the principal site of ovarian steroidogenesis during the luteal phase. Production begins approximately 1 week after conception and doubles in quantity every 2 days. The hormone is detectable in the blood by 8 days after conception and in the urine approximately 14 days after conception (around the time a woman would expect her next period). Plasma levels of β-hCG peak

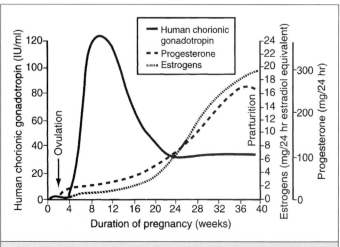

Figure 9-3. Human chorionic gonadotropin stimulates production of estrogen and progesterone by the corpus luteum. As the levels of this hormone drop, the placenta takes over as the major site of synthesis of ovarian steroids. (From Guyton AC, Hall J: Textbook of Medical Physiology, 11th ed. Philadelphia, WB Saunders, 2007.)

in the first trimester (by 10 weeks of gestation). Then, as the placenta begins to take over as the main site of maternal estrogen and progesterone secretion, β-hCG levels taper off (Fig. 9-3).

5. **Relative to a normal pregnancy, how would the β-human chorionic gonadotropin level differ for an ectopic pregnancy?**
    In ectopic pregnancy there is poor placentation (there are fewer syncytiotrophoblast cells to produce β-hCG), and therefore, the serum β-hCG is significantly lower than would be expected for normal pregnancy of the same gestational age. As a general rule of thumb, if β-hCG levels do not double appropriately and reach expected levels, you should suspect an abnormality with the pregnancy.

6. **Assuming the positive β-human chorionic gonadotropin test confirms a pregnancy in this woman, what was the approximate date of conception?**
    Because ovulation occurs approximately 2 weeks after the onset of menses, and her last menses began 9 weeks ago, the approximate date of conception was 7 weeks ago.

7. **What is the difference between the gestational age and the time since conception (developmental age)?**
    The gestational age is the period that has elapsed since the first day of her last menstrual period. It is not the time since conception, a mistake students commonly make. Because conception typically occurs 2 weeks later, the time since conception is 2 weeks shorter than the gestational age. Gestational age is most commonly used: She is 9 weeks by gestation.

8. **At what time during development is the embryo/fetus most susceptible to teratogens?**
    The fetus is most susceptible during the third to eighth weeks (days 15-56, the "embryonic period"), when organogenesis occurs. Common teratogens include alcohol, cocaine, nicotine, excessive vitamin A, lithium, warfarin, angiotensin-converting enzyme (ACE) inhibitors, alkylating agents, certain antibiotics, and valproic acid, to name a few.

9. **What is fetal alcohol syndrome?**
Fetal alcohol syndrome is the leading cause of congenital malformations in the United States and results from excessive alcohol intake during pregnancy. It is associated with a wide range of congenital defects including mental retardation, microcephaly, seizures, and motor disorders, all of which result from a disruption of neuroblast migration. Other defects include limb dislocation, heart abnormalities, and facial abnormalities (flat nasal bridge, upturned nose, "railroad track" ears, epicanthal folds, smooth philtrum, and small palpebral fissures) (Fig. 9-4).

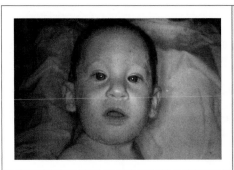

Figure 9-4. Infant with fetal alcohol syndrome. Note short palpebral fissures, mild ptosis, appearance of the nostrils, smooth philtral area, and narrow vermilion of the upper lip. (From Gilbert-Barness E: Potter's Pathology of the Fetus, Infant and Child, 2nd ed. Philadelphia, Mosby, 2007.)

10. **The risk of which fetal developmental abnormalities can be reduced by taking supplemental folic acid early during pregnancy?**
The risk of developmental abnormalities of the CNS and the spinal cord, which may cause neural tube defects such as spina bifida and anencephaly, may be reduced. Ideally, prenatal supplements are taken *prior* to pregnancy, because significant neural development may already have occurred by the time a woman realizes she is pregnant.

11. **Is the woman in Case 9-2 at high or low risk for having a baby with Down syndrome (trisomy 21)?**
The incidence of Down syndrome increases significantly with maternal age (as ova age, they acquire mutations), and because this woman is only 26, her risk is quite low. The risk increases with age from approximately 1 in 1500 for babies of 16-year-old mothers to approximately 1 in 25 babies for 45-year-old mothers.
   Note: Maternal serum α-fetoprotein (AFP) levels are often checked around the 16th week of pregnancy. High levels may indicate a neural tube defect such as spina bifida whereas low levels may indicate Down syndrome. Other laboratory findings associated with Down syndrome include decreased estriol and elevated β-hCG and inhibin A.

12. **Why should ergot alkaloids (e.g., ergonovine), triptans (e.g., sumatriptan), and synthetic prostaglandins (e.g., misoprostol) all be stringently avoided during pregnancy?**
These agents all cause powerful uterine contractions that can result in abortion. The effects of ergot alkaloids and triptans are principally mediated through serotonin receptors. Misoprostol is a synthetic prostaglandin that causes contractions in an analogous fashion to endogenous prostaglandins.

SUMMARY BOX: SECONDARY AMENORRHEA

- Most common cause: Pregnancy. Always check serum β-human chorionic gonadotropin (hCG) levels.

- β-hCG levels peak at 10 weeks gestation (approximately 100,000 mIU/mL).

- Ectopic pregnancies are associated with low β-hCG levels, and β-hCG levels do not double every 48 hours as they do in normal pregnancy.

- Gestational age is determined from the first day of the last menstrual period and is therefore 2 weeks earlier than the date of conception.

CASE 9-3

A 19-year-old G1P0 (gravida 1, para 0) woman who is 2 months pregnant by last menstrual period comes in for an urgent visit because of heavy vaginal bleeding.

1. **What is the differential diagnosis for first-trimester bleeding (<12-14 weeks)?**
   The differential diagnosis for first-trimester bleeding includes spontaneous abortion, ectopic pregnancy, molar pregnancy, and postcoital bleeding, as well as other non–pregnancy-related causes such as vaginal laceration or trauma.

CASE 9-3 continued:

She has not been seen in clinic, but she knows she is pregnant by a positive urine pregnancy test. She has had severe nausea and vomiting but thinks that is normal "morning sickness." You are concerned about a spontaneous abortion and ectopic pregnancy. A pelvic ultrasound (Fig. 9-5) reveals a "snowstorm" pattern and no discernible fetus. Serum β-hCG levels are elevated far and above what would be expected during pregnancy.

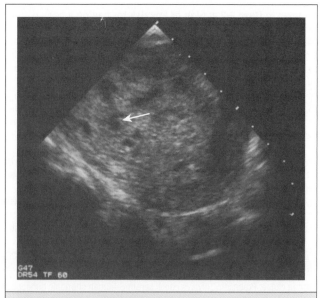

Figure 9-5. Pelvic ultrasound from patient in Case 9-3. (From Gabbe SG, Niebyl JR, Simpson JL: Obstetrics—Normal and Problem Pregnancies, 4th ed. Philadelphia, Churchill Livingstone, 2002.)

2. **What is the diagnosis?**
   Molar pregnancy (hydatidiform mole) is likely. Molar pregnancy is one subtype of gestational trophoblastic disease (GTD).

3. **How can β-human chorionic gonadotropin levels differentiate between a normal pregnancy and a molar pregnancy (complete or incomplete mole)?**
   Because these moles are made exclusively of trophoblastic (placental) tissue, the site of β-hCG synthesis, serum β-hCG levels are substantially elevated in comparison to a normal pregnancy of similar "gestational age." Other features that suggest a molar pregnancy include severe vaginal bleeding early in the pregnancy and vaginal passage of molar vesicles.

4. **What is the difference between an invasive mole and choriocarcinoma and from what does each generally arise?**
   An invasive mole invades the myometrium but does not normally metastasize. A majority of them arise from benign molar pregnancies. Choriocarcinoma, on the other hand, is often metastatic and spreads hematogenously. Half of these develop from benign molar pregnancies, one fourth after normal term pregnancy, and one fourth after miscarriage, abortion, or ectopic pregnancy. A key histologic distinction between invasive moles and choriocarcinomas is that choriocarcinomas are less differentiated and lack *a villous pattern.*

5. **Cover the columns on the right side of Table 9-2 and try to identify the characteristics of the different gestational trophoblastic diseases.**
   See Table 9-2 and Figure 9-6.

SUMMARY BOX: FIRST-TRIMESTER BLEEDING AND GESTATIONAL TROPHOBLASTIC DISEASE

- Molar pregnancy is characterized by heavy vaginal bleeding in the first trimester, passage of "grape like vesicles," snowstorm appearance on ultrasound, and increase in normal β-human chorionic gonadotropin (hCG) level.

- Gestational trophoblastic disease (GTD) refers to abnormal proliferation of placental tissue: mostly benign; molar pregnancies; and the malignant GTD: invasive moles, choriocarcinoma, and placental site trophoblastic tumor (PSTT).

- Complete moles are the most common molar pregnancy and have a higher percentage of persistent malignant disease.

CASE 9-4

A 32-year-old G2P1 (gravida 2, para 1) woman at 12 weeks' gestation by last known menstrual period complains of occasional palpitations, irritability, and heat intolerance.

1. **What is the differential diagnosis?**
   The differential diagnosis for palpitations and heat intolerance includes hyperthyroidism, normal pregnancy, anxiety, cardiac arrhythmia, and pheochromocytoma.

TABLE 9-2. GESTATIONAL TROPHOBLASTIC DISEASES

Type	Subclassification	Persistent Malignant Disease	Pathogenesis	Karyotype	Fetal Parts Present
Molar pregnancy/hyatidiform moles (80%) — Complete mole (90% of molar pregnancies)	Benign (in general)	15-25%	Sperm fertilizes empty egg, then duplicates	Diploid (46,XX)	No
Incomplete/partial mole	Benign (almost always)	Very low	Sperm fertilizes normal egg	Triploid (69,XXY or 69,XXX)	Yes
Invasive moles (10-15%)	Malignant		Months to years after molar pregnancy (50%), normal pregnancy (25%), after abortion, ectopic (25%)	Diploid	No
Choriocarcinoma (2-5%)	Malignant	Diploid	No		
Placental site trophoblastic tumor (rare)	Malignant	Diploid	No		

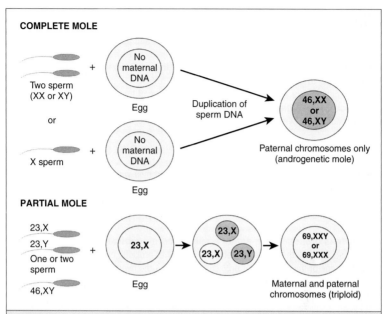

Figure 9-6. Patterns of fertilization to account for chromosomal origin of complete (46,XX) and triploid partial moles (XXY). In a complete mole, one or two sperm fertilize an egg that has lost its chromosomes. Partial moles are due to fertilization of an egg by one diploid or two haploid sperm, depicted in this example as one 23,X and one 23,Y. (From Kumar V, Abbas AK, Fausto N: Robbins and Cotran Pathologic Basis of Disease, 7th ed. Philadelphia, WB Saunders, 2005.)

CASE 9-4 continued:

Except for a gravid abdomen, physical examination is unremarkable. Cardiac auscultation reveals a regular rate and rhythm without murmurs or gallops, and an electrocardiogram (ECG) is normal.

2. What would you like to do for further workup?
   A thyroid panel to rule out hyperthyroidism would be helpful.

CASE 9-4 continued:

The results reveal elevated levels of total and free thyroid hormones (triiodothyronine [T_3] and thyroxine [T_4]) as well as reduced levels of TSH.

3. What is the diagnosis?
   These results suggest gestational hyperthyroidism. In pregnancy, the total T_4 is usually elevated because estrogen increases the synthesis of thyroxine-binding globulin by the liver. Notice, however, that this woman had elevated free T_4, levels as well and it is this elevated free T_4 (or free T_3) that causes hyperthyroidism.

4. How does the pregnant state predispose to hyperthyroidism?
   This effect is due to the presence of hCG in the maternal circulation. hCG is a glycoprotein synthesized and secreted by the placenta in large amounts. Owing to its similarity in structure to

TSH (TSH, FSH, LH, and β-hCG all share the same α-subunit), it often hyperstimulates the thyroid gland during pregnancy, resulting in gestational hyperthyroidism. This condition often spontaneously resolves following delivery of the fetus and placenta.

5. **How are maternal levels of follicle-stimulating hormone and luteinizing hormone likely to be affected in this woman, given that she is pregnant?**
They should be low and virtually undetectable because of the significant negative feedback that the high levels of estrogen and progesterone seen with pregnancy produce on the pituitary.

6. **Why is the decline in estrogen and progesterone after delivery beneficial for the beginning of lactation?**
Both estrogen and progesterone inhibit lactation, and their withdrawal allows the elevated prolactin present at the time of delivery to facilitate milk letdown and lactation. Recall that the placenta is the major site of progesterone and estrogen secretion, so its expulsion after delivery will reduce the levels of these hormones.

7. **How does breastfeeding act as a natural contraceptive?**
Nipple suckling by the baby stimulates the release of prolactin by the anterior pituitary gland. Because one of the functions of prolactin is to inhibit the hypothalamic secretion of GnRH, this results in reduced FSH and LH secretion by the pituitary. Reduced levels of these gonadotropins inhibit ovulation in the nursing mother and acts as a natural birth control pill. However, breastfeeding must be practiced continuously in order to be efficacious as a contraceptive method.

SUMMARY BOX: ENDOCRINOLOGY OF PREGNANCY

- In pregnancy the total thyroxine (T_4) is usually elevated because estrogen increases the synthesis of thyroxine-binding globulin by the liver.

- Increases in *free* T_4 and triiodothyronine (T_3) levels results in hyperthyroidism.

- High levels of prolactin in a nursing mother inhibit hypothalamic secretion of gonadotropin-releasing hormone (GnRH), resulting in reduced gonadotropin secretion and suppression of ovulation.

CASE 9-5

A 28-year-old woman in her 33rd week of pregnancy is complaining of increased fatigue and swelling of her hands and face. Urine dipstick testing shows 2+ proteinuria, and her blood pressure is elevated at 150/110 mm Hg (up from 130/90 mm Hg). Brisk deep tendon reflexes are also noted on examination.

1. **What is the diagnosis?**
Preeclampsia is defined by new-onset hypertension (>140/90 mm Hg) and proteinuria (>300 mg/day) occurring after 20 weeks' gestation. Although the definitive cause of preeclampsia is still unknown, the underlying cause is thought to be generalized arterial vasospasm.
    Note: The severity of preeclampsia is generally determined by the degree of proteinuria and blood pressure elevation.

2. **How should this patient be managed?**
This woman is classified as having mild preeclampsia. Because she is not yet at term (37 weeks), bed rest and expectant management would be appropriate, as one would not want to induce premature labor. She could also be given steroids such as betamethasone to enhance fetal lung maturity in the event that premature delivery is necessary.

CASE 9-5 continued:

The next week she develops right upper quadrant (RUQ) pain, her proteinuria worsens, and her blood pressure increases to 170/115 mm Hg.

3. **What is your primary concern at this point?**
The patient now has severe preeclampsia. The RUQ pain is concerning for HELLP syndrome, which can be a complication of severe preeclampsia. The HELLP syndrome consists of **H**emolysis, **E**levated **L**iver enzymes, and **L**ow **P**latelets. About 10% of patients with severe preeclampsia develop the HELLP syndrome.

4. **What changes occur in the spiral arteries in patients with preeclampsia?**
Preeclampsia is associated with mechanical or functional obstruction of the spiral arteries. The reason for this is multifold: Abnormal trophoblastic tissue invades the spiral arteries, and patients demonstrate increased levels of vasoconstrictors and decreased levels of vasodilators along with increased concentrations of growth factors. The end result is placental hypoperfusion with spiral artery atherosclerosis.

CASE 9-5 continued:

Laboratory tests reveal anemia, thrombocytopenia, and elevated liver enzymes, and a peripheral blood smear shows the presence of schistocytes.

5. **If this woman develops seizures also, how does that change the diagnosis?**
Then, assuming she does not have a preexisting seizure disorder or metabolic abnormality, she has eclampsia, which is defined by the presence of seizures in a patient with preeclampsia and without other known causes of seizures.

6. **What is the definitive treatment for preeclampsia, eclampsia, and the HELLP syndrome?**
Delivery of the fetus is the only definitive treatment. Supportive management includes magnesium sulfate ($MgSO_4$) for seizure prophylaxis in eclamptic patients. In preeclamptic patients, $MgSO_4$ is also often given as seizure prophylaxis during labor and delivery. Although $MgSO_4$ is considered to be the first-line treatment for seizures in these patients, diazepam can also be given. Patients should be placed on salt-restricted diets. If the baby must be delivered prematurely for the health of the mother, steroids should be given to improve fetal lung maturity.

7. **Why are angiotensin-converting enzyme inhibitors or angiotensin receptor blockers not used to treat hypertension in preeclampsia?**
ACE inhibitors and angiotensin receptor blockers (ARBs) should not be used to treat *any* pregnant woman because they carry the risk of causing fetal renal failure and even fetal death.

STEP 1 SECRET

Preeclampsia and eclampsia are high-yield subjects for boards. You should be able to recognize the findings associated with these diseases in pregnant patients and understand basic concepts regarding treatment.

SUMMARY BOX: PREECLAMPSIA, ECLAMPSIA, AND THE HELLP SYNDROME

- Preeclampsia is defined by hypertension (>140/90 mm Hg), proteinuria (>300 mg/24 hours), and nondependent edema after 20 weeks' gestation.

- Eclampsia is defined by the presence of preeclampsia with seizures.

- HELLP is **H**emolysis, **E**levated **L**iver enzymes, and **L**ow **P**latelets.

- Definitive treatment is delivery of the fetus.

CASE 9-6

A 26-year-old woman at 32 weeks' gestation has come to the hospital because she has been having contractions for the past 3 hours. Contractions are now occurring every 10 minutes. The diameter of her cervical canal is 2 cm. She is told she might be going into premature labor.

1. **What pharmacologic agents can be used to suppress labor in this woman?**
   Agents that inhibit uterine contractions are known as tocolytics. $MgSO_4$ is most widely used. Other classes of drugs include β_2-receptor agonists (usually terbutaline and ritodrine) and calcium channel blockers (nifedipine is most widely used). These latter two drug classes are smooth muscle relaxants. Additionally, indomethacin and other nonsteroidal anti-inflammatory drugs (NSAIDs) can decrease uterine contractions by inhibiting prostaglandin synthesis.
   Note: After approximately 32 weeks' gestation, there is concern about using NSAIDs because of their potential to cause premature constriction of the ductus arteriosus. Remember that prostaglandins are vasodilatory and that NSAIDs inhibit prostaglandin synthesis.

2. **What is the main source of risk to this woman's baby associated with premature delivery?**
   The principal concern with premature delivery is immature fetal lungs, which can cause neonatal respiratory distress syndrome. Fetal lung maturity is determined by the amount of surfactant present, which can be assessed with amniocentesis and evaluation of the lecithin-sphingomyelin ratio, which should be greater than 2 for mature lungs. Glucocorticoids can be given to a woman in premature labor to increase the production of surfactant. Typically, surfactant production begins by 28 weeks and is complete by 36 weeks.

RELATED QUESTIONS ON LABOR AND DELIVERY

3. **If placenta previa were present at term (or when delivery is necessary), why would a cesarean section be mandatory?**
   Placenta previa occurs when the placenta covers the internal cervical os. With a vaginal delivery, the placenta would have to rupture for the baby to pass through the cervix (a horrifying bloody mess).
   Note: Placenta previa can also present as *painless* bleeding during any trimester. Placental abruption, which occurs when the placenta loses its attachment to the uterus, is very *painful* and presents only in the third trimester.

4. **How can placenta accreta complicate the labor and delivery process?**
Placenta accreta occurs when the placenta has invaded into and attached firmly to the myometrium. In this situation, the placenta does not separate off the endometrial lining after delivery of the infant.

5. **What is oxytocin and how is it used to augment or induce labor?**
Oxytocin is a peptide hormone produced naturally by the posterior pituitary and is a stimulant for uterine contractions. Exogenous oxytocin (*pitocin*) enhances uterine contractions and accelerates the first stage of labor.
Note: During pregnancy, the number of oxytocin receptors on the uterus increases, which makes the uterus particularly sensitive to endogenous or exogenous oxytocin at the end of term.

6. **What pharmacologic agents could be used if delivery is complicated by postpartum hemorrhage?**
Several different pharmacologic agents, including the ergot alkaloids, oxytocin, and certain prostaglandins, all cause uterine contractions, which reduce postpartum bleeding by clamping down on bleeding vessels.
Note: Ischemic necrosis of the anterior pituitary gland, known as *Sheehan's syndrome*, is a potential complication of severe postpartum hemorrhage. It results from the enlargement of the pituitary during pregnancy that occurs without a proportional increase in vascular supply. This substantially increases the risk of infarction, especially after delivery when severe bleeding and hypoperfusion are likely to take place.

SUMMARY BOX: LABOR AND DELIVERY

- Tocolytics (used to stop contractions of premature labor): magnesium sulfate, β_2-agonists, calcium channel blockers, and nonsteroidal anti-inflammatory drugs (NSAIDs).

- Pitocin (exogenous oxytocin): used to stimulate or augment contractions.

- NSAIDs should not be used after 32 weeks because of the risk of premature closure of ductus arteriosus.

- Surfactant production begins by 28 weeks and is complete by 36 weeks.

- Placenta previa: Placenta covers the internal cervical os. Can present as painless bleeding in any trimester.

- Placental abruption: Placenta separates from wall of uterus. Presents as painful uterine bleeding during the third trimester (>24-28 weeks).

- Placenta accreta: Placenta invades into myometrium; may cause hemorrhage after delivery.

- Sheehan's syndrome—necrosis of the anterior pituitary gland—is a complication of postpartum hemorrhage.

CASE 9-7

A 26-year-old woman complains of fever and pelvic pain, neither of which is related to her menstrual cycle.

1. **What is the differential diagnosis for pelvic pain?**
There is a very broad differential diagnosis for pelvic pain:

Gynecologic causes:
- Uterine disease
    - Endometriosis
    - Adenomyosis
    - Leiomyomata (fibroids)
    - IUD, polyps
  - Extrauterine diseases
    - Adhesions
    - Pelvic inflammatory disease (PID)
    - Ovarian cysts
    - Abscess

Urologic causes:
- Chronic urinary tract infections (UTIs)
- Detrusor overactivity
- Interstitial cystitis
- Stone

Gastrointestinal (GI) causes:
- Chronic appendicitis
- Constipation
- Diverticular disease
- Irritable bowel disease
- Irritable bowel syndrome
- Malignancy

Musculoskeletal causes:
- Coccydynia
- Disk problems
- Degenerative joint disease (DJD)
- Low back pain
- Levator ani syndrome (spasm of pelvic floor)
- Nerve entrapment
- Osteoporosis

Psychiatric causes:
- Trauma/abuse
- Sexually transmitted disease
    - PID

CASE 9-7 continued:

She has multiple sexual partners and rarely uses any form of barrier contraception. Cervical examination is significant for bilateral adnexal tenderness and a purulent cervical discharge.

2. **Based on the preceding additional information, what is the most likely diagnosis?**
   PID secondary to infection with *Chlamydia trachomatis. Neisseria gonorrhoeae* is another common cause of PID. PID typically presents with fever, lower abdominal pain, abnormal uterine bleeding, vaginal discharge, and cervical motion tenderness.

CASE 9-7 continued:

Laboratory tests reveal a mild leukocytosis and a slightly elevated erythrocyte sedimentation rate (ESR). A quantitative β-hCG is negative, but a cervical smear is positive for *Chlamydia*, confirming the diagnosis.

3. **What long-term complications may possibly be prevented by treating this woman?**

   Tubal strictures can develop because of the inflammatory process, which can cause infertility or ectopic pregnancy. Tubes can also fill with pus, leading to hydrosalpinx. Adhesions between small bowel and pelvic structures can also develop, causing symptoms of bowel obstruction. An abscess can form around the tubes and ovaries (tubo-ovarian abscess). Rupture of a tubo-ovarian abscess can be a life-threatening event. Another potential complication of PID is Fitz-Hugh–Curtis syndrome, in which the infection spreads to the peritoneum and causes scar tissue formation on the surface of the liver. This manifests in the symptom of RUQ pain.

   Although treatment of PID cannot eliminate these complications, it can potentially reduce their frequency.

4. **How should she be treated?**

   She should be given antibiotics. *C. trachomatis*, an obligate intracellular parasite, is typically treated with the antibiotic doxycycline. However, endocervical culture will often reveal a polymicrobial infection, necessitating the additional use of a broad-spectrum antibiotic such as ceftriaxone (a third-generation cephalosporin). Additionally, *N. gonorrhoeae* is generally treated empirically in someone with chlamydial infection (it is susceptible to cephalosporins).

5. **If someone presented with similar signs and symptoms but also had acute onset of right knee pain and swelling without any recent trauma to the joint, what infecting organism should you suspect?**

   N. gonorrhoeae, a gram-negative intracellular diplococcus, should be suspected. In addition to being a common cause of PID, *N. gonorrhoeae* can also cause a septic arthritis if it disseminates.

6. **Is it sensible to recommend the use of an intrauterine device to this woman?**

   No. IUDs are specifically contraindicated in women who have had previous episodes of PID or multiple sexual partners because they may increase the risk of the subsequent development of PID. As with most implanted devices, these devices make it easier for bacteria to colonize and cause an infection.

   Note: You should suspect infection with *Actinomyces israelii* in a woman using an IUD who presents with symptoms of PID. This bacterium can be treated with penicillin.

SUMMARY BOX: PELVIC INFLAMMATORY DISEASE

- Pelvic inflammatory disease (PID) can be secondary to infection with *Chlamydia trachomatis*. *Neisseria gonorrhoeae* is another common cause of PID.

- PID is characterized by purulent discharge from cervical os, cervical motion tenderness, and cervical smear positive for chlamydial infection or gonorrhea.

- Treatment is with antibiotics doxycycline or ceftriaxone.

- Treatment reduces complications of tubo-ovarian abscess, infertility, and ectopic pregnancy.

RELATED QUESTION ON GYNECOLOGIC INFECTIONS

7. **What bacterium is responsible for maintaining the normal acidic pH of the vagina?**

   Lactobacillus acidophilus (acid loving) maintains the vaginal pH <4.5 (Table 9-3).

TABLE 9-3. INFECTIOUS CAUSES OF VAGINAL DISCHARGE

Feature	Bacterial Vaginosis	Trichomoniasis	Candidiasis
Chief complaint	Malodorous discharge	Thin yellowish-greenish frothy discharge; "strawberry cervix"	White cheesy exudate; itching
Pathogenesis	Overgrowth of normal vaginal flora	Sexually transmitted disease	Yeast infection
Tests	Saline preparation shows "clue cells"* KOH test produces a fishy odor pH 5-6	Motile protozoa on saline preparation smears[†] pH 6-7	KOH shows hyphae[†] pH 4-5
	Clue cells are vaginal epithelial cells that are "studded" with adherent bacteria		
Treatment	Metronidazole	Metronidazole	Nystatin or fluconazole

*From Holmes KK: Lower genital tract infections in women: cystitis/urethritis, vulvo-vaginitis, and cervicitis. In Holmes KK, Mardh PA, Sparling PF, et al (eds): Sexually Transmitted Diseases. New York, McGraw-Hill, 1984. Copyright © McGraw-Hill, Inc. Used by permission of McGraw-Hill Book Company.
[†]From Kaufman RH, Faro S, Brown D: Benign Diseases of the Vulva and Vagina, 5th ed, St. Louis, Mosby, 2004.

CASE 9-8

A 28-year-old woman who has never been pregnant with no history of prior surgeries complains of chronic pelvic pain.

1. **What is the differential diagnosis for pelvic pain?**
   The broad differential diagnosis for pelvic pain was discussed in the previous case:
   - *Gynecologic causes:*
     - Endometriosis
     - Adenomyosis leiomyomata (fibroids)
     - IUD
     - Polyps
     - Adhesions
     - PID
     - Ovarian cysts
     - Abscess
   - *Urologic causes*
     - Chronic UTIs
     - Detrusor overactivity
     - Interstitial cystitis
     - stone
   - *GI causes:*
     - Chronic appendicitis
     - Constipation
     - Diverticular disease
     - IBD
     - IBS
     - Malignancy
   - *Musculoskeletal causes:*
     - Coccydynia
     - Disk problems
     - DJD
     - Low back pain
     - Levator ani syndrome (spasm of pelvic floor)
     - Nerve entrapment
     - Osteoporosis
   - *Other causes:*
     - Psychiatric disorders
     - Abuse

   The pain would need to be characterized to narrow the differential diagnosis.

CASE 9-8 continued:

The pain is particularly severe during her menstrual period (dysmenorrhea). She also complains of significant pain during sexual intercourse (dyspareunia). Pelvic examination is significant for slight adnexal tenderness. Stains for *N. gonorrhoeae* and *C. trachomatis* are negative, and a β-hCG is also negative. A pelvic ultrasound does not reveal any cysts, fibroids, or structures suggestive of ovarian neoplasm.

2. **Now what is the likely diagnosis, what is its etiology, and how do we confirm?**
   The most likely diagnosis is endometriosis, given the history of severe pain during the menstrual period and negative workup for infectious and anatomic causes. Endometriosis is caused by the presence of endometrial tissue in ectopic (extrauterine) locations, such as the ovaries or uterine ligaments. Perhaps the most widely accepted theory to explain the presence of

endometrial tissue in extrauterine sites is the phenomenon of retrograde menstruation through the fallopian tubes, a process that is thought to occur in most women. Unfortunately, such retrograde flow does not completely explain the presence of ectopic endometrial tissues in distant anatomic sites such as the pleural cavity. An exploratory laparoscopy for direct visualization might help confirm the diagnosis.

CASE 9-8 continued:

Laparoscopy is performed and reveals the presence of "chocolate cysts" on both ovaries.

3. **What does the presence of these ovarian "chocolate cysts" indicate and why do they appear black?**
    Chocolate cysts are nonfunctional ovarian cysts (endometriomas) that develop from ectopic endometrial tissue present in advanced endometriosis. They appear black because they contain a blood-filled cavity.

4. **Why is pain worse during the menstrual period in this patient?**
    Ectopic endometrial tissue undergoes the same cycle of proliferation and breakdown as the normal endometrial lining in response to estrogen and progesterone. The resulting bleeding causes inflammation and pain. Over the long term, this inflammation can lead to tissue damage, fibrosis, adhesions, and compression of adjacent structures, resulting in signs and symptoms such as chronic pelvic pain and infertility. Because of these effects, it is important to diagnose and treat endometriosis early in its development.
    Note: Although ectopic endometrial tissue is most frequently found in the pelvis, it can also be found in various other anatomic sites, such as the upper abdomen or thorax and the colon, leading to rectal bleeding. These sites can also become painful during menstrual cycling. If ectopic tissue deposits in the fallopian tubes, it can result in infertility.

STEP 1 SECRET

Note that endometriosis results in *cyclic* bleeding because the ectopic tissue is also governed by hormonal regulation. In general, it will be helpful for you to classify gynecologic diseases according to these types of patterns (e.g., does the disease result in cyclic or noncyclic/anovulatory bleeding, is the disease associated with menstrual pain).

5. **What is first-line treatment in a 28-year-old woman?**
    NSAIDs or hormonal contraceptives are good first-line agents for mild endometriosis. The choice will depend on the symptoms and whether she is trying to conceive.

6. **What is the mechanism of action of leuprolide, a gonadotropin-releasing hormone analog, in treating endometriosis?**
    Because the pituitary gland normally releases gonadotropins in response to the *pulsatile* secretion of GnRH from the hypothalamus, the *continual* presence of leuprolide inhibits the pituitary release of LH and FSH. Suppression of FSH and LH secretion eliminates their stimulation of estrogen and progesterone production, essentially putting the woman in an artificial state of menopause. Without the estrogenic stimulation of the endometrial tissue for proliferation and the progesterone stimulation for maturation and eventual menses, there is no cycling with associated bleeding of ectopic endometrial tissue.
    Note 1: Because leuprolide causes an artificial state of menopause, it is used for only brief periods of time because of the risks of osteoporosis, hot flashes, and other "postmenopausal" problems.

Note 2: Danazol, a derivative of testosterone, which nonetheless has some progestational actions, is also used to treat endometriosis. It decreases pituitary FSH and LH secretion but has some unpleasant side effects (hirsutism, deepening of the voice) due to its androgenic actions.

7. **Another option for treating this woman is total abdominal hysterectomy with bilateral salpingo-oophorectomy. What is the value of excising the ovaries, in terms of treating endometriosis, if there are no endometrial implants on the ovaries?**
The estrogens produced by the ovaries are responsible for stimulating the cycling of any ectopic endometrial tissue that is not removed with hysterectomy.

8. **Another cause of dysmenorrhea is adenomyosis. What is this?**
Adenomyosis is ingrowth of the endometrial glands into the myometrium. In addition to dysmenorrhea, it can also cause heavy menstrual bleeding (menorrhagia).

SUMMARY BOX: ENDOMETRIOSIS

- Endometriosis is caused by the presence of endometrial tissue in ectopic (extrauterine) locations, such as the ovaries or uterine ligaments.

- The condition is characterized by severe pain with menstrual cycle and "chocolate cysts" on ovaries.

- Treatment can be with nonsteroidal anti-inflammatory drugs (NSAIDs), hormonal contraceptives, a gonadotropin-releasing hormone (GnRH) agonist (leuprolide), an androgen derivative (danazol), or surgery.

- Adenomyosis is growth of endometrial glands into myometrium and can cause heavy menstrual bleeding.

CASE 9-9

A 37-year-old African-American woman is being evaluated for abnormal uterine bleeding. She has regular periods, but they are heavy, and she also has some bleeding between her periods. Intercourse has become somewhat painful.

1. **What is the differential diagnosis for abnormal uterine bleeding in a premenopausal woman?**
The differential diagnosis for abnormal uterine bleeding in a premenopausal woman includes adenomyosis (invasion of the endometrium into the myometrium), endometriosis, endometrial polyps, uterine fibroids (leiomyomata), endometrial hyperplasia, and endometrial cancer.

CASE 9-9 continued:

Physical examination reveals the uterus to be enlarged and hardened, possibly with nodules. A pelvic ultrasound reveals an enlarged uterus with several tumorous growths within the myometrium.

2. **What is the probable diagnosis now?**
Leiomyomata (singular, leiomyoma), commonly referred to as uterine fibroids, is most likely. These tumors are benign, local proliferations of smooth muscle cells of the uterus that occur in whorled patterns, and are the most common of all tumor types in females. Uterine

fibroids are the most common gynecologic tumor, and African-American women have a significantly greater risk of developing them. As shown in Figure 9-7, uterine fibroids may be subserous, intramural, or submucosal depending on their location. Submucosal fibroids are a common cause of uterine bleeding.

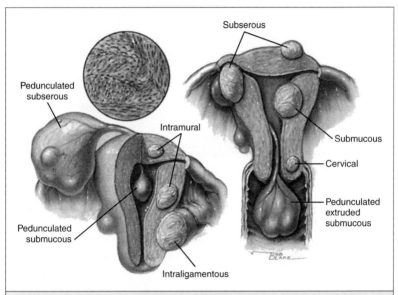

Figure 9-7. Histopathology of leiomyoma. Uterine fibroids are designated subserous, intramural, or submucosal depending on their location. Submucosal fibroids often cause abnormal uterine bleeding. (From Sabiston D: Textbook of Surgery, 16th ed. Philadelphia, WB Saunders, 2000.)

3. **What are the common symptoms associated with leiomyoma?**
   Although the condition is asymptomatic in a sizable proportion of patients, others may experience menorrhagia (if the location is submucosal) because the smooth muscle cells cannot properly clamp down on the spiral arteries during menses. Other symptoms include obstructive delivery, cramping with menses secondary to contraction of the smooth muscle cells, constipation secondary to pressure on the colon, and frequency and urgency secondary to pressure on the bladder.

4. **How do oral contraceptives affect uterine fibroids?**
   Because these are estrogen-sensitive tumors, exogenous estrogens in oral contraceptives may make them grow. Additionally, the substantial increase in estrogen that occurs during pregnancy can make these tumors grow to significant proportions. After menopause, when estrogen levels fall off, these tumors often shrink in size and become asymptomatic.
   Note: Pharmacologic agents that decrease plasma estrogen such as leuprolide, danazol, and progesterone can all be used to shrink uterine fibroids.

5. **Most fibroids are asymptomatic, but when is treatment with hysterectomy or myomectomy indicated?**
   If there is severe pain, rapid growth, very large or many leiomyomata, or urinary symptoms, hysterectomy is indicated. Recurrent miscarriage is also a rare complication of fibroids, so if future fertility is desired, myomectomy can be performed to resect just the tumor, leaving a viable uterus.

6. **What is a leiomyosarcoma?**
Leiomyosarcoma is a highly aggressive, malignant tumor derived from smooth muscle cells (of the uterus). It is not believed to arise from uterine fibroids. Leiomyosarcomas are very rare, but would be considered if there is very rapid growth of a mass in the uterus. Incidence is higher in black women than in white women.

SUMMARY BOX: ABNORMAL UTERINE BLEEDING, FIBROIDS

- Uterine fibroids (leiomyomata) are benign local proliferations of smooth muscle cells of the uterus, responsive to estrogen.

- They are three times more common in African-American women.

- Fibroids may be asymptomatic, but patients often experience menorrhagia, obstructive delivery, cramping, constipation, and frequency/urgency.

- Most fibroids do not require treatment. Drugs such as leuprolide and danazol decrease the amount of circulating estrogen and can shrink fibroids.

- Hysterectomy is definitive treatment. Myomectomy is indicated if future fertility is desired.

- Leiomyosarcoma is a rare malignant tumor of smooth muscle cells that does not arise from benign leiomyomata.

CASE 9-10

A 30-year-old woman presents to the free health care clinic complaining of postcoital bleeding for several months. She is otherwise healthy and denies any pain with intercourse (dyspareunia) or other gynecologic symptoms.

1. **Postcoital bleeding in a woman who does not see a doctor regularly is a red flag for malignancy. What risk factors for cervical cancer do you want to ask her about?**
   - Multiple sexual partners
   - Age at onset of sexual activity
   - Tobacco use

   Note: In utero diethylstilbestrol (DES) exposure of a fetus is a risk factor for the development of a rare cancer type called cervical or vaginal clear cell carcinoma.

CASE 9-10 continued:

She admits to becoming sexually active at an early age and having multiple male sexual partners. She has a 15-year history of cigarette smoking. A pelvic examination is performed and reveals an exophytic growth on the cervix. Colposcopy (light-powered magnification of the cervix) with cervical biopsy is performed, revealing stage I cervical cancer.

2. **Cervical cancer is most commonly what type of cancer?**
Squamous cell carcinoma makes up 90% of cervical cancers. Adenocarcinoma accounts for 10%.

3. **With what virus has she likely been infected?**
She is most likely infected with human papillomavirus (HPV), which is believed to cause the vast majority of cervical cancers. Subtypes 16, 18, 31, and 45 and many others are associated with cervical cancer.

Note: HPV types 6 and 11 are associated with condyloma accuminatum (genital wart) but curiously don't increase the risk of cervical cancer. The other genital "wart," condyloma latum, is due to secondary syphilis.

4. **What is the mechanism by which the human papillomavirus viral proteins E6 and E7 predispose to the development of cervical cancer?**
They interfere with functioning of the tumor suppressor proteins p53 and retinoblastoma (Rb). Specifically, the E6 protein binds p53 and increases its rate of proteolysis, in effect reducing levels of p53. The E7 protein prevents transcription of the Rb gene by binding and displacing bound transcription factors that are necessary for Rb transcription.

5. **What does cervical intraepithelial neoplasia (CIN) refer to? Differentiate among CIN I, CIN II, and CIN III.**
These diagnoses are made only by cervical biopsy (colposcopy with biopsy). CIN I corresponds to dysplasia of one third or less of the depth of the epithelium. CIN II corresponds to dysplasia of two thirds of the epithelium, and CIN III refers to dysplasia of the entire epithelial layer, which is also known as carcinoma in situ. CIN I, II, and III are also referred to as mild, moderate, and severe dysplasia, respectively. It typically takes about 7 years for CIN I to evolve into cervical cancer and 4 years for CIN II to evolve into cervical cancer.

6. **How can cervical cancer cause renal failure in this woman?**
The cancer can grow and obstruct the ureters (obstructive nephropathy). This is one of the most common causes of death from cervical cancer.

7. **Why might this woman have benefited from the human papillomavirus vaccine or annual Pap (Papanicolaou) smears?**
HPV vaccine against serotypes 6, 11, 16, and 18 was approved in 2006 for use among females aged 9 to 26 years for prevention of HPV-related cervical cancer; cervical, vaginal and vulvar cancer precursors; and anogenital warts. Approximately 70% of cervical cancers worldwide are caused by types 16 and 18, but because the vaccine does not cover all the serotypes that can lead to cancer, regular Pap smears are still recommended.

The Pap smear has been shown to effectively detect preinvasive and early cancerous cervical lesions after HPV infection. Recall that cervical cancers can have a prolonged "latent" period, so early detection via Pap smears and excision of premalignant lesions have been able to drastically reduce mortality risk associated with cervical cancer.

Note: Perhaps the largest risk factor for developing cervical cancer is simply the failure to have Pap smears on a regular basis.

8. **Where are cells sampled from during a Pap smear?**
Cells are taken from the squamocolumnar junction, the so-called transformation zone, where columnar cervical cells meet stratified squamous vaginal epithelium. Pap smears cannot diagnose cancer; a tissue biopsy is required for this.

SUMMARY BOX: CERVICAL CANCER

- Cervical cancer most commonly is squamous cell carcinoma.

- Cervical cancer risk factors include early intercourse, multiple partners, high-risk partners, low socioeconomic status, sexually transmitted diseases, tobacco use, diethylstilbestrol (DES) exposure.

- Human papillomavirus (HPV) vaccine, approved for women ages 11 to 26, is effective against serotypes 6, 11, 16, and 18.

- Papanicolaou (Pap) smears have been shown to reduce mortality risk associated with cervical cancer.

CASE 9-11

A 49-year-old asymptomatic woman seen for a routine examination is noted to have enlarged ovaries bilaterally on pelvic examination.

1. **What is the differential diagnosis for an ovarian mass?**
   - PCOS, multiple cysts bilaterally
   - Ovarian cyst (functional; follicular and corpus luteum cyst; "chocolate" cysts)
   - Primary ovarian tumor
   - Epithelial mass (benign or malignant)
   - Germ cell tumor (benign teratoma = dermoid cyst; yolk sac; choriocarcinoma)
   - Sex cord stroma
   - Metastasis commonly from breast or GI tract (Krukenberg tumor)

2. **What is polycystic ovary syndrome?**
   PCOS occurs as a result of increased pituitary production of LH out of proportion to FSH (LH/FSH ratio >2) and hyperandrogenism secondary to unregulated synthesis by theca cells. Hyperandrogenism can result in hirsutism and virilization (male secondary sex characteristics and clitoromegaly), but androgens are also aromatized to estrogen in adipose tissue, thus increasing the risk of endometrial carcinoma. PCOS is associated with anovulation, obesity, and insulin resistance. The condition is often diagnosed at a younger age, as symptoms generally appear at menarche. Polycystic ovaries have multiple 2- to 8-mm subcapsular cysts that can be visualized on ultrasound (Fig. 9-8). These cysts result in amenorrhea and infertility.

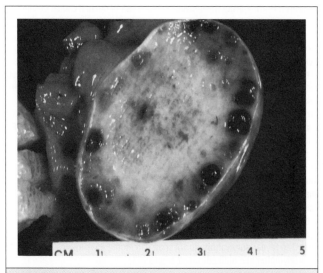

Figure 9-8. Sagittal section of a polycystic ovary illustrating a large number of follicular cysts and a thickened stroma. (From Stenchever MA: Comprehensive Gynecology, 4th ed. St. Louis, Mosby, 2001.)

STEP 1 SECRET

Expect to see a question on polycystic ovary syndrome (PCOS) on the USMLE Step 1.

CASE 9-11 continued:

Pelvic ultrasound shows a 10-cm cystic and solid mass with septations on the left and a 6-cm mass on the right. Given these ultrasound characteristics (>8 cm; solid; septations), it is thought to be highly suspicious for malignancy.

3. **What is the most likely diagnosis in this patient?**
   Although 80% of ovarian tumors are benign, age is a risk factor for malignancy. Germ cell tumors are common in women <20 years of age, whereas epithelial tumors are more common in those >20years.

4. **What is most common type of ovarian cancer?**
   Serous cystadenocarcinoma, an epithelial cell tumor, is most common.

5. **Is ovarian cancer hereditary?**
   About 90% of ovarian cancers are sporadic; 10% have a familial syndrome. Hereditary nonpolyposis colorectal cancer (HNPCC)–Lynch II syndrome is HNPCC syndrome in which there is a high rate of familial breast, ovarian, colon, and endometrial cancers. Breast cancers (*BRCA1* and *BRCA2* mutations) are also implicated in familial ovarian cancer.

6. **What are the major risk factors for ovarian cancer?**
   - Family history of ovarian cancer
   - Long periods of uninterrupted ovulation (low parity)
   - History of colon or breast cancer

   Remember: Hormonal contraceptives decrease risk of ovarian cancer because they suppress ovulation.

7. **Are there any effective screening tests for ovarian cancer?**
   Not really. Cancer antigen 125 (CA-125) is a tumor marker in some ovarian cancers and is used to follow response to treatment, but it is *not* an appropriate screening tool for the general population because CA125 is not specific for ovarian cancer. Routine pelvic examinations are the best screening tool we have for ovarian cancer.

   Germ cell tumors often are associated with elevated tumor markers (AFP, hCG, L-lactate dehydrogenase), which can be helpful in diagnosis and response to treatment. AFP is elevated in embryonic sinus and yolk sac tumors; hCG is elevated in choriocarcinoma.

   Dermoid cysts sometimes produce thyroid hormone if they contain thyroid tissue, called struma ovarii.

   Granulosa cell tumors secrete estrogen and can cause precocious puberty, endometrial hyperplasia, or carcinoma. They are characterized by "Call-Exner bodies," which are eosinophilic secretions.

8. **What is the prognosis for ovarian cancer?**
   Not great. The 5-year survival rate for ovarian carcinoma 25% to 30%, typically because the disease is asymptomatic until advanced stages.

SUMMARY BOX: OVARIAN CYSTS, OVARIAN CANCER

- Polycystic ovary syndrome (PCOS) is characterized by anovulation, hyperandrogenism, multiple cysts on the ovaries, and elevated luteinizing hormone (LH).

- Krukenberg tumor is a metastasis to the ovary from another source: commonly gastrointestinal tract or breast.

- Hormonal contraceptives decrease the risk of ovarian cancer.

- Cancer antigen 125 (CA-125) is elevated in many ovarian cancers but is NOT a screening marker for ovarian cancer.

CASE 9-12

A 58-year-old postmenopausal woman presents with abnormal uterine/vaginal bleeding. She has been postmenopausal for 6 years and has never experienced this problem previously.

1. **What is generally assumed to be the cause of postmenopausal bleeding until proven otherwise?**
   Until proved otherwise, postmenopausal bleeding indicates endometrial cancer, which is the most common gynecologic cancer in the United States.

2. **What else should be considered in the differential diagnosis for postmenopausal bleeding?**
   Other uterine sources of bleeding such as endometrial hyperplasia as well as vaginal sources of bleeding such as vaginal atrophy/laceration or cervical polyps would be considered.
   Note: Endometrial hyperplasia, which also commonly presents as postmenopausal bleeding, is a precursor to endometrial cancer.

CASE 9-12 continued:

A physical examination reveals the source of the bleeding to be the cervical os (i.e., uterine bleeding, not a vaginal source). There are no abnormal masses palpated on bimanual examination, and the uterus is of normal size and shape.

3. **What studies can be done to help with the diagnosis?**
   Pelvic ultrasound will show the anatomy—fibroids, polyps, or endometrial hyperplasia. Normally, a postmenopausal woman should have a very thin endometrial stripe because of lack of estrogen.

CASE 9-12 continued:

A pelvic ultrasound reveals a thickened endometrium, so an endometrial biopsy is done. The pathology report indicates malignancy.

4. **What is the most common type of endometrial cancer?**
   Adenocarcinoma (80%) is the most common type.

5. **Why does endometrial cancer, once detected, generally have a much better prognosis than newly diagnosed ovarian cancer?**
   Endometrial cancer is usually detected at a much earlier stage than ovarian cancer thanks to the fact that abnormal uterine bleeding is an early warning sign. In contrast, there are few warning signs of early ovarian cancer.

6. **What are the risk factors for endometrial carcinoma?**
   Abnormally increased estrogen levels (e.g., PCOS, granulosa cell tumor) or use of estrogen without progesterone (e.g., hormone replacement therapy), obesity (adipose tissue can convert androgens into estrogens), hypertension, diabetes, early menarche, late menopause, and Lynch syndrome are all risk factors.

7. **In pathophysiologic terms, why does it make sense that the risk factors for endometrial cancer are similar to those for breast cancer?**
Because estrogen plays an important role in the etiology of both types of cancer. This is why obesity (increased peripheral production of estrogen), unopposed estrogens, nulliparity (increased exposure to *cycling* estrogens), and late menopause (increased estrogen exposure) are common risk factors for the development of breast cancer and endometrial cancer.
   Remember: Hormonal contraceptives actually decrease risk of endometrial cancer because progesterone thins the uterine lining and prevents unopposed growth by estrogen.

8. **If this woman also has atrophic vaginitis, why should vaginal estrogen creams not be used to treat it?**
A significant percentage of the cream gets absorbed systemically, and because endometrial cancer is an estrogen-dependent cancer, the resulting elevated plasma estrogen can cause the cancer to progress.
   Remember: Estrogen-dependent tumors/cancers are an absolute contraindication to the use of exogenous estrogens.

SUMMARY BOX: POSTMENOPAUSAL BLEEDING AND ENDOMETRIAL CANCER

- Endometrial carcinoma is the most common, and most curable, gynecologic cancer in the United States.

- Postmenopausal bleeding should be considered endometrial cancer until proven otherwise.

- Risk factors for endometrial cancer include obesity, unopposed estrogens, nulliparity, late menopause, diabetes, and hypertension.

- Hormonal contraceptives decrease the risk of endometrial cancer.

CASE 9-13

A 22-year-old woman is being evaluated for a breast mass she detected while showering. She has never had a mammogram and is wondering if she should get one.

1. **What is the differential diagnosis for a breast mass?**
   - Fibrocystic disease
   - Benign: fibroadenoma, cystosarcoma phyllodes, intraductal papilloma
   - Malignant carcinoma

2. **What characteristics of a breast mass are more consistent with benign versus malignant disease?**
See Table 9-4 for these characteristics.

CASE 9-13 continued:

The mass is round, mobile, rubbery, and nontender. There is no family history of breast or ovarian cancer.

TABLE 9-4. CHARACTERISTICS OF BREAST MASSES

Benign: Fibroadenoma	Malignant: Carcinoma
Soft	Firm
Tender	Nontender
Round, distinct borders	Irregular indistinct borders
Mobile	Fixed
Changes seen during cycle	No changes seen during cycle
Affects women 20-35 years of age	Affects women older than 35 years of age

3. **Should a mammogram be ordered to evaluate this breast mass? What other study can be done?**
Mammogram can be used to further evaluate a suspicious mass, but ultrasound is useful in a less suspicious palpable mass to determine if it is cystic or solid. A fluid-filled cyst can be drained with a needle in the office.

CASE 9-13 continued:

An ultrasound reveals the mass to be solid, not cystic, so an excisional biopsy is performed.

4. **What is the most likely diagnosis?**
Fibroadenoma is the most common breast tumor in premenopausal women; it is benign.

5. **What is the difference between fibroadenoma and fibrocystic breast disease?**
Both are benign processes, but fibroadenoma is an encapsulated tumor, whereas fibrocystic breast disease encompasses a wide spectrum of abnormalities, all due to an excessive stromal response to hormones and growth factors. These changes can include cyst formation, nodule formation, and epithelial hyperplasia.
Fibroadenoma is NOT a precursor to breast carcinoma. Fibrocystic disease usually does not increase risk of carcinoma except in cases of fibrocystic disease with atypical hyperplasia.

6. **What is cystosarcoma phyllodes?**
Phyllodes tumors are a variant of fibroadenoma and present as a large bulky masses with rapid growth. Most are benign, but a few tumors do have malignant cells.

7. **If a woman presents with bloody nipple discharge, what should be done, and what are the two diseases that can cause this?**
The discharge should be sent for cytologic evaluation. A benign process, *intraductal papilloma*, which indicates local proliferation of the epithelial lining of the lactiferous ducts, is one possibility. The other possibility is *invasive papillary carcinoma*, a malignant process.

SUMMARY BOX: WORKUP OF PALPABLE BREAST MASS

- Soft, round, mobile mass suggests benign disease. Firm, irregular, and immobile mass is concerning for malignancy.

- Ultrasound is used to determine if a mass is cystic or solid.

- Fibroadenoma is the most common benign tumor of breast. It occurs in women aged 20 to 35.

- Cystosarcoma phyllodes is a variant of fibroadenoma with malignant potential.

- Intraductal papilloma is the most common cause of bloody nipple discharge, but invasive papillary carcinoma should be ruled out by sending discharge for cytologic evaluation.

CASE 9-14

A 59-year-old woman is being evaluated for a breast mass she detected while showering. She is concerned about breast cancer because her mother was diagnosed with breast cancer at the age of 72.

1. **Based solely on the family history and the known genetics of breast cancer, is this woman at high risk for developing a familial breast cancer?**
   No. The vast majority of breast cancers (~90%) are sporadic. Because her mother was elderly when she developed breast cancer, it is highly unlikely that this patient had a familial predisposition (e.g., *BRCA1* or *BRCA2* mutations) to develop breast cancer. A first-degree relative family history is a risk factor for sporadic breast cancer, but postmenopausal breast cancer in a first-degree relative only slightly increases risk.

CASE 9-14 continued:

History is significant for a nontender mass that does not change in size or shape with her menstrual cycle and a single episode of bloody nipple discharge. Her menstrual cycles began at age 13 and she entered menopause at 55. She has no children and has never been pregnant.

2. **What risk factors for breast cancer does she have?**
   - Female
   - Age (postmenopausal)
   - Late menopause
   - Nulliparity

3. **What is the significance of the age at menarche and age at menopause for the risk of developing breast cancer?**
   The younger the age at menarche and the older the age at menopause are both correlated with a higher risk of breast cancer. These relationships are explained by increased cumulative exposure to estrogen.

4. **Why does a woman who has been pregnant multiple times have a lower risk for developing breast cancer than a nulliparous woman, given that she has actually been exposed to larger amounts of circulating estrogen?**
   No one really knows, but there are several theories that are worth mentioning. Estrogen levels during pregnancy are higher than in the nonpregnant woman, but this estrogen is not *cycling* (as it does in the nonpregnant woman) and its actions are *opposed* by the high levels of progesterone associated with pregnancy.

CASE 9-14 continued:

On examination, her breasts are asymmetric; there is a firm, nontender, irregular mass in her right breast, with redness and dimpling of the skin, and her right nipple appears slightly retracted. All previous mammograms in this woman have been normal.

5. **Based on the physical examination findings, does this woman likely have breast cancer?**

   Yes, she has many of the classic signs: an irregular, firm breast mass causing retraction or dimpling of the skin or nipple (peau d'orange) and a bloody discharge.

   Remember: Intraductal papilloma, a benign process, is actually the most common cause of a bloody nipple discharge. Invasive papillary carcinoma is next.

CASE 9-14 continued:

A diagnostic mammogram is ordered, and she is referred to a surgeon for biopsy.

6. **Which type of breast cancer is this woman most likely to have?**

   Infiltrating (invasive) ductal carcinoma is the most common type of breast cancer and should be the presumed diagnosis pending a definitive pathology report.

7. **If biopsy reveals estrogen receptor–positive (ER+) and progesterone receptor–positive (PR+) cells, why might treatment with tamoxifen or anastrazole be useful?**

   Tamoxifen is a selective estrogen receptor modulator (SERM). It acts as an estrogen receptor agonist in certain tissues (e.g., bone, uterus) but as an estrogen antagonist at other tissues (e.g., breast). Anastrazole is an antiestrogen aromatase inhibitor that is also useful in ER+ and PR+ cancers. Because growth of ER+ and PR+ tumor cells is somewhat hormone-dependent, these cancers can be treated with agents such as tamoxifen or anastrazole.

RELATED QUESTIONS

8. **If an elderly woman presents with eczematous nipple changes, what should you suspect this is, what should you do, and why?**

   Paget disease of the nipple produces this finding, and a breast biopsy should be done because an underlying malignancy is found in the vast majority of patients with this disease.

9. **If a woman has a unilateral inflamed breast and orange peel (dimpled) appearance to the skin of that breast, what disease process should you suspect and what is the pathophysiology?**

   She probably has inflammatory breast carcinoma, which can be attributed to the tumor embolizing into the dermal lymphatics. This in turn causes the redness, swelling, and warmth. Because there has been tumor embolization, it is not surprising that there is axillary lymph node involvement. Distant metastases are frequent when this is found.

SUMMARY BOX: BREAST CANCER

- Most breast cancers are sporadic, with a minority due to genetic factors.

- Risk factors: sex, age, previous breast cancer, nulliparous, early menarche, late menopause, obesity, high dietary first-degree relative with breast cancer.

- Infiltrating ductal carcinoma is the most common breast malignancy.

- Tamoxifen, a selective estrogen receptor modulator, antagonizes estrogen in the breast tissue. Anastrazole is an aromatase inhibitor, which decreases estrogen production.

CASE 9-15

A 16-year-old boy visits the doctor because he worries that he has not yet gone through puberty. He has been unable to grow facial hair, and his voice has not become deep. Embarrassed, he admits that his genitals are smaller and less developed than what he thinks is normal for his age.

1. **What is the differential diagnosis for delayed puberty?**
   Because this vignette does not mention that the patient has ever had ambiguous or female external genitalia, for the purpose of boards we can tentatively rule out hermaphroditism, androgen insensitivity syndrome, and 5α-reductase deficiency (though as a general rule, you should never rule out a disease because the patient does not specifically mention something to you!). Consider constitutional delay, family history of delayed puberty, malnutrition, hypopituitarism, and Kallmann syndrome.

CASE 9-15 continued:

At birth, the patient presented with micropenis and cryptorchidism. He has also had a poor sense of smell for most of his life.

2. **What is the most likely diagnosis in this patient?**
   Kallmann syndrome, which is a genetic condition that leads to an absence of GnRH-producing neurons in the hypothalamus. This leads to lack of testosterone production and secondary sexual characteristics.

3. **Why do these patients often present with anosmia?**
   Kallmann syndrome can be associated with a lack of olfactory neurons in the brain as well. This results in a decreased or total loss of smell. Patients may also present with color blindness.

SUMMARY BOX: KALLMANN SYNDROME

- Kallmann syndrome results from a lack of gonadotropin-releasing hormone (GnRH) neurons in the brain.

- The triad for Kallmann syndrome is delayed puberty, anosmia, and color blindness.

CASE 9-16

A 15-year-old girl is examined by an endocrinologist in the hospital. She has short stature, a webbed neck, and a broad shield-like chest with widely spaced nipples. Secondary sexual characteristics, such as breast development, are absent, and her external genitalia are infantile-appearing. She has never had a period. She has normal intellect and seems to be a happy, healthy person. A pelvic ultrasound reveals streak ovaries. The laboratory findings include a normal growth hormone level and an elevated FSH. Her karyotype is 45,XO. There is an absence of Barr bodies observed in cells from a buccal smear.

1. **What disease do you suspect is responsible for this patient's amenorrhea?**
   Turner syndrome, which occurs in 1 in every 2500 females, is most likely.

2. **What causes the development of Turner syndrome?**
The presence of an incomplete sex genotype (45,XO) due to chromosomal nondisjunction (60%) or mosaicism (40%) is the cause. As a result, these women have decreased estrogen levels. About 80% of the cases are caused by meiotic error in the father; that is, the patient did not receive an X chromosome from the father.

This disease is characterized by a number of physical abnormalities, including short stature, webbed neck, and broad chest. Girls (women) with Turner syndrome also have ovarian dysgenesis, in which instead of normal ovaries they have "streaks" of connective tissue that do not produce normal quantities of estrogen or progesterone, hormones that are required for the development of secondary sexual characteristics. Because the ovaries are replaced by fibrous stroma and are devoid of oocytes by the age of 2, many of these women are infertile. However, a small percentage (5-10%) have sufficient ovarian development to support fertility.

Note: Turner syndrome is the most common cause of primary amenorrhea.

3. **What phenomenon is responsible for this patient's webbed neck?**
This condition is called cystic hygroma and is a form of lymphangioma commonly found in the neck. Although the condition is benign, it can be quite disfiguring in some patients.

4. **If this patient were to develop hypertension, what diagnostic test(s) should be performed?**
Patients with Turner syndrome are at increased risk for preductal coarctation of the aorta, which often results in hypertension limited to the upper extremities and cerebral vessels. In a manner analogous to renal artery stenosis, aortic coarctation causes hypertension because chronic underperfusion of the kidneys results in activation of the renin-angiotensin-aldosterone system and volume retention.

The easiest initial diagnostic test is a comparison of upper and lower extremity blood pressures to assess for a significant discrepancy. Coarctation results in a lower femoral artery pressure and a delayed femoral pulse relative to the pressure and pulse of the brachial artery. A chest x-ray study will often show the classic "rib notching" due to increased collateral blood flow through the intercostal arteries, which bypass the coarctation. Imaging or often echocardiogram is usually performed to confirm the diagnosis.

5. **What are some other complications of Turner syndrome?**
Other complications include bicuspid aortic valve, horseshoe kidney, and hypothyroidism.

6. **How might this patient be managed pharmacologically to correct the lack of secondary sexual characteristics?**
Estrogen therapy for teenage girls with Turner syndrome can help promote development of secondary sexual characteristics.

7. **What is Klinefelter's syndrome?**
The genotype of Klinefelter's syndrome is 47,XXY (sometimes 48,XXXY). Because these individuals have a Y chromosome, they are males who possess a Barr body. They undergo fibrosis of the seminiferous tubules, leading to azospermia, infertility, and loss of Sertoli cells. Decreased inhibin production secondary to Sertoli cell loss leads to increased production of FSH. Klinefelter patients also exhibit abnormal Leydig cell function, which results in decreased production of testosterone and testicular atrophy. Because testosterone is unavailable to exert negative feedback upon the pituitary, LH concentrations become high. This stimulates the production of estrogens, leading to gynecomastia, eunuchoid body shape, and female hair distribution. These patients tend to be tall with long extremities due to delayed closure of the epiphyseal plates that results from decreased androgen concentrations.

STEP 1 SECRET

Turner and Klinefelter syndromes appear very frequently on boards so be sure that you can recognize their presentations.

---

8. **How does the presentation of the XXY Klinefelter phenotype differ from the XYY phenotype?**

XYY or double Y males are phenotypically normal with normal fertility. They tend to be taller than normal males and often present with severe acne. It is also typical for these males to present with aggressive, antisocial, or even criminal behavior.

9. **What is trisomy X?**

Trisomy X refers to the genotype 47,XXX. These females often have no apparent abnormalities but may experience mild menstrual irregularities and exhibit mild mental retardation. They are frequently taller than normal females.

SUMMARY BOX: SEX CHROMOSOME DISORDERS

- Turner syndrome (45,XO) results in decreased estrogen levels and streaked ovaries. Patients typically present with short stature, webbed neck, and broadened chest. Turner syndrome is the most common cause of primary amenorrhea. It is associated with an increased risk of coarctation of the aorta.

- Coarctation of the aorta results in a discrepancy between upper and lower extremity pressures characterized by upper extremity hypertension. A chest x-ray film will classically show rib notching. Other complications of Turner syndrome include bicuspid aortic valve, horseshoe kidney, and hypothyroidism.

- Klinefelter syndrome (47,XXY or 48,XXXY) results in decreased levels of testosterone and increased levels of estrogen. Patients typically present with infertility, gynecomastia, female hair distribution, eunuchoid body shape, tall stature, and long extremities.

- Trisomy X (47,XXX) females are typically normal but may experience mild menstrual irregularities or exhibit mental retardation. They are generally tall.

- XYY individuals are phenotypically normal but may be taller and more aggressive than normal males.

CASE 9-17

A 16-year-old girl is concerned because she hasn't started having her period yet, whereas all of her friends have had periods for at least 2 years now. She additionally has no breast development. On physical examination she has scant axillary and pubic hair, and the uterus is not palpable. On speculum examination no cervix is visible (i.e., the vagina ends in a blind pouch). A pelvic ultrasound is performed, and she is found to have no uterus or ovaries but instead undescended testes. Consequently, a karyotype is performed, which comes back 46,XY.

1. **What is this patient's syndrome?**

This child likely has androgen insensitivity syndrome, which is also known as testicular feminization syndrome. These patients are genetically and gonadally male but phenotypically female.

2. What is the cause of this syndrome?
As mentioned in the basic concepts section of this chapter, genetic alterations in the androgen receptor make the tissues unresponsive to the androgenic effects of testosterone and other androgens. Testicles are present and functional (they produce testosterone) but the tissues do not respond.

3. Why does this patient have a vaginal pouch?
In a normal male, the potent androgen DHT, which is produced from testosterone by the action of the enzyme 5α-reductase, acts upon the androgen receptor in the tissues of the urogenital fold to stimulate the formation of the external genitalia (i.e., penis, prostate, and scrotum) during development.

   In the absence of androgen activity, either in a normal female or in a male with androgen insensitivity, the urogenital fold develops into a vaginal pouch.

   The effect of DHT on genital tissue has clinical relevance in the treatment of benign prostatic hyperplasia (BPH). Inhibitors of the enzyme 5α-reductase, (e.g. finasteride) have been shown to reduce prostate size, often resulting in symptomatic improvement in men with BPH.

4. Why does this patient have no pubic or axillary hair?
In both males and females, the initial development of secondary sexual characteristics, particularly pubic and axillary hair, adult body odor, and sebaceous gland activity, depends on adrenal androgen production. These changes usually occur before the hormonal changes of central puberty—that is, increased production of estrogen (specifically estradiol) in females and testosterone in males. In androgen insensitivity, lack of activity of adrenal or testicular androgens results in the lack of axillary and pubic hair.

   Recall that the major adrenal androgens include dehydroepiandrosterone (DHEA) and dehydroepiandrosterone sulfate (DHEA-S). In fact, DHEA-S is specific to the adrenal gland, and its levels will be increased in disorders of adrenal androgen overproduction such as rare hormone-producing adrenal carcinomas and the virilizing forms of congenital adrenal hyperplasia.

5. How can we explain the lack of uterus in this child?
Recall that the uterus is formed from the müllerian duct. In males these structures are dissolved by müllerian inhibiting substance (MIF), which is produced by the testes. As there is no abnormality in the testes themselves in this disease, this substance will be secreted and the duct will dissolve, resulting in the absence of an internal female reproductive tract (i.e., fallopian tubes, uterus, and cervix).

   Recall that the internal male genital tract (i.e., the seminiferous tubules, the epididymis, and vas deferens) develops from the wolffian duct, but this differentiation requires the activity of testosterone.

   Thus, because the testes are normal and produce müllerian inhibiting substance in androgen insensitivity syndrome but the activity of testosterone is absent, neither a male nor a female internal genital tract develops.

6. Would testosterone levels be low or high in this patient?
Testosterone levels would be high because the nonfunctional androgen receptors prevent negative feedback upon pituitary LH production. High LH levels in turn increase testosterone production by the testes. In other words, the lack of testosterone activity in the pituitary disinhibits LH release, which stimulates the testes to produce high levels of testosterone.

7. Why should this patient's testicles be removed?
Undescended (or cryptorchid) testes from any cause, whether spontaneously undescended or undescended as part of a syndrome, are at increased risk for giving rise to testicular cancer. If an undescended testis fails to spontaneously descend within about a year or so of birth, it should be surgically replaced within the scrotum (i.e., orchiopexy) or surgically removed (i.e., orchiectomy).

SUMMARY BOX: ANDROGEN INSENSITIVITY SYNDROME AND SEXUAL DEVELOPMENT

- Normally in females, in the absence of testes, internal and external female reproductive organs develop.

- Normally in males, the developing testes produce both testosterone and müllerian inhibiting substance (MIF). The male internal reproductive tract develops under the influence of testosterone, and the female internal reproductive organs involute under the influence of MIF.

- The male external genitalia, including the prostate, normally develop under the influence of dihydrotestosterone (DHT). The enzyme 5α-reductase converts testosterone into the more potent androgen DHT. Inhibitors of this enzyme (such as finasteride) are used to treat benign prostatic hyperplasia.

- Adrenal androgens, such as the adrenal-specific hormone dehydroepiandrosterone sulfate (DHEA-S), are normally responsible for the initial development of secondary sexual characteristics (such as adult body hair, adult body odor, and sebaceous gland activity) during puberty of both males and females.

- Androgen insensitivity syndrome (or testicular feminization syndrome) results from a defect in the androgen receptor. Patients have a male karyotype (46,XY) and undescended testes, but they fail to develop male external genitalia and phenotypically appear female. Because their testes are able to produce MIF they lack a female internal reproductive tract; however, because they lack testosterone activity, they also lack a male reproductive tract. Patients are left with female external genitalia, including a vagina that ends in a blind pouch. Lack of androgen activity also results in absence of secondary sex characteristics such as pubic and axillary hair or adult body odor.

- Undescended (or cryptorchid) testes of any cause should eventually be replaced within the scrotum or surgically removed because of increased risk of malignancy.

CHAPTER 10

ONCOLOGY

Douglas W. Jones, Thomas A. Brown, MD, and Sonali J. Shah

INSIDER'S GUIDE TO ONCOLOGY FOR THE USMLE STEP 1

It is no surprise that boards are big on oncology. As with pharmacology, almost every topic area has an oncology-related component. Yet before you can delve into these individual tumor types, you should develop a firm understanding of basic tumor biology. If you have the time to do so, we recommend that you read the "Neoplasia" chapter in *Robbins and Cotran Pathologic Basis of Disease*. Once you understand these concepts, you will see that every cancer type follows the same basic set of principles, and it will be much easier to focus on mastering specific facts.

BASIC CONCEPTS—CELL BIOLOGY OF CANCER

1. **What is the difference between an oncogene and a tumor suppressor gene?**
   An oncogene is a mutated form of a normal gene (proto-oncogene). Proto-oncogenes code for proteins that can lead to cellular proliferation and neoplasia. However, proto-oncogenes are normally silent (unexpressed). Activating mutations convert proto-oncogenes into oncogenes and predispose to neoplasia. Because only a single gene needs to be mutated, oncogenes are seen as dominant mutations. An example of a proto-oncogene is a gene for a growth factor receptor that, when mutated, could lead to inappropriate activation of the receptor, leading to uncontrolled cellular proliferation in the absence of excessive levels of that growth factor.

   A tumor suppressor gene is a normally active gene (in contrast with a proto-oncogene). Tumor suppressor genes encode proteins that suppress cellular proliferation; therefore, if its function is lost (*disinhibited*), cancerous cells are permitted to survive. Mutations in tumor suppressor genes are said to be recessive because mutation must occur in both alleles in order to completely knock out the function of the gene.

2. **Which type of mutation is more commonly involved in familial cancer syndromes?**
   Tumor suppressor genes are more commonly involved in familial cancer syndromes because an embryo with one mutated copy of a tumor suppressor gene is likely to develop normally. However, a second mutation may be acquired at a later date, leading to cancer (loss of heterozygosity). On the other hand, an embryo is less likely to survive if it has inherited an oncogene because the effects of this dominant negative mutation are typically much more disruptive to development.

3. **How does Knudson's "two-hit hypothesis" relate to tumor suppressor genes?**
   Alfred Knudson studied retinoblastoma, which was later found to be a form of cancer caused by the mutation of the retinoblastoma tumor suppressor gene. At the time, he observed that in familial forms of retinoblastoma, tumors formed in patients at a much younger age than was

typical for those arising in patients with no family history of the disease. He theorized that in familial cases, a germ-line mutation was inherited (the first hit) and that a second sporadic mutation occurred early in life (the second hit), thus deactivating both tumor suppressor genes and causing tumor formation. This theory was therefore called the two-hit hypothesis. In nonfamilial cases, however, mutations of both tumor suppressor genes (both hits) had to occur sporadically and thus took much longer to manifest as tumor formation.

4. **What are the phases of the cell cycle? Where is the restriction point?**
   Most cells in the human body are quiescent (i.e., not actively dividing). Exceptions include cells of the hematopoietic system, the integument, and the intestinal mucosa. However, those cells that divide follow a well-defined cyclic pattern. Major challenges in cell replication include high-fidelity DNA duplication (in the S phase) and segregation of chromosomes into daughter cells (during mitosis or the M phase). Different phases and checkpoints help address these issues (Fig. 10-1):
   - S phase: DNA synthesis
   - G_2 phase: gap period 2
   - M phase: mitosis
   - G_1 phase: gap period 1
   - R: restriction point

   The restriction point occurs just prior to the S phase; it is important because once the restriction point is passed, a cell is committed to complete the cell cycle. Multiple cellular factors interact to allow a cell to pass the restriction point.

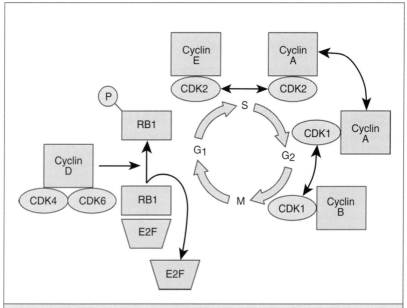

Figure 10-1. Regulation of the cell cycle. (From Hoffman R, Benz EJ Jr, Shattil SJ, et al: Hematology: Basic Principles and Practice, 4th ed. Philadelphia, Churchill Livingstone, 2005.)

5. **What is the function of checkpoints and cell cycle arrests?**
   The most important function of cell cycle arrest is to allow for the repair of cellular damage and DNA sequences. If improperly duplicated DNA were not repaired at cell cycle checkpoints, then DNA mutations would quickly propagate, and the integrity of cellular

homogeneity could not be maintained. A cell may also arrest in the absence of proper nutrients, growth factors, or hormones.

Cyclins are proteins that regulate progression from one phase of the cell cycle to the next. Cyclins phosphorylate cyclin-dependent kinases (CDKs) to form cyclin-CDK complexes that must be in either an activated or inactivated state for various cell cycle stages to commence or terminate. CDKs are regulated by CDK inhibitors such as p16, p21, and p27. If these CDK inhibitors are mutated, the cell cycle becomes deregulated and cancer can result. Table 10-1 lists the regulators of the cell cycle that you should know for boards.

TABLE 10-1. REGULATORS OF THE CELL CYCLE

Stage	Promoter(s)	Inhibitor
G_1 to S	Cyclin D/CDK4 and CDK6	p53
	Cyclin E-CDK2	Rb
S to G_2	Cyclin A-CDK2	—
G_2 to M	Cyclin B-CDK1	—
	CDc25	

6. **What is the importance of p53?**

The p53 protein ("guardian of the genome") is a tumor suppressor gene protein responsible for promoting apoptosis in cells that should not propagate because of excessive DNA mutations or cellular damage. p53 has a number of functions. It can activate DNA repair genes during DNA damage, initiate apoptosis in cells that cannot be repaired, activate the CDK inhibitor p21, and prevent the phosphorylation and inactivation of the retinoblastoma (Rb) protein. Loss of p53 can lead to loss of apoptotic regulation and thus to uncontrolled cellular proliferation. The p53 gene, TP53, is the most commonly mutated gene in human cancers.

7. **What is the function of the retinoblastoma protein?**

Like p53, Rb is a tumor suppressor protein that functions to prevent cell cycle progression from the G_1 to S phase by binding to and inhibiting the transcription factor E2F. It is heavily regulated via p53 and cyclin-CDK complexes. When in a hypophosphorylated state, Rb functions as an active tumor suppressor. As mentioned in the preceding question 6, p53 helps to maintain Rb in a hypophosphorylated state. During G_1 to S transition, increased levels of cyclin D/CDK4 and CDK6 and cyclin E/CDK2 phosphorylate Rb and prevent its binding to E2F. E2F then activates additional proteins which push the cell cycle to the S phase.

8. **When can a solid tumor be detected clinically?**

A tumor mass may be clinically detectable when it has reached 10^9 cells or when it weighs approximately 1 g. Assuming the mass began as a single cellular mutation, this equates to approximately 30 to 33 cell doublings. Once a tumor mass has achieved this number of doublings, only a few further doublings will lead to the death of the patient. As a result, the point in time when a tumor can be detected and an intervention offered is very late in the replicative life of the tumor mass. Unsurprisingly, approximately 70% of patients have distant metastases at the time of diagnosis of a solid tumor.

9. **What is the importance of angiogenesis in solid tumor growth?**

It is thought that a solid tumor must form new blood vessels in order for a mass to grow larger than a few millimeters in diameter. Otherwise a tumor would soon outstrip the physiologic blood supply and the tumor cells would die (this is sometimes seen in larger tumors without effective angiogenesis that develop a necrotic core). Solid tumors, then, must be able to allow for and encourage the formation of new blood vessels as the tumor mass expands.

Note: In some cases growth of solid tumor metastases is promoted by removal of the primary tumor. This phenomenon has led to the idea that in some settings a primary tumor secretes angiogenesis inhibitors that cause distant micrometastases to remain dormant. Removal of the primary tumor also eliminates these inhibitors, allowing the micrometastases to proliferate. Angiogenesis inhibitors are a promising chemotherapeutic field of study.

10. **What is dysplasia? What is anaplasia?**
Dysplasia refers to abnormal cell growth and is marked by loss of cell shape, orientation, and size compared to normal tissue. Dysplastic changes are commonly precursors to neoplastic conditions, although dysplasia is reversible. By contrast, anaplasia is an irreversible condition that is marked by lack of differentiation. It is difficult to identify the tissue of origin in an anaplastic lesion.

BASIC CONCEPTS—CANCER EPIDEMIOLOGY

11. **What are three leading causes of death in the United States?**
    1. Heart disease
    2. Cancer
    3. Stroke

12. **Aside from skin cancer, which cancers have the highest incidence in men and in women? Which cancers are the leading cause of death in men and in women?**
Cancers with the highest incidence in men:
   - Prostate cancer
   - Lung cancer
   - Colorectal cancer

Cancers with the highest incidence in women:
   - Breast cancer
   - Lung cancer
   - Colorectal cancer

Leading causes of cancer deaths in men:
   - Lung cancer
   - Prostate cancer
   - Colorectal cancer

Leading causes of cancer deaths in women:
   - Lung cancer
   - Breast cancer
   - Colorectal cancer

Note: The incidence of lung cancer and colorectal cancer both exceed incidence of prostate and breast cancer when data for men and women are combined.

BASIC CONCEPTS—CANCER CLASSIFICATION

13. **What is the difference between "grade" and "stage" of a neoplasm?**
Grade: The grade of a neoplasm is determined *pathologically*. This designation usually refers to cellular characteristics of the neoplasm, especially the degree of differentiation of the cells involved. Grading of a neoplasm requires tissue, usually from a biopsy. Grades are reported by roman numerals I to III or I to IV, with the higher numbers representing more poorly differentiating cellular patterns.

Stage: The stage of a cancer is determined *clinically* but often takes into account information provided by the pathologist (the grade). Stage is most frequently reported using the tumor-node-metastasis (TNM) system:

- **T**: Tumor size. T refers to local growth measured by the size of the primary tumor.
- **N**: Nodes. N refers to the involvement of regional lymph nodes and is an indication of the extent of tumor spread.
- **M**: Metastases. M refers to the presence or absence of distant metastases. Presence of metastases typically confers a high stage.

Staging is most helpful in determining prognosis. Higher stages indicate a poorer prognosis.

STEP 1 SECRET

You will not be asked to determine the grade or stage of a cancer on Step 1, but you should understand the general concepts.

14. What is the difference between a benign tumor and a malignant tumor?

The distinction between benign and malignant tumors is primarily based on invasiveness, although other characteristics are also evident.

Benign tumors remain localized and may be surrounded by a capsule (the exception to this rule is leiomyoma, which is a benign tumor that is not surrounded by a capsule). They grow slowly and do not metastasize. With reference to tumor grade, these tumors tend to be well differentiated but may undergo malignant transformation.

Malignant tumors are characterized by their invasive properties. They are not surrounded by a capsule, and tumor cells locally invade the tissues that surround them. They tend to grow rapidly and may metastasize. Histologically, these tumors can be poorly differentiated, indicating uncontrolled cellular proliferation.

Even though malignant tumors generally have a worse prognosis than benign tumors, you should not be fooled into thinking that benign tumors are harmless. Depending on location, benign tumors can cause major obstruction that can severely compromise the function of that organ. Brain tumors are great examples of this principle.

15. How are cancers named according to the cell type they originate from?

Epithelial cells are the most common cells that lead to the formation of cancers (likely due to their high levels of replication). Cancers may arise from glandular cells, squamous cells, or transitional cells. Benign epithelial tumors frequently end in the suffix -oma. Malignant tumors of epithelial origin are referred to as carcinomas. So a benign tumor of squamous cell origin may simply be called a papilloma, but when it becomes malignant it is called a squamous cell carcinoma.

Mesenchymal cells can lead to benign tumors (also typically ending in -oma), but their malignant counterparts are called sarcomas. So a benign tumor originating from skeletal muscle may be called a rhabdomyoma, whereas its malignant counterpart is called a rhabdomyosarcoma.

Other cancers may originate from cell types that are not completely differentiated and may be able to give rise to other cell types (i.e., totipotential cells/germ cells). Leukemias and lymphomas are classified in this way and have a unique naming system. Many variations exist in the naming of cancers, but the rules mentioned here are helpful to remember.

CASE 10-1

A 50-year-old man is evaluated for a 6-month history of mild upper abdominal pain. The pain is associated with mild nausea and bloating but is unrelated to meals. He denies a retrosternal burning sensation. His appetite has been poor, and he has unexplainably lost 10 lb in the last 3 months. He is otherwise feeling well and has been taking no medications.

1. **What is dyspepsia?**

   Dyspepsia refers to acute, chronic, or recurrent discomfort in the upper abdomen. It can be associated with abdominal fullness, early satiety, bloating, and nausea and vomiting. Dyspepsia is different from heartburn, which is a retrosternal burning sensation more commonly associated with esophageal reflux. However, dyspepsia and heartburn often coexist.

2. **What is the differential diagnosis for dyspepsia?**

   It is broad and includes gastric causes such as peptic ulcer disease, gastroesophageal reflux disease, and gastric cancer; pancreatic causes such as pancreatitis and pancreatic carcinoma; biliary tract diseases such as cholelithiasis and choledocholithiasis; and "functional dyspepsia" when no obvious organic cause is found. Functional dyspepsia is the most common cause of chronic dyspepsia. Finally, cardiac ischemia can also present with dyspepsia.

   ### CASE 10-1 continued:

   The patient is given a trial of omeprazole without relief of symptoms. He now notes early satiety and worsening fatigue. Physical examination reveals conjunctival pallor, and rectal examination reveals stool positive for blood. Laboratory workup reveals hemoglobin of 10.2 g/dL with a mean corpuscular volume (MCV) of 65 fL.

3. **How does this information change your differential diagnosis?**

   The patient is bleeding into his gastrointestinal tract, most likely from peptic ulcer disease or from a gastric adenocarcinoma. He needs to have upper endoscopy performed as soon as possible.

STEP 1 SECRET

Whenever a patient has unintentional weight loss, particularly if appetite is suppressed, you should consider cancer as part of your differential diagnosis.

---

4. **What is the significance of his anemia?**

   He has a microcytic anemia that is most likely an iron deficiency anemia related to ongoing blood loss. An anemia of chronic disease is also possible but less likely in the setting of ongoing blood loss.

   ### CASE 10-1 continued:

   The patient undergoes upper endoscopy, during which an ulcer is located in the distal antrum of the stomach. It is not actively bleeding at the time of endoscopy. Biopsies are taken of the ulcer margin and of the antrum.

5. **Why were biopsies taken at these sites?**

   Gastric ulcers are always biopsied on endoscopy due to the fact that approximately 3% to 5% of ulcers, often benign-appearing, are malignant. The antral biopsy is taken to test for *Helicobacter pylori* infection.

   ### CASE 10-1 continued:

   Biopsy of the ulcer margin shows gastric adenocarcinoma, and biopsy of the antrum is positive for *H. pylori*.

6. **What is the significance of the *Helicobacter pylori*–positive biopsy?**
   H. pylori is one of the two major etiologic agents for peptic ulcer disease (nonsteroidal
   anti-inflammatory drug [NSAID] use being the other), but it is also highly correlated with gastric
   adenocarcinoma. Chronic *H. pylori* gastritis of the distal stomach increases the relative risk for
   developing gastric adenocarcinoma 4- to 20-fold.

7. **What are the different pathologic types of gastric cancer?**
   - Adenocarcinoma accounts for 90% to 95% of the cases.
   - Lymphoma, gastrointestinal stromal tumor, carcinoid, adenocanthoma, and squamous cell
     carcinoma make up the rest.

8. **In gastric adenocarcinoma, what are the two histologic patterns in which
   neoplastic cells can distribute?**
   Diffuse type: In this pattern, there is no cellular cohesion. Neoplastic cells invade the wall of
   the stomach diffusely without producing a distinct lesion. This type tends to occur in
   younger patients and has a poor prognosis. **Note:** Diffuse gastric adenocarcinomas present
   with signet ring cells (Fig. 10-2).
   Intestinal type: In this pattern, cells do cohere and form glandular structures that often have
   an ulcerative appearance. Lesions are most often found in the antrum and lesser curvature of
   the stomach. This type tends to occur in older patients and has a better prognosis than
   the diffuse type.

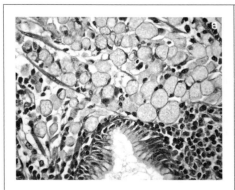

Figure 10-2. Diffuse type of gastric
carcinoma with signet ring tumor
cells. (From Kumar V, Cotran RS, Robbins
SL: Robbins Basic Pathology, 8th ed.
Philadelphia, WB Saunders, 2007.)

9. **What is linitis plastica?**
   Linitis plastica ("leather bottle") is a term used to describe involvement of the submucosa
   throughout the stomach, producing a rigid, atonic stomach. The histologic features are those of
   diffuse type adenocarcinoma.

10. **If the patient were to be examined again at a much later stage of disease, what
    specific signs might be found on physical examination that might indicate
    metastasis?**
    - Virchow's node: left supraclavicular lymphadenopathy
    - Sister Mary Joseph nodule: umbilical nodule
    - Krukenberg tumor (in women): ovarian tumors (often bilateral) that may be palpable on pelvic
      examination

11. **In retrospect, what aspects of this patient's presentation are most suspicious for gastric cancer?**
    - Onset of dyspepsia after age 40
    - Unintentional weight loss of 10 lb in 3 months
    - No response to proton pump inhibitor therapy
    - Development of early satiety
    - Iron deficiency anemia from occult intestinal bleeding

SUMMARY BOX: GASTRIC ADENOCARCINOMA

- The presentation of gastric adenocarcinoma is very similar to that of peptic ulcer disease and gastroesophageal reflux disease.

- From 60% to 90% of cases of distal gastric adenocarcinoma are attributed to chronic *Helicobacter pylori* infection.

- An ulcerated gastric lesion should always be biopsied because as many as 5% may harbor gastric cancer cells.

- Adenocarcinoma comprises almost all gastric cancers and can be classified by gross or microscopic pathologic appearance.

- Adenocarcinoma may produce distinct lesions or may infiltrate the stomach diffusely.

CASE 10-2

A 28-year-old woman presents with a lump in her left breast. She does monthly breast self-examinations and found this new lump 2 days ago. She has had no pain around the site of the lump and has noticed no nipple discharge. She is tearful and anxious. On examination, a 2-cm poorly localized, nontender mass is palpated in the upper left quadrant of the left breast. There are no skin changes in the area overlying the mass and no structural distortion of the breast. She has no lymphadenopathy.

1. **When examining a new breast lump, what findings may suggest breast cancer?**
   Nontender, firm or hard masses with poorly delineated margins can suggest breast cancer. There may be skin or nipple retraction and slight asymmetry.

2. **What is the most common presentation of breast cancer and where are most cancers found?**
   Approximately 70% of new cases of breast cancer present with a new lump in the breast. About 90% of all lumps are found by the patient. Up to 60% of breast carcinomas are found in the upper outer quadrant of the involved breast.

3. **What do the following physical examination findings indicate?**
   A. Bloody discharge from the nipple
      This can be a sign of breast cancer but is more commonly found in intraductal papilloma (a small benign tumor of the milk duct) when the discharge is found to be coming from a single duct.
   B. Small erosions (1-2 mm) of the nipple epithelium
      Dermatitis or Paget carcinoma is possible. Although nipple erosions most frequently represent a dermatitis or bacterial infection, this sign may also indicate an underlying ductal

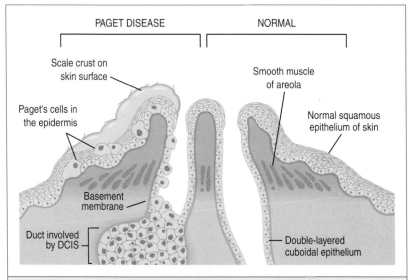

Figure 10-3. Paget disease of the nipple. DCIS, ductal carcinoma in situ. (From Kumar V, Abbas AK, Fausto N: Robbins and Cotran Pathologic Basis of Disease, 7th ed. Philadelphia, WB Saunders, 2005.)

carcinoma in situ (DCIS). As pictured in Figure 10-3, the neoplastic cells propagate toward the surface of the breast without violating the basement membrane. The presence of neoplastic cells does violate the epithelial barrier, allowing extrusion of extracellular fluid onto the nipple surface.

C. Rapidly growing breast with erythematous, edematous, and warm overlying skin
     Inflammatory carcinoma is possible. Invasion of the subdermal lymphatics by carcinoma can cause spreading erythema that can often be mistaken for infection. Resultant edema produces typical *peau d'orange* appearance (Fig. 10-4).

4. **What is the most common cause of a dominant breast mass for a woman in her 20s?**
    Fibroadenomas are typically described as round, rubbery, discrete, relatively mobile, and measuring 1 to 5 cm. No treatment is usually necessary. Diagnosis must be based on tissue biopsy or cytologic examination so as to avoid misdiagnosis of a malignancy.

CASE 10-2 continued:

During examination of the patient's right breast, a 1.5-cm discrete, nontender, mobile lump is found in the lower outer quadrant. The patient is very upset with the discovery of a lump in her right breast and reveals that her mother died of breast cancer at the age of 40 and that her older sister was diagnosed with breast cancer at the age of 27.

5. **What do bilateral breast lumps indicate with regard to a malignant or benign cause?**
    Fibroadenomas can occur at multiple sites in up to 10% to 15% of patients. Simultaneous bilateral breast cancers can also occur, so a bilateral malignant process is also a possibility.

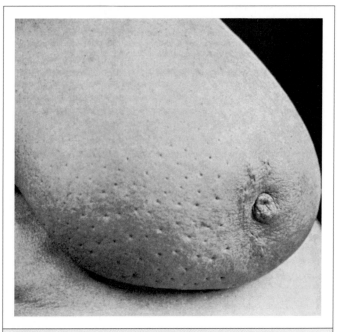

Figure 10-4. Peau d'orange ("skin of the orange") or edema of the skin of the breast. (From Townsend CM, Beauchamp RD, Evers BM, et al: Sabiston Textbook of Surgery, 17th ed. Philadelphia, WB Saunders, 2004.)

6. **What disease is she at risk for with the finding of bilateral breast masses and a family history of two first-degree relatives?**
   She is at risk for hereditary breast cancer. Up to 45% of familial cases of breast cancer are associated with a germ-line mutation, and in these syndromes, presentation with simultaneous bilateral breast lumps is common. A family history of breast cancer in more than one first-degree relative is highly suggestive of an inherited germ-line mutation.

7. **What specific genetic mutations confer a lifetime risk of 50% to 85% for developing breast cancer?**
   BRCA1 and *BRCA2* both are tumor suppressor genes whose gene products inhibit tumor growth. A single mutation is inherited and the second gene acquires a mutation (the "second hit") at some point in the patient's life. Multiple different inherited mutations to these genes have been identified. Though these genes have been well documented, they account for only approximately 25% of familial cases.

8. **If her tumor is found to be positive for *BRCA1*, for what other malignancy would this patient be at risk?**
   She would be at risk for ovarian cancer.

CASE 10-2 continued:

The lump in her left breast is biopsied and is found to harbor ductal carcinoma. Surgical excision is planned.

9. What are the common histologic types of breast cancer?

Carcinomas are divided into two broad categories: in situ and invasive carcinomas.

Breast cancers are also classified as ductal or lobular based on where they arise: Ductal origin refers to cancers arising from the epithelial lining of the large or intermediate-sized ducts, and lobular origin refers to cancers arising from the epithelium of the terminal ducts of the lobules (Fig. 10-5).

- *In situ carcinoma* describes a neoplastic population of cells that has not penetrated the basement membrane of the affected duct or lobule.
- DCIS makes up 80% of in situ carcinomas. Approximately half of mammographically detected cancers are DCIS because they tend to present with calcifications. DCIS is thought to progress to invasive ductal carcinoma in most women.
- Lobular carcinoma in situ (LCIS) never forms a density or calcifications and is therefore always an incidental finding on breast biopsy. It is found to be bilateral in 20% to 40% of women and turns into invasive cancer at a rate of approximately 1% per year; therefore, LCIS can be thought of as a risk factor for the development of invasive carcinoma.

Invasive carcinoma is characterized by neoplastic cells that have penetrated the basement membrane and may affect significant architectural distortion.

- Ductal carcinoma accounts for up to 80% of invasive carcinomas. Most histologic types of invasive cancer (colloid, medullary, etc.) are subtypes of invasive ductal carcinoma.
- Lobular carcinoma shows the classic histologic description of linear arrangements of cells (sometimes only one cell wide) invading surrounding tissue.
- Medullary carcinoma is found in women with the *BRCA1* gene; up to 13% of cancers are of this type.

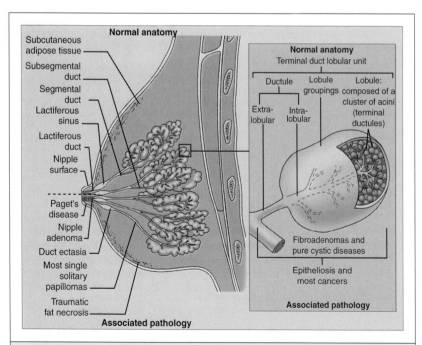

Figure 10-5. Anatomy of the breast. (From Hayes D: Breast cancer. In Skarin AT [ed]: Atlas of Diagnostic Oncology. Philadelphia, Lippincott, 1991.)

10. **What are two important biomarkers of a breast cancer that help guide treatment?**
    - *Estrogen receptor (ER)/progesterone receptor (PR):* If these receptors are present in the cytoplasm of cancer cells, then there is a better prognosis. After resection, patients are typically treated with tamoxifen (a selective estrogen receptor modulator [SERM]), which inhibits endogenous hormone stimulation of tumor cells. As a result, breast cancer is less likely to recur and mortality rate may be decreased by as much as 25% among women with receptor-positive tumors. Anastrazole (an aromatase inhibitor) is used when the patient has contraindications to tamoxifen use.
    - *HER2/neu* (also known as *ERBB2*): If a patient has a metastatic breast carcinoma that overexpresses this gene, trastuzumab (Herceptin) may be used. Trastuzumab is a monoclonal antibody directed against the HER-2 protein. When used with first-line chemotherapy following surgery, trastuzumab increases the time to disease progression.

SUMMARY BOX: BREAST CANCER

- Nontender, firm breast masses with poorly delineated margins are concerning for invasive breast cancer.

- Other findings concerning for breast cancer include nipple discharge, nipple scaling, breast asymmetry, nipple inversion, peau d'orange, erythema, and warmth.

- The most common cause of breast masses in young women is fibroadenoma.

- *BRCA1* and *BRCA2* mutations predispose to the development of breast cancer and account for approximately 25% of familial breast cancer syndromes.

- *BRCA1* mutations additionally confer increased risk for development of ovarian cancer.

- Most breast cancers arise from the intermediate ducts and are invasive (invasive ductal carcinoma).

- Ductal carcinoma in situ (DCIS) is thought to progress to invasive ductal carcinoma in most women.

- Lobular carcinoma in situ (LCIS) progresses to invasive lobular carcinoma in some women but not at the same rate of DCIS progression.

- Estrogen receptor/progesterone receptor (ER/PR) and *HER2/neu* (*ERBB2*) are important biomarkers and may guide adjuvant therapy for breast cancer following resection.

CASE 10-3

A 78-year-old man presents with a 2-month history of epigastric pain. He describes the pain as a vague pressure that occasionally radiates to his back. It does not reliably occur before or after meals. He has lost 20 lb in the last 2 months, though he attributes this to his recent lack of appetite. He has taken NSAIDs with no relief. The pain occasionally subsides when he leans forward while sitting up. He smoked two packs of cigarettes per day for 35 years but quit 2 years ago. Examination is significant for scleral icterus and a nontender palpable gallbladder.

1. **What diagnosis is suggested by this presentation and what are the key pieces of evidence?**
   Pancreatic carcinoma is likely. Pain is present in over 70% of cases of pancreatic carcinoma and often radiates to the back. Weight loss is suggestive of underlying neoplasm but may also be

related to depressive symptoms often seen in pancreatic cancer. Scleral icterus indicates obstruction of the biliary ductal system. Courvoisier's sign describes the finding of a nontender palpable gallbladder on abdominal examination and also indicates obstruction of the biliary ductal system. Courvoisier's sign is more commonly seen in obstruction by a neoplasm, whereas scleral icterus results from obstruction by any mechanism.

2. **Where would a pancreatic mass most likely be located in order to cause biliary obstruction?**
Pancreatic head. Two thirds of pancreatic cancers are located in the head of the pancreas, where they can easily obstruct the biliary ductal system. One third of pancreatic cancers occur in the body or tail.

3. **What are important acquired and hereditary risk factors for the development of pancreatic cancer?**
Acquired risk factors include cigarette smoking (note that this patient was a smoker), industrial chemical exposure, type 2 diabetes mellitus, and obesity.
   Hereditary risk factors include a family history of pancreatic cancer (7-8% of pancreatic cancer patients have a first-degree relative with pancreatic cancer, versus 0.6% of control subjects) and a familial form of chronic pancreatitis. The following familial cancer syndromes also confer an increased risk of developing pancreatic cancer:
   - Peutz-Jeghers syndrome
   - Ataxia-telangiectasia
   - Hereditary nonpolyposis colorectal cancer (HNPCC)
   - Familial breast cancer (*BRCA2-positive*)

4. **What is the prognosis with pancreatic adenocarcinoma?**
Prognosis is poor. Tumors located in the body or tail have an even poorer prognosis than those located in the head because they often do not produce signs and symptoms until they have invaded adjacent structures. Surgical resection offers a median survival time of 18 months and a 5-year survival rate of approximately 20%. When tumors are not resectable, median survival time is 4 to 8 months. Only 10% to 15% of all tumors are resectable at presentation.

CASE 10-3 continued:

An abdominal computed tomography (CT) scan reveals a mass at the head of the pancreas. The splenic vein is completely occluded by clot, and there is invasion of the superior mesenteric artery. No metastases are seen. The tumor is deemed unresectable, and he is offered palliative care.

5. **What serum cancer marker is likely to be elevated in this patient?**
CA 19-9. However, CA 19-9 lacks sufficient sensitivity (50-75%) and specificity (approximately 85%) to be used in the screening of asymptomatic individuals. However, it may be followed postoperatively by some physicians in order to assess disease progression or regression.

6. **What are the most common histologic types of pancreatic cancer?**
   - Pancreatic adenocarcinoma: >90%. Neoplastic cells arise from ductal cells of the pancreas. Neoplastic cells will form ductules and may even secrete mucin.
   - Neuroendocrine tumors: <5%. Arising from the neuroendocrine cells of the pancreas, these tumors tend to be less invasive and have a better prognosis.
   - Cystic tumors: <5%. These tumors may be benign or malignant. These tumors are also less aggressive than adenocarcinoma.

7. **What are the most frequent mutations in pancreatic cancer?**

The *KRAS* gene is activated by a point mutation in 80% to 90% of pancreatic cancers. These mutations cause a deactivation of the protein product's guanosine triphosphatase activity. As a result, the protein is constitutively active. *Ras* activates multiple other intracellular signaling pathways.

The p16 gene is the most frequently inactivated tumor suppressor gene, and it is inactivated in 95% of pancreatic cancers. It is important in cell cycle control.

Many other mutations also occur in pancreatic cancers.

CASE 10-3 continued:

The patient returns to the office 1 month later and is noted to have a random glucose of 180 mg/dL. He also complains of pain in his right calf. On examination of his leg, you note a superficial palpable cord that is tender. A fasting glucose drawn 2 days later is 124 mg/dL.

8. **What two processes have developed in this patient?**

Glucose intolerance tends to develop after the diagnosis of pancreatic cancer has been made and is presumably due to destruction of normal pancreatic beta cells and ducts by tumor.

Peripheral venous thrombosis (superficial thrombophlebitis) has developed. Patients with cancer are at an increased risk for clotting and frequently develop both deep and peripheral venous thromboses. When migratory peripheral venous thromboses are noted in a patient with pancreatic cancer, it is called *Trousseau's syndrome* or *Trousseau's sign*. Deep venous thrombosis and pulmonary embolism are the most common thrombotic conditions in patients with cancer.

Note: Of interest, Dr. Armand Trousseau first described the finding of migratory venous thromboses in himself; he was subsequently found to have pancreatic cancer.

SUMMARY BOX: PANCREATIC CANCER

- Pain is frequently present in patients with pancreatic adenocarcinoma and may radiate to the back. Painless jaundice is another important presentation for pancreatic adenocarcinoma.

- Courvoisier's sign refers to a nontender distended gallbladder palpable on examination.

- CA 19-9 levels are typically elevated in pancreatic adenocarcinoma. Although not helpful for screening asymptomatic patients, they may be helpful in diagnosing a patient suspected of having pancreatic cancer. They may also be helpful in following disease progression.

- *KRAS* and p16 are two common genetic mutations found in pancreatic adenocarcinoma.

- Glucose intolerance and Trousseau's syndrome are among the many complications of pancreatic cancer.

CASE 10-4

A 63-year-old man is evaluated for hemoptysis. He has a history of chronic obstructive pulmonary disease (COPD) and has been a smoker for 35 years. He used to smoke as many as three packs per day but has recently been able to decrease this amount to one pack per day. He has always had a dry, hacking cough but says that recently it has become more forceful and that over the last 2 weeks he began to produce small amounts of blood. His vital signs are within normal limits.

1. **What is the most common cause of hemoptysis?**
   Acute bronchitis. Other causes of hemoptysis include lung cancer, pulmonary infections such as tuberculosis, and sarcoidosis. Given this man's smoking history, lung cancer is a concern.

   CASE 10-4 continued:

   Chest x-ray film reveals a right hilar pulmonary nodule and right hilar lymphadenopathy. CT scan reveals a 2.2-cm intraluminal bronchial polypoid mass, multiple enlarged hilar lymph nodes, and no evidence of distant metastases.

2. **Aside from hemoptysis, how else might lung cancer clinically manifest?**
   Change in character of a "smoker's cough," persistent upper respiratory infections or "postobstructive" pneumonias, asymptomatic pulmonary nodule found on routine chest x-ray, hoarseness, signs and symptoms of metastatic disease, or paraneoplastic syndrome might occur.

3. **What percentage of lung cancer occurs in patients who are active smokers or who have stopped recently?**
   Approximately 90%. There is also an association between the frequency of lung cancer and these smoking characteristics:
   - Amount of daily smoking
   - Duration of smoking behavior
   - Tendency to inhale
   However, 10% to 15% of lung cancers occur in patients who don't smoke, and only 10% to 15% of patients with high-risk smoking activity develop lung cancer.

4. **What four histologic types of lung cancer are the most common, accounting for more than 90% of cases of primary lung cancer?**
   Squamous cell carcinoma, adenocarcinoma, small cell carcinoma, and large cell carcinoma. For purposes of staging and treatment, these categories of lung cancer are separated into two broad categories:
   - Small cell lung cancer (SCLC)
   - Non–small cell lung cancer (NSCLC)
   SCLC is considered separately from NSCLC because it has a different natural history and is therefore treated differently. Approximately 80% of new cases a year in North America are NSCLC.
   The remaining 10% of lung cancers that are not accounted for by the four major categories mentioned here are bronchoalveolar carcinoma (this is often considered to be a type of adenocarcinoma and is associated with nondestructive growth of the tumor along the alveolar architecture); adenosquamous carcinoma; carcinoma with pleomorphic, spindle, or sarcomatous elements; carcinoid tumors; and carcinomas of salivary gland type. Malignant mesothelioma is another type of lung cancer that is popularly tested on boards. This malignancy of the pleura occurs 25 to 40 years after exposure to asbestos and is associated with the formation of psammoma bodies (concentric calcium deposits).
   Note: All the above-mentioned types are carcinomas (i.e., of epidermal origin). Other types are more rare (lymphoproliferative disorders, mesothelial tumors, soft tissue tumors, etc.) and will not be discussed.

5. **How do small cell lung cancer and non–small cell lung cancer behave differently?**
   SCLC: Early hematogenous spread is typical. These cancers are rarely resectable or responsive to surgical therapy and are very aggressive with a median untreated survival time of 6 to 18 weeks. Chemotherapy and radiation therapy are commonly administered.
   NSCLC: This form tends to spread more slowly than SCLC and may even be cured if diagnosed in the early stages when local resection may be possible.

6. **Which two types are most strongly associated with cigarette smoking?**
   Squamous cell carcinoma and small cell carcinoma are located centrally within the lung tissue and are strongly associated with smoking; adenocarcinoma and large cell carcinoma are peripherally located.

7. **Describe how the following symptoms or symptom complexes might be produced by local tumor invasion or regional metastases:**
   A. Superior vena cava (SVC) syndrome
      SVC syndrome (neck vein distention and facial swelling) is produced by compression of the superior vena cava by an enlarging tumor. SVC syndrome is generally associated with SCLC and presents with puffiness and purple disocoloration of the face, arms, and shoulder regions. Fatal complications of SVC syndrome include retinal hemorrhage and stroke. Treatment for SVC syndrome includes radiation therapy and stents to bypass sites of obstruction.
   B. Horner syndrome
      Horner syndrome (ptosis, miosis, anhydrosis) can be caused by invasion of the cervical sympathetic nerves and ganglia. This is most often associated with squamous cell carcinoma (in which the finding will be ipsilateral) and is referred to as Pancoast tumor.
   C. Diaphragmatic paralysis
      Tumor invasion of the phrenic nerve can cause diaphragmatic paralysis.
   D. Hoarseness
      Tumor invasion of the recurrent laryngeal nerve on the left can cause hoarseness.
   E. Tamponade, congestive heart failure (CHF)
      Malignant pericardial effusion can produce these effects.

CASE 10-4 continued:

Sputum cytologic examination confirms squamous cell carcinoma (Fig. 10-6). A polypoid lesion is surgically resected, and the patient receives adjuvant chemotherapy. The patient dies of complications of metastatic disease 6 months later.

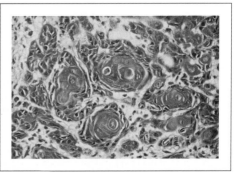

Figure 10-6. Squamous cell carcinoma. The many well-differentiated foci of eosinophilic-staining neoplastic cells produce keratin in layers (keratin pearls). (From Forbes C, Jackson W: Color Atlas and Text of Clinical Medicine, 3rd ed. St. Louis, Mosby, 2003, p 211, Fig. 4-184.)

Note: Squamous cell carcinoma can always be differentiated from other types of cancer by the presence of keratin pearls. Oat cell carcinoma is also easy to recognize from the presence of small, blue neuroendocrine cells (Fig. 10-7).

STEP 1 SECRET

USMLE test makers commonly include gross and histologic images of lung tumors on the examination.

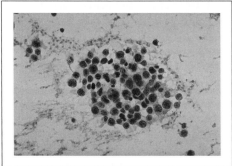

Figure 10-7. Small cell carcinoma, oat cell type. The characteristic features of oat cell carcinoma, including nuclear molding, hyperchromatic granular chromatin, and high nucleocytoplasmic ratios, are seen. Bronchial brushing (Papanicolaou). (From Bibbo M, Wilbur D: Comprehensive Cytopathology, 3rd ed. Philadelphia, Saunders, 2009.)

8. **To which distant sites does lung cancer commonly metastasize?**
   Lung cancer can metastasize almost anywhere, but there are four common sites where metastases are often found: brain, bone, liver, adrenal glands.

SUMMARY BOX: LUNG CANCER

- Acute bronchitis is the most common cause of hemoptysis. However, hemoptysis is also concerning for lung cancer and tuberculosis.

- The most common presentations of lung cancer are:

  □ Asymptomatic pulmonary nodule

  □ Change in "smoker's cough"

  □ Nonpurulent "pneumonia" in an adult

  □ Persistent upper respiratory infection

  □ Hemoptysis

  □ Hoarseness

  □ Signs and symptoms of metastatic disease

  □ Signs and symptoms of paraneoplastic syndrome

- Approximately 90% of lung cancers occur in smokers.

- The four most common histologic types of primary lung cancer are squamous cell carcinoma, adenocarcinoma, large cell carcinoma, and small cell carcinoma.

- Small cell lung cancer (SCLC) and non–small cell lung cancer (NSCLC) behave very differently and have markedly different prognoses.

- Lung cancer can produce symptoms by local tumor growth, regional spread, or metastatic disease.

CASE 10-5

A 50-year-old African-American man goes to his primary care provider (PCP) for his annual physical examination. Two years ago he was diagnosed with hypertension, and he is currently taking hydrochlorothiazide. Review of systems is unrevealing. On rectal examination, the patient's prostate is noted to be firm, without lesions or asymmetry, and appropriately sized for a 50-year-old man. The patient's prostate-specific antigen (PSA) returns at 5.4 ng/mL (normal <4.0 ng/mL).

1. **How is the anatomy of the prostate defined clinically (i.e., on digital rectal examination)?**
   On digital rectal examination, two lateral lobes separated by a central sulcus can be palpated. These lobes are felt for nodules and asymmetry. They make up the posterior portion of the posterior surface of the prostate gland, which is the only area accessible to digital rectal examination.

2. **Describe the zonal anatomy of the prostate and how the various zones relate to the development of prostatic cancer and benign prostatic hypertrophy**
   Transition zone accounts for only 5% to 10% of prostatic glandular tissue and surrounds the urethra. Approximately 20% of prostate cancers arise in the transition zone. This zone commonly gives rise to benign prostatic hypertrophy. This is why benign prostatic hyperplasia (BPH) commonly manifests with urinary symptoms: the zone of the prostate that is enlarging impinges on the prostatic urethra.
   Central zone accounts for 25% of prostatic glandular tissue, lies posterior to the transition zone, and extends up to the base of the bladder. Only 1% to 5% of prostate cancers arise in this zone.
   Peripheral zone makes up 70% of the prostatic glandular tissue and covers the posterior and lateral aspects of the prostate. This is the zone palpable on digital rectal examination. Up to 70% of prostatic cancer arises in this zone. It is also the area most commonly affected by chronic prostatitis (Fig. 10-8).

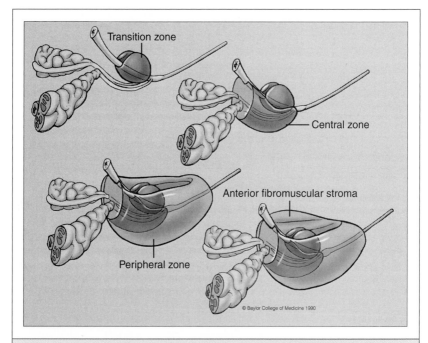

Figure 10-8. Zones of the prostate. (From Green DR, Shabsign R, Scardino PT: Urological ultrasonography. In Walsh PC, Rettic AB, Stamey CA, Vaughan ED Jr [eds]: Campbell's Textbook of Urology, 6th ed. Philadelphia, WB Saunders, 1992.)

3. **What is prostate-specific antigen and what does it indicate?**

   PSA is produced in the cytoplasm of both benign and malignant cells of the prostate. It therefore correlates with the volume of prostatic tissue in a patient and is not specific for prostate cancer. PSA values increase normally with age, so men 40 to 49 years of age normally have values <2.5 ng/mL, whereas men 70 to 79 years old can have PSA values as high as 6.5 ng/mL and still be considered normal (due to age-related benign enlargement of the prostate). Nonetheless, a PSA value of >4.0 ng/mL is generally considered abnormal.

   The degree of PSA elevation is important. Only 18% to 30% of men with an intermediate elevation in PSA (4.1-10.0 ng/mL) will be found to have prostatic cancer. However, 50% to 70% of men with a PSA of >10.0 ng/mL will be found to have prostatic cancer.

4. **What does an abnormal prostate-specific antigen level mean?**

   Because PSA indicates volume of prostatic tissue, it can be elevated in prostatic cancer (because of an increased volume of malignant prostatic cells) or benign prostatic hypertrophy (because of an increased volume of benign prostatic cells). It can also be elevated in cases of prostatitis.

   Note: Minor elevations in PSA values (4.1-10.0 ng/mL) can be associated with both BPH and prostate cancer. Always examine the values of free PSA. BPH is associated with elevations in free PSA values, but prostate cancer is not.

5. **What is a 50-year-old man's lifetime risk of developing prostate cancer and of dying from prostate cancer?**

   A 50-year-old man has a 40% chance of developing prostate cancer. However, he has only a 10% chance of developing clinical disease. This is because prostate cancer is most commonly asymptomatic. Furthermore, he has only a 3% risk of dying from prostate cancer. Of the large number of men who develop prostate cancer (including asymptomatic forms), about 1 in 13 will die from it. Because such a small percentage of men with prostate cancer die from prostate cancer, the use of PSA as a screening tool remains controversial.

   CASE 10-5 continued:

   The patient is referred to a urologist, who performs a transrectal ultrasound–guided biopsy. A hyperechoic area in the peripheral zone of the prostate is visualized and biopsied.

6. **What is the most commonly found histologic type of cancer?**

   Adenocarcinomas arising from the glandular acini make up the large majority of prostate cancers. However, the regions seen on biopsy are often heterogeneous (i.e., multiple patterns with varying degrees of differentiation can be seen). The Gleason grading system was developed to account for multiple patterns within a single biopsy. A score of 1 (most differentiated) to 5 (no glandular differentiation) is applied to the dominant histologic pattern. A second score of 1 through 5 is applied to the second most abundant histologic pattern. Adding the two scores together gives the Gleason grade (2-10). This is the best marker, along with TNM staging, for predicting prognosis.

7. **Why might a patient with prostate cancer present with urinary obstruction? with hematospermia?**

   Advanced local disease often presents with urinary obstruction as the tumor mass encroaches on the prostatic urethra. If the tumor invades the seminal vesicles, it can cause hematospermia or decrease in ejaculate volume.

8. **Where are the most common sites of metastasis? Which signs and symptoms might indicate metastases in this patient?**

   Bone and pelvic lymph nodes are the most common sites of metastases.

When affecting bone, prostate cancer most often metastasizes to axial skeleton including vertebral bodies. As a result, patients with advanced disease may present with lower back or pelvic pain. Osteoblastic metastases are virtually diagnostic for prostate cancer.

When affecting pelvic lymph nodes, metastases can cause unilateral lymphedema.

SUMMARY BOX: PROSTATE CANCER

- 70% of prostatic tissue is in the peripheral zone.

- 70% of prostate cancer cases arise in the peripheral zone.

- The peripheral zone is the only area accessible via digital rectal examination.

- Most cases of prostate cancer are asymptomatic and detected by abnormal findings on digital rectal examination or elevated prostate-specific antigen (PSA).

- PSA can be elevated in prostate cancer, benign prostatic hyperplasia (BPH), or prostatitis.

- Only a small number of men who develop prostate cancer will die as a result of it.

- Screening with annual PSA levels may allow detection of prostate cancer at earlier stages.

- Prognosis of prostate cancer is determined by Gleason grade (2-10) and tumor staging (TNM system).

- Prostate cancer spreads by local extension and metastases to bone (especially axial skeleton) and pelvic lymph nodes.

CASE 10-6

A 35-year-old woman presents to the emergency room complaining of postcoital bleeding. She has not had health care insurance for the last 5 years and does not have a gynecologist. Her history reveals that she has been sexually active since the age of 21 and has had two sexual partners. She has never been pregnant. She had a *Chlamydia* infection at age 29 that resolved with antibiotics. She does not smoke or take oral contraceptives. She has no family history of gynecologic cancer. Her vital signs are normal. Upon speculum examination a fungating lesion is visualized near the external os of the cervix in the 3 o'clock position.

1. What is the differential diagnosis for this lesion?
   - Carcinoma of the cervix: The most common presenting symptom for cervical cancer is irregular vaginal bleeding, particularly postcoital bleeding.
   - Endocervical polyp: These inflammatory polyps usually occur in the endocervical canal and may extrude from the external os and become visible. They occur in 2% to 5% of adult women and can also present with irregular vaginal bleeding.

2. What is the transformation zone of the cervix and how is it relevant to the development of cervical cancer?
   The surface of the cervix is composed of squamous epithelium and the endocervical canal is composed of columnar epithelium. The interface of these two types of epithelium is called the squamocolumnar junction and exists on the surface of the cervix until menarche (i.e., columnar cells extend out onto the surface of the cervix). With age, columnar cells on the surface of the cervix begin to change into squamous cells in a metaplastic process. The result is that the

squamocolumnar junction appears to migrate toward the endocervical canal, producing a new squamocolumnar junction. As this process is occurring, the site of the original squamocolumnar junction remains visible. The area between the original squamocolumnar junction and new squamocolumnar junction is known as the transformation zone and the cells within this zone are most susceptible to neoplastic changes. For this reason, squamous cell carcinoma of the cervix is most typically found in the transformation zone and this is the area that Papanicolaou (Pap) smears attempt to screen (Fig. 10-9).

3. **Why is it important that this patient has not seen her gynecologist in 5 years?**
Since the advent of the Pap smear, incidence of invasive cervical cancer and related mortality risk has fallen by approximately 70%. Owing to the proved efficacy of this screening method, women begin testing with Pap smears within 3 years of the onset of sexual activity or the age of 21. Had this patient been seen regularly by a gynecologist, it is likely that she would have had an abnormal Pap smear prior to developing cervical cancer (the time from development of carcinoma in situ to penetration of the basement membrane is 2-10 years).

4. **Why is a sexual history particularly important in this patient?**
Cervical cancer is a sexually transmitted disease. Nearly 90% of squamous cell carcinomas have identifiable associated human papillomavirus (HPV) type, and HPV has been shown to be transmitted sexually. HPV is very common and can be found in more than 50% of women who are sexually active between the ages of 16 and 21. However, only some of these women develop abnormal Pap smears.

    Other risk factors for cervical cancer include multiple partners, having sex from an early age, smoking, STDs, and immunosuppression.

5. **Which types of human papillomavirus are considered high risk for the development of cervical cancer?**
HPV-16 is associated with 46% to 63% of cervical squamous cell carcinoma and HPV-18 is associated with 10% to 14%. Thus, HPV-16 and HPV-18 are classified as high-risk types of HPV. Many other subtypes are associated with the remaining lesions (HPV-45, -31, -33). The recent HPV vaccine protects against HPV-16 and -18 as well as types -6 and -11, which cause genital warts.

6. **Which viral oncogenes are responsible for causing cervical cancer?**
E6 and E7 (both HPV-associated oncogenes). E6 binds to and inhibits p53 function, while E7 binds to Rb. This induces cervical intraepithelial neoplasia (CIN), which progresses over time.

CASE 10-6 continued:

The patient returns 1 week later for colposcopy (visual examination of the vaginal and cervical mucosa using a lighted colposcope) and biopsy of the lesion. Pathologic examination shows squamous cell carcinoma.

7. **What are the most common histologic types found in cervical cancer?**
- Squamous cell carcinoma: 75%
- Adenocarcinoma: 15% to 25%
- Adenosquamous carcinoma: <10%

    Recall that if you are given an image of squamous cell carcinoma of the cervix, you will be able to spot keratin pearls!

8. **Why are Pap smears effective in preventing the development of cervical cancer?**
A Pap smear is obtained by direct scraping of the cells in the transformation zone. If abnormal cells are seen, then the patient returns for colposcopy and biopsy to determine whether or not she

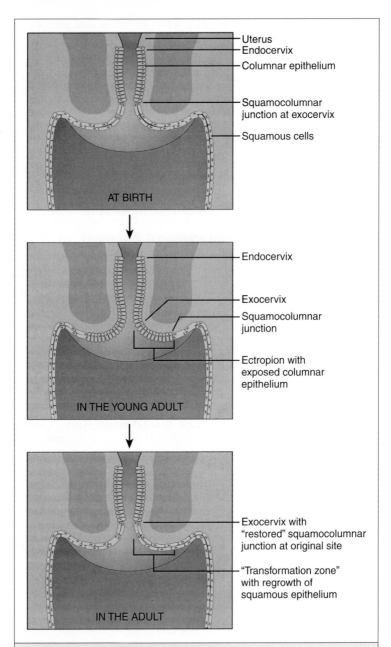

Figure 10-9. Schematic of the development of the cervical transformation zone. (From Kumar V, Abbas AK, Fausto N: Robbins and Cotran Pathologic Basis of Disease, 7th ed. Philadelphia, WB Saunders, 2005.)

has CIN. Even if she does have CIN, there are methods of treatment (excisional cone biopsy, loop electrosurgical excision procedure) that can excise the lesion and prevent the development of invasive cervical carcinoma.

The abnormal cells that we look for to detect cervical dysplasia are called koilocytes. Koilocytes are squamous epithelial cells that have undergone transformation secondary to papillomavirus infection. You should know how to recognize these cells for boards. They typically present with large, hyperchromatic nuclei with perinuclear halos (Fig. 10-10).

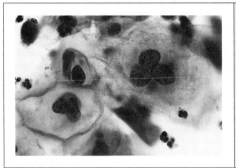

Figure 10-10. The cytologic appearance of cervical intraepithelial neoplasia as seen on the Papanicolaou smear. Normal cytoplasmic staining in superficial cells may be either red or blue. Image shows low-grade squamous intraepithelial lesion—koilocytes. (From Kumar V, Abbas AK, Fausto N, Aster J: Robbins and Cotran Pathologic Basis of Disease, 8th ed. Philadelphia, Saunders, 2010. Courtesy of Dr. Edmund S. Cibas, Brigham and Women's Hospital, Boston, MA.)

9. **Which symptoms are typically seen in a patient with cervical dysplasia or cervical carcinoma?**
    Many patients are asymptomatic, but some will present with vaginal bleeding (often postcoital), malodorous discharge, or dyspareunia.

SUMMARY BOX: CERVICAL CANCER

■ Invasive cervical carcinoma typically manifests with abnormal vaginal bleeding or postcoital spotting.

■ Invasive cervical carcinoma most often occurs in the transformation zone of the cervix, between the original squamocolumnar junction and the new squamocolumnar junction.

■ Cervical carcinoma is a sexually transmitted disease, the etiologic agent of which is human papillomavirus (HPV) (most frequently types 16 and 18); therefore, risk factors are primarily related to sexual behaviors.

■ Squamous cell carcinoma is the most frequent histologic type, occurring in 75% of cases.

■ The Papanicolaou (Pap) smear has markedly reduced the incidence of invasive cervical cancer in America as a result of its ability to screen for preinvasive lesions.

CASE 10-7

A 64-year-old man presents to the emergency room with vision changes and a fixed and dilated right pupil on examination. He was diagnosed with right-sided temporal glioblastoma multiforme 3 months ago following workup for persistent right-sided headaches.

1. **What are the three most common types of primary brain neoplasms in adults and what are their respective cells of origin?**
    - Meningioma: 27%
    - Glioblastoma: 21%
    - Other astrocytomas: 11%

    Meningiomas arise from arachnoidal cells in the meninges (arachnoidal fibroblasts). They do not arise from brain parenchyma. They are benign in 90% of cases and usually operable. However, malignant meningiomas can invade adjacent brain tissue.

    Glioblastomas arise from astrocytes, the supporting cells of the central nervous system (CNS). Tumor cells invade surrounding parenchyma and often have areas of necrosis.

    "Other" astrocytomas also arise from astrocytes. This category makes up grades I to III in the World Health Organization (WHO) system for grading astrocytomas (see following question).

2. **The World Health Organization system for grading astrocytomas is important for understanding the histologic patterns of this common brain tumor. How does glioblastoma multiforme fit into this grading system?**

    WHO grade I: Pilocytic tumors. Most are benign and are cured surgically. They are more common in children than adults.

    WHO grade II: Diffuse astrocytomas. In these tumors, invading cells can be found in the brain parenchyma in areas distant from the expanding mass, and gray/white matter boundaries may be eliminated. Other features include low cellularity, low nuclear pleomorphism, no endothelial proliferation, and no necrosis.

    WHO grade III: Anaplastic astrocytomas. These tumors are similar to grade II tumors except that there is much greater mitotic activity histologically. There is increased cellularity, nuclear pleomorphism, and mitotic activity.

    WHO grade IV: Glioblastoma multiforme. These tumors are distinguished from anaplastic astrocytomas by the presence of endothelial proliferation or necrosis. Gross specimens show discoloration and cystic changes that result from hemorrhage and necrosis.

3. **What does the histologic pattern of "pseudopalisading" represent?**

    In glioblastoma multiforme (Fig. 10-11), tumor cells can be seen to crowd around areas of necrosis, forming the appearance of palisades of cells rimming acellular/necrotic areas.

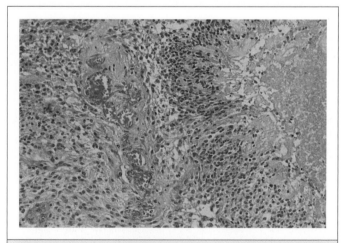

Figure 10-11. Glioblastoma with small, anaplastic tumor cells, vascular proliferation, and areas of necrosis with pseudopalisading of tumor cells. (From Goetz CG: Textbook of Clinical Neurology, 2nd ed. Philadelphia, WB Saunders, 2003.)

4. **Different histologic stains can be used to highlight different types of central nervous system cells. What is the protein expressed in the cytoplasm of astrocytes that pathologists direct antibodies against in order to visualize cells of astrocytic origin?**
Glial fibrillary acidic protein (GFAP) is expressed.

5. **In the patient in Case 10-7, compression of which cranial nerve is leading to his right-sided fixed and dilated pupil?**
Cranial nerve III (oculomotor nerve) has a somatic component and an autonomic component.
Somatic: Supplies four of the six extraocular muscles (superior rectus, inferior rectus, medial rectus, inferior oblique) and the levator palpebrae muscle
Autonomic: Parasympathetic innervation of the constrictor pupillae and ciliary muscles
Compression of cranial nerve III typically involves the autonomic as well as the somatic limb. Removal of parasympathetic tone causes fixed dilation of the pupil unresponsive to light or accommodation.

CASE 10-7 continued:

The patient's mental status begins to deteriorate. A limited neurologic examination reveals a right-sided homonymous hemianopia. Soon after the examination is completed, the patient becomes obtunded.

6. **What process is evolving in this patient?**
Uncal herniation. Space-occupying lesions lead to edema of the surrounding tissue and increased pressure in a particular cranial compartment. As this progresses, brain tissue may herniate into a compartment with lower pressure. Uncal herniation occurs when the hippocampal gyrus herniates through the tentorial notch. This may lead to compression of cranial nerve III and other effects (Fig. 10-12).

7. **What part of the herniation syndrome is responsible for the contralateral homonymous hemianopia?**
Compression of the posterior cerebral artery supplying the occipital lobe.

SUMMARY BOX: BRAIN CANCERS

- Meningiomas are the most common type of primary brain tumor, occurring in 27% of cases.

- Astrocytomas arise from astrocytes and are divided into four grades based on histologic appearance. Of these grades, glioblastoma multiforme has the worst prognosis.

- Glioblastoma multiforme is distinctive because of endothelial proliferation and necrosis.

- "Pseudopalisading" is often seen in glioblastoma multiforme.

- Uncal herniation syndrome results from hippocampal gyrus herniation through the tentorial notch. Herniation produces pressure on the posterior cerebral artery and brain stem.

- Herniation is caused by an increase in pressure in one intracranial compartment. This pressure increase is due not only to the presence of a space-occupying lesion but also to significant edema in the parenchyma surrounding the lesion.

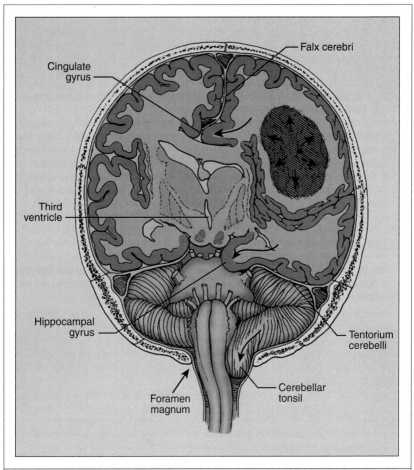

Figure 10-12. Intracranial herniation syndromes evoked by supratentorial masses. (From Abeloff MD, Armitage JO, Niederhuber JE, et al: Clinical Oncology, 3rd ed. Philadelphia, Churchill Livingstone, 2004.)

CASE 10-8

A 24-year-old man is evaluated for a small "lump" in his neck. He feels well but is concerned because his father, who died from a stroke at age 39 for unclear reasons, required neck surgery in the past. Examination reveals a 1-cm nodule in the right upper lobe of the thyroid. Laboratory workup reveals normal thyroid-stimulating hormone (TSH), moderately elevated calcium, and moderately reduced phosphate. Fine needle aspiration of the nodule reveals cells suggestive of medullary thyroid carcinoma.

1. **What is the cell of origin in the development of medullary thyroid carcinoma?**
   The parafollicular cells or C cells. This is a neuroendocrine tumor that elaborates calcitonin. As a result, measurement of calcitonin can be used in the diagnosis of this tumor and in postoperative follow-up if it is resected.

2. **What are the major histologic categories of thyroid cancer?**
   - Papillary carcinoma: 75% to 85%
   - Follicular carcinoma: 10% to 20%
   - Medullary carcinoma: 5%
   - Anaplastic carcinoma: <5%

   Papillary and follicular carcinomas develop from the follicular cells of the thyroid. Anaplastic carcinomas are very aggressive undifferentiated tumors of the follicular epithelium, with a mortality rate approaching 100%.

3. **What test should be ordered to evaluate the hypercalcemia and hypophosphatemia?**
   Parathyroid hormone (PTH) level should be tested. PTH levels are often included in the workup of hypercalcemia and are especially important in the context of a concurrent hypophosphatemia. Some cancers may even elaborate PTH-related peptide (PTHrP), causing bone resorption. This is considered to be one of the paraneoplastic syndromes and is known as humoral hypercalcemia of malignancy. PTH levels are suppressed when PTHrP is causing hypercalcemia.

   CASE 10-8 continued:

   A serum PTH level is elevated at a follow-up visit 2 weeks later. He is still asymptomatic, and his examination findings are unchanged.

4. **What unifying diagnosis could explain his medullary thyroid carcinoma and primary hyperparathyroidism?**
   Multiple endocrine neoplasia type IIA (MEN IIA).
   Medullary thyroid carcinoma is the most common manifestation of MEN IIA. Hyperparathyroidism also occurs in 15% to 20% of patients.

5. **What other neoplastic process accompanies medullary thyroid carcinoma and hyperparathyroidism in multiple endocrine neoplasia type IIA?**
   Pheochromocytoma is present in approximately 50% of patients with MEN IIA. Elaboration of epinephrine and norepinephrine causes hypertension with palpitations, nervousness, headaches, and flushing. These symptoms usually occur in episodes, and blood pressure can get high enough to cause hypertensive emergencies (such as hemorrhagic stroke).

6. **How are the multiple endocrine neoplasia syndromes inherited? What is the mutation in multiple endocrine neoplasia (MEN) type IIA?**
   Both MEN I and MEN II syndromes are inherited in an autosomal dominant manner. Both MEN IIA and MEN IIB can be caused by mutations of the *RET* proto-oncogene that encodes a tyrosine kinase receptor. MEN I is caused by mutations in a tumor suppressor gene (encoding the menin protein); as a result, only one mutation is inherited, and the "second hit" occurs later in life.
   Because MEN IIA is inherited in an autosomal dominant manner, it is likely that his father also had MEN IIA and died of a stroke resulting from a hypertensive crisis.

7. **Which disorders are typically present in multiple endocrine neoplasia type IIB?**
   - Medullary thyroid carcinoma
   - Pheochromocytoma
   - Ganglioneuromatosis (patients typically present with marfanoid habitus)

8. **Which disorders are typically present in multiple endocrine neoplasia type I?**
   - Hyperparathyroidism
   - Pancreatic islet cell neoplasia

- Gastrin production: Zollinger-Ellison syndrome
- Insulin production: insulinoma
- Glucagon production: glucagonoma
- Vasoactive intestinal peptide (VIP) production: Verner-Morrison syndrome or watery diarrhea syndrome (watery diarrhea, hypokalemia, hypochlorhydria, metabolic acidosis, all thought to be due to the overproduction of VIP)
- Pituitary tumors
  - Prolactinoma: most common
  - Growth hormone: acromegaly
  - Adrenocorticotropic hormone (ACTH): Cushing disease
  - Carcinoid tumors: a late, less frequent manifestation of MEN I

STEP 1 SECRET

You should expect to have at least one question on multiple endocrine neoplasia (MEN) syndromes on your examination. Know each component of the triads that are associated with MEN I, MEN IIA, and MEN IIB.

SUMMARY BOX: THYROID CANCER

- Medullary thyroid cancers may occur as an isolated thyroid cancer or may be part of multiple endocrine neoplasia type IIA (MEN IIA).

- Medullary thyroid cancers arise from C cells, which secrete calcitonin.

- Other types of thyroid cancer arise from follicular cells.

- The typical triad of MEN IIA is medullary thyroid carcinoma, pheochromocytoma, and primary hyperparathyroidism.

- The typical triad of MEN IIB is medullary thyroid carcinoma, pheochromocytoma, and ganglioneuromatosis.

- The typical triad of MEN I is hyperparathyroidism, pancreatic islet cell tumor, and pituitary tumor.

- Both MEN I and MEN II are inherited in an autosomal dominant fashion.

CASE 10-9

A 50-year-old man presents to his PCP for his annual physical. He tells his physician that he is feeling well and has no complaints except that he has had intermittent constipation over the last few months. Sometimes he notices small amounts of streaked blood in his stool. His vital signs and physical examination are completely normal. On rectal examination, there are no masses. His fecal occult blood test is positive. He has no family history of colon cancer or inflammatory bowel disease and has not been diagnosed with diverticulitis in the past. The patient is scheduled for a screening colonoscopy (his first), as his doctor recommends that all of his patients get a colonoscopy once they reach 50 years of age. The colonoscopy reveals a circumferential mass in the descending colon. Biopsies are taken.

1. **What is the predominant histologic type found in colon cancers?**
   - Adenocarcinoma accounts for approximately 98% of tumors in the large intestine.
   - Carcinoid tumors comprise approximately 2% large intestine tumors but almost 50% of small intestine malignant tumors.
   - Gastrointestinal lymphoma and mesenchymal tumors (gastrointestinal stromal tumors) are also found.

2. **In what part of the colon are most colon cancers found?**
   - Rectosigmoid colon: 55%
   - Cecum/ascending colon: 22%
   - Transverse colon: 11%
   - Descending colon: 6%
   - Other sites: 6%
     Ninety-nine percent of colon cancers appear at one site (i.e., no synchronous tumor).There has been a gradual increase in the percentage of tumors that appear proximal to the splenic flexure.

3. **What is the precursor lesion to adenocarcinoma of the colon?**
   Adenoma.

4. **What are the different types of adenomas and their morphologic features?**
   See Table 10-2.

TABLE 10-2.   ADENOMAS AND THEIR MORPHOLOGIC FEATURES

Adenoma	Morphology
Tubular adenomas	Small and pedunculated
>75% tubular architecture	Make up 90% of adenomas found in the colon
Villous adenomas	Large and sessile
>50% villous architecture	Make up 1% of adenomas found in the colon
Tubulovillous adenomas	Varying morphology
25-50% villous architecture	Make up 5-10% of adenomas found in the colon

5. **What type of adenoma has the highest risk of turning into cancer?**
   Cancer risk is highest with villous adenomas greater than 4 cm in diameter (approaching 40%). Cancer risk is much lower with tubular adenomas less than 1 cm in diameter.

6. **Which genes are typically altered in the development of colorectal adenocarcinoma?**
   There may be as many as nine genes altered for adenocarcinoma to develop but the first step is thought to be mutation of the *APC* gene on chromosome 5q. Because *APC* is a tumor-suppressor gene, a mutation must occur in both alleles in order to inactivate it. The second mutation is the so-called "second hit." After the second hit on *APC*, the sequence progresses with an activating mutation of the proto-oncogene *KRAS*. Because *KRAS* is a proto-oncogene, only one allele need be activated for tumor progression (i.e., only one mutation need occur). The final step appears to involve loss of function in the p53 tumor suppressor gene (Fig. 10-13).

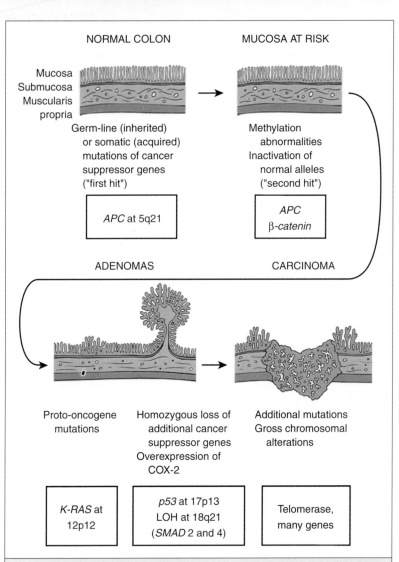

Figure 10-13. Schematic of the morphologic and molecular changes in the adenoma-carcinoma sequence. COX-2, cyclooxygenase-2; LOH, loss of heterozygosity. (From Kumar V, Abbas AK, Fausto N: Robbins and Cotran Pathologic Basis of Disease, 7th ed. Philadelphia, WB Saunders, 2005.)

STEP 1 SECRET

Genetic mutations involved in cancer are not often tested on boards, although you may randomly get one question on this. You should determine how much time you would like to dedicate to this topic depending on the limitations of your own study schedule. At the minimum, you may want to know which genes are oncogenes and which are tumor suppressor genes. We would also suggest that you briefly look at which tumors are associated with which genes. Test makers will occasionally throw in a difficult question regarding the product of an individual gene, but this is not common. It is unimportant to know the chromosomes on which these genes are located, so do not dwell on this topic.

7. **What is the importance of the p53 gene in human malignancy?**
It is the most commonly inactivated tumor suppressor gene in human malignancies. Normally p53 helps to recognize damaged DNA and acts to block cell cycle progression so as to allow DNA repair. It also functions in triggering apoptosis.

8. **Without taking into account familial cancer syndromes, what is the importance of family history in the development of colorectal cancer?**
A patient who has a first-degree family member who was diagnosed with colon cancer before 45 years of age has a relative risk 3.8 times that of the general population. This relative risk decreases to 2.2 if the family member was diagnosed at 45 to 59 years of age and 1.8 if the family member was diagnosed after 60 years of age.

9. **What is the association of colon cancer with familial cancer syndromes? with inflammatory bowel disease?**
Hereditary nonpolyposis colon cancer (HNPCC): Mutations in DNA mismatch repair genes (specifically microsatellite nucleotide sequences) lead to an 80% lifetime risk of developing colon cancer. These tumors are predominantly right-sided. These patients are also at an increased risk of tumors of endometrial origin (ovarian, stomach, small bowel cancers).
Familial adenomatous polyposis (FAP): Germ-line mutation of *APC* tumor suppressor leads to thousands of adenomatous polyps at a young age (i.e., the first hit is inherited). This confers a 100% lifetime risk of developing colon cancer, and there is an increased risk of thyroid, stomach, and small intestinal cancers.
Inflammatory bowel disease: Though the link has been more firmly established between ulcerative colitis and colon cancer, it is now evident that both ulcerative colitis and Crohn's disease confer an increased risk of colon cancer when compared to the general population. This risk begins to rise 7 to 10 years after disease onset and increases with duration of disease. Cancers tend to occur at a younger age than in the general population. There also has been an observed increased risk in small intestinal adenocarcinomas in patients with Crohn's disease.

CASE 10-9 continued:

Biopsies reveal adenocarcinoma. As part of a surgical workup, a CT scan of chest, abdomen, and pelvis is performed and reveals metastases to the liver.

10. **Why are colon cancers thought to metastasize to the liver? What are other common sites of metastasis?**
Venous drainage of the colon and upper rectum is through the portal vein. Therefore, metastases are often found in the liver of patients with colon cancer. Lymph nodes, lung, and peritoneal metastases are also seen.

SUMMARY BOX: COLON CANCER

- Adenocarcinomas make up 98% of primary colon cancers.

- The precursor lesion to adenocarcinoma is the colonic adenoma, of which the villous type is the most carcinogenic and has the lowest incidence.

- About half of primary colon cancers occur distal to the splenic flexure, though this pattern has been changing in recent years.

- The genetics of colon cancer progression are some of the best-studied in oncology. The tumor suppressor gene *APC* has to sustain two hits before the sequence can continue. The next step is usually a mutation of the proto-oncogene *KRAS*. The final step is inactivation of the ubiquitous p53 tumor suppressor gene.

- Familial adenomatous polyposis (FAP) and hereditary nonpolyposis colorectal cancer (HNPCC) confer 100% and 80% lifetime risk of developing colon cancer, respectively.

- Inflammatory bowel disease confers a higher risk of developing colon cancer than that in the general population and is directly related to duration of disease.

- Metastases to the liver often occur and can be attributed to venous drainage of the colon.

CASE 10-10

A 47-year-old man presents to his oncologist with persistent headaches for the past month. Six months prior, he had been treated with cisplatin and etoposide for limited-stage SCLC. He was told that his cancer had gone into remission and was asymptomatic until 1 month ago when he began developing headaches. His wife, who has accompanied him, says that he seems more confused lately. His vital signs are normal. On examination, he has no focal neurologic findings but does have trouble following some directions and seems confused.

1. **What is the most potentially serious explanation for this patient's headaches?**
Metastatic disease to the brain. The patient's cancer initially had been classified as limited-stage SCLC, yet it is assumed that micrometastases are present whenever SCLC is diagnosed. Although chemotherapy is quite successful in limited-stage disease (50-70% complete response), remissions tend to last only 6 to 8 months. When cancer recurs, the median survival time is 3 to 4 months.

2. **Which cancers commonly metastasize to brain?**
   - Lung cancer
   - Breast cancer
   - Melanoma
   - Renal cell carcinoma
   Approximately 50% of brain tumors are metastases.

CASE 10-10 continued:

The CT scan shows no brain metastases. The patient's laboratory tests reveal a serum Na 124 mmol/L and a urine Na 40 mEq/L. The patient is admitted to the hospital and is noted to have a blood pressure of 124/75 mm Hg that does not change significantly when taken lying down versus standing up. He has no edema. He says he drinks one to two glasses of water per day and stopped drinking alcohol 6 months ago when he was diagnosed with lung cancer.

3. **What basic electrolyte disturbance does this patient have?**
Hyponatremia.

4. **What is the likely cause of this patient's electrolyte disturbance?**
The patient has a euvolemic hyponatremia based on his lack of orthostatic hypotension. In the context of euvolemia, the kidneys' ability to excrete free water must be evaluated. The fact that this patient has a high urine sodium indicates that he is reabsorbing free water in the face of excess intravascular free water. This could easily be accounted for by inappropriately elevated levels of antidiuretic hormone (ADH) or syndrome of inappropriate secretion of antidiuretic hormone (SIADH). This is commonly seen in SCLC and is the likely cause of his hyponatremia.

5. **What are the causes of syndrome of inappropriate secretion of antidiuretic hormone?**
ADH secretion is normally regulated by baroreceptors and neural input at two sites: in the CNS and the chest. Therefore, SIADH may occur with CNS lesions (e.g., head trauma, stroke, subarachnoid hemorrhage, hydrocephalus) or with lung lesions (tuberculosis, bacterial pneumonia, aspergillosis, etc.). It is also seen in many malignancies as a paraneoplastic syndrome and may be the result of drug effects.

6. **What does the term "paraneoplastic syndrome" refer to?**
A paraneoplastic syndrome is a constellation of symptoms attributable to the secretion of peptides or antibodies by a neoplasm. In the setting of SCLC, the tumor may secrete ectopic ADH (a peptide), leading to SIADH, or may secrete autoantibodies to neural tissue, leading to Lambert-Eaton syndrome, which is characterized by proximal muscle weakness. The pathophysiology of paraneoplastic syndromes is incompletely understood.

7. **How could a paraneoplastic syndrome cause the following signs and symptoms, and which tumors are commonly associated with each?**
   A. Cushing syndrome
      Ectopic secretion of ACTH or ACTH-like peptide: small cell lung carcinoma (SCLC)
   B. SIADH
      Ectopic secretion of ADH: SCLC, intracranial neoplasms
   C. Polycythemia
      Ectopic erythropoietin: renal cell carcinoma, hemangioblastoma
   D. Lambert-Eaton syndrome
      Autoantibodies to presynaptic Ca^{2+} channels at neuromuscular junction: thymoma, SCLC
   E. Carcinoid syndrome (diarrhea, cutaneous flushing, asthmatic wheezing, right-sided valvular disease)
      Ectopic serotonin (5-HT) and bradykinin: carcinoid tumors most commonly found in the appendix
   F. Zollinger-Ellison syndrome
      Ectopic gastrin: found in pancreatic, duodenal tumors

STEP 1 SECRET

Paraneoplastic syndromes, especially those associated with various types of lung cancers, are among the highest-yield oncology topics for boards.

8. **What paraneoplastic syndromes are particularly important in lung cancer?**
From 10% to 30% of patients with SCLC will develop SIADH, and 10% of patients with squamous cell carcinoma (NSCLC) will develop hypercalcemia.

9. **If this patient were found to have hypercalcemia, what two causes could be attributed to the cancer?**
Most cases of hypercalcemia in cancer can be attributed to bone metastases leading to osteolysis. However, approximately 20% of cases are attributed to humoral hypercalcemia of malignancy (paraneoplastic PTHrP secretion).

10. **On what organs does parathyroid hormone act, and how does it cause increased serum calcium?**
    - Bone: Calcium is released from bone mineral compartment; PTH stimulates bone resorption and bone matrix degradation.
    - Kidney: PTH stimulates calcium reabsorption.
    - Gut: PTH stimulates intestinal calcium reabsorption.

11. **This patient was initially treated with cisplatin and etoposide. How do these chemotherapeutic agents work?**
    Cisplatin is thought to have action similar to alkylating agents. It kills cells in all stages of cell cycle, inhibits DNA biosynthesis, and binds DNA via interstrand cross-links. It has a synergistic effect with other chemotherapeutic agents.

    Etoposide inhibits topoisomerase II, thereby resulting in DNA damage through strand breakage. It is specific to late S phase and G_2 phase of the cell cycle.

STEP 1 SECRET

Students always want to know how much they should learn about chemotherapeutic drugs for boards. First Aid has an excellent list of these drugs, but the various uses for these drugs are quite detailed. We recommend that you approach chemotherapeutic drugs in the following manner:

- Begin by learning the various drug classes (antimetabolites, alkylating agents, etc.) and their mechanisms of action. Classify each individual drug according to these groups.

- Learn the toxicity of each individual chemotherapeutic agent. "Chemo man," which is available on the Internet, is a terrific resource to help you undertake this task. Step 1 is fond of testing students on toxicities of chemotherapeutic drugs.

- Briefly study the drugs that can help to neutralize the toxic effects of chemotherapeutic agents. By far the most important one to know is mesna, which can prevent hemorrhagic cystitis in patients receiving cyclophosphamide.

- Believe it or not, learning the clinical uses of chemotherapeutic agents is last on our list. You do not have to know which drugs are used for all types of cancers, but there are a few on which you should focus. We recommend knowing the drugs that are useful for testicular cancer (etoposide, bleomycin, and cisplatin), choriocarcinoma (methotrexate and vincristine/vinblastine), acute myelogenous leukemia (cytarabine), and brain tumors (nitrosoureas). You should also know that 5-fluorouracil can be given topically for actinic keratosis.

SUMMARY BOX: PARANEOPLASTIC SYNDROMES

- Small cell lung cancer (SCLC) is differentiated from non–small cell lung cancer (NSCLC) by its history of rapid spread. It is prone to early hematogenous spread and a very aggressive course.

- SCLC is not staged using the tumor-node-metastasis (TNM) system because micrometastases are assumed to be present on diagnosis.

- From 10% to 30% of patients with SCLC present with the syndrome of inappropriate secretion of antidiuretic hormone (SIADH).

- SIADH accounts for euvolemic hyponatremia with increased urinary sodium.

- Symptoms of hyponatremia include nausea/vomiting, headaches, confusion, lethargy, seizures, and coma. Symptoms are more pronounced with acute changes in serum sodium.

- Paraneoplastic syndromes are caused by ectopic secretion of peptides or autoimmune dysfunction leading to secretion of autoantibodies.

- There are many paraneoplastic syndromes and resulting symptoms may occur prior to, concurrent with, or after the diagnosis of a neoplasm.

CASE 10-11

A 45-year-old woman presents with concerns for her risk of developing ovarian cancer. Her mother died at age 60 of ovarian cancer, and she has a sister who was recently diagnosed with breast cancer. She smokes two packs of cigarettes per day and drinks alcohol occasionally. She has three children and had an intrauterine device (IUD) inserted 10 years ago. The patient wants to know what her chances of developing ovarian cancer are.

1. **What is the risk of an American woman developing ovarian cancer in her lifetime? How is this risk altered if the woman has a first-degree relative with ovarian cancer?**
   Ovarian cancer is the fifth leading cause of cancer death among women in the United States and is the leading cause of death among gynecologic malignancies. A woman's lifetime chance of developing ovarian cancer is roughly 1.6% but increases to 5% with an affected first-degree relative.

2. **Older age and a family history of ovarian cancer in a first-degree relative are major risk factors for the development of ovarian cancer. What is the third major risk factor for the development of epithelial ovarian cancer, and how does it relate to theories regarding the pathogenesis of epithelial ovarian cancer?**
   Nulligravity is a powerful risk factor for the development of epithelial ovarian cancer (EOC) and confers a relative risk of 1.6%. The predominant theory is that repeated ovulation leads to minor trauma to the epithelial surfaces of the ovaries and that this repeated trauma predisposes the epithelium to malignant transformation. In women who have had children, there have been significant periods in their lives during which they were not ovulating and the epithelial surfaces of their ovaries were not disturbed. Though this theory has not been proved, it is helpful in remembering that nulligravity is a major risk factor for the development of EOC and is consistent with the observation that birth control pills also decrease the rate of developing EOC because they inhibit ovulation. Protective factors are use of oral contraceptive pills, multiparity, tubal ligation, and breastfeeding.

3. **In a female patient with two first-degree relatives with diagnoses of ovarian and breast cancer, what genetic test is appropriate to determine her risk of developing ovarian or breast cancer?**
   Germ-line mutation of the *BRCA* genes is one of the few identified genetic risk factors for ovarian cancer and is associated with both ovarian and breast cancer. Women with a *BRCA1* mutation have a 45% lifetime risk of developing ovarian cancer, and those with a *BRCA2* mutation have a 25% risk. Though it would be inappropriate to use *BRCA* testing to screen for ovarian cancer risk, it is justified in this patient, who has two first-degree relatives with ovarian and breast cancer.

4. **What laboratory test might be used to follow an ovarian carcinoma once it has been diagnosed?**
   Cancer antigen 125 (CA-125). The use of both annual CA-125 and transvaginal ultrasonography has been advocated for early detection of ovarian cancer. However, these tests are not thought to be effective in screening the general population. CA-125 levels correlate well with disease progress, though, and are frequently used to assess response to treatment (Table 10-3).

TABLE 10-3. TUMOR MARKERS	
Marker	**Tumors/Conditions Monitored**
CA-125	Ovarian cancer
PSA	BPH
	Prostate cancer
α-Fetoprotein	Hepatocellular carcinoma
	Yolk sac tumor
CEA	Colorectal cancer
	Pancreatic cancer
β-hCG	Hydatidiform mole
	Choriocarcinoma
S-100	Neuroendocrine tumors
Bence Jones proteins	Multiple myeloma
	Waldenström's macroglobulinemia
TRAP	Hairy cell leukemia

BPH, benign prostatic hypertrophy; CEA, carcinoembryonic antigen; β-hCG, β-human chorionic gonadotropin; PSA, prostate-specific antigen; TRAP, tartrate-resistant acid phosphatase.

STEP 1 SECRET

You should expect at least one question on tumor markers. These are listed for you in Table 10-3.

CASE 10-11 continued:

The patient returns to the office to discuss results of the genetic testing that she requested. She is told that she has a *BRCA1* mutation and that as a result, she has a >50% risk of developing breast cancer and a 45% chance of developing ovarian cancer in her lifetime. She decides to undergo prophylactic bilateral mastectomy and oophorectomy. On pathologic examination of the resected ovaries, she is found to have a 1-cm serous cystadenocarcinoma of the right ovary that had not been seen on preoperative ultrasonography.

5. **What are the three pathologic classifications of ovarian cancer and their relative frequencies?**
   1. Epithelial ovarian carcinoma: 65% to 70%

Epithelial ovarian carcinomas (EOC) (or celomic epithelial carcinoma of the ovary) are seen as part of a spectrum of tumors that can arise from anywhere on the epithelial surface of the peritoneal cavity but tend to occur with the most frequency in the ovarian epithelium. The five major pathologic types of EOC are as follows:

- Serous
- Mucinous
- Endometrioid
- Clear cell tumor
- Brenner tumor

2. Germ cell neoplasms: 15% to 20%

Germ cell neoplasms occur much less frequently and are typically found in younger patients. Common types are teratoma, dysgerminoma, endodermal sinus tumor, and embryonal carcinoma. These tumors tend to behave aggressively and can often be cured with surgery and chemotherapy. There is much similarity between these tumors and male testicular cancers.

3. Stromal tumors: 5% to 10%

It is the sex cords in the embryonic gonad that eventually develop into the ovarian stroma in women. When undifferentiated, the sex cords can develop into either the specific cell types of men (Sertoli and Leydig cells) or women (granulosa and theca cells). Stromal tumors also follow this pattern with proliferation of different cell types: granulosa-theca cell tumors, Leydig cell tumors, and Sertoli cell tumors. These neoplastic cells tend to produce the same estrogens or androgens that their precursor cells produce. As a result, feminizing or virilizing effects may be seen (Fig. 10-14).

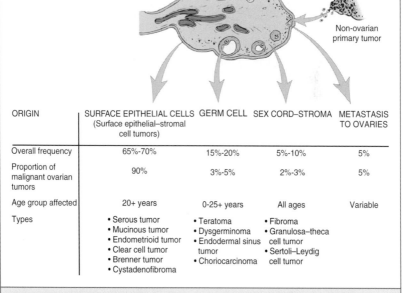

ORIGIN	SURFACE EPITHELIAL CELLS (Surface epithelial–stromal cell tumors)	GERM CELL	SEX CORD–STROMA	METASTASIS TO OVARIES
Overall frequency	65%-70%	15%-20%	5%-10%	5%
Proportion of malignant ovarian tumors	90%	3%-5%	2%-3%	5%
Age group affected	20+ years	0-25+ years	All ages	Variable
Types	• Serous tumor • Mucinous tumor • Endometrioid tumor • Clear cell tumor • Brenner tumor • Cystadenofibroma	• Teratoma • Dysgerminoma • Endodermal sinus tumor • Choriocarcinoma	• Fibroma • Granulosa–theca cell tumor • Sertoli–Leydig cell tumor	

Figure 10-14. Derivation of various ovarian neoplasms and some data on their frequency and age distribution. (From Kumar V, Abbas AK, Fausto N: Robbins and Cotran Pathologic Basis of Disease, 7th ed. Philadelphia, WB Saunders, 2005.)

6. **What is a Brenner tumor?**

   A Brenner tumor is a transitional cell tumor mimicking the epithelium found in the bladder. These rare tumors make up only 2% of all epithelial ovarian cancers (EOCs) and are mostly benign.

7. **In a patient with a granulosa cell tumor that secretes estrogen, what other malignancy would she be at risk for?**

   Unopposed excess estrogen exposure is a risk factor for endometrial carcinoma, which is in fact seen in 5% of patients with granulosa cell tumors.

8. **What types of cancers have been found to metastasize to the ovary? What is a Krukenberg tumor?**

   Breast, colon, gastric, and pancreatic cancers metastasize to the ovary. Krukenberg tumor is the name for a mucin-secreting gastrointestinal cancer that metastasizes to the ovaries. This typically occurs bilaterally. Look for the presence of signet ring cells in the ovary to confirm the diagnosis.

9. **What is the primary mode of spread in epithelial ovarian cancer?**

   Neoplasms tend to form within cysts and eventually rupture through the surface of the ovary and spread along the peritoneal surfaces. Tumor cells may also spread through the lymphatics or hematogenously, though these tumors occur after peritoneal spread. Because an ovarian cancer tends to be asymptomatic until it has spread outside the affected ovary, most women are diagnosed in the advanced stages of ovarian cancer when it finally becomes symptomatic.

CASE 10-11 continued:

The patient has no signs of peritoneal spread of the tumor and makes an uneventful recovery.

SUMMARY BOX: OVARIAN CANCER

- Ovarian cancer is the leading cause of death in gynecologic malignancies, primarily because it is usually diagnosed at such an advanced stage.

- Age, nulligravity, and family history of ovarian cancer in a first-degree relative are important risk factors for the development of epithelial ovarian carcinoma.

- CA-125 may be elevated in epithelial ovarian carcinoma and is used to follow the progress of a cancer once it has been diagnosed.

- Epithelial ovarian carcinomas make up a majority of ovarian cancers; germ cell neoplasms and stromal tumors are less common.

- A Krukenberg tumor is a gastrointestinal cancer that metastasizes to the ovaries.

- Ovarian cancer spreads first through the peritoneal cavity and then may metastasize hematogenously or through the lymphatics.

GENETIC AND METABOLIC DISEASE

J. Pedro Teixeira, Thomas A. Brown, MD, and Sonali J. Shah

CHAPTER 11

INSIDER'S GUIDE TO GENETIC AND METABOLIC DISEASE FOR THE USMLE STEP 1

Understanding biochemistry and genetics will be crucial to achieving a good score on the USMLE Step 1. These subjects lay the foundation for many of the diseases that you are expected to know for boards. This is an intimidating thought for many students who think that they will be expected to memorize a bunch of pathways, enzymes, and intermediates. Yet this is not the case. Although you are not expected to memorize every step of every biochemical pathway, you should understand the implications of abnormalities in these pathways and how they result in various disease symptoms. Focus on the rate-limiting steps and key enzymes of the pathways that you learn as well as where the reactions take place (e.g., cytosol, mitochondrial membrane, mitochondrial matrix, or a combination of the aforementioned locations). More importantly, you should know how these pathways are regulated. One final tip of advice: Do not ignore vitamins and other micronutrients when studying for boards. This is one of the highest-yield Step 1 topics!

BASIC CONCEPTS

1. **What is an enzymopathy and how does it result in clinical symptoms?**
   An enzymopathy is a genetic disease in which a deficiency in activity of an enzyme leads to a block in a metabolic pathway. The altered (usually reduced) enzymatic activity can be due to reduced cellular expression of the enzyme or to expression of a dysfunctional enzyme. The pathologic manifestations of the enzyme deficiency are a result of the accumulation of substrate (or its derivatives) prior to the blockage, a lack of the product(s), or a combination of both (Fig. 11-1).

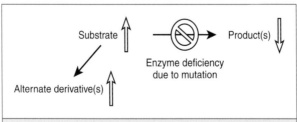

Figure 11-1. Mechanisms by which an enzymopathy produces clinical symptoms. ↑ = increased, ↓ = decreased. (From Brown TA, Brown D: USMLE Step 1 Secrets. Philadelphia, Hanley & Belfus, 2004.)

2. **What is the typical pattern of inheritance observed in enzymopathies?**
Almost all enzymes are produced in excess of minimal requirements. So although heterozygous carriers of an enzyme deficiency typically have only 50% of normal enzyme activity levels, usually they are phenotypically normal. Thus, almost all enzymopathies have an autosomal recessive pattern of inheritance, in which a phenotypic abnormality manifests only when there is nearly no enzyme activity. This generalization is extremely useful for the boards.

3. **Explain why the pathologic consequences of X-linked enzymopathies are manifested almost exclusively in males.**
Again, enzyme deficiencies generally require a near-total loss of enzyme activity to result in phenotypic abnormalities. As males have only a single X chromosome, inheritance of a single defective copy of an X-linked gene from the mother will result in the pathologic consequences of the enzyme deficiency/abnormality. Because females have two X chromosomes, they will generally exhibit the disease only if they are homozygous for the mutated alleles, which is far less likely. (For example, if the odds of a male inheriting a single defective gene is $1/p$, the odds of a female inheriting two defective copies will be approximately $1/p^2$.)

Important examples of X-linked recessive enzymopathies include hemophilia A (factor VIII deficiency), hemophilia B (factor IX deficiency), glucose-6-phosphate dehydrogenase deficiency, and Lesch-Nyhan syndrome (LNS) (hypoxanthine-guanine phosphoribosyltransferase [HGPRT] deficiency).

STEP 1 SECRET

The USMLE loves to ask students to calculate inheritance risk. This will require you to know the inheritance pattern of the disease in question and apply it to the Hardy-Weinberg principle. Recall that if a population is in Hardy-Weinberg equilibrium, and p is the frequency of the normal allele while q is the frequency of the abnormal allele, disease prevalence $= p^2 + 2pq + q^2$ where p^2 and q^2 represent the prevalence of homozygosity and $2pq$ is heterozygosity prevalence (see Case 11-2, q4).

4. **What is the process of lyonization and how may it cause the manifestation of X-linked diseases in females?**
Because females have two X chromosomes, they would have twice the level of expression of genes located on the X chromosome were it not for the random inactivation of one X chromosome that occurs in each somatic cell early in embryogenesis. This process is called lyonization (named after the scientist Lyon, who was the first to propose it). One of the manifestations of lyonization is the Barr body, a condensed, often drumstick-shaped body of DNA seen at the periphery of the nuclei of the cells of females, which corresponds to the inactivated X chromosome. Another nonpathologic manifestation of lyonization is the coloration pattern of calico cats.

Owing to the normally random nature of the X chromosome inactivation, some females may happen to have a mutated X-linked allele on the active X chromosome of a large number of cells and, as a result, may exhibit some pathologic features. These rare individuals are termed "mosaics" or "manifesting heterozygotes." For example, some female carriers of hemophilia A will have some degree of anemia if a large enough proportion of their bone marrow cells inactivate the X chromosome carrying the normal factor VIII allele.

5. **Why do some diseases show an autosomal dominant pattern of inheritance? Why do the genetic diseases of connective tissue usually fall within this category?**

In autosomal dominant diseases, the disease manifests even though there is a normal copy of the gene remaining that produces 50% of the normal amount of gene product. Dominance of a defective gene can be attributed to one of the following reasons: more than 50% of normal gene product is needed for a nondiseased physiologic state; the defective protein adversely affects the normal gene product (a dominant negative effect); or the defective protein has acquired a novel, detrimental property.

Most diseases caused by mutations in nonenzymatic structural proteins (e.g., collagen, fibrillin) or in membrane receptors (e.g., low-density lipoprotein [LDL] receptor) are inherited in an autosomal dominant manner. This again is a useful generalization for the boards.

6. **What is the general relationship between the function of a protein and its pattern of inheritance?**

Table 11-1 shows these relationships.

TABLE 11-1. PROTEINS IN ENZYME DEFICIENCY

Functional Category*	Inheritance Pattern	Example Disease(s)	Defective Protein
Enzymes	Autosomal recessive	Phenylketonuria (PKU)	Phenylalanine hydroxylase
		Galactosemia	Galactose-1-phosphate uridyltransferase
		Medium-chain acyl-CoA dehydrogenase (MCAD) deficiency	Medium-chain acyl-CoA dehydrogenase
		Tay-Sachs disease	Hexosaminidase A
Transport protein	Autosomal recessive	Thalassemias	α- or β-Hemoglobin
		Cystic fibrosis	Chloride channel
Structural proteins	Autosomal dominant	Osteogenesis imperfecta	Type I and type II collagen
		Marfan syndrome	Fibrillin
		Hereditary spherocytosis	Spectrin (found in the RBC membrane)
Developmental gene expression	Autosomal dominant	Achondroplasia	Fibroblast growth factor receptor 3 (FGFR3)
Metabolic receptors	Autosomal dominant	Familial hypercholesterolemia	LDL receptor

*The information presented conveys the general pattern, but a few exceptions can be found in each category. CoA, coenzyme A; LDL, low-density lipoprotein; RBC, red blood cell.

7. **What are the following molecular biology diagnostic methods used for? Explain briefly how they work.**

A. Southern blotting

This technique involves detecting the presence of a specific DNA sequence within a mixture of DNA by using a sequence-specific strand of complementary DNA or messenger RNA (a "probe") that is able to hybridize to the targeted DNA. The specific steps include separating the mixture of DNA fragments by gel electrophoresis, denaturing the DNA (i.e., altering the DNA solution so that the double-stranded DNA separates into single strands), transferring (i.e., blotting) the DNA onto a membrane, and mixing the blotted DNA mixture with radioactively labeled probes to allow for hybridization. In the laboratory, it is often used to detect the presence of large unique DNA sequences (such as a gene mutation) within a patient's genome.

B. Northern blotting

Northern blotting is very similar to Southern blotting, except that a specific sequence of RNA (rather than DNA) is detected using a nucleic acid probe. This technique is commonly used to measure expression of a gene in a patient, as determined by its production of messenger RNA (mRNA).

C. Polymerase chain reaction (PCR)

PCR allows for detection of a specific DNA sequence (such as a mutant allele) by making billions of copies of that allele from as little as a single DNA molecule. This test is performed by using two primers, which are complementary to the DNA regions at the ends of the sequence of interest that is to be amplified. The target DNA is amplified via multiple rounds of DNA denaturation, primer hybridization (or annealing), and extension catalyzed by a temperature-insensitive DNA polymerase.

D. Western blotting

This test is similar to Southern or Northern blotting, but rather than detecting a nucleic acid, it measures the level of a specific protein. First, the protein mixture is coated by a negatively charged detergent molecule that denatures the proteins (i.e., unfolds it into linear peptides) such that the proteins can be separated according to size using gel electrophoresis. Next, the proteins are blotted onto a membrane to which an antibody against the protein of interest (the primary antibody) is added. If the protein is present, the primary specific antibody will bind to the membrane and this binding, in turn, will be detected using a secondary antibody that is both directed against the first antibody and labeled in an assayable fashion. (For example, the primary antibody may be a specific sheep antibody, but the secondary antibody is an antisheep antibody linked to an enzyme that produces a colored product upon exposure to the reagents.) Western blots are used clinically to measure the degree of protein expression of a gene. This is important because diseases can be caused by translational problems, in which transcription of the gene into mRNA occurs normally but the translation of this mRNA is defective.

SUMMARY BOX: BASIC CONCEPTS IN BIOGENETICS

- Enzymopathies (enzyme deficiencies) are caused by a deficiency in activity of an enzyme, resulting in a toxic accumulation of intermediates, a lack of products, or both. Enzymopathies are usually autosomal recessive or X-linked recessive.

- Lyonization, the random inactivation of one of the two X chromosomes in the somatic cells in early female embryonic development, can result in mosaic females that exhibit pathologic symptoms of X-linked disorders.

- Defects in structural proteins typically exhibit autosomal dominant inheritance.

- Both Southern blotting and polymerase chain reaction can be used to detect specific sequences within mixtures of patient DNA. Northern and Western blotting similarly measure RNA and protein levels, respectively.

CASE 11-1

A 2-day-old infant boy tests positive for a relatively rare, but simply managed, medical condition. The diagnosis is based on the presence of markedly elevated serum levels of an essential amino acid. A second positive test result is obtained during his 2-week checkup visit. His family history is remarkable for mental retardation in a 45-year-old aunt.

1. **What is the most likely diagnosis in this baby and how is it inherited?**
    The most likely diagnosis is phenylketonuria (PKU), which, as with most enzymopathies, is inherited in an autosomal recessive manner.

2. **What is the major defect and underlying pathophysiology of this disorder?**
    PKU is caused by the defective conversion of phenylalanine to tyrosine resulting from mutations in the phenylalanine hydroxylase (PAH) gene (classic PKU). The PAH enzyme deficiency leads to both an accumulation of phenylalanine (substrate) and its derivatives phenylpyruvic acid and other phenylketones, as well as a decrease in the levels of tyrosine (product) and its derivatives (such as dopa and melanin). A rarer form of PKU involves a defect in the synthesis of tetrahydrobiopterin (BH_4), which serves as a cofactor for PAH. This cofactor is also required for the synthesis of L-dopa from tyrosine. L-Dopa is then converted to dopamine, which can be used to synthesize the catecholamines norepinephrine and epinephrine. In order to distinguish between the genetic causes of PKU, one can examine levels of dopamine and prolactin. Recall that dopamine is a negative inhibitor of prolactin release. Because classic PKU does not affect dopamine synthesis, prolactin levels should be relatively normal. BH_4 deficiency, on the other hand, will reduce dopamine synthesis and thus prolactin levels will be elevated in these patients.
    The pathology is primarily a result of substrate (phenylalanine) accumulation, which causes severe neuronal damage, mental retardation, growth retardation, and motor dysfunction. The lack of neurotransmitter compounds derived from tyrosine (particularly the catecholamines dopamine, norepinephrine, and epinephrine) may also contribute to damage of the central nervous system (CNS). Other manifestations include a predisposition to eczema, a "musty" odor (caused by phenylketone excretion into sweat), and fair skin coloring (due to tyrosine deficiency, which normally serves as a precursor to melanin) (Fig. 11-2).

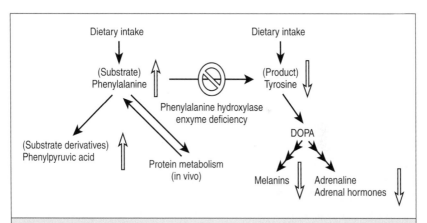

Figure 11-2. Pathologic mechanisms of phenylketonuria. (From Brown TA, Brown D: USMLE Step 1 Secrets. Philadelphia, Hanley & Belfus, 2004.)

STEP 1 SECRET

The biochemical pathway affected in patients with phenylketonuria (PKU) shows up quite frequently on Step 1. Be familiar with the functions of phenylalanine hydroxylase (PAH) and tetrahydrobiopterin and their relevance to this disease. You should also know every step of the catecholamine synthesis pathway.

3. **How is phenylketonuria treated?**
Patients with PKU need to follow a strict diet that restricts phenylalanine intake and is supplemented with tyrosine. If started within the first month of life, this diet is very effective in preventing mental retardation. Because phenylalanine is found in breast milk, most babies suffering from PKU must be placed on special phenylalanine-restricted formulas. Phenylalanine is also found in high concentrations in artificial sweeteners such as aspartame.

4. **Given the fact that phenylketonuria is a relatively rare condition (prevalence rates range from 1 in 2600 to 1 in 200,000 live births), why does it make sense to screen all neonates for this condition?**
The screening test (Guthrie test) is inexpensive (as it simply involves measuring plasma phenylalanine levels), and PKU is easily prevented by dietary modifications. Furthermore, early screening detects the disease before irreparable damage (particularly to the CNS) has occurred (i.e., early intervention affects outcome).

5. **If the parents have a female child with this disease, why is it crucial to advise the child about the risks to her baby if she becomes pregnant when she is older?**
As patients generally tolerate more dietary phenylalanine with age, most women with PKU abandon the diet therapy by their early teens, well before they reach childbearing age. This termination of dietary therapy generally has limited ill effects on the women themselves at this age but will cause irreparable harm to a developing fetus should they become pregnant. Specifically, high levels of phenylalanine can diffuse across the placenta, causing brain damage in the developing fetus. So, although these babies will (virtually always) be heterozygous for the PAH mutation and are thus born without PKU, they can exhibit severe mental retardation, a condition termed maternal PKU.

RELATED QUESTION

6. **Why is screening for congenital hypothyroidism (cretinism), congenital adrenal hyperplasia, and galactosemia also routinely performed in newborns?**
These diseases are similarly screened for because they are additional preventable causes of mental retardation or death. In general, screening is performed on diseases for which treatment is available, for which a rapid and low-cost laboratory test is available, and that are frequent and serious enough to justify the screening cost.

SUMMARY BOX: PHENYLKETONURIA AND NEONATAL SCREENING

- Phenylketonuria (PKU) is due to a defect in the phenylalanine hydroxylase gene that results in the accumulation of the phenylalanine substrate and its phenylketone derivatives as well as the lack of the tyrosine product and its derivatives (such as melanin or catecholamines).

- PKU can result in mental retardation, growth retardation, motor dysfunction, eczema, a "musty" odor, and fair skin coloring.

- The manifestations of PKU can be prevented by neonatal screening and early institution of a diet with low phenylalanine and high tyrosine levels. Women with a history of phenylalanine who are pregnant or may become pregnant should strictly follow such a diet regardless of their personal symptoms due to the risk of fetal neurologic damage (maternal PKU) resulting from embryonic exposure to high phenylalanine levels.

■ In addition to PKU, congenital hypothyroidism, congenital adrenal hyperplasia, and galactosemia are routinely screened for in newborns because their disease manifestations (such as mental retardation or death) can be prevented with early intervention.

CASE 11-2

A woman and her husband just gave birth to a child with cystic fibrosis (CF). Both the woman and her husband are in their 30s and are completely asymptomatic.

1. **If the parents decide to have another child, what is the probability of that child having cystic fibrosis?**
    Because CF is an autosomal recessive disease, the chance of the second child having CF remains at 25%. Each parent is a heterozygous carrier of the mutant allele such that each parent has a 50% chance of passing it on to their offspring, and the chance of the child receiving both mutant alleles is $0.5 \times 0.5 = 0.25$, or 25%.

    Note: Each birth is a completely independent event, such that the outcomes of prior pregnancies do not affect the odds of disease transmission in subsequent pregnancies.

STEP 1 SECRET

Students are frequently asked to calculate genetic probabilities on the USMLE.

2. **If the parents want to have another child, what kind of genetic screening methods are available for them to consider?**
    A few genetic screening methods are available:
    The first method involves preimplantation diagnosis using in vitro fertilization (IVF). The zygotes resulting from IVF are allowed to develop into an 8-cell or 16-cell blastomere, from which a single cell is removed. The DNA is isolated from this single cell and PCR is then used to screen for a mutation in the cystic fibrosis transmembrane regulator (*CFTR*) gene locus. Only the unaffected embryos (wild type or carrier status) are implanted.
    Other genetic screening methods involve prenatal diagnosis using either amniocentesis (the withdrawal of 20-30 mL of amniotic fluid at 15-17 weeks of gestation) or chorionic villus sampling (the aspiration of several milligrams of villus tissues at 10-11 weeks of gestation).

3. **Despite having mutations in the same gene, why do patients with cystic fibrosis exhibit significant variability in disease severity?**
    First, different patients may have different mutations of the same gene, with certain mutations causing less severe phenotypes. For example, mutations of the chloride channel gene that have a smaller detrimental effect on its function result in milder clinical manifestations. There are over a thousand mutations of CFTR that have been identified in patients with CF. This phenomenon of different mutations of the same allele resulting in differing disease manifestations is known as allelic heterogeneity. Interestingly, many patients with CF (>33%) are compound heterozygotes, with a different locus mutated on each copy of their *CFTR* genes.
    Second, even in patients with identical mutations, there is often some degree of clinical heterogeneity. This may be due to other genetic differences or to environmental variables that influence disease expression.

Note: Many genetic diseases have allelic heterogeneity, leading to significant heterogeneity in clinical manifestations.

4. **Assuming a cystic fibrosis prevalence rate of 1 in 2500, what is the carrier frequency for this disease?**
   Here, the Hardy-Weinberg law can be used to describe the genotypic distribution of an abnormal allele ($p + q = 1$) and the phenotypic distribution of the disorder:

$$p^2 + 2pq + q^2 = 1$$

p = frequency of normal allele
q = frequency of abnormal allele $(1 - p)$
p^2 = frequency of unaffected individuals
$2pq$ = frequency of carriers (usually asymptomatic in autosomal recessive diseases)
q^2 = frequency of disease
These equations are easy to remember if one realizes that the phenotype equation is simply the square of the genotype equation:

$$(p + q)^2 = p^2 + 2pq + q^2 = 1^2 = 1$$

Assuming a CF prevalence of 1 in 2500, $q^2 = 1/2500$ such that $q = 0.02$. Because $p + q = 1$, p is 0.98. Therefore, the carrier frequency for CF is $2pq = 2 (0.98) (0.2) = 0.039$, or approximately 4% of the population. Thus, in this example, 1 in every 25 is a carrier. This is roughly the carrier frequency in whites, whereas the mutation and the disease are less common in nonwhites.

The Hardy-Weinberg law can be applied to alleles and populations that are in "genetic equilibrium" (i.e., populations in which the allele frequency is not undergoing rapid change). For the purposes of the USMLE, usually such equilibrium can be assumed.

SUMMARY BOX: POPULATION GENETICS AND PRENATAL GENETIC SCREENING

- Children born to two carriers of an autosomal recessive mutation have a 25% chance of inheriting the mutation, regardless of the outcome of prior pregnancies.

- Genetic screening methods include preimplantation diagnosis using in vitro fertilization as well as amniocentesis (done at 15-17 weeks' gestation) or chorionic villus sampling (done at 10-11 weeks' gestation).

- The prevalence of various genotypes and phenotypes relating to an allele in genetic equilibrium in a population can be predicted using the Hardy-Weinberg equation.

CASE 11-3

A 9-month-old baby girl is brought to the hospital by her parents, both of whom are Ashkenazi Jews. The parents report that over the past 3 months the baby has been having trouble feeding and has become lethargic and "floppy" -appearing. They have also noticed that the child startles easily. More recently, the baby has developed worsening motor dysfunction, now with rigid and spastic movements. The parents are also concerned the baby girl is going blind. On examination, a cherry-red spot was observed at the center of the macula.

1. **What two diagnoses are top considerations in the differential diagnosis at this point?**

Progressive neurodegeneration and macular cherry-red spots in a child should automatically make you think of Tay-Sachs disease (TSD) and Niemann-Pick disease (NPD). Both are autosomal recessive lysosomal storage diseases and, more specifically, sphingolipidoses. TSD is caused by a deficiency of hexosaminidase A, and NPD is caused by a deficiency in sphingomyelinase. The prevalence of both these disorders is higher in Ashkenazi Jews.

Note: Many of the lysosomal storage diseases have multiple subtypes based on the underlying biochemical and molecular characteristics. The syndromes described here correspond to the most common subtype (i.e., type 1 or type A) of each disorder.

CASE 11-3 continued:

Cells from this child are isolated and examined under the electron microscope, revealing "onion-skinning" of lysosomes.

2. **Now what is the most likely diagnosis?**

This feature is associated with TSD but not NPD. On the other hand, "foamy histiocytes" (macrophages filled with sphingomyelin) are found the tissues of patients with NPD.

Note: The exaggerated startle reaction reported in the initial vignette was particularly suggestive of TSD. The startle reaction is caused by hyperacusis and, as it does not occur in NPD, can be a major clue to the early diagnosis of TSD.

3. **What is the pathogenesis of Tay-Sachs disease?**

Hexosaminidase A is a lysosomal enzyme that cleaves a cerebral ganglioside (G_{M2}, a sphingolipid). Mutations make this enzyme less effective, leading to massive accumulation of G_{M2} and its byproducts within the lysosomes of neurons. These lysosomes become enormously enlarged such that they begin to interfere with normal cell function and ultimately cause neuronal death. Neuronal death that overlies the fovea centralis of the retina is responsible for the cherry-red spot seen on funduscopic examination. More specifically, ganglion cells in the retina fill with lipid, which imparts an opaque gray color to the retina. Because the optic disk does not contain ganglion cells, it remains red on a gray background, giving the look of a cherry-red spot. This is a common buzzword used by USMLE test makers.

The pathogenesis of other sphingolipidoses such as NPD or Gaucher disease is similarly due to accumulation of substrates of lysosomal enzymes. The differing disease manifestations of these sphingolipidoses depend upon the organs in which the sphingolipids accumulate and the underlying organ sensitivities. For example, visceral sphingolipid accumulation and hepatosplenomegaly are prominent in NPD but not in TSD. TSD, in contrast, is characterized by relatively isolated central nervous system (CNS) sensitivity to G_{M2} accumulation.

4. **Which is the most common sphingolipidosis?**

Gaucher disease is not only the most common sphingolipidosis but also the most common lysosomal storage disease. The disease is caused by deficiency of glucocerebrosidase and is characterized by the presence of glucocerebroside-laden Gaucher cells, macrophages with characteristic "crumpled-tissue paper" appearance and nuclei displaced by lipid. It also more common among Ashkenazi Jews.

Unlike TSD and NPD, Gaucher disease usually spares neuronal tissue. Glucocerebroside instead accumulates in the reticuloendothelial system, namely, the spleen and liver (causing hepatosplenomegaly), bone (causing bone pain and fractures), and bone marrow (causing pancytopenia, with particularly prominent thrombocytopenia).

Note: Despite the characteristic histologic or cytologic findings of many storage diseases, virtually all of these disorders are today diagnosed using testing for the underlying specific genetic defects.

5. **What are the mucopolysaccharidoses?**

Mucopolysaccharidoses are a different type of lysosomal storage disease in which the substrates that accumulate in the lysosomes are extracellular matrix molecules called glycosaminoglycans (which were previously known as mucopolysaccharides). Like the sphingolipidoses, these diseases are caused by hereditary deficiency of lysosomal enzymes. The two main examples of this type of disease, Hurler syndrome and the similar but less severe Hunter syndrome, are both caused by accumulation of the glycosaminoglycans heparan sulfate and dermatan sulfate (Table 11-2).

To keep these two disorders straight, think of the hunter being male (X-linked) with aggressive behavior and great vision (no corneal clouding). The only other commonly tested lysosomal storage disease that is X-linked recessive is Fabry disease (α-galactosidase A deficiency). Look for peripheral neuropathy and cardiovascular/renal involvement in a patient presenting with Fabry disease on the USMLE Step 1.

TABLE 11-2. MUCOPOLYSACCHARIDOSES: HURLER SYNDROME AND HUNTER SYNDROME

Disorder	Deficient Enzyme	Inheritance Pattern	High-Yield Associations
Hurler syndrome (mucopolysaccharidosis type I H)	α-L-Iduronidase	Autosomal recessive	Coarse facial features (gargoylism), hepatosplenomegaly, mental retardation, joint and skeletal abnormalities, cardiac disease, corneal clouding
Hunter syndrome (mucopolysaccharidosis type II)	Iduronate sulfatase	X-linked recessive	Same features but with milder mental retardation with aggressive behavior and no corneal clouding

6. **Quick review: Cover the three columns on the right side of Table 11-3 and attempt to describe the enzyme deficiency, accumulated substrate, inheritance pattern, pathophysiology, and any high-yield associations for the listed lysosomal storage disorders.**

TABLE 11-3. LYSOSOMAL STORAGE DISEASES

Lysosomal Storage Disease	Enzyme Deficiency/ Accumulated Substrate	Inheritance Pattern	Pathophysiology and High-Yield Associations
Tay-Sachs disease	Hexosaminidase A/G_{M2} ganglioside	Autosomal recessive	Accumulation of cerebral ganglioside causes progressive psychomotor deterioration, macular cherry-red spot, lysosomes with onion-skinning

Continued

TABLE 11-3. LYSOSOMAL STORAGE DISEASES—continued

Lysosomal Storage Disease	Enzyme Deficiency/ Accumulated Substrate	Inheritance Pattern	Pathophysiology and High-Yield Associations
Gaucher disease	Glucocerebrosidase/ glucocerebroside	Autosomal recessive	Gaucher cells (enlarged lipid-laden histiocytes with "wrinkled tissue paper" cytoplasm) accumulate in bone, marrow, liver, and spleen causing bone pain and fractures (bone crises), osteonecrosis of femoral head, massive HSM, pancytopenia
Niemann-Pick disease	Sphingomyelinase/ sphingomyelin	Autosomal recessive	Sphingomyelin accumulation in neurons and liver/spleen causes progressive psychomotor dysfunction, macular cherry-red spots, "foamy histiocytes," and HSM
Fabry disease (angiokeratoma corporis diffusum)	α-Galactosidase A ceramide trihexoside	X-linked recessive	Accumulation in the vascular endothelium results in "Maltese crosses" (fat bodies) in urine and renal disease, angiokeratomas, burning peripheral neuropathy, stroke, and cardiovascular disease
Krabbe disease (globoid cell leukodystrophy)	β-Galactosidase/ ceramide galactoside (i.e., galactocerebroside)	Autosomal recessive	Demyelination and accumulation of globoid cells in CNS result in optic atrophy, peripheral neuropathy, and psychomotor retardation
Metachromatic leukodystrophy	Arylsulfatase A/cerebroside sulfatides	Autosomal recessive	Sulfatide accumulation and central and peripheral demyelination result in ataxia and psychomotor degeneration; dementia in adults

CNS, central nervous system; HSM, hepatosplenomegaly.

SUMMARY BOX: LYSOSOMAL STORAGE DISEASES

- Both Tay-Sachs disease and Niemann-Pick disease are lysosomal storage diseases and sphingolipidoses that are characterized by progressive neurodegeneration along with macular cherry-red spots and blindness. Both disorders are more common among Ashkenazi Jews.

- Tay-Sachs is characterized by easy startling (due to hyperacusis), while Niemann-Pick patients usually have hepatosplenomegaly. Pathologically, Tay-Sachs is characterized by lysosomal "onion-skinning," whereas the tissues of Niemann-Pick patients contain "foamy histiocytes."

- Gaucher disease is the most common sphingolipidosis and lysosomal storage disease. It results in hepatosplenomegaly, bone pain and fractures, and marrow failure but spares neuronal tissue. Pathologically it is characterized by lipid-laden Gaucher cells (macrophages) in these organs of the reticuloendothelial system.

- The most common mucopolysaccharidoses are Hurler syndrome and the X-linked Hunter syndrome. They both result in retardation, hepatosplenomegaly, and coarse facial features but differ in severity (Hurler syndrome is more severe) and in the presence of corneal clouding (seen only in Hurler syndrome).

CASE 11-4

A 2-year-old boy was brought to the clinic with choreoathetosis (constant and involuntary writhing movements of the legs and arms), spasticity (muscular hypertonicity with increased tendon reflexes), impaired cognitive development, and self-mutilation (compulsive biting of the fingers, lips, tongue, and inside of the mouth). The parents also observed the presence of orange "sand" in the child's diapers when the boy was a few months old.

1. **What is the most likely diagnosis?**
   Lesch-Nyhan syndrome (LNS), a rare X-linked recessive disease, is caused by a defective HPRT (hypoxanthine phosphoribosyltransferase) enzyme. The HPRT enzyme is present in most cell types and is involved in the salvage pathway of purine metabolism. The most striking and characteristic neurologic symptom of this disease is self-mutilation.
   Recall that the purine bases are adenine and guanine and the respective nucleosides are adenosine and guanosine. A nitrogenous base linked to a sugar ribose or deoxyribose is referred to as a nucleoside, whereas a phosphorylated nucleoside is referred to as a nucleotide.
   The mnemonics "PURe As Gold" and "CUT the PY" can be used to remember that **A**denine and **G**uanine are **Pur**ine bases, whereas **C**ytosine, **U**racil, and **T**hymine are **PY**rimidines. Likewise, although addition of sugar to a base produces a nucleoside, nucleotides are nucleosides that are "tied" to a phosphate.

2. **What is the normal function of the purine "salvage" pathway?**
   The purine salvage pathway functions to "salvage" purine metabolites such as hypoxanthine and guanine, preventing them from being unnecessarily degraded and then renally excreted as uric acid. (Hypoxanthine is another purine that is an intermediate in the synthesis or degradation of adenosine monophosphate [AMP] or guanosine monophosphate [GMP]; Fig. 11-3). As shown in Figure 11-3, the salvage pathway recycles these metabolites to replenish the purine bases guanine and adenine by the action of the HGPRT enzyme. Normally, the de novo pathway (smaller dark arrows) provides only about 10% of the daily purine requirement, whereas the salvage pathway (large curved arrows) provides the remaining 90%. The amount of net degradation to

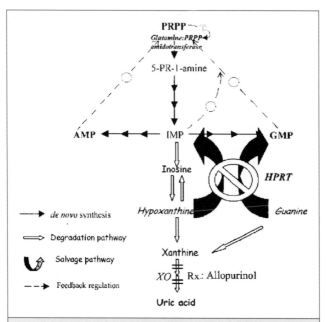

Figure 11-3. The purine salvage pathway. See additional discussion in text. AMP, adenosine monophosphate; GMP, guanosine monophosphate; HPRT, hypoxanthine phosphoribosyltransferase; IMP, inosine monophosphate; PRPP, 5'-phosphoribosyl-1-pyrophosphate; XO, xanthine oxidase. (From Brown TA, Brown D: USMLE Step 1 Secrets. Philadelphia, Hanley & Belfus, 2004.)

uric acid (open arrows) is always balanced with the amount of purines synthesized via the de novo pathway. It follows that the loss of the salvage pathway would result in a dramatic increase in de novo purine synthesis and a similarly dramatic increase in uric acid generation.

3. **How do defects in the purine salvage pathway cause hyperuricemia?**
   In LNS, HGPRT activity is less than 1% of normal. Owing to the absence of HGPRT, the ability to reutilize hypoxanthine and guanine to make the purine nucleotides inosine monophosphate (IMP) and GMP is lost, so these intermediates are degraded to uric acid. As explained already in the preceding question, the purine requirements in this case must be met by increased de novo synthesis. Additionally, because of the reduced levels of IMP and GMP, the feedback inhibition normally exerted by IMP and GMP upon the de novo pathway is lost (broken arrows in Fig. 11-3), even further promoting the activity of the de novo synthesis pathway. Because purine synthesis via the de novo pathway must be balanced by purine degradation into to uric acid, the dramatic increase in de novo synthesis results in severe hyperuricemia.

   In other words, both excessive activation of the de novo pathway and insufficient HGPRT salvage of purine metabolites contribute to the hyperuricemia in LNS.

4. **What was the orange "sand" in his diapers observed by his parents?**
   The sand represents uric acid crystals. Uric acid has limited solubility such that in conditions of extreme hyperuricemia, it will precipitate from urine, forming visible orange "sand." It can also precipitate from the plasma and accumulate in the joints, causing gouty arthritis. Interestingly, most patients with LNS do not develop gout, presumably because of the patients'

short life span (of about 20 years). However, patients with only a partial deficiency of HPRT (with 1-20% of normal activity) have a normal life span but are susceptible to developing severe tophaceous gout.

5. **Why do boys with Lesch-Nyhan syndrome typically present with renal dysfunction?**

Patients with LNS develop kidney disease primarily from repeated uric acid kidney stones and urinary tract obstruction. In addition to nephrolithiasis, chronic hyperuricemia (from any cause) can result in renal insufficiency caused by urate deposition in the renal parenchyma, a process referred to as urate nephropathy.

Note: In contrast with the renal and joint disease, the cause of the neurologic symptoms in LNS is not well-established.

6. **How might this patient be managed pharmacologically?**

Allopurinol is useful in the treatment of hyperuricemia of any cause. It works by preventing uric acid production by inhibiting the enzyme xanthine oxidase (XO) (see Fig. 11-3). The xanthine and hypoxanthine that accumulate instead are more soluble and readily excreted than uric acid.

Other, more common uses of allopurinol include the treatment or (more commonly) the prevention of urate nephropathy, uric acid stones, gouty arthritis, and tumor lysis syndrome (which is caused by treatment of acute leukemias or disseminated lymphomas).

SUMMARY BOX: LESCH-NYHAN SYNDROME AND PURINE METABOLISM

- Lesch-Nyhan syndrome is caused by a defect in the purine salvage pathway, resulting in both overactivity of the de novo purine synthesis pathway and excess generation of the purine metabolite uric acid.

- This X-linked disorder is clinically characterized by retardation, motor dysfunction (choreoathetosis and spasticity), and very characteristic self-mutilating behavior. Patients also can exhibit the manifestations of severe hyperuricemia, including severe tophaceous gout, frequent uric acid kidney stones, and urate nephropathy.

- The production of uric acid can be controlled to some degree in Lesch-Nyhan syndrome using the xanthine oxidase inhibitor allopurinol. This agent is more commonly used in patients without Lesch-Nyhan syndrome to prevent complications of hyperuricemia or uric acid deposition, including attacks of gout, uric acid kidney stones, or urate nephropathy, and tumor lysis syndrome in patients being treated for leukemia or lymphoma.

CASE 11-5

A 4-year-old boy is evaluated for profound hypoglycemia and seizures. Examination is remarkable for nontender hepatomegaly. He has a history of multiple hospitalizations for seizures and hypoglycemia since he was 6 months old. His parents have noticed that he has never tolerated even short periods of fasting well. In his previous hospital stays, low blood sugar levels were consistently observed within a few hours after each feeding. He has also repeatedly had lactic acidosis, hyperlipidemia, and hyperuricemia. A liver biopsy indicates excessive accumulation of glycogen and fat.

1. **What is the diagnosis?**
   Type 1 glycogen storage disease (or von Gierke disease), an autosomal recessive disorder, is caused by deficiency of the enzyme G6Pase.

2. **What type of enzymatic deficiency is present in all types of glycogen storage diseases?**
   These disorders are caused by a defect in either an enzyme required for glycogen synthesis or an enzyme required for glycogen catabolism (i.e., glycogenolysis) called glucose-6-phosphatase (G6Pase). Glycogen storage diseases principally affect either the liver or skeletal muscle, which are the main sites where glycogen is stored. When they affect the liver, they can lead to hepatomegaly and can predispose to hypoglycemia and its attendant complications (e.g., seizures and, with repeated episodes of hypoglycemia, neurologic impairment). When they affect the skeletal muscles, they can cause muscle pain and exercise intolerance, but they do not result in hypoglycemic episodes, as skeletal muscle plays no role in maintaining plasma glucose. Recall that skeletal muscle lacks G6Pase, so it cannot deliver glucose to the bloodstream, as glucose-6-phosphate (G6P) is unable to cross the plasma membrane (see question 10).

3. **How is glycogen normally synthesized and degraded in the liver?**
   Upon entry into a liver cell, glucose is prevented from diffusing out by phosphorylation to G6P, a reaction catalyzed by the enzyme glucokinase (this function is served by hexokinase in nonhepatic tissues). G6P is then converted into glucose-1-phosphate by phosphoglucomutase and then uridine diphosphoglucose (UDP-glucose) prior to attachment to glycogen by the enzyme glycogen synthetase.

   Glycogen degradation is primarily dependent on the activity of the enzyme glycogen phosphorylase (Fig. 11-4).

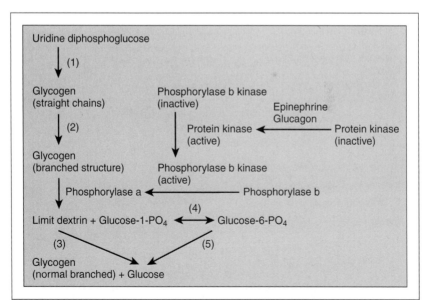

Figure 11-4. Glycogen synthesis and degradation. *1*, Glycogen synthetase; *2*, brancher enzyme; *3*, debrancher enzyme; *4*, phosphoglucomutase; *5*, glucose-6-phosphatase. (From Kliegman RM, Marcdante KJ, Jenson HB, Behrman RE: Nelson Essentials of Pediatrics, 5th ed. Philadelphia, WB Saunders, 2006.)

4. **What is the function of glucose-6-phosphatase?**
   This hepatic enzyme cleaves phosphate off glucose, which then enables glucose to diffuse out of the cell. This reaction is important in the maintenance of blood glucose because the final product of both glycogenolysis and gluconeogenesis is G6P.

5. **Why is hepatomegaly seen on examination?**
   The deficiency of G6Pase causes G6P to accumulate, which stimulates glycogen synthesis, which in turn enlarges the liver.

6. **What is the explanation for his severe fasting hypoglycemia and lactic acidosis?**
   During short-term fasting, liver glycogenolysis is the major pathway that maintains blood glucose. When G6Pase is deficient, glycogenolysis is not effective at releasing glucose into the bloodstream, leading to hypoglycemia. In addition, the release of glucose made by gluconeogenesis during fasting is also impaired because this process is also dependent upon the enzyme G6Pase. This further contributes to hypoglycemia. Excessive accumulation of G6P greatly promotes glycolysis, resulting in high levels of pyruvate production. The pyruvate is then converted into lactate when the mitochondrial uptake of pyruvate is saturated, resulting in lactic acidosis (see Fig. 11-4).

   For your own review, recall that the production of lactic acid from pyruvate does not cause any additional increase in production of adenosine triphosphate (ATP). The function of this pathway is to simply regenerate the electron carrier NAD^+ from NADH.

7. **Why is this patient susceptible to hypertriglyceridemia?**
   Excessive accumulation of G6P overstimulates hepatic glycolysis, supplying substrate for downstream pathways. In addition to lactate synthesis, these pathways also include de novo fatty acid and triacylglycerol (i.e., triglyceride) synthesis. Because the hypoglycemia stimulates glucagon production over insulin release, lipolysis is promoted, providing abundant fatty acids to other tissues for energy production (i.e., β-oxidation). A substantial portion of these fatty acids enters the mitochondria of various tissues to be oxidized, but the excess is repackaged in the liver to form triglyceride-rich, very low density lipoprotein (VLDL) particles to be released into the circulation. High insulin levels normally prevent formation and release of VLDL particles from triglycerides, but in states of profound hypoglycemia, this inhibitory signal is not present.

   You should know how glucagon permits β-oxidation to occur (Fig. 11-5). Note in Figure 11-5 that glucagon stimulates activity of malonyl-CoA decarboxylase, which catalyzes the breakdown

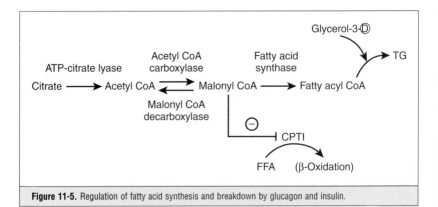

Figure 11-5. Regulation of fatty acid synthesis and breakdown by glucagon and insulin.

of malonyl-CoA into acetyl-CoA. Insulin, on the other hand, stimulates the production of malonyl-CoA along the pathway of triglyceride synthesis. Malonyl-CoA provides an inhibitory signal to carnitine palmitoyltransferase I (CPTI), a mitochondrial enzyme that shuttles long-chain fatty acids into the mitochondrial matrix for β-oxidation. Without CPTI activity, β-oxidation cannot occur. It makes sense that insulin would prevent β-oxidation from occurring, because it would be a waste of energy for the body to oxidize newly synthesized triglycerides in the fed state. At the same time, it would be advantageous to promote β-oxidation when glucagon is present in the fasting state. See how important it is to know the biochemistry behind the diseases that you study?

STEP 1 SECRET

Notice that we did not suggest that you should memorize every step of the pathways that we depicted throughout the case. By simply understanding the major steps, key enzymes, and regulators of the pathways that you learn, you can better reason through disease findings. This is how the USMLE will expect you to think on the examination.

---

8. **What causes the hyperuricemia in this patient?**

As previously mentioned, a lack of G6Pase activity leads to an accumulation of G6P in the cell. G6P is shunted into the hexose monophosphate shunt (also known as the pentose phosphate pathway), leading to accumulation of both ribose 5-phosphate and PRPP (5′-phosphoribosyl-1-pyrophosphate). PRPP is the major allosteric activator of the rate-limiting enzyme (glutamine-PRPP amidotransferase) (see Figure 11-3 in Case 11-4) of the de novo purine synthetic pathway. As discussed in Case 11-4, an increase in de novo purine synthesis leads to an increase in purine degradation, leading to increased uric acid production.

Hypoglycemia also makes cells less able to resynthesize the high-energy molecules adenosine triphosphate (ATP) and adenosine diphosphate (ADP) from adenosine monophosphate (AMP). The resulting increase in cytosolic AMP drives an increase in uric acid production.

Finally, the excess plasma lactate competes with uric acid for urinary excretion, further exacerbating the hyperuricemia.

9. **Quick review: Cover the columns on the right side of Table 11-4 and explain how these diseases affect the activity of the rate-limiting enzymes in the pathways listed in the table.**

TABLE 11-4. METABOLIC PATHWAYS IN GLYCOGEN STORAGE DISEASES			
Pathway	**Rate-Limiting Enzyme**	**Effect**	**Basis of Effect**
Glycolysis	Phosphofructokinase-1	Increase	Increased substrate (G6P)
Glycogen synthesis	Glycogen synthetase	Increase	Increased substrate (G6P)

Continued

TABLE 11-4. METABOLIC PATHWAYS IN GLYCOGEN STORAGE DISEASES—continued

Pathway	Rate-Limiting Enzyme	Effect	Basis of Effect
Fatty acid synthesis	Acetyl-CoA carboxylase	Increase	Increased substrate (G6P is converted using pyruvate to acetyl-CoA) through exaggerated glycolysis
Hexose monophosphate shunt	G6P dehydrogenase	Increase	Increased substrate (G6P)
Triacylglycerol (triglyceride) synthesis		Increase	Increased substrate (glycerol and fatty acids from de novo synthesis or from lipolysis)

CoA, coenzyme A; G6P, glucose-6-phosphate.

RELATED QUESTIONS

10. **Why does a deficiency of muscle glycogen phosphorylase (seen in type V glycogen storage disease, or McArdle disease) not result in hypoglycemia?**
    Muscle glycogen phosphorylase is required for glycogenolysis (breakdown of glycogen into G6P) in muscle. There is a similar enzyme, encoded by a different gene, in the liver. However, unlike in the liver, there is no G6Pase present in muscle to dephosphorylate glucose. As such, glucose is unable to diffuse out of the muscle cell. Similarly, when glucose enters a muscle cell and is phosphorylated by hexokinase, it remains permanently trapped. In other words, glucose that enters a muscle cell cannot be released and, instead, must be consumed by that cell. For this reason, muscle normally makes no contribution to the maintenance of blood glucose.

    In McArdle disease, only muscle glycogen phosphorylase is lost. The corresponding liver enzyme is unaffected. The abnormal accumulation of G6P in muscle results in symptoms such as cramps and muscle fatigue, but there is no impairment in the maintenance of blood sugar. You may also see myoglobinuria associated with this condition as a result of muscle damage.

11. **Review the high-yield glycogen storage diseases.**
    See Table 11-5 for a summary of these diseases.
    Note: Although the liver accounts for the majority (about 90%) of gluconeogenesis and blood glucose maintenance, the kidney contributes about 10%. As such, type I disease can also result in less severe renal disease (with kidney enlargement, proteinuria, and renal insufficiency).

TABLE 11–5. SUMMARY OF HIGH-YIELD GLYCOGEN STORAGE DISEASES

Glycogen Storage Disease	Enzyme Deficiency	Clinical Hallmarks
Type I (von Gierke disease)	Hepatic and renal glucose-6-phosphatase	Massive hepatomegaly and liver dysfunction, renal enlargement, severe hypoglycemia, growth failure
Type II (Pompe disease)	Lysosomal glucosidase	Cardiomegaly leading to cardiac failure; skeletal muscle weakness leading to respiratory muscle failure
Type III (Cori disease)	Amylo-1,6-glucosidase (debranching enzyme)	Milder disease leading to stunted growth, hepatomegaly, and hypoglycemia
Type V (McArdle disease)	Muscle glycogen phosphorylase	Exercise-induced muscle cramps, myoglobinuria with strenuous exercise

Also note that type II (Pompe) disease is both a glycogen storage disease and a lysosomal α-1,4 storage disease. Normally a small percentage (about 2%) of cellular glycogen breakdown is carried out by lysosomal glucosidase. As hepatic and renal glycogen phosphorylase are still functional, deficiency in the enzyme does not result in hypoglycemia but, instead, causes accumulation of glycogen within the lysosomes. This occurs most significantly in the cardiac and skeletal muscles.

SUMMARY BOX: GLYCOGEN STORAGE DISEASES

- Type I glycogen storage disease (von Gierke disease) is caused by a defect in glucose-6-phosphatase, the enzyme required for the release of glucose (generated either from glycogen breakdown or gluconeogenesis) from the liver or kidneys. The lack of this enzyme results in increased synthesis of glycogen, fatty acids, and triglycerides as well as increased activity of the hexose monophosphate shunt. The disorder is clinically characterized by profound hypoglycemia (resulting in seizures, poor growth, or neurologic impairment); lactic acidosis, hyperlipidemia, and hyperuricemia; and massive hepatomegaly, liver dysfunction, and renal enlargement due to glycogen and fat accumulation.

- Type V glycogen storage disease (McArdle disease) is due to absent muscle glycogen phosphorylase activity. This results in muscle symptoms (such as cramps, fatigue, or myoglobinuria with exercise) due to abnormal accumulation of glycogen in muscle. The maintenance of blood sugar, however, is normal.

- Type II glycogen storage disease (Pompe disease), due to deficient lysosomal glucosidase, is a lysosomal storage disease. It is characterized by prominent cardiac and skeletal muscle involvement, with cardiomegaly, which can result in heart failure, as well as skeletal muscle weakness, which can result in respiratory muscle failure.

- Type III glycogen storage disease (Cori disease), due to absent debranching enzyme, is similar to type I disease but is milder. Patients exhibit stunted growth, hepatomegaly, and hypoglycemia.

CASE 11-6

An 8-month-old baby girl is brought to the emergency room by her parents. The baby has been vomiting and irritable over the past 2 days, and in the past 8 hours she has become very lethargic. On examination, her liver is mildly enlarged. Laboratory findings indicate hypoglycemia, moderate hyperammonemia, and abnormally low urine ketones (given the degree of hypoglycemia present). Analysis of the patient's urine reveals a mixture of organic acids ranging between 6 and 12 carbons long.

1. **What is the most likely diagnosis?**
   This baby likely has medium-chain fatty acyl-CoA dehydrogenase (MCAD) deficiency, the most common genetic disorder of fatty acid oxidation.

2. **What are the three length classifications of fatty acids?**
   Most edible fats contain a mixture of three types of fatty acids: short-chain, medium-chain (with 6-12 carbons), and long-chain fatty acids. These fatty acids (in fatty acyl-CoA form) are oxidized in the mitochondria of the peripheral cells, which metabolize fatty acids by the enzymes LCAD (long-chain acyl-CoA dehydrogenase), MCAD (medium-chain AD), and SCAD (short-chain AD), respectively.

3. **What are the reasons for the clinical and laboratory findings exhibited by this patient?**
   Many tissues (especially heart and skeletal muscle) rely heavily on fatty acid oxidation as the primary fuel source for ATP production during fasting or during times of metabolic stress, such as exercise or illness, especially illness that results in decreased oral intake. In addition, a substantial amount of these fatty acids undergo β-oxidation in the liver, which uses the resulting acetyl-CoA to produce ketone bodies that are released to provide energy for the brain (which is unable to directly oxidize fatty acids) (Fig. 11-6).
   When MCAD is deficient, medium-chain fatty acyl-CoA molecules are unable to undergo β-oxidation in these tissues. In addition, although long-chain fatty acyl-CoA compounds can be oxidized into medium chain acyl-CoA molecules, β-oxidation is arrested at the 12-carbon fatty acyl-CoA stage. As a result, medium-chain fatty acyl CoA molecules accumulate in the

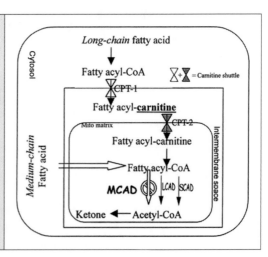

Figure 11-6. Summary of metabolism of fatty acids. CoA, coenzyme A; CPT, carnitine palmitoyltransferase; LCAD, long-chain acyl-CoA dehydrogenase; MCAD, medium-chain acyl-CoA dehydrogenase; SCAD, short-chain acyl-CoA dehydrogenase. (From Brown TA, Brown D: USMLE Step 1 Secrets. Philadelphia, Hanley & Belfus, 2004.)

cytosol and mitochondrial matrix. Some of these medium-chain compounds are converted to the organic acid derivatives that can be detected in the urine. These derivatives may also be toxic to tissues that carry out β-oxidation. In the liver, a substantial portion of these medium-chain fatty acyl CoA molecules is used in cytosolic resynthesis of triglycerides, resulting in liver enlargement from fatty infiltration.

MCAD deficiency also causes ATP production and ketogenesis to be greatly decreased. Without an adequate supply of energy, the rate of the urea cycle is decreased, leading to hyperammonemia. The rate of gluconeogenesis is similarly reduced, and the endogenous glucose supply (liver glycogen) is rapidly exhausted, resulting in hypoglycemia. Loss of MCAD function also results in decreased production of acetyl-CoA, which, in turn, leads to decreased ketone production despite the hypoglycemia. This distinctive hypoketotic hypoglycemia pattern is characteristic of MCAD deficiency.

Other clinical features of MCAD deficiency reflect the involvement of organs that are (directly or indirectly) dependent on β-oxidation. These findings include liver damage and liver function test (LFT) elevation; muscle enzyme elevation, hypotonia, and rhabdomyolysis; congestive heart failure; and neurologic impairment and cerebral edema. Interestingly, this constellation of features is similar to that seen in Reye syndrome (which occurs rarely in children after treatment of a viral illness with aspirin).

4. **How should this child be treated?**
   Avoidance of fasting and of medium-chain fatty acids in the diet is essential. By not allowing this child to rely on peripheral lipolysis and β-oxidation for energy needs, hypoglycemia and accumulation of intermediates caused by the metabolic block will be minimized. Frequent small meals high in carbohydrate and protein and low in fat (<20% of calories) are recommended. Patients with MCAD deficiency should take carnitine supplements to promote efficient long-chain fatty acyl-CoA transport into the mitochondria. Because the carnitine shuttle (i.e., mitochondrial uptake of long-chain fatty acids) is the rate-limiting step for long-chain fatty acid oxidation, promoting this pathway by supplementing carnitine may reduce the energy deficit caused by MCAD deficiency.

5. **How are the pathways/cycles listed in Table 11-6 affected by medium-chain fatty acyl-CoA dehydrogenase deficiency?**

TABLE 11-6.   MEDIUM-CHAIN ACYL-COENZYME A (CoA) DEHYDROGENASE DEFICIENCY

Pathway or Cycle	Activity of Pathway	Cause
Hepatic gluconeogenesis	Decreased, causing hypoglycemia	Low ATP levels
Hepatic urea cycle	Decreased, causing hyperammonemia	Low ATP levels
β-Oxidation of medium-chain fatty acids	Decreased	Enzyme deficiency
Hepatic ketogenesis	Decreased	Low acetyl-CoA production

ATP, adenosine triphosphate.

SUMMARY BOX: MEDIUM-CHAIN ACYL-CoA DEHYDROGENASE DEFICIENCY AND FATTY ACID METABOLISM

- Medium-chain acyl-CoA dehydrogenase (MCAD) deficiency, the most common inherited defect of fatty acid oxidation, results in arrest of β-oxidation at the 12-carbon stage with resultant hypoglycemia, hyperammonemia, increased triglyceride synthesis, impaired ketogenesis, and the build-up of organic acids in the urine.

- Possible clinical manifestations include hypoketotic hypoglycemia; hepatomegaly from fatty infiltration along with liver damage and liver function test (LFT) elevation; muscle enzyme elevation, hypotonia, and rhabdomyolysis; congestive heart failure (CHF); and neurologic impairment and cerebral edema.

- Treatment requires dietary modification. Specifically, patients should avoid fasting and the intake of medium-chain fatty acids and instead should eat frequent small meals high in carbohydrate and protein and low in fat.

CASE 11-7

A woman with acute intermittent porphyria (AIP) is seeking advice on how to avoid exacerbations of her disease.

1. **What are the porphyrias?**
   The porphyrias are a series of disorders caused by enzymatic defects in heme biosynthesis. The enzymatic block leads to the accumulation of intermediates, porphyrins, in the heme biosynthetic pathway that have toxic effects when present at high serum levels. The various forms of porphyria can be diagnosed by detecting the presence of these porphyrin intermediates in the urine, serum, or stool. Each form of porphyria is associated with a particular pattern of porphyrin accumulation, with the pattern depending on the specific location of the block in the heme synthetic pathway.

   In contrast with a majority of enzymopathies, most of the porphyrias have an autosomal dominant mode of inheritance with reduced, but not altogether absent, heme synthesis. Complete absence of heme synthesis is presumably lethal.

2. **What are the types of porphyria?**
   The three major types of porphyria are acute, chronic (hemolytic), and cutaneous. In acute porphyrias, patients usually experience disease exacerbations following specific triggers, which include certain drugs and chemicals, hormones (i.e., estrogens and progestins), smoking, and various forms of stress (such as illness, fasting, infection, or surgery). The acute porphyrias tend to cause neurotoxicity, with prominent autonomic nervous system involvement, resulting in so-called neurovisceral symptoms, such as abdominal pain, vomiting, constipation, muscle weakness, and confusion. AIP, caused by a defect in porphobilinogen (PBG) deaminase, is the most common acute porphyria.

   Defects in the later steps of heme biosynthesis cause accumulation of photoreactive intermediates, resulting in the photosensitivity characteristic of cutaneous porphyrias. Porphyria cutanea tarda (PCT) is both the most common cutaneous porphyria and the most common porphyria overall. PCT is caused by a defect in the enzyme uroporphyrinogen decarboxylase and results in chronic, blistering lesions of sun-exposed skin and, over time, scarring, pigment changes, and increased hair growth (hypertrichosis).

The last (and least common) group of porphyrias are the hemolytic porphyrias. Significant heme synthesis occurs not only in the liver but also in red blood cell precursors. In these disorders, red blood cells are lysed when their accumulated photoreactive porphyrin intermediates are exposed to light as the red blood cells pass through capillaries in the skin.

3. **Why may cigarette smoking or anticonvulsants such as phenytoin and phenobarbital trigger acute porphyrias?**
   Cigarette smoke and many anticonvulsants are potent inducers of hepatic cytochrome P-450 enzymes. These P-450 enzymes contain heme, and consequently their induction increases the demand for heme and increases its biosynthesis. In patients with acute porphyria, a drug- or stress-induced increase in activity of the heme biosynthesis pathway results in an increased accumulation of the toxic porphyrin intermediates. In patients with AIP, acute attacks are often heralded by the development of red urine.

   Interestingly, PCT is not triggered by inducers of P-450. However, it is strongly associated with various hepatotoxic agents such as alcohol, cigarette smoke, hepatitis C infection, and hemochromatosis or iron overload. In women, it is also associated with estrogen exposure, both exogenous (e.g., oral contraceptives or hormone replacement) and endogenous (i.e., pregnancy).

4. **Why is hemin or glucose given to patients with acute porphyrias?**
   Hemin, an oxidized form of heme, acts via negative feedback to decrease the synthesis of aminolevulinic acid (ALA) synthase, the rate-limiting enzyme of heme biosynthesis. This negative feedback mechanism is exploited therapeutically in the treatment of acute porphyrias as intravenous hemin is the most effective way of reducing porphyrin accumulation and the neurovisceral attacks. Glucose infusion (the opposite of fasting) can also be useful because glucose exerts a similar negative feedback upon ALA synthase.

   PCT, interestingly, is effectively treated by phlebotomy. It is thought that blood loss decreases porphyrin production in the liver by decreasing total body and, most importantly, liver iron stores.

   Avoidance of triggers and treatment of exacerbating factors is important in the treatment of all forms of porphyria.

RELATED QUESTIONS

5. **How does lead poisoning affect heme synthesis?**
   Lead poisoning inhibits the heme synthesis enzymes ALA dehydrase and ferrochelatase, resulting in anemia. For Step 1, know that red blood cells (RBCs) on a peripheral blood smear in patients with lead poisoning will demonstrate basophilic stippling.

6. **What are the sideroblastic anemias?**
   These anemias are due to defects in the heme biosynthesis pathway. Unlike the porphyrias, the clinically apparent pathology results from insufficient heme production rather than the accumulation of toxic heme precursors. Because a substantial amount of the body's iron is stored in heme, defects in heme synthesis can lead to abnormal iron accumulation. In the bone marrow of patients with sideroblastic anemia, iron will deposit within mitochondria to form "siderotic" granules in a ring pattern around the nucleus of some of the red blood cell precursors, so-called ringed sideroblasts.

   Use the **TAILS** mnemonic for microcytic anemias: Because **T**halassemia, **A**nemia of chronic disease, **I**ron deficiency, **L**ead poisoning, and **S**ideroblastic anemias involve a defect in heme or hemoglobin synthesis, they are all often microcytic and hypochromic.

SUMMARY BOX: THE PORPHYRIAS AND DISORDERS OF HEME SYNTHESIS

- The porphyrias are caused by enzymatic defects in heme biosynthesis. They are diagnosed by the pattern of buildup of porphyrin intermediates in the urine, serum, or stool. They tend to be autosomal dominant and associated with reduced (but not altogether absent) heme synthesis.

- The acute porphyrias, of which acute intermittent porphyria (AIP) is most common, are characterized by acute episodes of "neurovisceral" symptoms following exposure to inducers of the P-450 enzyme system, such as estrogen, smoking, certain anticonvulsants, and physiologic stress.

- The cutaneous porphyrias, of which porphyria cutanea tarda (PCT) is the most common, result in photosensitivity due to the accumulation of photoreactive porphyrin intermediates in the skin.

- PCT is the most common porphyria and results in blistering, scarring, dyspigmentation, and hypertrichosis (hairiness) of sun-exposed skin. PCT is associated with various hepatotoxic agents or processes such as alcohol, smoking, hepatitis C, or hemochromatosis.

- The hemolytic porphyrias are uncommon and are characterized by the buildup of photoreactive intermediates within red blood cells, resulting in hemolysis as red blood cells pass through skin capillaries.

- Lead poisoning inhibits heme synthesis, resulting in a microcytic anemia with basophilic stippling of peripheral red blood cells.

- The sideroblastic anemias are defects in heme biosynthesis that similarly result in microcytic anemia (rather than the toxic accumulation of intermediates); they are characterized by the presence in the bone marrow of ringed sideroblasts.

CASE 11-8

A 7-week-old baby girl is brought to the office and presents with vomiting, diarrhea, poor feeding, and failure to thrive. The mother has recently noticed that the baby vomits or has diarrhea after nursing. Findings on examination include jaundice, dry skin, pallor, hepatomegaly, and poor tone. The laboratory findings include hypoglycemia, elevation in serum galactose and RBC galactose-1-phosphate (Gal-1-P), galactosuria, albuminuria, and indirect hyperbilirubinemia.

1. **What is the diagnosis?**
   This baby likely has galactosemia, which is a disease that, if left untreated, can lead to severe mental retardation. It is due to defective galactose metabolism and elevated levels of serum galactose (recall that lactose, the sugar present in milk, is metabolized to glucose and galactose). Typically, disorders of galactose metabolism result from deficiencies in galactokinase, a condition called galactokinase deficiency, or galactose-1-phosphate uridyltransferase, termed classic galactosemia (Fig. 11-7). Because both serum galactose and Gal-1-P were elevated this child, she likely suffers from a deficiency of Gal-1-P uridyltransferase (GALT) or "classical galactosemia."

   As demonstrated in Figure 11-6, galactose is metabolized by galactokinase into Gal-1-P. If GALT is not present to metabolize Gal-1-P into glucose 1-phosphate, Gal-1-P can accumulate to toxic levels.

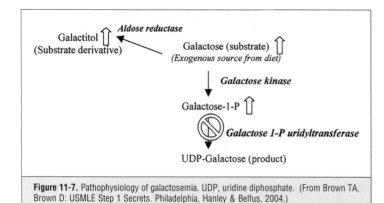

Figure 11-7. Pathophysiology of galactosemia. UDP, uridine diphosphate. (From Brown TA, Brown D: USMLE Step 1 Secrets. Philadelphia, Hanley & Belfus, 2004.)

2. **Why does galactose-1-phosphate uridyltransferase deficiency manifest with jaundice?**
   As in other tissues such as nervous tissue, the lens, and kidney, the pathologic manifestations of galactosemia in the liver and RBCs are due to the accumulation of Gal-1-P and galactitol. This accumulation results in the premature destruction of RBCs (i.e., hemolysis), which results, via the breakdown of hemoglobin, in increased release of unconjugated bilirubin into the circulation. Prehepatic jaundice develops because, if the degree of hemolysis is significant enough, the liver will be incapable of conjugating the entire bilirubin load, leading to buildup of unconjugated bilirubin. The pathologic effect upon the liver can result in liver function test (LFT) abnormalities and liver dysfunction, further contributing to the hyperbilirubinemia.
   Recall that unconjugated bilirubin is indirect whereas conjugated bilirubin is direct. These terms reflect how conjugated bilirubin is water-soluble (i.e., charged) and can be measured directly, whereas in order to measure total bilirubin, a serum sample must be treated such that the water-insoluble (i.e., uncharged) unconjugated bilirubin is brought into solution.

3. **Why do infants with galactosemia tend to develop cataracts if left untreated?**
   When galactose (the substrate) accumulates due to the metabolic block, it enters an alternate reaction catalyzed by aldose reductase (refer to Fig. 11-6), leading to production of the sugar alcohol galactitol (the substrate derivative). Accumulation of galactitol in the lens leads to increased osmolarity, resulting in cataract formation as water is drawn into the lens tissue.
   Note: The classical explanation for cataract formation in diabetes invokes the same mechanism of osmotic damage, with prolonged or repetitive hyperglycemia resulting in deposition in the lens of sorbitol (the sugar alcohol created by the activity of aldose reductase upon glucose).
   Any newborn with cataracts (especially if bilateral) should be evaluated for galactokinase deficiency, classic galactosemia, and other metabolic disorders. Other causes of neonatal cataracts include trisomies (i.e., Down, Edwards', and Patau syndromes) and other genetic disorders as well as intrauterine infections (i.e., toxoplasmosis, other agents, rubella, cytomegalovirus, herpes simplex [TORCH] infections), particularly rubella.

4. **What is the treatment for classical galactosemia?**
   The patient needs to follow a strict diet that eliminates all galactose-containing compounds, including lactose (milk and dairy products) and galactose-containing supplements. Recall that lactose is the disaccharide formed from galactose and glucose. Avoidance of dietary galactose intake quickly eliminates the risk of developing the complications of mental retardation, poor growth, jaundice, anemia, liver disease, and cataracts and may help reverse any complications already present.

STEP 1 SECRET

Be able to recognize the signs and symptoms of classic galactosemia for the USMLE. These symptoms include Infantile cataracts, Jaundice, Failure to thrive, Hepatomegaly, and Mental retardation. An easy way to recall these is to think of the mother in this case telling the doctor that her baby's symptoms appeared after "I Just Fed Her Milk."

SUMMARY BOX: GALACTOSEMIA

- Galactosemia is due to a defect in galactose metabolism, usually deficiency of galactose kinase or galactose-1-phosphate uridyltransferase (GALT), which results in elevated serum and urine galactose levels.

- The disorder results in milk intolerance, hypoglycemia, and poor growth as well as accumulation of galactose derivatives (galactitol and galactose-1-phosphate) in neurons (ultimately leading to mental retardation), in the kidneys (resulting in proteinuria and renal dysfunction), in red blood cells (causing hemolytic anemia and jaundice), in liver (with abnormalities on liver function tests [LFTs], hepatomegaly, liver dysfunction, and worsening jaundice), and in lens tissue (causing cataracts).

- The treatment is avoidance of dietary galactose (including lactose).

- The differential diagnosis for neonatal cataracts includes galactosemia and other metabolic disorders, genetic disorders such as Down syndrome and other trisomies, and rubella and other intrauterine (i.e., TORCH) infections.

CASE 11-9

A tall, slim 14-year-old boy is referred to the genetic disorders clinic by his ophthalmologist. He has ectopia lentis (detached lens), flat corneas, and hypoplastic irides. His mother, who was a tall, thin woman, died suddenly while jogging. An autopsy revealed aortic dissection to be her cause of death. On physical examination, the boy has an arm span–height ratio of 1.15 (normal <1.05), pectus excavatum (sunken chest), scoliosis, joint hypermobility, arachnodactyly (spider fingers), and stretch marks on his shoulders and thighs. He has positive thumb and wrist signs. An early diastolic decrescendo murmur heard best at the left sternal border is appreciated on cardiac examination.

1. **What is the diagnosis?**
   The patient likely has Marfan syndrome, an autosomal dominant disorder caused by mutations of the fibrillin gene. Fibrillin is a glycoprotein that serves as a scaffold for elastic fibers around connective tissue.

2. **Why does this patient exhibit multiple pathologic presentations in the ocular, skeletal, and cardiovascular systems?**
   Fibrillin is a component of microfibrils, which are part of the extracellular matrix of eye tissue, aorta, skin, and periosteum. Microfibrils combine with elastin to form elastic fibers, which convey structural support and elasticity to many tissues. Detached or malpositioned lenses (ectopia lentis), aortic dilation, and abnormally stretchy skin are all pathologic consequences of defective

fibrillin. Progressive aortic dilation often results in separation of the leaflets of the aortic valve, resulting in aortic regurgitation and the corresponding diastolic murmur. The skeletal defects such as arachnodactyly (long, skinny, "spider-like" fingers and toes), tall stature, pectus excavatum, scoliosis, and joint hypermobility are caused by the periosteum's inability to provide the normal oppositional force to bone growth. Overgrowth of bone occurs when the periosteum has become too "flexible" as a result of defective fibrillin. The thumb and wrist signs are useful in demonstrating arachnodactyly. The thumb sign is positive when the thumb, when completely enclosed within a clenched fist, protrudes beyond the fist's ulnar border; the wrist sign is positive when the thumb and pinky overlap when wrapped around the opposite wrist.

3. **What pathologic condition would you suspect in a patient with Marfan syndrome who complains about "the worst headache of my life?"**
    Rupture of a berry aneurysm is likely. Patients with Marfan syndrome are prone to berry (saccular) aneurysms, which are arterial aneurysms that occur at bifurcations in the circle of Willis (the most common site is the bifurcation of the anterior communicating artery). These junctions are common sites for aneurysm formation because they lack internal elastic lamina and smooth muscle, thus weakening them. Because Marfan syndrome already results in weakened vessels, these patients are especially susceptible to berry aneurysms.

    The most common complication of berry aneurysms is rupture, which results in subarachnoid hemorrhage. Spinal tap will reveal blood or yellow fluid, which results from the breakdown of oxyhemoglobin into bilirubin. Blood breakdown products can lead to vasospasm, so patients should be placed on calcium channel blockers.

4. **What are the major cause(s) of death in this disorder?**
    The major causes of death in patients with Marfan syndrome are progressive heart failure from aortic regurgitation and sudden death from aortic dissection. Pregnancy or heavy exercise increases cardiac output greatly, thus elevating the risk of these major cardiovascular complications.

RELATED QUESTIONS

5. **What hereditary skeletal disease predisposes to bone fractures from minor stress? What structural protein defect underlies the disorder?**
    Osteogenesis imperfecta (OI), caused by defects in type I collagen, is an inherited disorder of bone fragility. The most common form of the disorder (type I) is autosomal dominant, but, interestingly, most cases are sporadic (i.e., due to a new mutation). Type I collagen is the predominant collagen type in the extracellular matrix of bone, but it is also found in other structures such as teeth, sclerae, ligaments, skin, and blood vessels. Type I OI is the least severe form, associated with fewer fractures and limited skeletal deformity. Distinct features of OI include blue sclerae, hearing loss (from involvement of middle ear ossicles), and abnormal teeth (i.e., dentinogenesis imperfecta, discolored teeth that wear easily). The reduced collagen content of the sclerae allows the dark choroid layer of the eye to show through the sclerae. Other, less specific features of OI include ligamentous laxity and joint hypermobility; kyphoscoliosis; smooth, thin, and lax skin; and easy bruising (from vessel fragility).

6. **What is the genetic defect in Ehlers-Danlos syndrome?**
    Ehlers-Danlos syndrome can develop from multiple different genetic abnormalities in one of the collagen types. There are many types of Ehlers-Danlos syndrome, with most common being autosomal dominant. Most forms are characterized by extreme skin hyperextensibility and joint hypermobility; tissue fragility; poor wound healing leading to thin, wide, atrophic scars; and easy bruising. The most common form (type I) is due to a defect in collagen V. There is a vascular or ecchymotic form of the disorder (type IV), which is due to a defect in type III collagen,

which is the major component of reticular fibers found in various organs and found along the lining of blood vessels. This form of disease is important to diagnose because, in addition to ecchymoses, these patients are prone to catastrophic rupture of medium-sized arteries, bowel, or uterus (during pregnancy).

SUMMARY BOX: MARFAN SYNDROME AND GENETIC CONNECTIVE TISSUE DEFECTS

- Marfan syndrome is an inherited autosomal dominant defect in fibrillin, a component of the microfibrils found within elastic fibers.

- Marfan patients often exhibit skeletal deformity, with tall thin stature, arachnodactyly (with positive wrist and thumb signs), pectus excavatum, scoliosis, and joint hypermobility; stretchy skin; ectopia lentis (detached lens); and aortic dilation, aortic valve regurgitation, and risk of developing berry aneurysms, heart failure, or sudden death from aortic dissection.

- Osteogenesis imperfecta is a genetic defect in type I collagen, resulting in bone fragility and frequent fractures of varying severity, often with abnormal teeth, blue sclerae, and hearing loss. Less specific features include ligamentous laxity, joint hypermobility, kyphoscoliosis, lax skin, and easy bruising.

- The various types of Ehlers-Danlos syndrome are defects, generally autosomal dominant, in various collagen types. Patients typically exhibit extreme skin hyperextensibility, joint hypermobility, tissue fragility, poor wound healing with atrophic scarring, and easy bruising.

CASE 11-10

A 6-year-old boy is brought to the hospital by his mother because of severe shortness of breath. He has fever and leukocytosis, and a chest x-ray study shows a right lower lobe infiltrate. His mother is really worried because he has had pneumonia already three times as a child. A sputum culture grows *Pseudomonas aeruginosa*. A sweat test shows significantly elevated sodium and chloride.

1. **What is the most likely diagnosis?**
   Cystic fibrosis (CF) is most likely.

2. **What is the etiology of this disease?**
   The defect underlying CF is found in the *CFTR* gene, which codes for a chloride channel found in exocrine glands throughout the body. More specifically, the mutation associated with CF results in defective protein folding of the chloride channel so that it is degraded before it ever reaches the surface of the cell membrane. This channel allows for active reabsorption of chloride from sweat and active secretion of chloride in the lungs, liver, and pancreas. As discussed in Case 11-2, CF is inherited in an autosomal recessive manner.

3. **How does the cystic fibrosis transmembrane regulator (*CFTR*) mutation lead to disease?**
   The lack of active chloride secretion normally carried out by this channel prevents passive secretion of sodium and water because water normally flows down its osmotic gradient. The consequence is abnormally thick secretions in the respiratory tract, pancreas, gastrointestinal (GI) tract, and biliary tree.

4. **Why does this child develop respiratory infections so easily?**
In CF, the abnormally viscous secretions of the tracheobronchial mucous glands impair mucociliary action and predispose to recurrent pulmonary infections. In addition to increased susceptibility to the respiratory pathogens seen in normal hosts, patients with CF frequently become colonized and infected with organisms such as *Staphylococcus aureus*, *P. aeruginosa* and other gram-negative rods, and *Burkholderia cepacia*. Repeated pulmonary infections frequently lead to progressive lung disease, which is the major cause of CF-related death. Chronic infection and inflammation of airways damage the airways, ultimately resulting in airway obstruction, air-trapping, and hyperinflation, which are physiologic changes similar to those seen in chronic obstructive pulmonary disease (COPD).

5. **Why might this child be susceptible to developing pancreatitis as he grows older?**
There is also increased viscosity of pancreatic exocrine secretions, which impairs pancreatic secretion and predisposes to plugging and obstruction of the pancreatic ductules. Such plugging can cause pancreatitis. Most common is pancreatic insufficiency, often resulting in failure to thrive in children, weight loss or poor weight gain, and fat malabsorption (often with frequent, floating, greasy, malodorous stools and flatulence). Fat malabsorption can lead to deficiencies in the fat-soluble vitamins A, D, E, and K.

Abnormal secretions occur in multiple organs and exocrine glands throughout the body. Other possible manifestations of this include high rates of meconium ileus at birth and poor intestinal motility in adults, as well as impaired bile secretion (which in some cases can lead to cholestatic liver disease or even obstructive cirrhosis). In the sweat glands, loss of CFTR function results in impaired reabsorption of chloride, allowing for the diagnosis of CF on the basis of elevated sweat chloride levels.

6. **What is bronchiectasis and why does it commonly develop in cystic fibrosis?**
Ectasis or ectasia means dilation. Bronchiectasis is an irreversible dilation of one or more bronchi. The primary cause for the dilation is usually a combination of inflammation and obstruction (often subtotal obstruction) of the airways. In CF, repeated infection and poor mucus flow contribute to inflammation and airway obstruction.

Other clinical syndromes in which bronchiectasis occurs include obstructing tumors, mucus impaction, foreign body aspiration, necrotizing pulmonary infections (such as *Klebsiella*, *S. aureus* pneumonia or tuberculosis), or certain rheumatic and systemic diseases (such as rheumatoid arthritis). The dilated bronchi are easily collapsible, which causes or aggravates expiratory airflow obstruction and impaired secretion clearance, resulting in the clinical symptoms of dyspnea, cough (which is often severe), and occasionally hemoptysis.

STEP 1 SECRET

Expect to see at least one question on cystic fibrosis and its complications on the USMLE Step 1.

7. **Why is *N*-acetylcysteine used as a treatment for cystic fibrosis?**
N-acetylcysteine cleaves disulfide bonds in the glycoproteins that form mucus. This reduces the thickness of the mucus seen in patients with CF and loosens mucous plugs. *N*-acetylcysteine is also used as an antidote for acetaminophen toxicity and to prevent radiocontrast-induced nephropathy.

RELATED QUESTIONS

8. **Why does Kartagener's syndrome produce clinical manifestations similar to those of cystic fibrosis?**

In Kartagener's syndrome (which is also known as primary ciliary dyskinesia or immotile cilia syndrome), there is a primary disturbance in ciliary function and mucociliary clearance due to dysfunction of the dynein arm of microtubules. Recall that microtubules are found within cilia of the upper respiratory epithelial cells and flagella of sperm. This defective mucociliary clearance compromises sputum expectoration, leading to repeated sinus and pulmonary infections. Patients often have chronic cough, and bronchiectasis can develop in some. It also leads to infertility due to sperm dysmotility.

Interestingly, in CF ciliary dysfunction is secondary to increased secretion viscosity, whereas in Kartagener's syndrome it results from an intrinsic defect in the microtubules. In both diseases there are recurrent sinopulmonary infections as well as infertility in men. Note that the infertility that occurs in each disorder has a different cause. Infertility in CF is not due to abnormal secretions but, instead, is usually due to congenital absence of the vas deferens (presumably because the *CFTR* gene is involved in the embryonic development of the vas). Many women with CF have difficulties conceiving due to thickened cervical mucus. Malnutrition secondary to impaired fat absorption may also disrupt ovulation in these women.

Note: *Situs inversus* is observed in 50% of patients with primary cilia dyskinesia. The classic definition of Kartagener's syndrome is the triad of sinusitis, bronchiectasis, and situs inversus. Situs inversus is characterized by complete left-to-right reversal of all organs and vessels of the body. For example, the heart would on the right side of the thorax (i.e., dextrocardia) and the liver would be in the left upper quadrant of the abdomen. This is distinct from isolated dextrocardia, which can occur in the setting of congenital heart disease. It is felt that situs inversus occurs in ciliary dyskinesia because microtubules are involved in the normal polarization of the body that occurs early in embryogenesis. Without functional microtubules, the polarization of the body occurs randomly such that 50% of patients exhibit normal polarization and 50% exhibit complete reversal.

SUMMARY BOX: CYSTIC FIBROSIS AND DISORDERS OF CILIARY DYSFUNCTION

- Cystic fibrosis (CF) is caused by an inherited, autosomal recessive defect in the CFTR (cystic fibrosis transmembrane regulator) chloride channel that results in abnormally thick secretions of exocrine glands.

- CF can be diagnosed with genetic testing or by documenting an elevated sweat chloride level.

- Thick respiratory secretions and poor mucociliary clearance lead to repeated respiratory infections by characteristic organisms such as *Staphylococcus aureus*, *Pseudomonas aeruginosa*, and *Burkholderia cepacia*. These infections lead to progressive, obstructive lung disease, bronchiectasis, and significant rates of morbidity and mortality.

- Patients with CF can develop pancreatitis and pancreatic insufficiency and, less commonly, meconium ileus at birth or poor intestinal motility in adults as well as cholestatic liver disease.

- Infertility in CF results from congenital absence of the vas deferens.

- *N*-acetylcysteine is used as a treatment for CF to loosen mucous plugs.

- Kartagener's syndrome (or primary ciliary dyskinesia) is classically characterized by the triad of sinusitis, bronchiectasis, and situs inversus. It is due to an intrinsic defect of ciliary function (dysfunction of the dynein arm of microtubules). Infertility results secondary to immotile sperm.

CASE 11-11

While playing basketball over the weekend, a 35-year-old college professor experiences severe chest pain that radiates to his left jaw and left arm. He is taken by ambulance to the emergency room, where an electrocardiogram confirms that he has suffered a myocardial infarction (MI). Physical examination is significant for the presence of xanthelasma and several tendinous xanthomas. His family history is remarkable for coronary heart disease in two first-degree relatives diagnosed when they were in their mid-40s. Blood work reveals plasma total cholesterol of 420 mg/dL (Table 11-7), and a coronary angiogram reveals 90% occlusion of the right coronary artery and 50% occlusion of the left anterior descending artery. He responds well to coronary angioplasty and stenting and is discharged home after only 3 days.

TABLE 11-7. BLOOD WORKUP FOR CASE 11-11

Lipid	Measured Values	
	Patient's Level (mg/dL)	Reference Range (mg/dL)
Triacylglycerol	150	60-160
Total cholesterol	420	<200
HDL cholesterol	31	≥35
VLDL cholesterol	30	20-40
LDL cholesterol	359	<100

HDL, high-density lipoprotein; LDL, low-density lipoprotein; VLDL, very low-density lipoprotein.

1. **What is your diagnosis based on this patient's family history and fasting lipid profile?**

   He most likely has familial hypercholesterolemia (FH). His MI at a young age, his family history of premature cardiovascular disease, his elevated total cholesterol almost entirely in the LDL fraction, his normal triacylglycerol (triglyceride) levels, and the presence of xanthelasma and tendinous xanthomas on examination are all consistent with FH. Xanthomas are pathologic depositions of lipids in nonvascular tissues. In heterozygous FH, xanthomas are often detectable as palpable nodules along tendons such as the Achilles or extensor tendons of the hand. Xanthelasmas are yellow-orange plaques on the eyelids and medial canthi that result from cholesterol deposition into these skinfolds around the eye.

   FH is caused by a defective LDL receptor. This receptor is found on peripheral tissues that utilize lipids found in LDL particles, and on the liver, which plays an important role in the clearance of cholesterol from the blood.

2. **Based on his clinical presentations, is this patient likely to be heterozygous or homozygous for this deficiency?**

   This patient is likely a heterozygote. FH is usually inherited in an autosomal dominant fashion in which a single abnormal LDL receptor gene leads to disease. However, there is a gene dosage effect in that patients who are homozygous for the abnormal LDL receptor have more severe disease.

   Homozygotes typically suffer their first heart attack before age 20, and their total cholesterol levels usually range between 500 and 1000 mg/dL. Prominent presence of cutaneous planar xanthomas is another telltale sign of homozygous FH. Heterozygotes typically have cholesterol levels between 300 and 500 mg/dL, and they do not suffer heart attacks until later in life. Occasionally a few xanthomas can be found on the Achilles tendon in heterozygous FH.

3. **What is the primary mechanism by which mutations in the low-density lipoprotein receptor impair low-density lipoprotein uptake from the plasma?**
   Physiologically, serum LDL is continually made from IDL (intermediate-density lipoprotein), which in turn is derived from VLDL degradation. About 75% of LDL is cleared via LDL receptor-mediated endocytosis, which occurs primarily in the liver and, to a lesser degree, in cholesterol-requiring tissues such as the adrenal cortex (where cholesterol is used as a substrate for steroid hormones). The remainder of LDL is cleared via poorly understood LDL receptor–independent mechanisms, which include, among others, endocytosis of oxidized LDL by macrophages.

   Note: Five classes of mutations of the LDL receptor result in impairment of receptor-mediated uptake of LDL from the circulation. These mutations include (1) null mutations (which prevent LDL receptor protein synthesis), (2) defective transport mutations (which prevent normal insertion of the receptor into the plasma membrane), abnormal clathrin-mediated endocytosis due to (3) defective ligand receptor–binding mutations, or (4) defective internalization mutations, and (5) defective recycling mutations (which result in an inability of the LDL receptor to be recycled back to the membrane).

4. **What is the pathologic consequence of elevated plasma low-density lipoprotein?**
   The mechanism by which excess plasma LDL can result in atherosclerosis is briefly described next:

   In the setting of a defective LDL receptor or of excess serum LDL of any cause, plasma LDL clearance occurs via other mechanisms, including scavenger receptors on macrophages that "scavenge" (endocytose) oxidized LDL. Oxidized LDL levels are proportional to the levels of LDL, but LDL levels may be increased by other cardiac risk factors such as smoking or systemic inflammation. These macrophages then form foam cells and release cytokines, causing proliferation of arterial smooth muscle cells at the site of cholesterol plaque formation. Initially, the smooth muscle cells produce enough extracellular matrix proteins to form a fibrous cap over the foam cells, forming a stable fibrous plaque. However, because the scavenger receptors are not downregulated by intracellular cholesterol concentration, the foam cells continue to accumulate, to endocytose oxidized LDL, and to release inflammatory mediators. In some cases, the inflammatory process erodes the fibrous cap, resulting in the formation of a thinly covered unstable plaque that can eventually rupture, resulting in acute thrombus formation. It is the process of unstable plaque rupture that underlies many strokes and most acute coronary syndromes (i.e., unstable angina and MI). Progressive luminal occlusion by growing stable fibrous plaques can result in chronic ischemic symptoms such as stable angina or claudication.

5. **How might this patient be managed medically and pharmacologically to decrease his risk of future cardiovascular complications?**
   This patient should be managed the same as any other patient with cardiovascular disease and associated risk factors. He would be encouraged to undertake dietary and lifestyle modification, such as increased exercise and smoking cessation, and would likely be treated pharmacologically with HMG-CoA (3-hydroxy-3-methylglutaryl coenzyme A) reductase inhibitors (i.e., statins), possibly in combination with other antilipid drugs such as bile sequestrants (such as cholestyramine) or ezetimibe (an inhibitor of dietary cholesterol uptake).

   Along with statins, aspirin, beta blockers, and angiotensin-converting enzyme (ACE) inhibitors have also been proved to be effective in the secondary prevention of MI (i.e., in patients with a history of MI, they decrease the risk of another MI).

RELATED QUESTION

6. **How do HMG-CoA reductase inhibitors specifically reduce serum low-density lipoprotein levels?**

   HMG-CoA reductase is the rate-limiting enzyme in cholesterol synthesis. Statins lower LDL levels by decreasing intracellular levels of cholesterol within hepatocytes. Statins do so by decreasing de novo cholesterol synthesis. Hepatocytes and other tissues require free cytosolic cholesterol for synthesis of the plasma membrane, steroid hormones, and bile acids. The hepatocytes thus compensate for the decreased cytosolic cholesterol levels by increasing expression of their surface LDL receptors (the same receptors that are mutated in FH) in an attempt to replenish the cytosolic cholesterol supply.

   Bile acid sequestrants such as cholestyramine or colestipol act in a similar fashion. The loss of bile acids in the gut results in a compensatory increase in bile acid synthesis, which tends to consume cytosolic free cholesterol within hepatocytes. Again, this results in a compensatory increase in hepatocyte expression of surface LDL receptors.

SUMMARY BOX: FAMILIAL HYPERCHOLESTEROLEMIA AND LIPOPROTEIN METABOLISM

- Familial hypercholesterolemia (FH) is due to a defect in the low-density lipoprotein (LDL) receptor. Patients exhibit elevation of total cholesterol and, specifically, of LDL with normal triglyceride levels; signs of pathologic lipid deposition, such as xanthelasma and tendinous xanthomas; and a personal or family history of premature atherosclerosis or coronary artery disease.

- High levels of LDL of any cause result in increased clearance of LDL via scavenger receptors on macrophages that recognize oxidized LDL. These macrophages accumulate as "foam cells" within atherosclerotic plaques, and they release inflammatory mediators that drive smooth muscle cell proliferation and fibrous cap formation. Ultimately, inflammation within plaques can lead to fibrous cap erosion and the formation of the unstable plaques that underlie acute coronary syndromes.

- Statins (i.e., HMG-CoA reductase inhibitors) inhibit the rate-limiting step of cholesterol synthesis in the liver. Low cytosolic cholesterol levels within hepatocytes lead to compensatory upregulation of surface LDL receptors and enhanced clearance of LDL from plasma.

CASE 11-12

A 15-year-old boy is sent to a developmental pediatric clinic for evaluation of intellectual delay and hyperactivity. His examination is notable for an unusually long face with a prominent jaw and large ears and large testes (macro-orchidism). His 17-year-old sister was diagnosed with mild mental retardation and a learning disability last year. His family history is also notable for learning disabilities in a maternal aunt diagnosed when she was young and a maternal great uncle. His mother and maternal grandfather, however, both had normal intellect. Neither his father nor any of his paternal relatives had learning disabilities or retardation.

1. **What is the most likely diagnosis?**

   This child likely has fragile X syndrome, an X-linked dominant disorder. It is associated with mental retardation and autistic spectrum behaviors such as attention-deficit/hyperactivity disorder, perseveration, and social avoidance. The characteristic physical features such as long face, protruding jaw (prognathism), and large testes usually become apparent around puberty.

Fragile X syndrome is the most common form of inherited mental retardation. Among genetic disorders, it is the second most common cause of mental retardation (after Down syndrome, which can be inherited but usually is not).

2. **What is the pathogenesis of this disorder?**
Fragile X is caused by expansion of a trinucleotide repeat in the *FMR1* (familial mental retardation-1) gene. The *FMR1* gene normally contains a limited number of repeats (less than 40). However, patients with fragile X syndrome have an expanded number of repeats (usually over 200). The expansion results in a proportional decrease in expression of the fragile X mental retardation (FXMR) protein.

The decreased expression occurs because the repeat region is a site of gene methylation. Recall that gene methylation is a normal regulatory mechanism for silencing gene expression. In this case, expansion of the repeat region results in hypermethylation of *FMR1* and abnormally low levels of expression.

The disease pathogenesis is poorly understood. The FXMR protein is thought to play an important role in transporting nuclear mRNA from the nucleus into the cytoplasm prior to translation, but it is not clear how deficient levels of FXMR protein result in clinical disease. However, disease severity clearly correlates inversely with protein expression levels.

3. **Southern blot analysis indicates that his mother has 90 CGG trinucleotide repeats, whereas he has 350 CGG repeats. What accounts for this finding and what is its clinical significance?**
Fragile X syndrome and other trinucleotide repeat disorders exhibit genetic anticipation due to germ-line expansion of the trinucleotide repeat.

The normal unexpanded *FMR1* gene is transmitted in a stable fashion. However, an expanded *FMR1* gene (with over 40 repeats) is unstable and is subject to further expansion. Furthermore, the longer the gene, the more unstable it is. However, in the case of the *FMR1* gene, this expansion occurs during oogenesis but not spermatogenesis. In other words, instability occurs only in meiosis in women. The result is that a female carrier of an expanded fragile X gene will often transmit an *FMR1* gene that is further expanded. As mentioned earlier, longer repeat regions result in more severe protein deficiency and more severe disease. As a result, subsequent generations experience more severe symptoms and earlier-onset disease, a phenomenon referred to as genetic anticipation. Genetic anticipation is uncommon in genetic disorders and usually results from expansion of trinucleotide repeats (Fig. 11-8).

Note: Because the disorder is X-linked dominant, females with one normal *FMR1* gene and one mutated (expanded) gene will often have some disease features. However, the normal functioning *FMR1* gene usually attenuates the disease to some extent, such that females usually have milder intellectual impairment rather than severe retardation, even in the setting of a full mutation (i.e., >200 repeats).

These two features, genetic anticipation and X-linked dominance, result in the significant but predictable variability of disease severity seen in families with fragile X syndrome.

Figure 11-8. Anticipation due to expansion of trinucleotide repeats (amplification). (From Brown TA, Brown D: USMLE Step 1 Secrets. Philadelphia, Hanley & Belfus, 2004.)

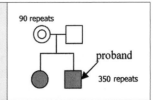

RELATED QUESTION

4. What other relatively common inherited disorder exhibits genetic anticipation?
Huntington's disease is also due to a trinucleotide repeat expansion and exhibits genetic anticipation because of progressive expansion of the trinucleotide repeat in subsequent generations. The disorder is characterized by the triad of motor dysfunction with choreoathetosis, behavior and personality changes (including aggression and depression), and dementia. The disorder is often suspected on the basis of family history and findings from head computed tomography (CT) or magnetic resonance imaging (MRI), specifically, prominent atrophy of the caudate nucleus. The diagnosis can be confirmed with genetic testing.

Huntington's disease is the most common of a group of inherited neurodegenerative disorders (so-called CAG repeat disorders) which, like fragile X, all exhibit genetic anticipation due to expansion of a trinucleotide repeat. However, unlike fragile X, they share autosomal dominant inheritance. Also unlike fragile X, the germ-line expansion occurs in both males and females (i.e., in both oogenesis and spermatogenesis), as one might expect for autosomal disorders. In the case of Huntington's disease, expansion of the CAG repeat results an abnormally long Huntington protein within neurons and other tissues. This elongated protein exhibits a toxic gain of function, such that a normal gene copy is unable to mask a mutated gene.

SUMMARY BOX: FRAGILE X SYNDROME AND TRINUCLEOTIDE REPEAT DISORDERS

- Fragile X syndrome is an X-linked dominant disorder caused by expansion of a region of trinucleotide repeats within the familial mental retardation (*FMR1*) gene. The expansion leads to gene hypermethylation and abnormal silencing of gene expression.

- Fragile X is the most common cause of inherited mental retardation.

- Fragile X is clinically characterized by mental retardation and autistic-like behaviors (inattentiveness, hyperactivity, social avoidance, etc.) as well as characteristic physical features, including protruding jaw (prognathism), long face, and macro-orchidism (large testes), that appear around puberty.

- Fragile X exhibits genetic anticipation, which is the process by which subsequent generations experience more severe symptoms or earlier-onset disease due to germ-line expansion of the trinucleotide repeat.

- Huntington's disease is characterized by the triad of choreoathetosis, behavior and personality changes (including aggression and depression), and dementia. Pathologically, it is associated with prominent atrophy of the caudate nucleus. It belongs to a group of neurodegenerative CAG repeat disorders that, like fragile X, exhibit genetic anticipation due to trinucleotide repeat expansion. Because the CAG repeats result in toxic gain of protein function, these disorders exhibit autosomal dominant inheritance.

CASE 11-13

A newborn boy, born to a 42-year-old woman, presents with upslanting palpebral fissures, excess skin of the inner eyelid (epicanthal folds) and at the back of the neck, a flattened maxillary and malar region, and a single palmar crease (simian crease). The child also exhibits poor muscle tone. Cytologic testing reveals an abnormal karyotype.

1. **What is the most likely diagnosis?**

   The child has Down syndrome, or trisomy 21, an aneuploid condition that leads to the most common genetic cause of mental retardation. Aneuploidy refers to an abnormal chromosome number (that is not a multiple of 23), which is typically due to either a missing chromosome or an extra chromosome (i.e., monosomy or trisomy, respectively). Generally speaking, maternal age older than 35 (so-called advanced maternal age) greatly increases the incidence rate of Down syndrome and other chromosomal abnormalities.

   Note that although Down syndrome is the most common cause of congenital mental retardation, it is not the most common hereditary cause of mental retardation, because most cases of Down syndrome are due to meiotic nondisjunction during oocyte development (during meiosis I of oogenesis). A smaller percentage of cases can be attributed to robertsonian translocation and mosaicism

   Also note that although advanced maternal age is an important risk factor for Down syndrome, most children with Down syndrome are born to mothers younger than 35 years of age. On one hand, this may simply reflect the fact that women under 35 years old become pregnant more often than women over the age of 35. On the other hand, it illustrates that errors of meiosis are fairly common in younger and older women alike. Nondisjunction events can result in viable states such as Down syndrome, but they often result in nonviable states. In fact, chromosomal abnormalities account for about half of all first-trimester spontaneous abortions.

2. **What is a robertsonian translocation and how does a robertsonian translocation in a parent result in Down syndrome in the offspring?**

   A robertsonian translocation causes trisomy 21 via a different mechanism than the meiotic nondisjunction events that give rise to a majority of Down syndrome cases. It results in a familial form of Down syndrome that is unrelated to maternal age and accounts for 2% to 4% of all cases.

   A robertsonian translocation is caused by a translocation event in the germ line of either parent. During meiosis, the long arm of chromosome 21 may attach to the long arm of another chromosome, usually chromosome 14 (with loss of the negligible short arms of both chromosomes). This can result in the offspring having the equivalent of trisomy 21, with two normal copies of chromosome 21 and an additional copy of chromosome 21 fused to chromosome 14.

   A second possible outcome is a balanced translocation, which results in a phenotypically normal individual who has a single normal copy of each of chromosomes 14 and 21 as well the translocation product containing the fused long arms of chromosomes 14 and 21. Any patient with a robertsonian translocation, regardless of whether that patient is affected by Down syndrome due to functional trisomy 21 or whether the patient appears normal due to the presence of a balanced translocation, has a chance of transmitting Down syndrome to offspring.

3. **What is the mechanism that gives rise to mosaic Down syndrome, whereby only select tissues express the trisomy 21?**

   Mosaic Down syndrome (which accounts for 1-3% of cases) is caused by a mitotic nondisjunction event that occurs early in embryonic development. Thus, mosaic Down syndrome is entirely independent of maternal events. This contrasts with the typical meiotic nondisjunction event responsible for a majority of Down syndrome cases (and with the robertsonian translocation, which is also due to an error in meiosis). As one would expect, the earlier during fetal life that the nondisjunction occurs, the more tissues that are affected and the greater the severity of disease.

4. **If the child were to fail to initiate proper feeding, what abnormality should be suspected?**

   Children with Down syndrome are at risk for GI tract abnormalities such as congenital bowel obstruction caused by duodenal atresia. Duodenal atresia is caused by failure of normal recanalization of the GI tract during fetal development. It can be suspected on the basis of the "double-bubble" sign on abdominal radiographs caused by gaseous distention of both the stomach and duodenum proximal to the atretic segment. Patients with Down syndrome are also at risk for other GI abnormalities such as imperforate anus or Hirschsprung disease (aganglionic megacolon). Annular pancreatitis is also more common in patients with Down syndrome.

5. **What causes most of the deaths in infancy and in childhood in Down syndrome?**
Patients with Down syndrome are at increased risk for various congenital heart defects, which are the major cause of early death.
   The most common cardiac abnormalities are endocardial cushion defects, which include defects of the atrioventricular canal (i.e., atrioventricular valve abnormalities and atrial and ventricular septal defects). Patent ductus arteriosus and tetralogy of Fallot can also occur.

6. **Which cancer types are associated with Down syndrome?**
Patients with Down syndrome are at substantially increased risk for developing acute leukemia (both acute lymphoblastic and, to a lesser extent, acute myelogenous leukemias).

7. **What characteristic neuropathologic changes are seen in brains of older people (i.e., >40 years of age) with Down syndrome?**
Almost all patients with Down syndrome in this age group develop the characteristic manifestations of Alzheimer's disease, including neurofibrillary tangles and amyloid deposits in brain tissue. This predisposition to early-onset Alzheimer's disease may relate to the fact that the gene for the protein found in the amyloid deposits (amyloid precursor protein [APP]) is found on chromosome 21.

STEP 1 SECRET

The complications of Down syndrome are frequently tested on the USMLE Step 1.

RELATED QUESTIONS

8. **What other two autosomal trisomies can sometimes produce live-born infants?**
Trisomy 18 (Edwards' syndrome) and trisomy 13 (Patau syndrome) are both viable conditions. However, both trisomies produce more severe disease than in trisomy 21, causing death within the first few months or years of life. As with Down syndrome, most cases result from maternal nondisjunction during meiosis I of the respective chromosome pair.
   Both Edwards' syndrome and Patau syndrome often result in rocker-bottom feet, cardiac defects, and renal defects. An important distinction is that Edwards' syndrome often causes micrognathia (small lower jaw), whereas Patau syndrome results in microphthalmia (small eyes) and cleft lip and palate.

9. **What two diseases result from microdeletion of the same section of chromosome 15?**
Angelman syndrome and Prader-Willi syndrome.

10. Why is the parental source of the chromosome significant in the aforementioned microdeletion syndromes?

It had once been a central dogma of genetics that phenotype is the same whether a given allele is from a paternal or a maternal source. Like most dogmas, however, this idea has not stood the test of time and it appears that the expression of a select number of genes depends on whether they are maternally derived or paternally derived. This phenomenon of gene expression based on parental origin is known as *genomic imprinting*. Genomic imprinting is felt to be due to differential methylation of chromosome regions in female and in male gonads, resulting in different patterns of gene silencing depending on the parental source of the chromosomes.

Angelman syndrome results from a microdeletion in the maternally derived chromosome 15, leading to a loss of function of many genes located in that region (Fig. 11-9). Patients with this disease often exhibit uncontrollable and inappropriate laughter ("happy puppet syndrome"), as well as mental retardation, ataxia, and seizures.

Prader-Willi syndrome is usually due to a microdeletion of the paternally derived chromosome 15. Patients often exhibit uncontrolled appetite, frequently resulting in obesity, as well as mental retardation, hypogonadism, hypotonia, and behavioral problems.

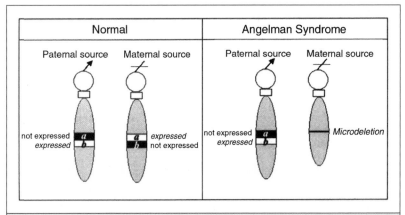

Figure 11-9. Maternal microdeletion in Angelman syndrome. (From Brown TA, Brown D: USMLE Step 1 Secrets. Philadelphia, Hanley & Belfus, 2004.)

SUMMARY BOX: DOWN SYNDROME, CHROMOSOMAL DISORDERS, AND GENOMIC IMPRINTING

- Down syndrome (trisomy 21) is usually due to nondisjunction of chromosome 21 occurring during meiosis I of oogenesis. Such meiotic nondisjunction events occur more commonly as women age.

- Down syndrome is less commonly due to a robertsonian translocation, usually involving chromosomes 14 and 21. It results in a familial (i.e., inherited) form of trisomy 21 that accounts for 2% to 4% of Down syndrome cases.

- Mosaic Down syndrome, accounting for 1% to 3% of cases, is the least common form of trisomy 21. It results from a mitotic nondisjunction event early in embryonic development.

- The characteristic physical findings in Down syndrome include upslanting palpebral fissures, exaggerated epicanthal folds, single palmar (simian) crease, and hypotonia.

- Complications of Down syndrome include gastrointestinal (GI) tract anomalies (such as duodenal atresia, imperforate anus, or Hirschsprung disease), congenital heart disease (usually endocardial cushion defects such as defects of the atrioventricular valves or septa), early-onset Alzheimer's disease, and increased risk of acute leukemia.

- Edwards' syndrome (trisomy 18) and Patau syndrome (trisomy 13) are the two other viable trisomies. They are both associated with rocker bottom feet, cardiac defects, and renal defects. Edwards' syndrome, however, is associated with micrognathia (small jaw), whereas Patau syndrome is associated with microphthalmia (small eyes) and cleft lip and palate.

- Angelman syndrome and Prader-Willi syndrome result from a microdeletion of chromosome 15; Angelman syndrome results from microdeletion of the maternally derived chromosome, whereas Prader-Willi syndrome results when the microdeletion is paternally inherited.

- The differential expression of parentally derived genes, a phenomenon referred to as genomic imprinting, is thought to be due to differential methylation.

CASE 11-14

A 54-year-old male smoker is sent to the emergency room with complaints of severe chest pain. Serial cardiac enzyme levels show no evidence of MI after 24 hours, but an angiogram is performed and reveals severe atherosclerotic coronary artery disease. A triple coronary bypass is then performed. Postoperatively, he remains hospitalized for 2½ weeks because the healing of his sternal wound is progressing slowly. He has been eating a normal diet, though his appetite has been somewhat poor. On examination, he has obvious skin peeling on the back and buttocks and pitting edema. His hair is light colored at the base and can be plucked painlessly. Laboratory findings are remarkable for serum albumin of 1.9 g/dL (normal range is 3.4-5.0 g/dL). His daily urinary urea excretion is about 15 g/day (normal is less than 5 g/day).

1. **What is the (noncardiac) diagnosis in this patient?**
   This patient has kwashiorkor, which results from inadequate protein intake despite fair or overall adequate overall caloric intake. It is a maladaptive state caused by protein calorie malnourishment or severely increased catabolic rate. In developed nations, it is typically caused by acute, life-threatening illnesses such as trauma and sepsis. It is also seen after major surgical operations.
   In developing nations, kwashiorkor usually occurs in young children who are being weaned off breast milk (a good protein source) and started on a high-carbohydrate, very low-protein diet.

2. **What is the reason for his elevated urinary urea nitrogen excretion?**
   Critical illness dramatically elevates one's calorie and, even more so, one's protein requirements. Thus, despite fairly normal intake, his body is in a hypercatabolic state and is breaking down endogenous protein in an attempt to supply his liver with precursors for gluconeogenesis. Because urea is formed exclusively from amino acid metabolism and is exclusively excreted by the kidneys, elevated protein catabolism results in a proportional increase in both urea synthesis and urea excretion.

Patients with critical illness should have these increased protein requirements provided. As many intensive care unit (ICU) patients are intubated and unable to eat, the protein often must be given in the form of amino acid– or protein-enriched total parenteral nutrition or enteric feeds (i.e., tube feeds).

3. **What is the reason for the low serum albumin level?**
This patient's dramatic serum albumin decrease is a result of catabolism of albumin (amid a generalized increase in protein catabolism) caused by the severe stress (bypass surgery) and, to a lesser extent, by poor feeding. Additionally, inflammatory mediators may also reduce hepatic albumin production. Hepatic albumin production is unable to compensate for the degree of catabolism. The low albumin level contributes significantly to his edema.

This edema is the primary clinical distinction between kwashiorkor and marasmus (in which edema does not occur). Patients with kwashiorkor often have anasarca, severe diffuse edema of the entire body, due to low oncotic pressure. The edema affects the face and periorbital area, producing a rounded face with puffy eyes. Patients, particularly children, also often have a characteristic abdominal distention, or "pot belly," due to a combination of ascitic fluid accumulation and hepatomegaly (from fatty infiltration). Other characteristic features include dry atrophic, peeling, hyperkeratotic skin and dry, hypopigmented hair that either spontaneously falls out or is easily plucked out. The decreased hair pigmentation results from a lack of melanin, which is derived from amino acids (specifically tyrosine, a derivative of the essential amino acid phenylalanine). The hair hypopigmentation, after restoration of adequate protein intake, will result in the so-called "flag sign" with interspersed bands of normal pigmentation and hypopigmentation.

4. **Would you expect this patient to have an obviously emaciated appearance and muscle wasting?**
No. In fact, it is typically noted that people with kwashiorkor usually have relatively preserved peripheral muscle mass with increased fat reserves. The most dramatic deficit is the loss of visceral (i.e., organ-associated) protein, which is more difficult to appreciate. The anasarca also prevents patients from appearing emaciated. This lack of emaciation can be very deceiving because it will often mask the severity of a patient's malnutrition.

These findings are in contrast with those in marasmus, in which there is severe muscle wasting and "broomstick" extremities as a result of total calorie malnutrition.

5. **What are some potential dangers if this condition is left treated?**
Kwashiorkor, in addition to the foregoing description, results in poor wound healing and impaired immune function. This, in turn, results in increased susceptibility to infections, particularly sepsis, pneumonia, and gastroenteritis.

6. **Compare and contrast marasmus and kwashiorkor**
Table 11-8 compares the features of marasmus and kwashiorkor.

TABLE 11–8. KWASHIORKOR AND MARASMUS		
Feature	**Kwashiorkor**	**Marasmus**
Cause	Stress-induced protein catabolism and/or low protein intake (develops over only weeks)	Chronic low total calorie intake (develops over months to years)

Continued

TABLE 11-8. KWASHIORKOR AND MARASMUS—continued

Feature	Kwashiorkor	Marasmus
Basic characteristic	Loss of visceral protein with increased visceral fat and relatively preserved peripheral protein	Severe loss of peripheral protein
Clinical presentation	Poorly pigmented, easily plucked hair; anasarca (severe diffuse edema), increased infection risk, poor wound healing	Emaciated appearance, often with weight lower than 80% of ideal weight
Laboratory test results	Very low serum albumin (<2.8 mg/dL)	Low creatinine (from decreased muscle mass)

SUMMARY BOX: KWASHIORKOR AND MARASMUS

- Kwashiorkor results from inadequate protein intake despite fair or adequate overall calorie intake. It results from lack of protein intake or severely increased catabolic rate (as in critical illness or after major surgery).

- Excess protein catabolism can be detected by measuring urinary urea nitrogen excretion.

- Kwashiorkor is characterized by severe hypoalbuminemia; edema, often with ascites or anasarca; hepatomegaly from fatty infiltration; abdominal distention or "pot belly" appearance; atrophic scaly skin; and hypopigmented, easily plucked hair. In contrast with marasmus, there is relative preservation of peripheral muscle mass and fat reserves with severe depletion of visceral protein. Most relevant to hospitalized patients are poor wound healing and impaired immune function. The latter results in an increased risk of infections such as sepsis or pneumonia.

- Marasmus results from total calorie malnutrition and is characterized by severe generalized wasting with severe depletion of muscle mass (and low creatinine).

CASE 11-15

A 20-year-old woman comes to the office because of new-onset headaches and joint pain. She also notes that her hair has been falling out. Physical examination reveals dry, peeling skin and brittle nails. You believe that her signs and symptoms may be related to a new medication that she has been taking for severe acne.

1. **What is the likely diagnosis in this patient?**
   Hypervitaminosis A (vitamin A toxicity) is likely. Because vitamin A is fat-soluble (along with vitamins D, E, and K), it can accumulate in adipose tissue and has the potential to reach toxic levels if consumed in excess. Isotretinoin, a drug used to treat severe acne, is a vitamin A derivative that can cause toxicity in patients who do not adhere to their doctor's instructions when taking this medication.

Other potential sources of vitamin A toxicity include overconsumption of vitamin A–containing foods (egg yolk, butter, milk, bear liver) or vitamin A/multivitamin megadoses.

2. **What are the symptoms of vitamin A toxicity?**
   Vitamin A toxicity results in **H**eadache, **A**rthralgias, **S**ore throat, **S**kin changes, **A**lopecia, **F**atigue, and **T**eratogenicity (cardiac problems, cleft palate, and spontaneous abortions). Owing to the high potential for teratogenicity that results from hypervitaminosis A, women treated with isotretinoin must not become pregnant when taking this medication.
   Remember: Vitamin A **HAS-SAF-T** (safety) issues.

3. **What are the symptoms associated with vitamin A deficiency?**
   Because vitamin A is an essential component of visual pigments (e.g., rhodopsin), deficiency results in night blindness. It is also required for differentiation of epithelial cells into specialized tissues and prevents squamous metaplasia. Deficiency can result in dry skin and squamous metaplasia of the conjunctiva (Bitot's spots).

STEP 1 SECRET

As mentioned in the introduction to this chapter, nutrition is an extremely important subject to understand for boards and when discussing health and diet-related issues with patients. Most students will have multiple questions on this topic on their USMLE examination. Spend a great deal of time learning the symptoms associated with deficiency (and toxicity, when relevant) of the different water-soluble and fat-soluble vitamins. The best resource for this information is your copy of First Aid.

SUMMARY BOX: HYPERVITAMINOSIS A

- Fat-soluble vitamins include vitamin A, D, E, and K. Water-soluble vitamins include the B vitamins and vitamin C.

- Vitamin A toxicity can result from overconsumption of vitamin A–containing foods, multivitamin abuse, or treatment of severe acne with isotretinoin. Toxicity signs and symptoms include headache, arthralgias, sore throat, skin changes, alopecia, fatigue, and teratogenicity.

- Vitamin A deficiency results in night blindess, dry skin, and squamous metaplasia.

CHAPTER 12

ANEMIAS

Allyson M. Reid, Thomas A. Brown, MD, and Sonali J. Shah

INSIDER'S GUIDE TO ANEMIAS FOR THE USMLE STEP 1

Hematology on the USMLE Step 1 is divided into three major subjects: anemias, bleeding disorders, and hematologic malignancies. We will be covering each of these subjects in a series of three chapters because of the sheer volume and immense importance of all these topics. Anemias themselves are commonly tested on boards, and as you may have figured out, there are *many* different causes. The USMLE will expect you to reason through the cause of a patient's anemia based on clinical history and laboratory values. Images of blood smears will often be provided to aid you in your diagnosis. You should know the different cell morphologies associated with various types of anemia (e.g., sickled cells, bite cells, spherocytes, Heinz bodies) and what these cells look like on a blood smear. You should also know the various clinical tests and laboratory parameters used to classify and diagnose different anemias. These are discussed later in the chapter.

It will be of enormous benefit to you to group the causes of anemia according to their findings (e.g., intravascular vs. extravascular, hemolytic vs. nonhemolytic) as you study. If you develop a systematic approach to tackling anemias, you can make a complicated subject much simpler. We will attempt to demonstrate this practice within this chapter.

BASIC CONCEPTS

1. **What is anemia and how is it defined?**
   Anemia is the lack of normally formed, properly functioning red blood cells (RBCs) in the circulation, which impairs the body's ability to oxygenate the tissues at optimal levels. Anemia may be quantitative (decreased RBC count), qualitative (disordered cellular morphology or hemoglobin structure), or a combination of both. These abnormalities can be shown on a complete blood count (CBC), hemoglobin electrophoresis, peripheral blood smear, or rarely, a bone marrow aspirate if necessary.

STEP 1 SECRET

Normal reference ranges for all important laboratory parameters (including hematologic parameters) will be provided to you, so do not waste time memorizing all of these numbers. Instead, focus on specific clues in the clinical presentation, laboratory tests, and histologic findings that are diagnostic for each particular condition, as well as the major treatments and complications associated with each.

Although not required, it may be helpful to familiarize yourself with the most common laboratory values to save yourself precious time on the examination. Both USMLE World and Kaplan Qbank provide these values in charts that closely resemble those you will find on your actual examination.

2. **What are the three pathophysiologic mechanisms resulting in anemia?**
   Simply put, anemia can result from decreased production of RBCs, increased premature destruction of RBCs, or loss of RBCs from leakage out of the circulation, as in bleeding.

   Impaired marrow production is seen in substrate deficiency states (iron/folate deficiency), disorders of heme synthesis (sideroblastic anemias), disorders of hemoglobin synthesis (thalassemias), impaired marrow responsiveness to erythropoietin (anemia of chronic disease), bone marrow–infiltrative conditions (malignancies), and conditions associated with reduced erythropoietin production (renal failure).

   Increased RBC destruction can be seen in a variety of inherited and acquired conditions. Some of these are associated with abnormalities in RBC structure and function, such as hereditary spherocytosis, sickle cell anemia, glucose-6-phosphate dehydrogenase (G6PD) deficiency, and paroxysmal nocturnal hemoglobinuria (PNH). Others are associated with autoimmune and drug reactions, often leading to hypersplenism as the damaged cells are removed from the circulation.

   Chronic blood loss (as in a slow intestinal bleed) typically causes an underproduction anemia by depleting the body's iron stores. This loss can also occur in a menstruating woman with heavy menstrual bleeding, endometriosis, or uterine fibroids.

2. **What are reticulocytes? What is a normal reticulocyte count?**
   Reticulocytes are immature RBCs produced by the bone marrow and released into the blood. The number of reticulocytes present in the peripheral blood provides an indication of how effectively the bone marrow is producing RBCs, and thus responding to an anemia.

   A normal reticulocyte count varies between approximately 0.5% and 1.5%. A low or normal reticulocyte count *in a setting of anemia* typically indicates an underproduction anemia. However, calculation of the reticulocyte index (RI) can help determine whether or not the marrow compensation is appropriate for the severity of the anemia. The RI can be calculated by correcting the reticulocyte count for the degree of anemia:

$$RI = \text{Reticulocyte count} \times (\text{Patient's hematocrit/Normal hematocrit})$$

   With severe anemia (hematocrit <25%), reticulocyte precursors are released from the marrow earlier than normal reticulocytes. These must be accounted for when determining RI. Simply divide the calculated RI by a factor of 2 to yield the percentage of reticulocytes.

   Example: Assuming a severe anemia with a hematocrit of 10% and a reticulocyte count of 2.5%, we have

$$RI = (2.5\% \times 10/40)/2 = 0.625$$

   Here, we had to divide by 2 to account for the proreticulocytes found in circulation during severe anemia. Although this is useful to know for your clinical years, it is unlikely that you will be expected to make this calculation on boards. At the minimum, know how to calculate RI without worrying about the severity of anemia.

   A normal RI is 1. In the preceding example, the bone marrow (BM) is not appropriately compensating for the severe anemia by increasing reticulocyte release into the circulation. We would expect the reticulocyte count to exceed 3% in cases of anemia. In this situation, we can say that the bone marrow is unable to produce enough RBC precursors to ameliorate the anemia.

   Note: An *absolute reticulocyte count* can be obtained by multiplying the reticulocyte count by the concentration of RBCs. For example, in a normal patient with a reticulocyte count of 1% and a RBC count of $5 \times 10^6/\mu L$, the absolute reticulocyte count is 50,000 RBCs/μL.

3. **What are the hemolytic anemias and how are they typically classified?**
   Hemolytic anemias are anemias in which RBC destruction (hemolysis) is the cause of the anemia. The cause may be either hereditary or acquired. Hereditary causes include hereditary spherocytosis, PNH, G6PD deficiency, and sickle cell anemia. Acquired hemolytic anemias can be further classified as autoimmune (e.g., autoimmune hemolytic anemia), drug-induced, or traumatic (e.g., mechanical prosthetic heart valves).

4. **Regarding hemolytic anemia, what is the difference between intravascular and extravascular hemolysis?**

Intravascular hemolysis occurs when RBCs are directly lysed within blood vessels. Causative factors range from complement-mediated hemolysis in PNH to mechanical fragmentation of RBCs by mechanical prosthetic valves or by fibrin clot products, as in microangiopathic hemolytic anemias, which often occur in the setting of disseminated intravascular coagulation (DIC). Extravascular hemolysis, as the name implies, takes place outside the vasculature. In extravascular hemolysis, splenic macrophages or Kupffer cells in the liver destroy RBCs due to structural or morphologic abnormalities of the RBCs (e.g., hereditary spherocytosis, hypersplenism).

5. **Why is there a greater degree of hemoglobinemia and hemoglobinuria in intravascular hemolysis than in extravascular hemolysis?**

In intravascular hemolysis, lysed RBCs spill their hemoglobin directly into the bloodstream (hemoglobinemia), which may then be filtered out into the urine (hemoglobinuria). In extravascular hemolysis, the hemoglobin in phagocytosed RBCs is metabolized intracellularly to bilirubin, reducing the amount of hemoglobin that ends up in the blood or urine (Table 12-1).

Haptoglobin, a serum protein that sops up free heme in the circulation, will attempt to reduce the free heme secondary to hemolysis regardless of etiology, causing its levels to decrease. For reasons just explained, haptoglobin will be more greatly reduced in the setting of intravascular hemolysis than in extravascular hemolysis. You should keep this in mind for boards!

TABLE 12-1. CHARACTERISTICS OF HEMOLYSIS

Hematologic Feature	Intravascular Hemolysis	Extravascular Hemolysis
Hemoglobinemia	Yes	None or slight
Hemoglobinuria	Yes	None or slight
Plasma haptoglobin	Large decrease	Normal or slight decrease
Anemia	Yes	Yes
Jaundice	Yes	Yes
Hepatosplenomegaly	No	Often
Example disorders	Microangiopathic hemolytic anemia, disseminated intravascular coagulation, thrombotic thrombocytopenic purpura, paroxysmal nocturnal hemoglobinuria	Immune-mediated (ABO mismatch), hypersplenism

6. **How are microcytic, macrocytic, and normocytic anemias defined?**

This classification scheme used to categorize anemias is based on the size of the RBCs found in the patient's bloodstream. RBC size is generally determined by mean corpuscular volume (MCV), which is calculated by dividing hematocrit by RBC count per liter. Normal reference range is 80 to 100 fL. Anemias that remain in this range are classified as normocytic. Those that fall below this range are microcytic, and those above the range are termed macrocytic. Various causes of these three types of anemias will be explored throughout the cases presented in this chapter.

7. **What is the usual cause of anemia in end-stage renal failure?**
   In the setting of end-stage renal failure, anemia is principally due to reduced production of erythropoietin by the diseased kidneys. However, uremia from renal failure can also make the bone marrow less responsive to erythropoietin. Anemia caused by renal failure typically responds well to exogenously administered erythropoietin.

CASE 12-1

An 8-year-old Kenyan immigrant boy presents to his pediatrician complaining of generalized fatigue and mild yellow tinge to his scleras for the past several months. He has no family history of anemia. The remainder of his physical examination is normal. Concerned about elevated bilirubin levels, you suggest to your attending to obtain a CBC to check for anemia, as well as liver function tests and hepatitis serologic testing to rule out liver failure as a cause of jaundice. Pertinent laboratory findings are as follows: CBC reveals hemoglobin of 9.0 g/dL (normal 12–15), hematocrit of 27% (normal 35–42%), and a normal MCV.

1. **What is the differential diagnosis for normocytic anemia?**
   - Aplastic anemia
   - Hemolytic anemias
     - Hereditary
       - Spherocytosis
       - PNH
       - Sickle cell anemia
       - G6PD deficiency
       - Pyruvate kinase deficiency
     - Acquired
       - Autoimmune
       - Drug-induced
       - Traumatic
   - Myelodysplasia
   - Renal disease
   - Anemia of chronic disease
   - Blood loss

CASE 12-1 continued:

A peripheral blood smear reveals sickled RBCs and Howell-Jolly bodies (Fig. 12-1).

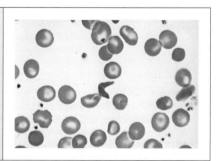

Figure 12-1. Peripheral blood smear for patient in Case 12-1. (From Stein JH: Internal Medicine, 4th ed. St. Louis, Mosby, 1998.)

2. **What is the expected diagnosis now and what is the confirmatory test?**
Sickle cell anemia, a hereditary hemoglobinopathy caused by a point mutation in position 6 of the β-globin chain, is expected. Hemoglobin electrophoresis can provide definitive evidence to make a diagnosis of sickle cell anemia. In this test, RBCs are obtained from the patient, lysed to free up the hemoglobin proteins, and separated by size and charge on a gel. A banding pattern develops that corresponds with the size of the hemoglobin proteins. Each specific type of hemoglobin has an identical banding pattern based on the hemoglobin variant present. Therefore, a patient with sickle cell anemia should show a hemoglobin electrophoresis banding pattern consistent with hemoglobin S (HbS) (the sickle cell variant).
   Note: The presence of sickled cells on peripheral smear is diagnostic of sickle cell anemia but is not the confirmatory test. Electrophoresis is the gold standard.

CASE 12-1 continued:

Hemoglobin electrophoresis of the patient's blood shows the presence of abnormal HbS.

3. **What are the three main types of hemoglobin found within normal adult red blood cells? How does this expression pattern differ in sickle cell anemia?**
The three primary types of hemoglobin in adult RBCs are hemoglobin A ($\alpha_2\beta_2$), hemoglobin A_2 ($\alpha_2\delta_2$), and fetal hemoglobin F (HbF) ($\alpha_2\gamma_2$). The vast majority (>95%) of hemoglobin in adult RBCs is normally of the hemoglobin A (HbA) type. Because sickle cell anemia is caused by a substitution of the hydrophobic valine for the hydrophilic glutamic acid in the β-globin protein, there is deficient production of HbA with increased expression of abnormal HbS.

4. **What causes "sickling" of red blood cells in this disease?**
In the deoxygenated form, HbS is significantly less soluble than HbA and is therefore predisposed to precipitate from the cytoplasm under conditions that cause higher concentrations of deoxyhemoglobin (e.g., hypoxemia, acidosis, hyperosmolarity/dehydration). Although the effects of hemoglobin precipitation are initially reversible, repeated bouts of hemoglobin precipitation lead to irreversible defects in structure and function of the RBC membrane, resulting in chronically sickled cells.

CASE 12-1 continued:

Physical examination reveals mild scleral icterus and no splenomegaly, and is otherwise unremarkable. Liver function tests reveal a total bilirubin of 1.4 mg/dL and direct bilirubin of 0.3 mg/dL.

5. **What is the mechanism of anemia in sickle cell anemia?**
Anemia results from increased intravascular hemolysis due to mechanical fragmentation, although there is also a small component of impaired erythropoiesis at the level of the bone marrow.

6. **If there is hemolysis producing the anemia, why is the spleen not palpable?**
By the age of 5 years, 94% of sickle cell patients will have experienced autoinfarction of the spleen as a result of the tortuous circulation that the misshapen RBCs must pass through. Lacking adequate oxygenation, the spleen becomes small, dense, and fibrotic. Calification may be seen on abdominal x-ray films.
   Note: Prior to autoinfarction, splenomegaly may occur. Splenomegaly occurs when RBCs occlude the efferent splenic vessels, leading to accumulation of blood within the spleen and consequent engorgement of the organ. This can sometimes lead to a splenic sequestration crisis, in which RBCs and platelets normally found within the general circulation pool in the

enlarged spleen. Platelet counts and plasma levels of hemoglobin and hematocrit may fall below normal, causing hypovolemic shock and death.

7. **Why are parents of children with sickle cell disease taught how to palpate the spleen whenever their children develop a febrile illness?**
Various infections predispose to "splenic sequestration crises" in which the spleen enlarges acutely to aid in the immunologic response against the infection. This in massive RBC sequestration and hemolysis in sickle cell patients as the splenic cords are compressed, making it even more difficult for the rigid sickled cells to pass through. Such splenic sequestration causes a rapid drop in the hematocrit and may cause symptoms of intravascular depletion and hypovolemic shock. If access to medical care (e.g., RBC transfusion) is not available, the mortality rate for these sequestration crises can approach 15%.

CASE 12-1 continued:

On further questioning, the patient admits to intermittent episodes of sharp abdominal pain.

8. **What are vaso-occlusive crises?**
This is a term to describe conditions under which increased RBC sickling occurs. The increased sickling of RBC occludes blood vessels, resulting in local lactic acidosis and pain secondary to tissue hypoxia.

9. **What factors are thought to increase the risk of experiencing these crises?**
The aforementioned factors that increase deoxyhemoglobin concentrations, such as dehydration, hypoxemia, and acidosis, may all "trigger" these crises.

CASE 12-1 continued:

Past medical history is remarkable for two previous hospital admissions for sepsis caused by encapsulated bacteria.

10. **Why should this boy receive vaccinations against encapsulated bacteria?**
Recurrent vaso-occlusive crises in the spleen typically lead to fibrotic scarring of the spleen (referred to as autosplenectomy), which significantly increases susceptibility to infection by encapsulated bacteria such as *Streptococcus pneumoniae* and *Haemophilus influenzae*.
   Note: Just as the lymph nodes filter bacteria from lymphatic fluid, the spleen filters encapsulated bacteria from the blood.

11. **This boy has one brother who does not have the disease. Neither of his parents are affected. How would you describe the genetics of this disease?**
The fact that no other members of his family are affected suggests autosomal recessive inheritance. Both parents must be unaffected carriers of sickle cell trait to pass the trait on to their son. Approximately 25% of the offspring generated by two carriers will be affected with sickle cell disease. This boy's brother may also be a carrier of sickle cell trait, having gotten one copy of the mutation from one parent and a normal copy from the other, or he may be completely unaffected, having gotten normal copies of the gene from both parents.

12. **How does sickle cell trait differ from sickle cell disease?**
The heterozygous carrier of the sickle cell mutation is said to have the sickle cell trait, genotypically referred to as HbAS. These patients are relatively asymptomatic, with very minimal symptoms of anemia, and typically do not experience episodes of pain from vaso-occlusive crises. The predominant hemoglobin in sickle cell carriers is HbA, just as in unaffected individuals.

13. **What is the evolutionary pressure for sickle cell trait?**
    The sickle cell mutation is more common in African Americans because in its heterozygous form it provides protection from infection with *Plasmodium falciparum*. In fact, in regions of Africa where malaria is common, up to 25% to 30% of the population is heterozygous for this mutation.

    CASE 12-1 continued:

    Two weeks later this patient's mother brings him in because of a significant increase in fatigue (evidenced by decreased desire to play), irritability, and a facial rash with a "slapped cheek" appearance.

14. **What infection do you suspect and what serious complication should be considered?**
    The slapped cheek appearance is characteristic of parvovirus infection. Parvovirus is known to infect erythrocyte progenitor cells and cause aplastic crisis in sickle cell anemia. The combination of increased RBC hemolysis (sickled cells have a severely reduced life span) and impaired erythropoiesis in sickle cell anemia can precipitate a severe state of anemia.

    CASE 12-1 continued:

    Four months later, this patient presents to his local emergency room with chest pain and shortness of breath that developed as he was playing outdoors. Oxygen saturation is 84% on room air, and chest x-ray study reveals perihilar infiltrates.

15. **What is the likely diagnosis and why does it occur in sickle cell anemia?**
    Acute chest syndrome is caused by occlusion of the pulmonary vasculature by sickled cells. This can also cause pulmonary edema and elevated white blood cell (WBC) count and may be indistinguishable from pneumonia on chest x-ray film. Treatment includes respiratory support, exchange transfusion, and empiric antibiotics for pneumonia due to fluid stasis in the lungs.

STEP 1 SECRET

A child experiencing chest pain during play is a commonly used clinical vignette on boards. Whenever you see this, consider acute chest syndrome in a sickle cell patient. Additional medical history to support your diagnosis will be provided to you.

16. **What are the indications for exchange transfusion in sickle cell disease?**
    Stroke or transient ischemic attack (TIA), acute chest syndrome, priapism, third-trimester pregnancy, and intractable vaso-occlusive crisis are all indications for exchange transfusion.

17. **Why is this boy is at risk for papillary necrosis of the kidneys?**
    The conditions of hypoxemia, acidosis, and hyperosmolarity specifically present in the renal medulla (an area that is especially prone to hypoxia) increases sickling of RBCs, resulting in vaso-occlusion of the vasa recta in the renal papillae. This result eventually leads to papillary necrosis.

CASE 12-1 continued:

As his physician, you recommend prophylactic cholecystectomy once he is stable.

18. **Why are patients with sickle cell disease at an increased risk for gallstones?**
About 70% of patients with sickle cell disease will get symptomatic cholelithiasis. Recall that these gallstones will be pigmented due to hyperbilirubinemia secondary to chronic hemolysis. Having a prophylactic cholecystectomy can also help distinguish gallbladder pain from cholelithiasis and abdominal pain secondary to vaso-occlusive crises.

19. **Patients with sickle cell disease can develop complications in many other organ systems as well. What two bone "diseases" are these patients predisposed to and why? To which other conditions are patients with sickle cell disease prone?**
Vaso-occlusive phenomena in sickle cell anemia can cause avascular necrosis of bones, particularly avascular necrosis of the femoral head. These avascular areas of bone are then more susceptible to the development of infection (osteomyelitis). *Salmonella* osteomyelitis is seen more frequently in sickle cell anemia, yet *Staphylococcus aureus* is the most frequent cause of osteomyelitis in the general population.
    Note: The reason for this discrepancy is attributed to the fact that *Salmonella* is an encapsulated organism. Patients with sickle cell crisis who undergo autosplenectomy are at risk for infection by encapsulated organisms.
    Other conditions affecting sickle cell patients include the following:
    - Enlarged heart/congestive heart failure (CHF)
    - Ischemic retinopathy
    - Priapism

20. **Some patients with sickle cell disease are treated with the chemotherapeutic drug hydroxyurea. What would be your rationale for starting this patient on this treatment?**
Hydroxyurea is a chemotherapeutic drug that increases the production of fetal hemoglobin (HbF), which presumably decreases the amount of HbS expression and therefore decreases HbS polymerization and RBC sickling. However, the precise mechanism of action of hydroxyurea remains poorly understood. Some authors believe that its main mechanism of action is through stabilizing RBC membranes. Nevertheless, students should know that it is an important therapeutic agent for sickle cell disease.

21. **What are sickle cell trait and Hemoglobin C (HbC)?**
Sickle cell trait occurs when a person has one abnormal sickle cell allele (HbS) but is not homozygous for the mutation. Because the alleles are codominant, heterozygous patients produce normal and abnormal hemoglobin. Approximately 90% abnormal hemoglobin product is required to produce sickle cell symptoms, so individuals with sickle cell trait are often asymptomatic.
    HbC is the product of an alternative mutation in position 6 of the β-globin gene in which glutamic acid is substituted for lysine. In the same fashion as for the sickle cell mutation, individuals who are heterozygous for the mutation often do not have any anemia, and homozygous individuals have a mild hemolytic anemia. Individuals who are HbSC have a milder form of sickle cell disease than HbSS patients.

SUMMARY BOX: SICKLE CELL DISEASE

- Sickle cell disease is inherited in an autosomal recessive manner.

- Carriers of sickle cell trait are usually asymptomatic and are protected from falciparum malaria. Africans are more often affected.

- Examination may show scleral icterus, mild jaundice, and hepatosplenomegaly in patients younger than 5 years.

- Blood tests show normocytic anemia, reticulocytosis, and elevated indirect bilirubin.

- Blood smear shows sickled cells, Howell-Jolly bodies, and reticulocytosis.

- Hemoglobin electrophoresis shows hemoglobin S (HbS).

- Treatment includes hydroxyurea, pneumococcal and *Haemophilus influenzae* vaccines, and analgesia and hydration for treatment of acute crises.

- Sickle cell crises are precipitated by infection, dehydration, and hypoxemia.

- Complications include the following:

  □ Cholelithiasis

  □ Renal papillary necrosis

  □ Aseptic necrosis of femoral head

  □ Infection with encapsulated bacteria: *H. influenzae, Streptococcus pneumoniae, Salmonella*

  □ Parvovirus infection causing aplastic anemia

  □ Priapism

  □ Splenic sequestration crisis

CASE 12-2

A 6-month-old boy of Greek descent is brought to the office by his parents because over the past 2 weeks he has been sleeping much more than usual. The examination reveals conjunctival pallor, scleral icterus, and hepatosplenomegaly. Concerned about a possible anemia, the pediatrician obtains an initial CBC to check for anemia and infection. The CBC reveals hemoglobin of 4.5 g/dL, MCV of 73 fL, and increased reticulocyte distribution width (RDW).

1. **What is the differential diagnosis for a microcytic anemia?**
   Iron deficiency, anemia of chronic disease, thalassemia, sideroblastic anemia, and lead poisoning are considerations.

CASE 12-2 continued:

Serum iron, ferritin, and total iron-binding capacity (TIBC) are all normal. A peripheral smear shows many nucleated RBCs and target cells.

2. **How does this change your differential diagnosis?**
   This largely rules out the two most common causes of hypochromic, microcytic anemia—iron deficiency and anemia of chronic disease. Both of these conditions demonstrate decreased serum iron.

CASE 12-2 continued:

Gel electrophoresis reveals elevated hemoglobin A$_2$ (HbA$_2$) and HbF and the complete absence of β-globin subunits.

3. **What is the diagnosis?**
Thalassemia major, also known as Cooley's anemia. If there was partial expression of β-globin, then the diagnosis would be thalassemia minor, but this is usually either very mild or completely asymptomatic.

4. **What is the pathogenesis of thalessemia major?**
Impaired synthesis of the β-subunit of hemoglobin due to a homozygous mutation. Normally, HbA is a tetramer made of two α chains and two β chains. Impaired production of the β chains leads to polymerization of the α chains within RBCs. These aggregates are insoluble and precipitate and damage the RBC membrane, causing premature hemolysis within the spleen and ineffective erythropoiesis in the bone marrow. The combination of the accelerated destruction and the impaired production of RBCs explains the severe anemia.

5. **Why did it not manifest until the age of 6 months?**
For the first 6 months, this boy was asymptomatic, because he still had large amounts of HbF, fetal hemoglobin, present in his circulation. Remember, HbF contains two α chains and two δ chains and does not require β-globin synthesis at all for proper functioning. As he transitioned to synthesis of adult hemoglobin (HbA contains two α and two β chains), the symptoms began to manifest as he became reliant on hemoglobin A production.

CASE 12-2 continued:

The examination reveals conjunctival pallor, scleral icterus, and hepatosplenomegaly.

6. **Why do you see scleral icterus and organomegaly?**
RBC hemolysis releases heme, which is degraded into bilirubin. The unconjugated bilirubin accumulates and deposits in the sclera, causing icterus. This eventually results in generalized jaundice.
    Hepatosplenomegaly occurs for two reasons. First, there is increased hemolysis of abnormal RBCs by macrophages in the spleen and liver. Second, there is extramedullary erythropoiesis in response to impaired bone marrow erythropoiesis. (However, this is no more effective than in the bone marrow because of the genetic defect in β-globin.)

STEP 1 SECRET

You may be given a radiograph of a skull that demonstrates a "crew cut" appearance (see Fig. 12-2). This is a sign of bone marrow expansion and is associated with thalassemia and sickle cell disease.

CASE 12-2 continued:

You tell the parents that their son will need frequent blood transfusions for the rest of his life. At the age of 4, the boy is seen in the emergency department because he is unable to walk after falling off his tricycle. The x-ray study shows a fracture of the right tibia.

7. **Why might this boy be more susceptible to fractures?**
Ineffective erythropoiesis in the bone marrow results in markedly hyperplastic bone marrow and bone marrow expansion (Fig. 12-2). This bone marrow expansion erodes away the cancellous and cortical bone, resulting in significant structural weakness.

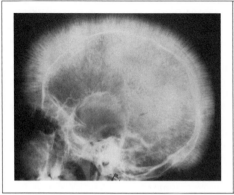

Figure 12-2. Thalassemia: x-ray film of the skull showing new bone formation on the outer table, producing perpendicular radiations resembling a crewcut. (Courtesy of Dr. Jack Reynolds, Department of Radiology, University of Texas Southwestern Medical School, Dallas, TX.)

CASE 12-2 continued:

This patient does well for many years, receiving frequent blood transfusions. At the age of 35, he is seen for a routine checkup and is found to have a fasting glucose level of 130 mg/dL. His skin is noted to be tanned although he spends little time in the sun. The electrocardiogram (ECG) shows some nonspecific ST-T wave changes.

8. **What is the diagnosis and why did it occur in this patient?**
Secondary (acquired) hemochromatosis is a common complication of repeated transfusions in these patients. Excess iron is delivered in the transfused RBCs and can deposit in organs such as the heart, pancreas, and skin, leading to restrictive cardiomyopathy and so-called bronze diabetes.
   Keep in mind that thalassemia is a disorder of globin chain deficiency, so iron studies will be completely normal. The boards exam loves to test students on their understanding of various disorders, so you should expect to be asked conceptual questions like this on your examination.

STEP 1 SECRET

The following type of *question format* commonly appears on boards:
   Example: Which of the following laboratory findings would be expected in a patient with β-thalassemia major who is receiving blood transfusions (compared with values for a normal patient)?

	β-Hemoglobin	Hemoglobin F	Serum Iron
A.	↓/normal	↓	Normal
B.	↓/normal	↓	↑
C.	↓/normal	↑	↑
D.	↑	Normal	↓

   The correct answer choice is C. Hematology, cardiology, nephrology, and pulmonology questions are especially suitable for this "↑/↓/normal" format. Thus, when you study these subjects, you should be thinking along comparative terms. Purchasing question bank software will give you some additional practice with handling these types of questions.

9. **How could it have been prevented?**
Treatment with iron-chelating agents such as deferoxamine can reduce the incidence of hemochromatosis. Obviously, phlebotomy to reduce iron stores (the usual treatment for hereditary hemochromatosis) would be counterproductive for someone receiving transfusions for anemia.

10. **If this patient had presented in his early 20s with similar symptoms and blood tests but β-globin is present on gel electrophoresis, what would be your diagnosis? What is the pathogenesis?**
α-Thalassemia is caused by impaired production of the α-subunit of hemoglobin. There are two genes for the α-subunit on each chromosome for a total of four genes. Unless someone is missing all four copies of the α chain gene, that person will still synthesize some α chains. For this reason, α-thalassemia patients typically present later in life with milder symptoms than in β-thalassemia. People missing one copy of the gene are asymptomatic, as enough α chain is produced by the remaining three copies of the normal gene. Missing two copies can cause a mild anemia that generally does not require treatment. Missing three copies results in a condition called HbH disease. The gel electrophoresis will show normal β-globin and decreased α-globin subunits. HbH precipitates on staining with brilliant cresyl blue. Typically, this occurs in people of Asian or African descent. Those of African descent are more likely to have received one bad copy from each parent, leading to an α−/α− genotype. Those of Asian descent are more likely to have gotten two bad copies from one parent, leading to an αα/− genotype.

11. **α-Thalassemia, in its most severe form, is called hydrops fetalis and can be fatal in utero. What is hydrops fetalis and why is it fatal?**
Hydrops fetalis occurs when the fetus is missing all four copies of the α-globin gene. HbA, HbA₂, and HbF all require the α-subunits to form, so in its complete absence, none of these can be made. The fetus instead produces hemoglobin consisting of four γ chains (hemoglobin Barts). This form of hemoglobin has an extremely high affinity for oxygen and hinders the ability of RBCs to deliver this oxygen to tissues. Fetuses affected with this disease are born with profound anemia due to tissue asphyxia as well as CHF from this asphyxia. This is often fatal *in utero*, as proper growth and development cannot occur in the setting of profound hypoxia. This is similar to the condition of babies afflicted with hemolytic disease of the newborn (Rh-positive babies born to Rh-negative sensitized mothers).

STEP 1 SECRET

Pay close attention to age, racial, and ethnic clues provided in question stems. Boards will commonly present "textbook cases" in their clinical vignettes, so these clues may aid you in prioritizing the considerations in your differential diagnosis. For instance, α-thalassemia is most common in Africans and Asians, but β-thalassemia is most common in African and Mediterranean populations. Notice that the patient in this case is of Mediterranean heritage.

12. **Why is sickle cell disease less severe than normal in a patient who is a hemoglobin S/β-thalassemia heterozygote?**
Patients with β-thalassemia produce high levels of HbF, which decreases sickling of RBCs.

SUMMARY BOX: THALASSEMIAS

α-Thalassemia

■ Caused by decreased α-globin synthesis

- Africans: $\alpha-/\alpha-$
- Asians: $\alpha\alpha/-$
- Symptoms based on the number of genes deleted
  - Asymptomatic
  - Mild anemia
  - HbH disease: splenomegaly
  - Hb Barts: hydrops fetalis—incompatible with life
- Diagnosis
  - Smear: microcytic anemia, hypochromia, target cells, Heinz bodies
  - HbH inclusion bodies seen on brilliant cresyl blue stain
- Treatment: blood transfusions

β-Thalassemia

- Caused by decreased β-globin synthesis
- Epidemiology: Mediterranean
- Symptoms
  - β-Thalassemia major: anemia, jaundice, and splenomegaly at 6 months due to switch from fetal to adult hemoglobin
  - β-Thalassemia minor: no symptoms
- Diagnosis: increased fetal hemoglobin (HbF) and hemoglobin A_2 (HbA$_2$) and decreased hemoglobin A (HbA) on gel electrophoresis
- Treatment
  - Transfusions + deferoxamine to increase iron excretion
  - Splenectomy
  - Possible bone marrow transplant

CASE 12-3

A 68-year-old woman is evaluated in a routine physical examination. She notes increasing fatigue and shortness of breath over the past few months. CBC reveals a microcytic anemia.

1. **What is the differential diagnosis for a microcytic anemia?**
   Iron deficiency anemia, sideroblastic anemia, thalassemia, lead poisoning, and anemia of chronic disease are all considered.

CASE 12-3 continued:

You order iron studies because iron deficiency is the most common cause of microcytic anemia. Serum iron and ferritin are both decreased. TIBC is increased, indicating an iron deficiency anemia. A smear shows hypochromic RBCs and a low recticulocyte index.

2. **Why is the anemia microcytic and hypochromic?**

    Iron is required for hemoglobin synthesis. Reduced cytoplasmic hemoglobin results in smaller (microcytic) cells that have less color (hypochromia).

3. **Why are there fewer reticulocytes?**

    Decreased ability to produce hemoglobin due to low iron results in less RBC production. Any anemia resulting from decreased erythropoiesis will result in a low reticulocyte count (see question 2 from Basic Concepts for further discussion).

4. **Why is total iron-binding capacity increased? Why is ferritin decreased?**

    TIBC is the amount of free serum transferrin that is available to bind iron. In iron deficiency, not only is the low serum iron contributing to an increased proportion of unbound transferrin, but the liver is also producing more transferrin.

    Ferritin is the storage form of iron, particularly in the liver and bone marrow. Ferritin levels closely parallel the body stores of iron, such that in conditions of iron deficiency, ferritin is low, whereas in conditions of iron overload (e.g., hemochromatosis), ferritin is high.

CASE 12-3 continued:

This woman has not had a colonoscopy in 15 years. When asked, she admits to seeing some blood in her stool recently but had assumed it had been from hemorrhoids. You do a rectal examination but find no hemorrhoids. Fecal occult blood test is positive.

5. **What is the cause of her iron deficiency anemia?**

    Blood loss through the intestinal tract is the cause. In any older patient with iron deficiency anemia, you should always consider an intestinal bleed with colon cancer as the cause until proven otherwise.

CASE 12-3 continued:

A colonoscopy is performed, and a necrotic mass is visualized and removed. Pathologic diagnosis is reported as adenocarcinoma.

6. **Suppose this woman were 30 years old and workup was negative for intestinal bleeding. What would be the most likely cause of her anemia?**

    In a woman of reproductive age, iron deficiency is usually due to menorrhagia (severe bleeding during menstruation) or pregnancy (though this is physiologic and due to expansion of plasma volume to greater than that of RBCs).

7. **Iron exists in many forms in the body and is used from heme synthesis for red blood cells. How is dietary iron absorbed?**

    Dietary iron is primarily absorbed in the proximal duodenum, where the acidic pH and presence of ferric reductase enzyme facilitate the conversion of ferric iron (Fe^{3+}) to ferrous iron (Fe^{2+}), which is more rapidly absorbed by enterocytes. Dietary iron is then transported into the circulation by the transmembrane protein ferroportin. Within the circulation, iron is complexed with transferrin, which is secreted by the liver. Transferrin delivers iron to all cells of the body where iron is then stored intracellularly complexed to the iron-storage protein ferritin. You may see this storage form of iron referred to as hemosiderin.

8. **Which factors increase or decrease dietary iron absorption?**

    Increased absorption: organic iron, ferrous iron, acids (e.g., citrate), low iron stores, high erythropoietin, pregnancy

    Decreased absorption: inorganic iron, ferric iron, alkali (e.g., phosphates), high iron stores, low erythropoietin, infection, tannins (i.e., excessive tea drinking)

Iron absorption is regulated by the protein hepcidin, which is encoded by a gene involved in the maintenance of iron homeostasis. Hepcidin downregulates ferroportin expression on enterocytes. When iron stores in the body are high, hepcidin expression increases and iron absorption decreases secondary to ferroportin downregulation. When iron stores are low, hepcidin production is decreased.

CASE 12-3 continued:

Suppose this woman had a history of *Helicobacter pylori* infection and came to the emergency department with a rapidly bleeding peptic ulcer. She is found to have a hemoglobin of 8.1 g/dL with an MCV of 81 fL.

9. **How would the temporal course of an intestinal bleed affect whether the anemia will be normocytic or microcytic?**
   With a significant intestinal bleed that rapidly changes the hematocrit (without depressing bodily iron stores), the anemia will initially be normochromic and normocytic, but as enough iron is lost, it will evolve to hypochromic and microcytic.

CASE 12-3 continued:

Now suppose a different woman was brought in by ambulance from the scene of an auto accident. Heart rate is 120 beats/min and blood pressure is 80/50 mm Hg. An ultrasound shows splenic rupture and intra-abdominal bleeding, and the woman is taken to the operating room for laparotomy.

10. **Would you expect her hematocrit to be low, normal, or high and why?**
    Hematocrit is the percentage of blood volume occupied by RBCs, and with a rapid bleed, this remains unchanged. The hematocrit would be normal because with a rapid hemorrhage, she is losing plasma and RBCs together.

SUMMARY BOX: IRON DEFICIENCY ANEMIA

Anemia is due to decreased iron stores because iron is needed for hemoglobin synthesis.

- Common causes: blood loss from (slow) intestinal bleeding or menorrhagia, malnutrition (iron deficiency in diet), pregnancy
- Symptoms: increased fatigue and dyspnea
- Physical examination findings in severe deficiency:
  - Glossitis: redness, swelling, and loss of papillae on the tongue*
  - Angular cheilosis: cracks at the corners of the mouth
  - Koilonychia: spoon nails
  - Esophageal web*
  - Pica: eating clay or ice
- Laboratory tests: low hemoglobin, low mean corpuscular volume (MCV), low serum iron, low ferritin, high total iron-binding capacity (TIBC)
- Treatment: iron replacement

*Note that the triad of iron deficiency, esophageal web, and atrophic glossitis is referred to as Plummer-Vinson syndrome.

CASE 12-4

A 42-year-old woman with rheumatoid arthritis comes into your office complaining of increasing fatigue and shortness of breath with exertion. Her CBC shows a microcytic anemia.

1. **What is the differential diagnosis for microcytic anemia?**
Iron deficiency anemia, sideroblastic anemia, lead poisoning, thalassemia, and anemia of chronic disease are all considered.

CASE 12-4 continued:

Iron studies reveal low serum Fe, elevated serum ferritin, and reduced TIBC.

2. **What is your diagnosis now?**
Anemia of chronic disease secondary to rheumatoid arthritis typically presents as a mild hypochromic anemia, although it can also be normochromic and normocytic.

3. **Why is ferritin elevated in this woman while serum iron is low?**
The chronic inflammatory response results in large amounts of hepcidin, which sequesters iron, resulting in reduced levels of plasma iron. Bodily stores of iron are normal but unavailable for erythropoiesis. This is shown by the normal ferritin levels. Ferritin is an intracellular storage form of iron. Ferritin levels closely parallel body stores of iron. Therefore, ferritin levels are low in iron deficiency anemia but normal to high in anemia of chronic disease. Ferritin levels may be elevated above normal in anemia of chronic disease because ferritin is an acute phase reactant that is secreted by the liver in inflammatory conditions.
   Note: The postulated reason for iron sequestration in states of chronic inflammation is that this is the body's automatic attempt to prevent microbes that have potentially invaded the host from acquiring iron required for their growth.

CASE 12-4 continued:

Transferrin saturation is reduced.

4. **Why are transferrin saturation *and* total iron-binding capacity reduced?**
Transferrin is secreted by the liver and binds iron in the bloodstream. TIBC is actually a measure of transferrin that is not bound to iron. The mechanism of low TIBC in anemia of chronic disease is not actually known but it is postulated that the chronic inflammatory response decreases transferrin production by the liver. In addition, the elevated levels of hepcidin sequesters iron in the bloodstream resulting in reduced transferrin saturation with iron.

CASE 12-4 continued:

Further history reveals that she has had rheumatoid arthritis for 10 years that has been moderately controlled on methotrexate and nonsteroidal anti-inflammatory drugs (NSAIDs).

5. **What do you have to rule out as a cause for her anemia based on this additional information?**
NSAIDs can cause gastric ulcers and upper intestinal bleeding. In a patient chronically on NSAIDs, you have to rule out bleeding and resultant iron deficiency as a cause for her anemia. This can be done with an occult blood test or upper endoscopy if suspicion is high enough. Methotrexate can suppress the bone marrow, resulting in a pancytopenia. This can be ruled out with a CBC by looking at all three cell lines (i.e., RBCs, WBCs, and platelets).

6. **Why does her long-standing inflammatory condition predispose her to developing anemia?**

Chronic inflammatory disorders with systemic involvement result in elevated plasma levels of many cytokines. These cytokines increase the phagocytic activity of immune cells, particularly in the spleen, resulting in increased phagocytic destruction of RBCs and a decrease in RBC life span. Additionally, these cytokines inhibit the secretion of erythropoietin, which normally stimulates erythropoiesis in the bone marrow. Another contributing factor is that hepcidin, which is released by inflammatory cells, binds serum iron and makes it unavailable for erythropoiesis. Although anemia of chronic disease is typically mild, if it is severe, these patients respond well to exogenously-administered erythropoietin.

7. **If this woman had heavy menses or heme-positive stool, you would be worried about iron deficiency anemia. How would you differentiate between anemia of chronic disease and iron deficiency anemia on the basis of serum iron, TIBC, ferritin, transferrin saturation, and bone marrow iron stores?**

Table 12-2 compares the values of these tests for both types of anemia.

TABLE 12-2. DIFFERENTIATION OF ANEMIA OF CHRONIC DISEASE AND IRON DEFICIENCY ANEMIA

Study	Characteristic Result	
	Anemia of Chronic Disease	Iron Deficiency Anemia
Serum iron	Low	Low
TIBC	Low to normal	High
Ferritin	Normal to high	Low
Percent transferrin saturation	Low	Low
Bone marrow iron stores	High	Low

STEP 1 SECRET

The information listed in Table 12-2 is particularly high yield for boards.

SUMMARY BOX: ANEMIA OF CHRONIC DISEASE

- Typically, seen as mild anemia in patients with chronic inflammatory conditions including rheumatologic diseases, malignancy, and infections such as tuberculosis and endocarditis

- Characterized by a functional iron deficiency: impairment of iron mobilization despite sufficient iron stores

- Symptoms: fatigue, dyspnea on exertion, symptoms of the underlying condition

- Laboratory tests: low serum iron and low total iron-binding capacity (TIBC), elevated ferritin

- Treatment: severe anemia (rare) responds well to exogenous erythropoietin; treat underlying condition

CASE 12-5

A 65-year-old man with a history of chronic gastritis presents with increasing fatigue and a tingling sensation in his toes for the last few months. CBC reveals hemoglobin of 9.5 g/dL and an MCV of 110 fL.

1. **What is the differential diagnosis for a macrocytic anemia?**
   Vitamin B_{12} deficiency, folate deficiency, liver disease, alcohol, drugs, and myelodysplastic syndromes are considered in this situation.

CASE 12-5 continued:

Further workup reveals a low reticulocyte count and a peripheral smear showing hypersegmented neutrophils (Fig. 12-3).

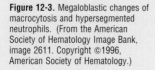

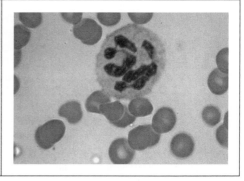

Figure 12-3. Megaloblastic changes of macrocytosis and hypersegmented neutrophils. (From the American Society of Hematology Image Bank, image 2611. Copyright ©1996, American Society of Hematology.)

2. **What is the probable diagnosis and what is the underlying disorder in this man's case?**
   He has vitamin B_{12} deficiency secondary to chronic gastritis.

STEP 1 SECRET

Figure 12-3 is particularly high-yield for boards. You should automatically associate hypersegmented neutrophils with vitamin B_{12} or folate deficiency.

3. **What are the some of the other causes of this deficiency?**
   Strict vegan diets are generally lacking in vitamin B_{12}. Also, malabsorption of vitamin B_{12} may be due to ileal resection, bacterial overgrowth, celiac sprue, Crohn's disease, or *Diphyllobothrium latum* (fish tapeworm) infection.

4. **Why are there hypersegmented neutrophils? Low reticulocyte count?**
   Remember from biochemistry that vitamin B_{12} (cyanocobalamin) is required for nucleic acid synthesis and recycling of tetrahydrofolate (THF). Why, then, do the neutrophils appear to have more genetric material than normal? Without proper DNA synthesis, the cells cannot progress

through the cell cycle from the G_2 (growth) phase to the mitosis phase. Therefore, the cells continually grow without division, leading to macrocytosis and hypersegmentation of the nuclear material. This is particularly prominent (and diagnostic!) in megaloblastic anemia. Beware, however, that this is not specific for only vitamin B_{12} deficiency, as folate deficiency will present with identical histologic findings!

Because the cells cannot progress through mitosis, rapidly dividing cell lines, especially the erythrocyte lineage, will be unable to keep up a normal synthesis rate. Reticulocytosis, the normal physiologic response to anemia, cannot occur. Remember, vitamin B_{12} is important for precursor cell synthesis, too! Thus, the reticulocyte count is low.

STEP 1 SECRET

Review the role of vitamin B_{12} and folate in biochemical pathways how and pay particular attention to defects in the pathways lead to disease. The USMLE loves crossovers from biochemistry into pathophysiology. Remember that most questions on your exam will be second- and third-order as well as interdisciplinary!

CASE 12-5 continued:

An upper endoscopy and gastric biopsy show chronic inflammation of the mucosal lining of the gastric fundus.

6. **What is the pathogenesis of this man's vitamin B_{12} deficiency?**
Chronic gastritis, either autoimmune or idiopathic in origin, results in destruction of gastric parietal cells that are found primarily in the fundus of the stomach (i.e., atrophic gastritis). Parietal cells normally produce intrinsic factor, which facilitates vitamin B_{12} absorption from the terminal ileum. Loss of parietal cells and thus intrinsic factor prevents adequate vitamin B_{12} absorption.

7. **Explain how vitamin B_{12} is absorbed from the intestine.**
Intrinsic factor produced by parietal cells of the gastric fundus binds dietary vitamin B_{12} in the intestinal tract. Pancreatic enzymes facilitate the absorption of vitamin B_{12} bound to intrinsic factor in the terminal ileum.

8. **What are the normal functions of vitamin B_{12} and how do these functions relate to the clinical signs and symptoms of vitamin B_{12} deficiency?**
Vitamin B_{12} is involved in two enzymatic reactions, one that catalyzes the conversion of both homocysteine to methionine and of methyltetrahydrofolate to THF, and another that catalyzes the conversion of methylmalonic acid to succinyl coenzyme A. The anemia is believed to be due to reduced levels of THF, the form of folic acid involved in DNA synthesis. The neuropathy that develops in vitamin B_{12} deficiency is thought to be due to a deficiency of methionine, because methionine serves as a precursor for S-adenosylmethionine, which is involved in the synthesis of various myelin proteins and phospholipids. Decreased myelination of the dorsal and lateral columns results in decreased vibration sense, decreased proprioception, gait apraxia, paresthesias, incontinence, and impotence. Anemia always precedes neurologic symptoms in vitamin B_{12} deficiency (Fig. 12-4).
Note: Any patient, particularly an elderly patient, presenting with symptoms of anemia and neurologic disturbance (either peripheral neural symptoms or altered mental status) must be evaluated for vitamin B_{12} deficiency. Though folate deficiency presents with an identical histologic picture, folate deficiency is not associated with neurologic dysfunction in patients after

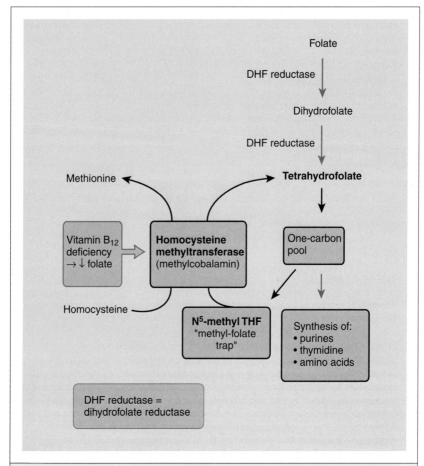

Figure 12-4. Role of folate and vitamin B_{12}. The only way to re-form tetrahydrofolate is via vitamin B_{12}–dependent synthesis of methionine: the methionine salvage pathway. (From Clark A: Crash Course: Metabolism and Nutrition. Philadelphia, WB Saunders, 2005.)

birth. Remember, folate deficiency is associated with defects in neural tube closure in utero and may present as spina bifida, myelomeningocele, or rarely anencephaly.

CASE 12-5 continued:

You do a Schilling test, which confirms your diagnosis of pernicious anemia.

9. **What is pernicious anemia? How does the Schilling test work?**
   Pernicious anemia is the autoimmune destruction of parietal cells in the gastric fundus. This leads to decreased production of intrinsic factor and therefore decreased vitamin B_{12} absorption in the terminal ileum.
   The Schilling test is no longer widely used owing to concerns about use of radiation. However, this test nicely demonstrates the pathophysiology of vitamin B_{12} deficiency due to inadequate intrinsic factor production:

- Step 1: Unlabeled vitamin B_{12} is given parenterally to saturate the cobalamin receptors such that when vitamin B_{12} is given orally a significant portion that is absorbed will be excreted in the urine.
- Step 2: Radioactively labeled vitamin B_{12} is given orally.
- Step 3: The amount of labeled vitamin B_{12} is measured in a 24-hour urine sample. If less than 10% of the amount that was administered orally is found in the urine, this indicates poor absorption of vitamin B_{12} in the intestine, as the vitamin B_{12} must be absorbed into the body in the small intestine to be later excreted by the kidney.
- Step 4: Repeat the test with the addition of exogenous intrinsic factor. If pernicious anemia is the cause of vitamin B_{12} deficiency, intrinsic factor will correct vitamin B_{12} absorption.

10. **What is the treatment for pernicious anemia?**
For serious deficiencies, vitamin B_{12} is given in weekly intramuscular injections in dosages as high as 1000 μg. This regimen may need to be continued or may be tapered to less frequent injections if the patient's vitamin B_{12} level normalizes. Oral therapy requires dosages of 1000 μg to 2000 μg to ensure adequate absorption. Remember, oral therapy must not be used for patients with autoimmune pernicious anemia because vitamin B_{12} will not be absorbed without intrinsic factor! Also, because vitamin B_{12} is water-soluble, overdose is not usually a concern.

11. **Suppose this man had a history of chronic pancreatitis and the addition of intrinsic factor did not increase vitamin B_{12} absorption. What would you do now to confirm a diagnosis?**
The next step would be to deliver exogenous pancreatic enzymes and see if this corrected the vitamin B_{12} absorption. Finally, if this did not work, you could treat the patient with 4 weeks of tetracycline and readminister the test. If this helped to increase vitamin B_{12} absorption, the presumed diagnosis would be bacterial overgrowth.

12. **Folate deficiency can present similarly to vitamin B_{12} deficiency but with some key differences. Which symptoms of vitamin B_{12} deficiency are *not* found with folate deficiency?**
Folate deficiency does *not* cause neurologic symptoms. Both vitamin B_{12} and folate deficiency show a macrocytic anemia with large, hypersegmented neutrophils, low reticulocyte count, and increased L-lactate dehydrogenase (LDH).

13. **What are some of the causes of folate deficiency?**
Deficient intake (common in alcoholics and the elderly who typically lack green, leafy vegetables in their diets), pregnancy (due to increased folate requirement), and certain drugs (methotrexate, phenytoin) that interfere with folate-dependent biochemical pathways can cause folate deficiency.

14. **What is the best blood test to determine folate deficiency?**
The best indicator of chronic folate deficiency is the total RBC folate level. This test indicates overall storage levels of folate, whereas serum folate is just a snapshot in time. For example, if the patient just ate a big spinach salad (rich in folate), serum folate could be normal because of the meal, but the storage level may still be depleted.

16. Cover each column of Table 12-3 and try to fill in the remaining information for yourself.

TABLE 12-3. VITAMIN B₁₂ AND FOLATE DEFICIENCY

Feature	Vitamin B₁₂	Folate
Food sources	Animal products	Vegetables
Stores	Long term, 2-12 years	Short term, 4-5 months
Water-soluble	Yes	Yes
Site and mechanism of absorption	Terminal ileum Absorbed with intrinsic factor	Duodenum and proximal jejunum Deconjugation of polyglutamate
Function	Cofactor for enzymatic reactions important for DNA synthesis and myelination	1-carbon carrier
Dietary deficiency	Uncommon—occurs with vegan diet	Common—occurs in alcoholics; a leafy green salad will increase serum levels but not RBC folate, so testing for both is required
Neurologic damage	Yes—dorsal columns–medial lemniscus, leading to decreased vibratory and joint position sense	No

SUMMARY BOX: VITAMIN B₁₂ AND FOLATE DEFICIENCIES

Vitamin B₁₂ Deficiency

- Megaloblastic anemia

- Etiology: inadequate intake, pernicious anemia, malabsorption

- Pathophysiology: deficiency of intrinsic factor prevents adequate vitamin B₁₂ absorption

- Symptoms: glossitis, gastric atrophy, neurologic symptoms (decreased vibratory and joint position sense)

- Laboratory tests/diagnosis: macrocytosis, large hypersegmented neutrophils, increased L-lactate dehydrogenase (LDH), positive Schilling test

- Treatment: parenteral or intramuscular vitamin B₁₂ weekly until levels are normal

Folate Deficiency

- Megaloblastic anemia

- Etiology: deficiency intake, pregnancy, drugs

- Symptoms: fatigue, pallor, dyspnea on exertion

- Laboratory tests/diagnosis: macrocytosis with low reticulocyte count, increased LDH, neutropenia, hypersegmented neutrophils, thrombocytopenia

- Treatment: parenteral folic acid after confirmation of the diagnosis. Folic acid is contraindicated in vitamin B_{12} deficiency because it masks the anemia although the neurologic symptoms will progress.

CASE 12-6

An 8-year-old white boy is brought to your office by his mother for evaluation of fatigue and pallor. CBC shows hemoglobin of 7.2 g/dL, MCV of 80 fL, and a reticulocyte count of 11%. Total bilirubin is 2.0 mg/dL.

1. **What is the differential diagnosis for a normocytic anemia?**
   Hemolytic anemia (autoimmune, drug-induced, traumatic, hereditary), hemoglobinopathies, aplastic anemia, myelodysplasia, hypothyroidism, and anemia of chronic disease could cause normocytic anemia.

CASE 12-6 continued:

Both of the boy's parents are currently healthy, but the father did have a splenectomy years ago for "some type of anemia."

2. **How does this change your differential diagnosis?**
   With a possible family history of anemia, you should focus your diagnosis on genetic causes of anemia. Hereditary spherocytosis, G6PD deficiency, sickle cell anemia, and pyruvate kinase deficiency are all options. To help navigate the many genetic causes of anemia, identify the inheritance pattern presented in the family. G6PD is X-linked. Remember, by definition, X-linked diseases are never passed from father to son! Pyruvate kinase deficiency is autosomal recessive, so even though his father is "affected," his mother would also have had to be a carrier of this rare condition. This seems unlikely, although not impossible. Sickle cell anemia, another autosomal recessive condition, presents similar genetic implausibility. Also, the boy is white, making this a much more rare possibility. Hereditary spherocytosis, an autosomal dominant condition, would typically present with this pedigree of affected father and son. Also, this disease is quite common among individuals of Northern European descent. Hereditary spherocytosis just jumped to the top of the differential diagnosis list!

STEP 1 SECRET

Inheritance patterns of genetic diseases are very important (and high-yield!) for Step 1. Taking the time to distinguish between diseases with similar presentations but different genetic pedigrees may often unlock a diagnosis for you. Once again, pay special attention to diseases that affect particular ethnic, racial, or age groups. Although never an absolute, these demographic clues may also point you in the right direction of diagnosis. You are expected to know the inheritance patterns of diseases commonly tested on the USMLE. This information is nicely organized in First Aid.

CASE 12-6 continued:

A peripheral blood smear shows spherical RBCs that lack central pallor as well as Howell-Jolly bodies (Fig. 12-5). A laboratory test using test tubes filled with solutions of increasing salt concentration reveals an abnormally increased osmotic fragility of RBCs.

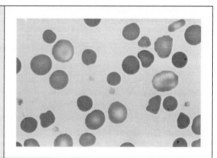

Figure 12-5. Hereditary spherocytosis (peripheral smear). (Courtesy of Dr. Robert W. McKenna, Department of Pathology, University of Texas Southwestern Medical School, Dallas, TX.)

3. **What is the diagnosis?**
   The boy has hereditary spherocytosis.

4. **What is the etiology of this condition and why do the red blood cells assume a spherical conformation?**
   Most commonly, hereditary spherocytosis is caused by dysfunction of the protein spectrin, a cytoskeletal protein that provides stability and plasticity to the plasma membrane of RBCs. In order for spectrin to function appropriately, it must interact with other cytoskeletal proteins, such as ankyrin and protein 4.1. Therefore, mutations in genes other than the spectrin can also compromise spectrin function. Any of these mutations can destabilize the RBC membrane and cause the cells to assume a spherical shape. In the absence of the normal biconcave shape, the degree of central pallor created by hemoglobin displacement to the periphery (normally ~⅓ of the diameter of the RBC) is markedly reduced. This spherical conformation minimizes the surface area to volume ratio of the RBCs. This shape is not as easily distorted in small capillaries as the biconcave shape, making these cells prone to mechanical hemolysis when squeezing through small vessels. Also as a result of the unstable membrane, these RBCs swell and burst when placed in increasingly hypotonic salt solutions as water rushes intracellularly. This is the basis for the positive osmotic fragility test, which is diagnostic for hereditary spherocytosis.

CASE 12-6 continued:

Physical examination is notable for pallor, mild jaundice, and splenomegaly. You perform both direct and indirect Coombs' tests on this patient's blood. As expected, both are negative.

5. **How do these Coombs' tests work? Why are they both negative?**
   The direct Coombs' test looks for antigens *on* the patient's RBCs. The indirect Coombs' test checks for antibodies to RBCs in the patient's serum. Both Coombs' tests are assays for antibodies in the plasma or antigens on the RBC surface that lead to an intravascular hemolysis due to antigen-antibody interaction. In hereditary spherocytosis, you would not expect an immune process

to be a primary cause of RBC destruction. Instead, the abnormal RBCs are sequestered in the spleen due to their lack of distensibility and as a result are subject to extravascular hemolysis.

More detailed information about direct and indirect Coombs' tests can be found in Chapter 15.

6. **Why is splenomegaly seen in this condition?**
   During their normal course through the spleen, RBCs must undergo impressive conformational changes in order to exit the splenic cords (i.e., cords of Billroth) and enter the splenic sinusoids. Spherical RBCs are much less able to undergo this conformational change than are normal biconcave RBCs. As a result, spherocytes obstruct the splenic cords, resulting in splenomegaly. They are ultimately phagocytosed by the splenic macrophages at an abnormally high rate, leading to anemia.

7. **You refer this boy to a pediatric surgeon for a therapeutic splenectomy to treat his anemia. Why does taking out his spleen help with his symptoms?**
   Although splenectomy does not fix the fundamental defect in these RBCs, it does prevent the anemia. Removing the spleen prevents the high rate of extravascular hemolysis that causes the anemia seen in this condition.

8. **What infections is this boy at risk for after splenectomy and how would you help to prevent them?**
   Infections by encapsulated bacteria (e.g., *S. pneumoniae, H. influenzae, Neisseria meningitidis*). Infection by all three of these bacteria can be prevented with vaccinations, which this boy should receive after splenectomy.

CASE 12-6 continued:

About 20 years later, this same patient is seen in a local emergency department with colicky right upper quadrant pain that increases after eating. He has a positive Murphy's sign.

9. **What is your diagnosis? Why is this patient at increased risk for this condition?**
   Cholecystitis. Patients with hereditary spherocytosis are at increased risk for gallstones due to hemolysis and development of bilirubin (pigment) stones in the bile duct system. As expected, the incidence of bilirubin stone formation will be much lower if a splenectomy is performed to decrease the rate of hemolysis. However, given the relative fragility of spherocytes, postsplenectomy patients still have a moderately increased rate of hemolysis. Thus, elevated indirect bilirubin can predispose to bilirubin (pigmented) gallstones.

SUMMARY BOX: HEREDITARY SPHEROCYTOSIS

- Defect in red blood cell membrane protein (spectrin or ankyrin) causing abnormally shaped erythrocytes. Red blood cells (RBCs) become sequestered in the spleen and hemolyzed.

- Genetics: autosomal dominant

- Symptoms: hemolysis (elevated bilirubin and haptoglobin, jaundice), splenomegaly, gallstones, family history

- Laboratory tests: increased osmotic fragility, spherocytes on peripheral smear, reticulocytosis, hyperbilirubinemia

- Treatment: splenectomy + vaccination for *Streptococcus pneumoniae, Haemophilus influenzae, Neisseria meningitidis*

CASE 12-7

A 28-year-old African-American man is planning to travel to India for work. He is given quinidine for antimalarial prophylaxis. Several days later he becomes fatigued, and a workup reveals a normocytic anemia.

1. **What is the differential diagnosis for a normocytic anemia?**
   Hemolytic anemia (autoimmune, drug-induced, traumatic, hereditary), hemoglobinopathies, aplastic anemia, myelodysplasia, and hypothyroidism should be considered.

CASE 12-7 continued:

Peripheral smear is notable for Heinz bodies (Fig. 12-6).

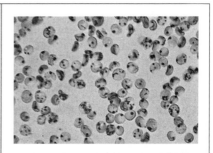

Figure 12-6. Heinz bodies. (From McPherson RA, Pincus MR: Henry's Clinical Diagnosis and Management by Laboratory Methods, 21st ed. Philadelphia, WB Saunders, 2006.)

2. **What is the likely diagnosis?**
   G6PD deficiency is caused by reduced activity of G6PD, which catalyzes the rate-limiting step in the hexose monophosphate pathway. G6PD deficiency is an inherited, X-linked recessive disorder. It most commonly affects men of African, Asian, and Mediterranean descent. It is the most common inherited hemolytic anemia and it is thought that, as in sickle cell anemia, mutations in the G6PD gene create a selective advantage to heterozygotes by creating a poor habitat in RBCs for the malarial merozoite.

3. **What are Heinz bodies and how are they formed?**
   Oxidation of the sulfhydryl groups on hemoglobin results in clumping and precipitation of hemoglobin within the cytoplasm of RBCs. These deposits of insoluble hemoglobin are referred to as inclusion bodies or Heinz bodies. These inclusion bodies are then removed by splenic macrophages as these RBCs pass through the splenic cords, producing so-called bite cells (Fig. 12-7).

4. **What is the normal function of the hexose monophosphate shunt in red blood cells?**
   In RBCs, the hexose monophosphate shunt (pentose phosphate pathway) is used primarily to generate the reduced form of nicotinamide adenine dinucleotide phosphate (NADPH). The NADPH generated recycles glutathione (via reduction of oxidized glutathione), and the glutathione is involved in combating oxidative damage by reactive oxygen species. Failure of this pathway results in the inability of RBCs to handle increased oxidative stresses and predisposes RBCs to intravascular hemolysis.

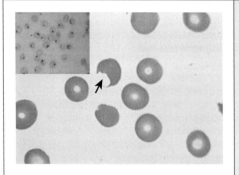

Figure 12-7. Peripheral blood smear in glucose-6-phosphate dehydrogenase deficiency. The arrow shows a bite cell with part of the red blood cell membrane removed. The inset shows a peripheral blood smear with a supravital stain visualizing punctate inclusions representing denatured hemoglobin (Heinz bodies). (From Kumar V, Fausto N, Abbas A: Robbins and Cotran Pathologic Basis of Disease, 7th ed. Philadelphia, WB Saunders, 2004, Fig. 13-8; inset from Wickramasinghe SN, McCullough J: Blood and Bone Marrow Pathology. London, Churchill Livingstone, 2003, Fig. 8-8.)

CASE 12–7 continued:

On examination you note scleral icterus and splenomegaly. Total bilirubin is elevated. Urinalysis is notable for gross blood, high urine sodium, and muddy brown granular casts.

5. **Is this man's hyperbilirubinemia most likely caused by conjugated or unconjugated bilirubin?**
   Hyperbilirubinemia can be broken down into prehepatic, hepatic, or posthepatic origin. Hemolytic anemia is a prehepatic cause of elevated bilirubin and would therefore be expected to be composed largely of unconjugated (indirect) bilirubin. The increased RBC breakdown results in the release of greater than average amounts of hemoglobin breakdown products, bilirubin, into the blood. This hemoglobin must circulate to the liver to be processed by the liver. This processing includes conjugating the bilirubin to protein, making the compound water-soluble and therefore easily excreted by the kidneys.
   For more information about causes of hyperbilirubinemia, refer to Chapter 7.

6. **Are his haptoglobin levels likely to be high or low?**
   Haptoglobin is a plasma protein that sequesters free heme in the circulation. Therefore, levels of haptoglobin would be reduced as it gets consumed by the large amount of free heme generated via oxidative damage and intravascular RBC lysis.

7. **What renal diagnosis does his urinalysis reveal and why is this occurring? What is his prognosis?**
   Gross blood, high urine sodium, and muddy brown casts are red flags for damage to the renal architecture. Specifically, muddy brown casts on urinalysis (UA) are diagnostic for acute tubular necrosis (ATN). In ATN, the acute drop in hemoglobin due to hemolysis causes ischemia and necrosis of the epithelial lining of the renal tubules. Without the epithelial lining, gross blood escapes into the urinary space and concentrating ability is lost, leading to high urine sodium. The muddy brown casts are composed of the necrosed, sloughed-off tubular epithelial cells passed into the urine. Prognosis is very good as long as the tubular basement membrane is intact. His renal function would be expected to recover within 1 to 2 weeks as the epithelial lining regenerates.

CASE 12-7 continued:

You obtain some further history and discover that the patient once remembers having blood in his urine when he was a child after eating some fava beans.

8. **What is the offending agent in this situation? What are some other offenders?**
    Many agents and compounds can trigger a hemolytic event in an individual with G6PD due to increased reactive oxygen species and oxidative stress. Many drugs can precipitate hemolysis because of oxidant stress, including isoniazid, sulfonamides, primaquine, ciprofloxacin, NSAIDs, nitrofurantoin, vitamin C (acids), and trimethoprim-sulfamethoxazole. Certain foods, such as fava beans, and infections can also precipitate hemolysis. Individuals with G6PD must be very closely monitored during infections, especially urinary tract infections, as many of the commonly prescribed medications for *Escherichia coli* cystitis are included in the preceding list of contraindicated medications due to increased risk of hemolysis.

STEP 1 SECRET

The classic clinical vignette on boards for glucose-6-phosphate dehydrogenase (G6PD) deficiency is a black individual who serves as a missionary worker in a remote area and is treated for malaria prior to the appearance of hemolytic anemia. However, be on the lookout for some of these other pharmacologic triggers of hemolysis in G6PD-deficient patients.

9. **What is the treatment for this man's condition?**
    For the USMLE, always consider the least invasive intervention first. In this case, the oxidant stressor (quinidine) must be immediately discontinued to prevent additional hemolysis. Hydration with normal saline may be necessary to keep intravascular volume up. Consider a packed RBC transfusion if the patient is hypoxemic *and* symptomatic. Acute crises will resolve spontaneously in about 1 week as new erythrocytes are produced with increased G6PD activity.

CASE 12-7 continued:

Two days later this man's hemoglobin is still 9.7 g/dL, but his MCV is now 95 fL.

10. **Why might the mean corpuscular volume be slightly elevated in this man and how does this reflect the self-limited nature of this hemolytic anemia?**
    A compensatory erythrocytosis in response to hemolysis produces increased numbers of circulating reticulocytes, which are premature RBCs that are much larger than mature RBCs. This explains the increased MCV, which is a reflection of RBC size. Furthermore, it turns out that G6PD activity in reticulocytes is much higher than in mature RBCs. A somewhat selective destruction of older RBCs therefore occurs in G6PD-deficient patients who are exposed to oxidative stress. This helps to limit the nature of the hemolytic crisis, even if mild exposure to the oxidative stressor continues.

11. **Suppose this man presented with a similar episode but also complained of severe back and abdominal pain. What would you be concerned about in this case and why?**
    Mesenteric ischemia and renal ischemia can often be complications of acute hemolytic crises in G6PD-deficient patients because their hemoglobin drops too rapidly for compensation to take

place. Treatment is supportive unless signs of peritonitis develop, in which case the patient may require surgery to remove potentially necrotic bowel.

SUMMARY BOX: GLUCOSE-6-PHOSPHATE DEHYDROGENASE DEFICIENCY

- Cause: enzyme defect in the hexose monophosphate pathway resulting in hemolysis when exposed to oxidant stresses

- The most common metabolic disorder of red blood cells (RBCs)

- X-linked disorder; affects Asian, African, Mediterranean men

- Precipitants: infection, acidosis, antimalarial drugs, sulfa drugs, fava beans

- Symptoms: jaundice, dark urine, acute tubular necrosis (ATN), anemia, organomegaly from chronic hemolysis

- Complications: mesenteric and renal ischemia

- Laboratory tests: low hemoglobin and increased reticulocytes, low haptoglobin, high L-lactate dehydrogenase (LDH), elevated bilirubin (indirect), negative Coombs' tests, urinalysis (UA) showing hemoglobinuria and muddy brown granular casts

- Treatment: supportive—removal of the offending agent, administration of fluids and transfusion if necessary

CASE 12-8

A 1-day-old newborn has jaundice that started on his face and spread to his body. Physical examination reveals scleral icterus and conjunctival pallor and hepatosplenomegaly. There is no cephalohematoma. Delivery was uneventful except for the finding that the placenta was moderately enlarged.

1. What are some causes of jaundice in the neonate?
   Infection, physiologic jaundice, intestinal obstruction, inborn errors of metabolism, and hemolytic disease of the newborn can cause jaundice.

2. What is the most serious complication of neonatal jaundice and how does it develop?
   Kernicterus is the deposition of insoluble unconjugated bilirubin in the brain, which can cause brain damage (particularly in the basal ganglia and hippocampus). Early signs include lethargy, poor feeding, vomiting, and hypotonia. Later symptoms include irritability, hypertonia, seizures, and deafness. Infants with their first case of jaundice are at highest risk for kernicterus. Risk factors include prematurity, sepsis, Asian ancestry, hemolytic disease, and high altitude.

CASE 12-8 continued:

Laboratory tests are significant for a hemoglobin of 12 g/dL (low for a newborn!) and a marked reticulocytosis and elevated indirect bilirubin. A direct Coombs' test is positive. Blood typing reveals that the mother is Rh-negative, the father is Rh-positive, and the baby is Rh-positive.

3. **What is your diagnosis? What is the pathophysiology of this disease?**
   Hemolytic disease of the newborn due to Rh incompatibility. Parental heterozygosity allows an Rh-positive infant to be carried by an Rh-negative mother. Maternal blood comes into contact with fetal blood cells, and maternal antibodies are produced against the Rh antigen present on the fetal blood cell surface. During a subsequent pregnancy with an Rh-positive fetus, maternal IgG antibodies can cross the placenta and bind to fetal RBCs, leading to hemolysis via opsonization and complement-mediated destruction. Destruction of fetal RBCs causes increased unconjugated bilirubin in the fetal circulation, which is metabolized by the placenta while the fetus is still in utero. After delivery, however, the infant must process the unconjugated bilirubin in his own immature hepatocytes. Because the uridine diphosphate (UDP) glucuronyltransferase activity is not yet maximal at time of delivery, the infant is functionally incapable of handling the high bilirubin level created by the hemolytic anemia of Rh incompatibility. Severe anemia leads to extramedullary erythropoiesis, which results in hepatosplenomegaly that is potentially visible on prenatal ultrasound.

CASE 12-8 continued:

This baby has a 3-year-old sister who is also Rh-positive. She was asymptomatic as a newborn.

4. **Why was the older sister unaffected?**
   The sister was the first child and probably sensitized the mother to the Rh antigen when there was mixing of maternal and fetal blood during delivery. Sensitization caused the mother to produce anti-Rh antibodies, which can cross the placenta. Prior to her first pregnancy, the mother did not make anti-Rh antibodies, so none could cross the placenta and cause hemolysis in the first child.

5. **What should have been given to the mother prior to delivery of her first child?**
   Anti-Rh immune globulin (RhoGAM) can be given to provide the mother with passive immunity against the Rh antigen. This antibody binds to any fetal Rh antigens that may enter the maternal circulation during delivery and so prevents the mother's immune system from ever recognizing the Rh antigen. Without so-called "sensitization" of the immune system to the Rh antigen, no anti-Rh antibodies are ever synthesized. Thus, there is no anti-Rh IgG available to cross the placenta and opsonize the fetal RBCs.
   Note: RhoGAM should be given to an Rh-negative woman in any situation in which there is potential for mixing of maternal and fetal blood, including spontaneous abortions, elective abortions, and abruptio placentae (abruption placenta).

CASE 12-8 continued:

The baby is treated with phototherapy and exchange transfusions. Further testing reveals that the mother's blood type is O, the father's is A, and the baby's is A.

6. **Why is ABO incompatibility so unlikely to be the cause of hemolytic disease of the newborn?**
   Anti-A and anti-B antibodies are predominantly IgM antibodies, which cannot cross the placenta. There are also multiple other cells that express the A and B antigens in the fetus, and these cells "mop up" most of any anti-A or anti-B antibodies that cross the placenta.

7. **Suppose an Rh-positive baby born to an Rh-positive mother developed jaundice on the third day of life. What is your diagnosis now?**
   Physiologic jaundice.

8. **What is physiologic jaundice and why does it develop?**

   Physiologic jaundice results from the increased destruction of RBCs with fetal hemoglobin during the newborn period. These cells are slowly being replaced by cells with adult hemoglobin over the first 6 months of life. Normal hemoglobin in the newborn is normally 14 to 20 g/dL, which helps to compensate for the decreased partial pressure of O_2 available to fetal RBCs in utero. At birth, with the onset of respirations, erythropoiesis slows down as the relative hypoxemia is reduced. The fetal RBC also has a decreased survival rate compared with the adult RBC. Within the first 3 months, blood volume increases markedly. All of these factors lead to increased RBC destruction, a decreased hemoglobin concentration and clinically visible jaundice that peaks on days 3 to 4 of life and starts to improve by days 4 to 5. It is thought that infants who develop physiologic jaundice do not yet have the hepatic capacity to clear the excess bilirubin that forms during this period. As the activity of UDP glucuronyltransferase increases over the first weeks of life, the jaundice usually becomes self-limited. Also note that though this is a clinical condition, nearly every newborn will demonstrate a mild degree of physiologic jaundice. Phototherapy is indicated for those newborns who develop bilirubin levels >25 mg/dL, to prevent kernicterus. Specific ultraviolet (UV) wavelength light directed at the skin of these newborns allows for a conformational change in the unconjugated bilirubin that allows it to be more water-soluble, effectively "skipping" the hepatic metabolism to allow for renal excretion of the bilirubin.

SUMMARY BOX: HEMOLYTIC DISEASE OF THE NEWBORN

- Erythroblastosis fetalis

- Caused by maternal sensitization to Rh antigens in an Rh-negative mother with the production of anti-Rh antibodies, which can cross the placenta and cause hemolysis of fetal red blood cells (RBCs) in an Rh-positive infant

- Sensitization: requires previous exposure to Rh-positive blood from a first pregnancy, abortion, placental abruption, or previous transfusion

- Symptoms: large placenta, elevated indirect bilirubin, rapidly progressive jaundice after birth, hepatosplenomegaly, generalized edema (ascites, scalp fluid, purpura, cyanosis, abduction of limbs, loss of limb flexion)

- Laboratory tests: positive direct Coombs' test, hyperbilirubinemia

- Treatment: exchange transfusions to the infant

- Prophylaxis: testing the mother's blood type early in pregnancy and administering RhoGAM during and immediately after delivery to prevent alloimmunization

CASE 12-9

A 2-year-old boy is brought to your office by his mother for recurrent stomach pain that comes and goes but has been worsening over the past few weeks. Upon taking a full social history, you learn that the boy and his family recently moved into the area and are living in his grandmother's home. Because he is a new patient, you perform a full physical examination, including a CBC to rule out infection or inflammation. Pertinent findings include guaiac-negative stool. Hemoglobin is 8.5 g/dL. MCV is 75 fL. A peripheral blood smear is shown in Figure 12-8.

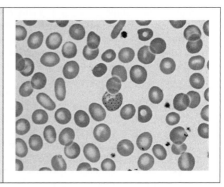

Figure 12-8. Peripheral blood smear of patient in Case 12-9. (From McPherson RA, Pincus MR: Henry's Clinical Diagnosis and Management by Laboratory Methods, 21st ed. Philadelphia, WB Saunders, 2006.)

1. **What is the likely diagnosis?**

   Lead poisoning must be ruled out in the workup of recurrent abdominal pain with anemia in a pediatric patient. In this case, we can assume that the source of the lead is from lead-based paint in the patient's new home. Remember that homes built before 1978 typically contained lead-based paint. Though the age of the house is not specifically stated, you do not need this information to suspect lead poisoning, given the laboratory tests and peripheral smear findings. The blood smear shows basophilic stippling, which is seen in lead toxicity due to accumulation of lead in the RBCs. Also, remember the general developmental milestones. A boy this age (24 months) will put everything in his mouth, including chips of paint that may be peeling.

   CASE 12-9 continued:

   The child started walking at 12 months, but recently he has become unsteady on his feet. His speech has also regressed. An x-ray film of his leg shows a thick transverse radiodense line in the metaphysis.

2. **Why is this boy ataxic?**

   Acute encephalopathy caused by the lead accumulation in neurons can lead to his unsteady gait and loss of speech. Lead poisoning blocks the function of porphobilinogen synthase leading to the accumulation of δ-aminolevulinic acid in the heme synthesis pathway. This δ-aminolevulinic acid is thought to be neurotoxic by mimicry of the function of γ-aminobutyric acid (GABA). These symptoms may be reversible with chelation of lead from the child's body if caught early, but may become irreversible if left untreated.

3. **What are the radiographic findings?**

   Lead lines are visible in areas of growth including the metaphysis of bones (Fig. 12-9). Remember, lead accumulates in rapidly dividing cells such as the metaphyses of long bones and RBCs.

4. **How does lead toxicity cause anemia?**

   Lead is a nonessential metal that binds irreversibly to sulfhydryl groups of proteins, including hemoglobin. Lead interferes with enzymes involved in heme production (porphobilinogen synthase) and impairs proper iron utilization. If functional hemoglobin cannot be produced, the patient will be functionally anemic. Treatment includes environmental control and chelation at higher lead levels with ethylenediaminetetraacetic acid (EDTA) or succimer.

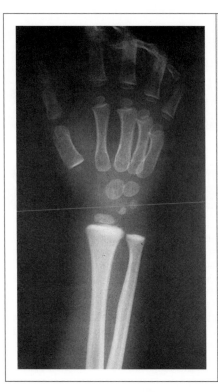

Figure 12-9. Lead lines in the distal radius. (From Ford MD, Delaney K, Ling L, Erickson T: Clinical Toxicology. Philadelphia, WB Saunders, 2001.)

STEP 1 SECRET

Signs of lead poisoning can be remembered using the mnemonic **ABCDEFG**:

Anemia
Basophilic stippling
Colicky pain
Diarrhea
Encephalopathy
Foot drop
Gums (lead line)

SUMMARY BOX: LEAD POISONING

- Variant of iron deficiency: interferes with iron utilization and hemoglobin synthesis

- Etiology: lead-containing paint, pica

- Symptoms: abdominal pain, acute encephalopathy, lead lines

- Laboratory tests: microcytic hypochromic anemia, basophilic stippling, increased serum lead level and protoporphyrin

CHAPTER 13

BLEEDING DISORDERS

Allyson M. Reid, Thomas A. Brown, MD, and Sonali J. Shah

INSIDER'S GUIDE TO BLEEDING DISORDERS FOR THE USMLE STEP 1

Bleeding disorders on the USMLE Step 1 are relatively straightforward if you understand the pathophysiology behind the diseases and correlate them with clinical findings. The best way to study for this section is to review the disorders mentioned in First Aid and be sure that you can reason through all the listed clinical findings and laboratory parameters. You should then attempt to go through these cases and create your own differential diagnosis before reviewing the answers. This will be great practice for the types of questions you will see and the thought processes that will be expected of you on boards.

In addition, pharmacology is especially important in this section. Many of the drugs that you are accountable for on boards and their associated mechanisms are listed for you in this chapter. Be sure to pay attention to pharmacologic antidotes whenever they are mentioned.

BASIC CONCEPTS

1. **Differentiate between the processes of primary and secondary hemostasis.**
   Primary hemostasis involves the formation of a temporary platelet "plug" following binding of platelets to exposed collagen, platelet secretion of procoagulant substances (e.g., adenosine diphosphate [ADP], Ca^{2+}), and platelet aggregation. This platelet plug is referred to as temporary because it is readily reversible at this stage. Secondary hemostasis involves the covalent cross-linking of fibrin between platelets, resulting in the formation of an irreversible platelet plug. This process is dependent on activation of the coagulation cascade (Table 13-1).
   Note: Disorders affecting platelet function will impair primary hemostasis, whereas disorders affecting the coagulation cascade will impair secondary hemostasis.

2. **What molecule is responsible for the binding of platelets to collagen?**
   Von Willebrand factor (vWF), which is synthesized by vascular endothelium and attaches to both collagen and platelet receptors (specifically glycoprotein Ib [GPIb]), is responsible for the binding of platelets to collagen.

3. **What constitutes the extrinsic, intrinsic, and common pathways in the coagulation cascade that forms the fibrin clot (secondary hemostasis)?**
   The extrinsic and intrinsic pathways are separate biochemical pathways that activate the coagulation cascade. Both the extrinsic and intrinsic pathways lead into the common pathway to cause formation of the fibrin clot.

TABLE 13-1. PRIMARY AND SECONDARY HEMOSTASIS

Feature	Primary Hemostasis	Secondary Hemostasis
Definition	Temporary platelet plug	Permanent platelet plug
Example disease(s)	Von Willebrand disease	Hemophilia A and B
Laboratory testing	Bleeding time, platelet aggregation studies	Prothrombin time (PT), partial thromboplastin time (PTT)
Clinical manifestations of disturbed mechanism	Relatively mild (e.g., excessive bleeding after dental work or surgery), mucocutaneous petechiae	Relatively severe (e.g., hemarthrosis)

The extrinsic pathway is referred to as "extrinsic" because the factor that activates it (tissue factor) is normally *extrinsic* to the vascular space and is exposed to the vascular space only when there is damage to the vascular endothelium that allows extracellular fluid and cells to enter. The extrinsic pathway includes tissue factor (factor III) and factor VII.

The intrinsic pathway has all of its constituents in the blood; hence, it is "intrinsic." It is activated by exposure to negatively charged foreign substances. The intrinsic pathway includes factors XII, XI, IX, and VIII.

As mentioned, the common pathway is activated by either the extrinsic pathway or intrinsic pathway, and it eventuates in the formation of a fibrin clot. This pathway includes factors X, V, II, and I (Fig. 13-1).

4. **What information can be provided by measuring the prothrombin time and activated partial thromboplastin time?**
   The prothrombin time (PT) reflects the time required for formation of a fibrin clot in a particular assay system (essentially, tissue factor is added to a sample of the patient's plasma). Because the extrinsic pathway must activate the common pathway to form a fibrin clot, the PT really reflects the time it takes for the extrinsic pathway *and* the common pathway to form the clot. The PT can be prolonged by clotting factor deficiencies in either pathway.

   The activated partial thromboplastin time (aPTT) also reflects the time required for formation of a fibrin clot in a particular assay system (in this case an activator of the intrinsic pathway is added to a sample of the patient's plasma). In other words, this value measures the time it takes the intrinsic pathway and common pathway to form a clot. The aPTT can be prolonged by clotting factor deficiencies in either the intrinsic or common pathway.

5. **What is the bleeding time? What is its clinical significance?**
   The bleeding time reflects the time required to form the platelet plug (primary hemostasis) and so reflects platelet function rather than functioning of the coagulation cascade. More commonly, however, in vitro platelet function tests are performed in place of measuring the bleeding time.

6. **What is the mechanism of action of the following drugs? How do they affect the times just discussed?**
   A. Aspirin
   Aspirin inhibits platelet function by irreversibly inhibiting the enzyme cyclooxygenase (COX), which normally functions to synthesize thromboxane A_2. Thromboxane A_2 normally functions to stimulate platelet aggregation and constriction of blood vessels, both of which act to limit bleeding

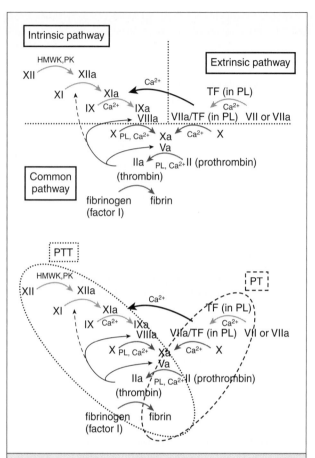

Figure 13-1. Simplified coagulation cascade. HMWK, high-molecular-weight kininogen; PK, prekallikrein; PL, plasminogen; PT, prothrombin time; PTT, partial thromboplastin time; TF, tissue factor. (From Ferri F: Ferri's Best Test: A Practical Guide to Clinical Laboratory Medicine and Diagnostic Imaging. St. Louis, Mosby, 2004.)

following vessel trauma. Consequently, inhibition of thromboxane A_2 by aspirin results in a prolonged bleeding time.

Note: Because aspirin is an irreversible inhibitor of platelet COX, its effect on platelet function lasts as long as the affected platelets remain in the circulation, ∼7 days.

B. Heparin

Heparin stimulates the activity of antithrombin III (ATIII), which is a potent inhibitor of thrombin (factor II), as well as several other factors in the intrinsic pathway. Because of this preferential inhibition of the intrinsic pathway, heparin acts rapidly to prolong the aPTT but will do so only at higher doses. It has no effect on the bleeding time because it does not affect platelet function (except in cases of heparin-induced thrombocytopenia [HIT]).

Note: Excessive bleeding from heparin toxicity can be rapidly reversed by administering protamine sulfate.

C. Warfarin

Warfarin inhibits the production of vitamin K–dependent clotting factors in the liver (factors II, VII, IX, and X) by antagonizing the action of vitamin K. It preferentially prolongs the PT more than the aPTT.

Because warfarin inhibits the *synthesis* of these clotting factors, and not their activity in the blood, there is a delay between its administration and its onset of action (typically a few days). For this reason, patients who require long-term anticoagulation are usually started on heparin and warfarin simultaneously, and once the patient is sufficiently well anticoagulated with warfarin, the heparin can be discontinued and the prothrombin time maintained within a therapeutic range.

Note: The effects of warfarin can be reversed by administering vitamin K, and this takes about a day or two. For emergent surgical procedures, fresh frozen plasma can be given to immediately replace the deficient clotting factors. Warfarin also inhibits the production of protein C and protein S, both vitamin K–dependent proteins secreted by the liver that exert *anti*coagulant effects. Consequently, inhibition of protein C and protein S synthesis by warfarin can initially result in a hypercoagulable state (in which the patient is prone to clotting). For this reason, "loading" doses of warfarin are not recommended. Instead, warfarin should be administered with heparin during the first week of therapy.

7. **What is the mechanism of action of tissue plasminogen activator?**
As its name suggests, tissue plasminogen activator (tPA) is an enzyme that activates the plasma enzyme plasminogen by converting it into its active form, plasmin. Plasmin is an enzyme that proteolytically cleaves fibrin strands, thereby degrading fibrin clots that may obstruct vessels. In addition to tPA, streptokinase and urokinase are sometimes referred to as "clot busters" (Table 13-2).

TABLE 13-2. PHARMACOTHERAPY FOR HEMOSTASIS			
Agent	Mechanism of Action	Effect on Clotting Profile	Antidote
Aspirin	Irreversibly inhibits platelet function by inhibiting thromboxane A_2 synthesis (mediated by COX)	↑ bleeding time	
Heparin	Stimulates ATIII, which inhibits the intrinsic pathway	↑ aPTT	Protamine sulfate
Warfarin	Antagonizes vitamin K, thereby interfering with production of clotting factors II, VII, IX, and X as well as the anticoagulant proteins C and S	↑ PT	Vitamin K, fresh frozen plasma
tPA	Stimulates production of plasmin, which degrades fibrin clot		Aminocaproic acid

aPTT, activated partial thromboplastin time; ATIII, antithrombin III; COX, cyclooxygenase; PT, prothrombin time; tPA, tissue plasminogen activator.

SUMMARY BOX: HEMOSTASIS, COAGULATION CASCADE, PHARMACOTHERAPY

- Primary hemostasis is the process whereby platelets adhere to the underlying collagen of damaged vascular endothelium and form a temporary platelet "plug."

- Secondary hemostasis is the process whereby these platelets are covalently cross-linked to form an *irreversible* platelet plug, a process that requires clotting factors.

- Disorders affecting platelet function will impair primary hemostasis. Platelet function can be tested by checking bleeding time (rarely done) or in vitro platelet function tests (more commonly done).

- Both the extrinsic and intrinsic pathways lead into the common pathway to cause formation of the fibrin clot.

- The prothrombin time (PT) reflects the time it takes for the extrinsic and common pathways to form a fibrin clot. The PT can be prolonged by clotting factor deficiencies in either pathway.

- The activated partial thromboplastin time (aPTT) reflects the time it takes for the intrinsic and common pathways to form a fibrin clot. The aPTT can be prolonged by clotting factor deficiencies in either pathway.

- Aspirin *irreversibly* inhibits platelets by inhibiting cyclooxygenase (COX), preventing the formation of thromboxane A_2, which normally promotes platelet aggregation and vasoconstriction in response to endothelial damage. Aspirin therapy results in a prolonged bleeding time.

- Heparin stimulates antithrombin III activity, thereby inhibiting the intrinsic pathway and prolonging the aPTT. Heparin has no effect on bleeding time because it does not (typically) affect platelet function. Heparin toxicity can be reversed with protamine sulfate.

- Warfarin (Coumadin) inhibits the synthesis of vitamin K–dependent clotting factors (II, VII, IX, and X) by antagonizing the action of vitamin K. It preferentially prolongs the PT. There is typically a delay of several days before patients achieve a therapeutic international normalized ratio (INR) on warfarin because warfarin inhibits the synthesis of further clotting factors but does not inhibit the activity of existing plasma clotting factors.

- Warfarin toxicity can be reversed by administering vitamin K (takes 1-2 days) or fresh frozen plasma (rapid).

- Tissue plasminogen activator (tPA), streptokinase, and urokinase are "clot-busting" drugs that can be used in particular clinical scenarios such as ST-segment elevation myocardial infarction or acute ischemic cerebrovascular accident.

CASE 13-1

A 7-year-old boy is brought to your office by his mother because of a swollen right knee. When questioned, she states that this has happened in the absence of significant trauma several times over the past few years. He does not appear febrile, and a complete blood count (CBC) is normal. Both parents are healthy, although the mother says that her father (the boy's maternal grandfather) had "some type of bleeding disorder."

1. **What is the most likely diagnosis?**
   Hemophilia typically presents with spontaneous bleeding into joints (hemarthrosis) and soft tissues or prolonged bleeding following dental procedures or minor surgery. Because hemophilia A is more common than hemophilia B, this boy most likely has hemophilia A.

2. **What is the cause of this disorder and how is it inherited?**
   Hemophilia A is caused by a hereditary deficiency of factor VIII and is inherited in an X-linked recessive manner. Females are very rarely affected because the approximate 50% factor levels in

most carriers are sufficient to prevent excessive bleeding. In rare circumstances, females may be affected due to unequal inactivation (lyonization) of factor VIII or factor IX alleles (see Chapter 11, Genetic and Metabolic Disease, for more information).

In this case study, in which the maternal grandfather was affected, the boy's mother is an asymptomatic female carrier who transmitted the "bad" X chromosome (from her father) to the child.

Note: Hemophilia B is an X-linked recessive disease in which factor IX of the coagulation cascade is deficient.

3. **Which measure of coagulation will be abnormal in hemophilia A?**
   A deficiency of factor VIII (hemophilia A) or factor IX (hemophilia B) impairs thrombin production by the factor IXa/factor VIIIa complex, resulting in dysfunction of the intrinsic pathway and prolonged bleeding from increased aPTT.

4. **What is the mainstay of medical treatment for this disease?**
   Treatment consists of infusion of the missing factor (factor VIII for hemophilia A or factor IX for hemophilia B).
   Note: Historically, isolation of clotting factors from pooled collections of blood resulted in human immunodeficiency virus (HIV)-contaminated fractions. This problem was most pronounced before the beginning of HIV screening of the blood supply. Currently, factors VIII and IX can also be produced by recombinant DNA methods, which obviates this problem.

SUMMARY BOX: HEMOPHILIA

- Hemophilia A and B are hereditary coagulopathies caused by deficiencies in factors VIII and factor IX, respectively. They are inherited in an X-linked recessive manner, so male offspring are much more commonly affected.

- Because factors VIII and IX are components of the intrinsic pathway, the activated partial thromboplastin time (aPTT) is prolonged in hemophilia.

- Hemophilia A and B are typically diagnosed following spontaneous bleeding into joints (hemarthrosis) and soft tissues or prolonged bleeding with trauma or minor surgery.

- Treatment of hemophilia involves replacement of the missing clotting factor.

CASE 13-2

A 35-year-old woman who is having a missed abortion (fetus dies but conceptus is retained in utero for a few months) develops petechiae on her skin and buccal mucosa, begins coughing up some blood (hemoptysis), and observes blood in her stool. While it is being arranged for her uterus to be evacuated, a CBC is done and reveals anemia and thrombocytopenia. A peripheral smear reveals schistocytes, the PT and PTT are elevated (although she is not taking any anticoagulants), and the D-dimer level is increased. Fresh frozen plasma and platelets are ordered.

1. **What is the most likely diagnosis?**
   She appears to be going into disseminated intravascular coagulation (DIC), which is characterized by thrombocytopenia, elevated PT and PTT, and an elevated D-dimer level.

2. **What is the pathogenesis of disseminated intravascular coagulation?**
   Procoagulant (thromboplastic) substances such as tissue factor and fibrin are released throughout the circulation and activate the clotting mechanism. This depletes clotting factors and platelets ("consumptive coagulopathy"), which then causes excessive bleeding. DIC is therefore characterized by excessive clotting and bleeding *occurring simultaneously* throughout the body. Laboratory values will show decreased platelet count and increased bleeding time in addition to the findings mentioned in question 1. The main disease states in which DIC occurs are obstetric complications (missed abortion, abruptio placentae), gram-negative sepsis, and malignancies.

3. **What are schistocytes and why do they form in disseminated intravascular coagulation?**
   Schistocytes are fragmented red blood cells (RBCs) that have been "clothes-lined" by fibrin strands that streak across blood vessels, tearing off part of the RBC membrane as the RBCs pass by (Fig. 13-2). The widespread fibrin deposition that occurs in DIC can lead to this condition.
   Note: Schistocytes are a hallmark of *microangiopathic hemolytic anemia* (hemolytic anemia due to intravascular fragmentation of RBCs).

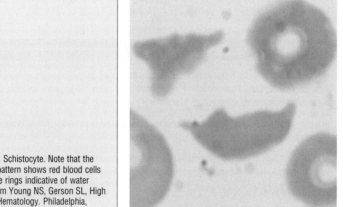

Figure 13-2. Schistocyte. Note that the schistocyte pattern shows red blood cells with refractile rings indicative of water artifact. (From Young NS, Gerson SL, High KA: Clinical Hematology. Philadelphia, Mosby, 2005.)

4. **How does the pathophysiology of thrombotic thrombocytopenic purpura differ from that of disseminated intravascular coagulation?**
   Thrombotic thrombocytopenic purpura (TTP) is marked by deficiency of ADAMTS13, a metalloprotease that is responsible for the degradation of vWF multimers. Absence of ADAMTS13 prevents vWF breakdown and promotes a hypercoagulable state.
   TTP involves *t*hrombosis, *t*hrombocytopenia, and abnormal bleeding as evidenced by *p*urpura on examination. It is precipitated by widespread damage to the endothelium. Because platelets adhere to the exposed subendothelial collagen of damaged vessels, massive activation of platelet binding and aggregation can cause thrombocytopenia, resulting in bleeding (purpura) and prolonged bleeding time. However, the clotting factors are not consumed as they are in DIC. Additionally, the cause of most cases of TTP is unknown. Both TTP and DIC show evidence of a microangiopathic hemolytic anemia.

5. **What is the pentad of thrombotic thrombocytopenic purpura and how does this disorder differ from hemolytic uremic syndrome?**
The pentad of TTP consists of microangiopathic hemolytic anemia, thrombocytopenia, neurologic symptoms, fever, and renal dysfunction. Most of the manifestations are explained on the basis of clot formation, with fibrin strands causing the microangiopathic hemolytic anemia. The neurologic symptoms and renal dysfunction are due to clots and occlusion of the cerebral circulation and glomerular capillaries, respectively. Hemolytic uremic syndrome (HUS) is very similar to TTP and involves most of the same symptoms and laboratory findings. The distinction to make for boards is that HUS does not involve neurologic manifestations.
   Note: Enterohemorrhagic *Escherichia coli* O157 and *Shigella* are both well-established causative agents of HUS.

6. **Quick review: Cover the two columns at the right in Table 13-3 and try to differentiate thrombotic thrombocytopenic purpura and disseminated intravascular coagulation on the basis of pathogenesis, changes in blood elements, bleeding time, and changes in prothrombin time, activated partial thromboplastin time, and D-dimer levels.**

TABLE 13-3.	THROMBOTIC THROMBOCYTOPENIC PURPURA/HEMOLYTIC UREMIC SYNDROME (TTP/HUS) AND DISSEMINATED INTRAVASCULAR COAGULATION (DIC)	
Feature	TTP/HUS	DIC
Pathogenesis	Endothelial damage leads to platelet consumption	Release of procoagulants or endothelial damage
Changes in formed blood elements	Thrombocytopenia, schistocytes microangiopathic hemolytic anemia	Thrombocytopenia, schistocytes, microangiopathic hemolytic anemia
Bleeding time	Increased	Increased
PT	Normal	Increased
PTT	Normal	Increased
D-dimer	Normal	Increased

PT, prothrombin time; PTT, partial thromboplastin time.

STEP 1 SECRET

As mentioned in Chapter 12, hematology is a great subject for "↑/↓/normal" questions. We recommend that you thoroughly understand laboratory parameters for bleeding disorders. They are a favorite USMLE test topic because, as you may have guessed, they fit in very nicely with this popular, multiple-choice question format.

SUMMARY BOX: DISSEMINATED INTRAVASCULAR COAGULATION

- Disseminated intravascular coagulation (DIC) is associated with obstetric complications (missed abortion, abruptio placentae), gram-negative sepsis, and malignancy.

- DIC is characterized by thrombocytopenia, prolonged prothrombin time (PT) and activated partial thromboplastin time (aPTT), elevated D-dimer level, and the presence of schistocytes.

- Schistocytes are fragmented red blood cell (RBCs) that have been "clothes-lined" by fibrin strands that streak across blood vessels. The widespread fibrin deposition that occurs in DIC can lead to this condition. Schistocytes are indicative of a microangiopathic hemolytic anemia.

- Thrombotic thrombocytopenic purpura (TTP) is precipitated by widespread damage to the endothelium, although the precise cause in most cases of TTP is unknown. It is characterized by thrombosis, thrombocytopenia, and abnormal bleeding as evidenced by purpura on examination.

- TTP and hemolytic uremic syndrome (HUS) are essentially the same entity.

- The pentad of TTP consists of microangiopathic hemolytic anemia, thrombocytopenia, neurologic symptoms, fever, and renal dysfunction. HUS consists of all of these symptoms except neurologic damage.

CASE 13-3

A 27-year-old man is evaluated for persistent bleeding from the gums since a dental cleaning the prior afternoon. On examination, his gums appear to be bleeding profusely, and his mouth requires packing with gauze pads to limit the bleeding. He denies any history of abnormal bleeding or any family history of bleeding disorders. He is not taking aspirin or other nonsteroidal anti-inflammatory drugs (NSAIDs). Review of systems is significant only for intermittent painful swelling of his right knee over the past 10 years. Suspecting a diagnosis of hemophilia, the clinician orders PT and aPTT, both of which are checked and return normal. However, bleeding time is prolonged at 15 minutes.

1. **What is the most likely diagnosis?**
   The prolonged bleeding time indicates platelet dysfunction, and the normal PT and aPTT argue against hemophilia. Given his additional history of hemarthrosis of the knee for the past 10 years, this man likely has von Willebrand disease, which is the most commonly inherited disorder of platelet dysfunction.

2. **What is the normal function of von Willebrand factor and what is the pathogenesis of this man's disease?**
   The high-molecular-weight protein vWF "links" platelets to exposed subendothelial collagen, one of the first steps required for clotting to occur. The vWF is secreted by vascular endothelial cells. A quantitative or qualitative deficiency in vWF causes von Willebrand disease.

3. **Why may someone with von Willebrand disease be mistakenly diagnosed with hemophilia A?**
Hemophilia A is caused by low levels of factor VIII. Because vWF acts as a carrier protein for factor VIII, patients with von Willebrand disease commonly have low levels of factor VIII as well. Although this patient's clinical presentation was consistent with hemophilia, the normal PT and aPTT largely rule out this possibility.

STEP 1 SECRET

Hemophilia and von Willebrand factor (vWF) deficiency appear with similar clinical findings. Both may present with elevated activated partial thromboplastin time (aPTT) and prolonged bleeding time, but hemophilia is often associated with hemarthroses (vWF deficiency does not do this). This is a good example of why it is important to read question stems carefully. The USMLE Step 1 exam often provides these giveaway details!

---

4. **What is the mechanism of action whereby administration of desmopressin acetate might help this man's symptoms?**
Desmopressin acetate (DDAVP) is useful in many of the bleeding disorders, as it induces the hepatic production of plasma clotting factors. It is effective in von Willebrand disease because it stimulates the release of vWF from endothelial cells. However, DDAVP may not be effective in variants of von Willebrand disease caused by *qualitative* defects in vWF function.

DIFFERENTIAL DIAGNOSIS

5. **If this man had normal levels of functional von Willebrand factor, and platelet function studies revealed a defect in platelet adherence to collagen, what rare disorder of platelet function might you suspect?**
You might suspect Bernard-Soulier syndrome, which is caused by a lack of or abnormal function of the platelet GPIb-IX receptor. The GPIb-IX receptor functions in platelet adherence to subendothelial collagen by binding to vWF (which is bound to subendothelial collagen).

6. **If platelet function studies demonstrated platelets capable of adhering to collagen but unable to aggregate with other platelets, what other rare disorder of platelet function might you suspect?**
Glanzmann's thrombasthenia is a possibility. This rare disease is caused by a lack of the GPIIb-IIIa receptor on platelets, which mediates platelet aggregation via a "fibrinogen bridge."
   Note: It may be difficult to differentiate clinically between von Willebrand disease, Bernard-Soulier disease, and Glanzmann's thrombasthenia, so the ristocetin assay is often used. Ristocetin is a molecule that allows vWF to bind to GPIb, resulting in agglutination. In the absence of either of these components (von Willebrand disease and Bernard-Soulier syndrome), ristocetin assay will be abnormal. In the case of Glanzmann's thrombasthenia, normal aggregation will occur after ristocetin is added. Boards will expect you to understand the principles behind the ristocetin assay and how it can be used to differentiate between the aforementioned diseases. You should also keep in mind that von Willebrand disease will affect PTT because vWF aids in carrying factor VIII in the blood, whereas Bernard-Soulier disease and Glanzmann's thrombasthenia will not.

7. **Given the previously mentioned function of the GPIIb-IIIa receptor, why are drugs such as abciximab (Integrilin) given to patients with cardiovascular disease?**
These drugs prevent platelet aggregation by antagonizing the GPIIb-IIIa receptors on platelets; therefore, they lower the risk for thromboembolic events in high-risk patients.

8. **Why might you suspect an abnormal bleeding time in this man if he suffered from diabetic nephropathy and osteoarthritis for which he routinely takes aspirin?**
Uremia and NSAIDs are common causes of acquired platelet dysfunction.

9. **Quick review: Cover the two columns on the right side of Table 13-4 and try to describe the mechanisms of action for the listed antiplatelet drugs.**

TABLE 13-4. ANTIPLATELET DRUGS		
Agent	**Mechanism of Action**	**Comments**
Aspirin	*Irreversible* inhibition of COX-1 and COX-2 (inhibits thromboxane A_2 synthesis)	Most common cause of platelet dysfunction
Clopidogrel (Plavix)	Inhibits platelet ADP receptor activation	
Abciximab (ReoPro) Eptifibatide (Integrilin) Tirofiban (Aggrastat)	Platelet GPIIb-IIIa inhibitors	Mimics Glanzmann's thrombasthenia
ADP, adenosine diphosphate; COX-1, -2, cyclooxygenase-1, -2.		

SUMMARY BOX: VON WILLEBRAND DISEASE

- The most commonly inherited disorder of platelet dysfunction is von Willebrand disease; von Willebrand factor (vWF) functions to link platelets (via the glycoprotein Ib [GPIb-IX] receptor) to exposed subendothelial collagen.

- Patients with von Willebrand disease may be mistakenly diagnosed as having hemophilia A because vWF is a carrier protein for factor VIII. A normal activated partial thromboplastin time (aPTT), however, should argue against a diagnosis of hemophilia A.

- Desmopressin acetate (DDAVP) may be useful in treating von Willebrand disease caused by a *quantitative* deficiency in vWF because it stimulates the release of vWF from endothelial cells.

- Bernard-Soulier syndrome and Glanzmann's thrombasthenia are rare disorders of platelet function.

- Bernard-Soulier syndrome is caused by lack/dysfunction of the GPIb-IX platelet receptor, which mediates binding of platelets to collagen via vWF.

- Glanzmann's thrombasthenia is caused by lack/dysfunction of the GPIIb-IIIa platelet receptor, which mediates platelet aggregation via a "fibrinogen bridge."

- Drugs such as abciximab (Integrilin) prevent platelet aggregation by antagonizing the GPIIb-IIIa platelet receptor; they therefore decrease the risk for thromboembolic phenomena in high-risk cardiovascular patients.

CASE 13-4

A previously healthy 35-year-old woman complains of easy bruising and occasional nosebleeds over the last few months. She does not take any medications. Physical examination reveals diffuse petechiae and ecchymoses. Laboratory tests show a platelet count of 5000/μL, white blood cell (WBC) count of 7200/μL, RBC count of 4.6×10^6/μL, and a normal PT and aPTT. A peripheral blood smear is unremarkable. Specialized testing reveals the presence of antiplatelet antibodies.

1. **What is the most likely diagnosis in this woman?**
   This sounds like immune thrombocytopenic purpura (ITP). However, it should be realized that ITP is a diagnosis of exclusion. Therefore, the myriad of other causes of thrombocytopenia (e.g., marrow-infiltrative processes such as cancer, infections such as rubella, folate or vitamin B_{12} deficiency, DIC, TTP) must be considered.

2. **What is the etiology of immune thrombocytopenic purpura?**
   ITP is caused by the production of immunoglobulin G (IgG) autoantibodies to platelets, resulting in destruction of antibody-coated platelets in the spleen. In children, ITP is often preceded by an upper respiratory tract infection.
   Note: The spleen is also the primary site for synthesis of antiplatelet antibodies in ITP. For this reason, a splenectomy can often be therapeutic in refractory cases.

3. **Would a bone marrow biopsy in this woman likely reveal increased or decreased numbers of megakaryocytes and why?**
   Normal to increased megakaryocytes, the precursors to platelets, would be revealed. This finding indicates that the thrombocytopenia is due to increased platelet destruction, not reduced production.

4. **What anticoagulant is well known for causing thrombocytopenia?**
   Heparin can cause thrombocytopenia. As many as 1% to 3% of patients receiving heparin may develop heparin-induced thrombocytopenia (HIT), which, oddly enough, can present with either excessive bleeding or excessive thrombosis. Thrombocytopenia in HIT is thought to be caused by the production of an IgG antibody against heparin. These anti-heparin antibodies bind to both heparin and a protein called platelet factor 4 (PF4). Upon initiation of this binding, the Fc region of the antibody binds to the platelet surface, resulting in widespread platelet activation and subsequent platelet depletion (i.e., thrombocytopenia).

5. **Why is the absence of splenomegaly important and therefore helpful in determining the cause of thrombocytopenia?**
   Splenomegaly/hypersplenism can result in increased platelet sequestration and thrombocytopenia. Splenomegaly most commonly results from congestion due to portal hypertension, but may also result from leukemia, lymphoma, and several other disease processes. Splenomegaly is *not* typically seen in ITP, although it is occasionally seen in children with ITP following a viral infection.

6. **Can pregnant women with this disease affect the platelet count of their fetuses?**
   Yes, ITP can cause neonatal thrombocytopenia because the autoantibodies, predominantly IgG, are able to cross the placenta and attack fetal platelets.

7. **What is the treatment strategy for this disease?**
   Corticosteroids such as prednisone will suppress the immunologically mediated destruction of platelets. If steroids fail, intravenous immunoglobulin (IVIG) may be helpful. Other agents with some efficacy include cyclophosphamide, azathioprine, and danazol. If necessary, a splenectomy is often helpful.

SUMMARY BOX: IMMUNE THROMBOCYTOPENIC PURPURA

- Immune thrombocytopenic purpura (ITP) is an autoimmune thrombocytopenia caused by the production of antibodies to platelets resulting in splenic destruction of circulating platelets.

- In children, ITP is often preceded by an upper respiratory tract infection.

- ITP is a diagnosis of exclusion. Other causes of thrombocytopenia such as marrow infiltrative processes, infections, drugs, and folate and vitamin B_{12} deficiency need to be considered.

- Bone marrow biopsy in ITP will show normal to increased large megakaryocytes.

- Heparin-induced thrombocytopenia is a concern in hospitalized patients receiving heparin. It occurs as a result of the synthesis of an IgG antibody against heparin and this antibody also reacts with platelets.

- Splenomegaly is not normally present in ITP; in an adult with splenomegaly, one therefore has to question the diagnosis of ITP.

- Treatment options include corticosteroids, intravenous immunoglobulin, danazol, immunosuppressants such as cyclophosphamide and azathioprine, and splenectomy.

CASE 13-5

A 58-year-old woman complains of a swollen and painful right leg since returning from a trip to Europe 2 days ago. Past medical history is significant for metastatic breast cancer, for which she is currently between chemotherapy regimens. On examination, her right calf is warm and tender to palpation and measures 20 cm in diameter, compared with her left calf, which is nontender to palpation and measures 16 cm in diameter. Compression ultrasonography reveals a clot in the right femoral vein.

1. **What is the diagnosis?**
   She has deep venous thrombosis (DVT). Risk factors for DVT include prolonged immobilization (e.g., recent surgery, transcontinental flight), malignancy, estrogen and oral contraceptives, obesity, heart failure, and a hereditary predisposition.
   Note: For completeness, other risk factors include the factor V Leiden mutation (which results in activated protein C resistance), prothrombin mutant, homocysteinemia, antiphospholipid syndrome, and HIT.

2. **From what site do deep venous thromboses, which give rise to pulmonary embolisms, typically arise?**
They arise from the deep veins of the calf muscles originally, but calf DVTs need to propagate into the deep veins of the proximal leg (popliteal, femoral, or iliac) to become large enough to cause clinically significant pulmonary emboli.

3. **What is Virchow's triad and how does this relate to this patient?**
Virchow's triad includes the three general causes of increased clotting, which are *abnormalities of the vessel wall* (as in vasculitis and atherosclerosis), *abnormalities of blood flow* (e.g., stasis), and *abnormalities of blood coagulability* (e.g., deficiencies of anticoagulants, presence of procoagulants). Of these, this patient had a recent history of immobilization from her long flight, which can cause hemostasis. Additionally, she likely has a hypercoagulable state secondary to her malignancy.

4. **How do deficiencies of proteins C and S and antithrombin III predispose to deep venous thrombosis?**
Proteins C, protein S and ATIII are all inhibitors of various clotting factors. Deficiencies therefore results in a hypercoagulable state.
   Note: Protein C normally functions to degrade factor V (among other actions). Patients with the factor V Leiden mutation synthesize a factor V that is resistant to degradation by activated protein C, resulting in a hypercoagulable state.

5. **What is antiphospholipid syndrome?**
Antiphospholipid syndrome is an autoimmune coagulation disorder that results from antibody production against phospholipids, which are often bound to plasma proteins. It has a high association with other autoimmune conditions (particularly systemic lupus erythematosus and HIV) and predisposes patients to arterior and venous thrombosis syndromes. You should consider this diagnosis in a woman with an autoimmune condition who experiences stroke, DVT, or hepatic vein thrombosis. In addition, the woman may have experienced a spontaneous abortion due to placental thrombosis.

SUMMARY BOX: DEEP VENOUS THROMBOSIS

- Risk factors for deep venous thrombosis (DVT) include prolonged immobilization (e.g., recent surgery, transcontinental flight), malignancy, estrogen and oral contraceptives, obesity, heart failure, and a hereditary predisposition.

- Still other risk factors include the factor V Leiden mutation, prothrombin mutant, homocysteinemia, antiphospholipid syndrome, and heparin-induced thrombocytopenia.

- DVTs, which give rise to pulmonary embolisms, most commonly arise from the deep veins of the proximal leg. DVTs in the calf are typically too small to cause clinically significant pulmonary emboli.

- Virchow's triad refers to the three general conditions that predispose to clotting: vascular damage, venous stasis, and clotting factor deficiencies/abnormalities.

- Deficiencies in protein C, protein S, and antithrombin III as well as the factor V Leiden mutation may result in a hypercoagulable state.

CHAPTER 14

HEMATOLOGIC MALIGNANCIES

Dana M. Carne, Thomas A. Brown, MD, and Sonali J. Shah

INSIDER'S GUIDE TO HEMATOLOGIC MALIGNANCIES FOR THE USMLE STEP 1

Hematologic malignancies are easy points on Step 1 if you study for these topics correctly. This chapter is included to focus you on the most high-yield points to take away for boards. Before you read through this chapter, you should skim the following list of tips to help you gain the maximum number of points on your examination:

- Know all of the chromosomal translocations mentioned in this chapter and First Aid. Board exams love to test students on these points.

- Pay careful attention to patient ages whenever they are given in the clinical history. Age can be very helpful in distinguishing various types of hematologic malignancies. You should especially memorize the age ranges for the most common types of leukemias. Acute lymphoblastic leukemia (ALL) occurs between the ages of 0 to 15, acute myelogenous leukemia (AML) occurs between the ages of 15 to 59, chronic myelogenous leukemia (CML) occurs between the ages of 40 to 59, and chronic lymphocytic leukemia (CLL) occurs after the age of 60 years. Keep in mind that boards will provide you with classic presentations for diseases, so memorizing particular rules like this one for the USMLE can be extremely helpful.

- Many high-yield images derive from this section. You should know how to diagnose different leukemias and lymphomas from images of peripheral blood smears or bone marrow aspirates. You should also know how to recognize Auer rods and Reed-Sternberg cells, two especially high-yield images covered in this section.

- When learning the various hematologic malignancies, focus on the information that helps you differentiate these cancers from one another. Sometimes, this is all you need to know for boards. A great example is hairy cell leukemia, for which you should know that these cells have hairlike projections and stain positively with tartrate-resistant acid phosphatase (TRAP). These are the two most unique facts about hairy cell leukemia, and at least one of them is guaranteed to be provided in any question stem you may receive on this topic. It's as simple as that. Use the information in this chapter (especially the tables) to guide what you should take away from each individual disease.

BASIC CONCEPTS

1. **What are the two principal lineages along which leukocytes differentiate?**
    The *lymphoid lineage* gives rise to B and T lymphocytes as well as natural killer (NK) cells, and the *myeloid lineage* gives rise to the granulocytes (eosinophils, basophils, neutrophils), monocytes, platelets, and erythrocytes (i.e., the nonlymphoid cells). Cells of the innate immune

system derive from the myeloid lineage, but cells of the adaptive immune system derive from the lymphoid lineage. The exception to this rule is NK cells, which are considered to be players in the innate immune system.

2. **What categories of hematologic malignancy arise from the lymphoid lineage?**
   - The lymphomas, including Hodgkin's lymphoma and the various types of non-Hodgkin's lymphoma (NHL)
   - The lymphocytic leukemias, including acute lymphoblastic leukemia (ALL) and chronic lymphocytic leukemia (CLL)
   - Tumors of plasma cells (antibody-secreting B cells), which include multiple myeloma and lymphoplasmacytic lymphoma
   Note: All lymphoid neoplasms arise from a single transformed cell and are consequently phenotypically monoclonal.

3. **What is the general distinction between lymphoma and leukemia?**
   Leukemia generally indicates significant bone marrow involvement with neoplastic cells (and often significant peripheral blood involvement). Lymphoma indicates a *mass* originating in the peripheral tissues (lymph nodes). However, this line is often blurred because lymphomas can evolve to infiltrate the marrow (a leukemic picture), and malignancies otherwise identical to leukemias may start out as peripheral tissue masses similar to lymphomas. Currently, leukemia or lymphoma refers to the usual tissue distribution of neoplasms of a particular cell type.

4. **What is the distinction between small cell lymphocytic lymphoma (SLL) and (B-cell) chronic lymphocytic leukemia (B-CLL)?**
   B-CLL and SLL are essentially the same entity with the exact same cell type, immunophenotype, and genetic alteration. They are therefore typically referred to as simply SLL/B-CLL, without designating a specific diagnosis. The distinction is that when the peripheral blood lymphocytes reach a certain level, then the disease is considered "leukemic." This is a fantastic example of the blur between leukemias and lymphoma.
   Note: Smudge cells are a characteristic feature of CLL on a peripheral smear.

5. **What categories of hematologic neoplasms arise from the myeloid lineage?**
   - Acute myelogenous leukemia (AML), which has multiple subclassifications
   - Myelodysplastic syndromes, all potential precursors of AML
   - Myeloproliferative disorders, including polycythemia vera (PV), chronic myelogenous leukemia (CML), and essential thrombocythemia
   - Histiocytoses (of monocyte-macrophage origin)
   Note: All myeloid neoplasms arise from a transformed hematopoietic progenitor cell. Features of these neoplasms often overlap, confusing medical students and physicians alike. They may also infiltrate the bone marrow, resulting in anemia, thrombocytopenia, and leukopenia. Additionally, both ALL and CLL, as well as many types of lymphoma, can have significant bone marrow involvement.

6. **What is the distinctive feature of acute myelogenous leukemia on bone marrow biopsy?**
   A substantial amount of the bone marrow is replaced by relatively undifferentiated blast cells that resemble one (or more) of the early steps of myeloid differentiation. Consequently, there are multiple subclassifications of AML, depending on which early cell type predominates (e.g., acute promyelocytic leukemia, acute myelomonocytic leukemia, acute megakaryocytic leukemia).

STEP 1 SECRET

The most important form of acute myelogenous leukemia (AML) to know for boards is the M3 subtype, which is characterized by circulating granulocytes and myeloblasts containing Auer rods. Auer rods are peroxidase-positive inclusion bodies in the cytoplasm of the neoplastic cells that are pathognomonic for this condition. Release of these Auer rods can result in disseminated intravascular coagulation (DIC), which is associated with the M3 subtype of AML.

The M3 form of AML is marked by a characteristic t(15,17) translocation that involves the retinoic acid receptor. Fortunately, this disease responds to treatment with all-*trans*-retinoic acid.

7. **What is the distinctive feature of myelodysplastic syndromes?**

In these diseases, a mutant stem cell that can give rise to all cell types of the myeloid lineage replaces the bone marrow (partly or wholly). However, this mutant stem cell produces cells of the myeloid lineage in an ineffective manner. Consequently, anemia, thrombocytopenia, and leukopenia are seen, from both ineffective hematopoiesis and replacement of bone marrow. Moreover, the myelodysplastic syndromes may evolve into AML.

Dysplastic changes of myelodysplastic syndrome include Pelger-Huet cells with "aviator" nuclei (bilobed polymorphonuclear cells) and ring sideroblasts. This syndrome is associated with *BCL2* mutation as well as methylation (and inactivation) of tumor suppressor genes.

8. **What is the distinct feature of the myeloproliferative disorders?**

In these diseases, a transformed hematopoietic progenitor cell causes a pathologically increased production of one of the final products of the myeloid lineage (granulocytes, erythrocytes, platelets). In other words, myeloproliferative disorders differ from other neoplastic leukocytic disorders in that they cause an overproduction of *mature* cells. Examples are polycythemia vera (increased red blood cell [RBC] production), essential thrombocytosis (increased platelet production), and CML, which results in an increased number of granulocytes.

Note: CML is unique among the myeloproliferative disorders in that it has a characteristic genetic defect: a chromosomal translocation (t9:22), known as the Philadelphia chromosome.

9. **What are the histiocytoses?**

A histiocyte is a tissue macrophage found within the interstitium. The histiocytoses are disorders involving uncontrolled proliferation of histiocytes. For Step 1, students need be familiar only with Langerhans cell histiocytosis (also known as histiocytosis X), which, depending on age at presentation and clinical course, is classified as Letterer-Siwe disease, Hand-Schüller-Christian disease, or eosinophilic granuloma. A characteristic feature of histiocytosis X is *Birbeck granules* in the cytoplasm, which you can easily recognize on Step 1 because they look like miniature intracellular tennis rackets.

Note: The term "eosinophilic" refers to the characteristic pink protein staining and not the cell type.

10. **What is the relationship between myelofibrosis and the myeloproliferative diseases?**

Myelofibrosis is simply fibrosis of the bone marrow with collagen. It has multiple causes, such as radiation, drugs, and chemicals, but is most commonly idiopathic. It can also occur as a result of the myeloproliferative disorders. Myelofibrosis is most likely due to signaling by abnormal megakaryocytes. The resulting fibrosis can impair hematopoiesis, resulting in hypocellular bone marrow and pancytopenia, which can unfortunately be rapidly fatal. The body tries to compensate for this deficiency with extramedullary hematopoiesis.

Myelofibrosis is marked by "teardrop RBCs," which result from damage to the RBC structure as these cells try to escape the fibrotic bone marrow. If you see these cells on a peripheral blood smear, you should immediately associate this finding with myelofibrosis.

11. **How does the leukocyte alkaline phosphatase level help differentiate reactive leukocytosis from a true leukemia?**
Reactive leukocytosis (leukemoid reaction; left shift) is a pronounced increase in white blood cell (WBC) count with infection and is associated with high levels of leukocyte alkaline phosphatase (LAP). In contrast, the abnormally large increase in WBCs seen in leukemia is typically associated with low levels of LAP because the neoplastic cells cannot produce this enzyme. This is an important distinction to look out for on boards.

12. **Quick review! Cover the right column in Table 14-1 and attempt to list the cell type and pertinent high-yield facts regarding the hematologic malignancies in the left column.**

TABLE 14-1. LEUKEMIA LINEAGES	
Disorder	**Cell Type/Comments**
Lymphoid Lineage	
Acute lymphoblastic leukemia	Precursor B or T lymphocytes (lymphoblasts)
Chronic lymphocytic leukemia/ small lymphocytic lymphoma	B cells, smudge cells on peripheral smear
Hodgkin's lymphoma	Reed-Sternberg cells
Lymphoplasmacytoma	Plasma cells (mature B cells—IgM-secreting); a common cause of Waldenström's macroglobulinemia
Multiple myeloma	Plasma cells (mature B cells—IgG- and IgA-secreting)
Non-Hodgkin's lymphoma	Multiple types, which generally are classified according to site in lymph node they resemble (e.g., follicular, mantle zone, marginal zone)
Myeloid Lineage	
Acute myelogenous leukemia	Cells of early myeloid lineage
Histiocytosis	Langerhans cell (of monocyte-macrophage origin)
Myelodysplastic syndromes	Hematopoietic stem cell with ineffective hematopoiesis that replaces bone marrow
Myeloproliferative syndromes	Clonal expansion of a multipotent hematopoietic stem cell, ultimately giving rise to excess numbers of one or more final products of the myeloid lineage

IgA, IgG, IgM, immunoglobulins A, G, and M.

13. **Quick review! Cover the right column in Table 14-2 and attempt to define the hematologic terms in the left column.**

TABLE 14-2.	HEMATOLOGIC TERMINOLOGY
Term	**Definition**
Leukemia	Malignant proliferation of blood cells within the bone marrow and circulatory system
Leukemoid reaction	Abnormally high WBC count, similar to that occurring in various forms of leukemia, but not as the result of leukemia (typically in response to infection)
Lymphoma	Proliferating mass of lymphocytic cells: B cells (most common), T cells, NK cells
Myelofibrosis	Fibrosis of bone marrow, often causing extramedullary hematopoiesis that results in hepatosplenomegaly
Myelophthisic anemia	Anemia that arises from a space-occupying lesion that displaces normal hematopoietic elements

NK, natural killer; WBC, white blood cell.

14. **What are the genetic alterations in the following non-Hodgkin's lymphomas?**
See Table 14-3.

TABLE 14-3.	GENETIC ALTERATIONS IN NON–HODGKIN'S LYMPHOMA
Non-Hodgkin's Lymphoma	**Genetic Alterations**
Burkitt's lymphoma	Translocation between chromosomes 8 and 14, involves c-*myc* activation on chromosome 8; often associated with HIV infection; EBV infection common in African Burkitt's (patients present with jaw mass) Sporadic form is associated with pelvic and abdominal lesions Look for characteristic "starry sky" appearance of Burkitt's type, due to sheets of neoplastic lymphocytes infiltrated with occasional macrophages
Follicular lymphoma	Translocation between chromosomes 14 and 18 involving *BCL2* activation (antiapoptosis gene) Associated with painless, generalized lymphadenopathy, primarily in adults
Mantle cell lymphoma	Translocation between chromosomes 11 and 14, which increases cyclin D expression and promotes cell cycle progression Associated with CD5 expression Usually fatal, occurs in adults Cells resemble mantle zone cells that surround follicular centers

EBV, Epstein-Barr virus; HIV, human immunodeficiency virus.

15. **What are some characteristics of the other non-Hodgkin's lymphomas?**
See Table 14-4.

TABLE 14-4. CHARACTERISTICS OF NON-HODGKIN'S LYMPHOMA (NHL)	
NHL Type	**Description**
Cutaneous T-cell lymphoma	Caused by a T-cell dyscrasia, unlike most NHLs, which are B cell in origin
	Examples are mycosis fungoides and Sézary syndrome
	T-cell lymphomas are associated with cutaneous lesions
Diffuse large B-cell lymphoma	Very aggressive lymphoma occurring mostly in older adults but sometimes in children
	Associated with *BCL6* overexpression, which silences p53
	Early stage is responsive to treatment
Marginal zone lymphoma (MALToma)	Begins as reactive polyclonal B cell proliferation, culminating in monoclonal B-cell neoplasm

16. **Quick review with high-yield word associations: Cover the right column of Table 14-5 and attempt to list the associated diseases.**

TABLE 14-5. HIGH-YIELD WORD ASSOCIATIONS	
Description	**Disease**
>30% myeloid blasts in bone marrow	Acute myelogenous leukemia (AML)
8:14 translocation	Burkitt's lymphoma
14:18 translocation involving *BCL2*	Follicular lymphoma
Auer bodies	Acute myelogenous leukemia
Bence Jones proteinuria	Multiple myeloma
Massive splenomegaly, B-cell proliferation, and presence of tartrate-resistant acid phosphatase in B cells	Hairy cell leukemia
Philadelphia chromosome	Chronic myelogenous leukemia (CML)
Reed-Sternberg (lacunar) cells	Hodgkin's lymphoma
Smudge cells on peripheral blood smear	Chronic lymphocytic leukemia (CLL)

CASE 14-1

A 65-year-old man is evaluated for recent-onset of low back pain, despite a negative history of trauma or injury to the back. The pain is moderately severe and has been waking him at night. He also reports a 10-lb weight loss in recent months as well as fatigue and recurrent sinus infections. The physical examination is significant only for focal tenderness to palpation at the level of the T12 vertebra.

1. **What is the differential diagnosis for back pain in an older patient?**

   The differential diagnosis is quite broad and includes musculoskeletal back pain (muscle strain, herniated disk), vertebral compression fracture, malignancies (primary or metastatic), abdominal aortic aneurysm, and an infectious cause such as osteomyelitis, abscess, or tuberculosis (Pott's disease).

   For boards, you need to have a high index of suspicion for malignancy, particularly in an older individual with constitutional complaints such as unintentional weight loss and fatigue, back pain that is waking the patient at night (one of the "alarm" symptoms of back pain), and recurrent infections. Malignancies to consider in an older man include metastatic prostate cancer and multiple myeloma.

   ## CASE 14-1 continued:

   An x-ray film of the skull for evaluation of his sinus infections is shown in Figure 14-1. Serum protein electrophoresis reveals an M spike. A urine dipstick test is negative for proteinuria, but a 24-hour urine protein collection reveals marked proteinuria.

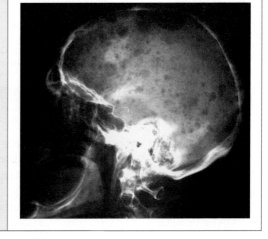

Figure 14-1. X-ray film of skull from patient in Case 14-1. (From Abeloff MD, Armitage JO, Niederhuber JE, et al: Clinical Oncology, 3rd ed. Philadelphia, Churchill Livingstone, 2004.)

2. **What is the expected diagnosis?**

   This is a classic presentation for a patient with multiple myeloma. The "punched-out" lytic lesions are caused by cytokines released by the myeloma cells, which promote osteolysis. The M spike on serum protein electrophoresis indicates the overproduction of a monoclonal antibody. The 24-hour urine collection showing increased protein represents the renal excretion of λ light chains (Bence Jones proteins). Note that the urine dipstick test, which detects negatively charged proteins such as albumin, does not show proteinuria, whereas a 24-hour urine protein collection reveals marked proteinuria because of the detection of the positively-charged light chains.

3. **What blood abnormalities often present with multiple myeloma and why?**

   Anemia, increased creatinine ("renal insufficiency"), and hypercalcemia often accompany multiple myeloma.

   The anemia occurs as a result of suppressed erythropoiesis. The reason for this is twofold: (1) cytokine secretion, particularly IL-6 by plasma cells, inhibits normal RBC production, and (2) widespread marrow infiltration by the plasma cells inhibits RBC formation.

The renal insufficiency can occur for a variety of reasons, but the primary causes are myeloma of the kidney and hypercalcemia. Light chains are directly toxic to the tubular epithelial cells of the nephron, can deposit within the tubular lumen causing obstruction, and can also deposit within the renal interstitium. In addition, myeloma patients are at increased risk of developing amyloidosis, which can further damage the kidneys.

The hypercalcemia can occur as a result of increased bone breakdown both from bony metastasis and from the elaboration of osteoclast-stimulating cytokines by tumor cells (primarily IL-1). This bone breakdown explains why myeloma patients are predisposed to pathologic fractures. Recall that symptoms of hypercalcemia include confusion, muscle weakness, polyuria, and constipation.

CASE 14-1 continued:

Blood work reveals the following:
Hematocrit: 29%
Hemoglobin: 9.2 g/dL
Albumin: 2.2 g/dL (normal 3.1-4.3 g/dL)
Total plasma protein: 8.6 g/dL (normal 6.3-8.2 g/dL)
Blood urea nitrogen (BUN): 22 mg/dL (normal 7-20 mg/dL)
Creatinine: 3.2 mg/dL (normal 0.7-1.4 mg/dL)
Plasma calcium: 12.4 mg/dL (normal 8.5-10.5 mg/dL)
A bone marrow aspiration sample is shown in Figure 14-2.

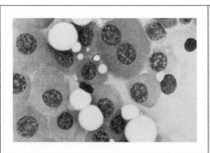

Figure 14-2. Bone marrow aspiration from patient in Case 14-1. (From Hoffman R, Benz EJ, Shattil SJ, et al: Hematology: Basic Principles and Practice, 4th ed. Philadelphia, Churchill Livingstone, 2005.)

4. **What cell type abnormally proliferates in multiple myeloma?**
Plasma cells, which are terminally differentiated antibody-secreting B cells. These malignant cells continuously secrete excessive amounts of a single monoclonal immunoglobulin, explaining the presence of the M (for monoclonal) spike seen on serum protein electrophoresis. This secretion of excessive amounts of a single immunoglobulin is referred to as a *monoclonal gammopathy*. The resulting hypergammaglobulinemia explains the elevated total plasma protein levels commonly seen in multiple myeloma. Hypoalbuminemia is also typical of multiple myeloma, and is thought to be secondary to elevated cytokine levels (e.g., IL-6) that reduce the hepatic synthesis of albumin.

5. **What is the association between Bence Jones proteinuria and the previously mentioned monoclonal gammopathy?**
Bence Jones proteins are immunoglobulin light chain subunits (most commonly of the λ isotype) that are filtered by the kidney and excreted in the urine. The malignant plasma cells also secrete heavy chain immunoglobulin subunits, but these are of high enough molecular weight that they are not typically excreted in the urine.

6. **What is amyloidosis and why is this man at risk for developing it?**
   Amyloidosis is a clinical syndrome caused by the deposition of insoluble fibrillar protein in various tissues. In amyloidosis caused by multiple myeloma, the monoclonal gammopathy results in elevated levels of free light chains in the blood, which can undergo processing and be pathologically deposited in tissues throughout the body as amyloid. Histologic staining of involved tissues with Congo red will reveal the classic apple-green birefringence when visualized under polarized light.

   Note: Among the numerous complications of amyloidosis is carpal tunnel syndrome, which can occur as a result of amyloid deposition in the carpal tunnel, causing compression of the median nerve.

7. **Explain why this man is at an increased risk for infection even though plasma levels of immunoglobulins are abnormally elevated.**
   Although total immunoglobulins are high, this is predominantly due to the M protein. The remaining immunoglobulins are low, predisposing the patient to infection.

8. **This patient's anemia can be characterized as myelophthisis. Why?**
   The suffix-phthisis refers to wasting away or atrophy of a body part. In this case the myeloma has infiltrated into the bone marrow and caused it to waste away, thus reducing production of RBCs.

9. **What is the characteristic finding on a peripheral blood smear, as shown in Figure 14-3, and why does this occur?**
   Rouleaux formation, in which RBCs are stacked on each other like a row of coins, occurs due to the agglutination of RBCs that is mediated by M protein.

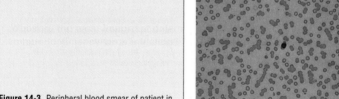

Figure 14-3. Peripheral blood smear of patient in Case 14-1 (×100). (Courtesy of Jean Shafer.)

10. **How might the presence of elevated serum κ light chains and amyloidosis affect kidney function in this patient?**
    They can seriously impair renal function, making renal failure a major cause of death in multiple myeloma. Elevated serum κ light chains get filtered and secreted by the kidney. These proteins are toxic to renal tubular epithelial cells and may also combine with a urinary glycoprotein, the Tamm-Horsfall protein, to form casts that obstruct the tubules. Renal deposition of amyloid, which may occur in primary amyloidosis, can also seriously compromise renal function.

11. **What is the pharmacologic basis for giving this patient allopurinol prior to and during chemotherapy?**
    Allopurinol inhibits the enzyme xanthine oxidase, which catalyzes the conversion of the purine metabolite xanthine to the relatively insoluble uric acid. In patients receiving toxic chemotherapy, DNA catabolism secondary to increased cell death results in the excessive

production of purine metabolites and, ultimately, uric acid. These patients are therefore at increased risk for developing painful gout uric acid kidney stones, but allopurinol reduces this risk by decreasing the production of uric acid.

DIFFERENTIAL DIAGNOSIS

12. **If workup reveals an IgM monoclonal gammopathy rather than an IgG or IgA gammopathy, what disease might you suspect?**
Waldenström's macroglobulinemia ("macro" for the large pentameric IgM molecule) is most commonly due to lymphoplasmacytic lymphoma, a plasma cell tumor that secretes IgM. The increased concentration of IgM increases plasma viscosity, which impairs blood flow and causes sludging in the retinal vessels and the cerebral vasculature (and elsewhere), predisposing to visual disturbances and neurologic problems.
    Note: Although Waldenström's macroglobulinemia is associated with an M spike and neoplastic cells, it differs from multiple myeloma in that there are no lytic bone lesions or hypercalcemia.

SUMMARY BOX: MULTIPLE MYELOMA

- Multiple myeloma often presents with anemia, renal insufficiency, hypercalcemia, and rouleaux formation on a blood smear.

- Suspect multiple myeloma in an older patient with unexplained back pain or a pathologic fracture.

- Multiple myeloma is caused by an abnormal clonal proliferation of antibody-secreting plasma cells, resulting in a monoclonal gammopathy.

- Renal failure in multiple myeloma can be caused by light chain toxicity and deposition within the tubules, hypercalcemia leading to nephrocalcinosis, and renal amyloidosis.

- Primary amyloidosis can occur as a result of processing of the light chains with deposition in various tissues, including the kidneys and carpal tunnel.

- Allopurinol is given with chemotherapy for multiple myeloma to prevent the release of large amounts of uric acid that can be seen in tumor lysis syndrome.

- Waldenström's macroglobulinemia is similar to multiple myeloma but is associated with secretion of IgM. This should not be confused with the M spike of multiple myeloma. Waldenström's macroglobulinemia is not associated with lytic bone lesions or hypercalcemia.

CASE 14-2

A 4-year-old girl is evaluated for fatigue, night sweats, anorexia, and a 10-lb weight loss over the past month. She also complains of pain in her lower back that she is unable to localize precisely. Because of this pain, she has started walking with a limp and, whenever possible, tries to avoid walking at all.

1. **Her parents are worried she might have cancer. What is the most common cancer in children?**
ALL, caused by a malignant proliferation of immature precursor B or T lymphocytes (i.e., pre–B or pre–T cells).

CASE 14-2 continued:

Physical examination is significant for conjunctival pallor, hepatosplenomegaly, painless lymphadenopathy, and diffuse petechiae.

2. **Why are fatigue, petechiae, and fever commonly seen in patients with acute lymphoblastic leukemias and myeloproliferative diseases?**
   The pancytopenia that occurs in these diseases as a consequence of marrow replacement is responsible, with the anemia causing fatigue, thrombocytopenia causing petechiae, and leukopenia predisposing to infection and fever.

3. **How does lymphadenopathy from infection differ from lymphadenopathy due to malignancy?**
   Tender lymph nodes often indicate a reactive (infective) process, whereas painless lymphadenopathy may indicate cancer, particularly when associated with constitutional symptoms such as fatigue, anorexia, weight loss, night sweats, and fever.

CASE 14-2 continued:

A complete blood count (CBC) reveals a marked lymphocytosis, thrombocytopenia, and anemia. A bone marrow biopsy is performed and reveals >50% lymphoblasts, karyotype analysis of which reveals multiple chromosomal translocations. Immunostaining of the abnormal marrow cells is positive for terminal deoxytransferase (TdT).

4. **How does the preceding information affect the differential diagnosis?**
   A diagnosis of ALL is much more likely. TdT is an enzyme involved in the normal gene rearrangement of immature lymphocytes (lymphoblasts) that creates unique antigen specificity. It is present in the vast majority of patients with ALL. Note that ALL is most common in children younger than 15 years of age.

5. **How does the presentation classically differ if the acute lymphoblastic leukemia is caused by a malignancy of pre–T cells rather than pre–B cells?**
   ALL caused by pre–B cells has a peak age of incidence of 3 to 4 years. This type of ALL is primarily a leukemia, with predominant bone marrow and peripheral blood involvement. However, the less frequent ALL caused by pre–T cells typically occurs in adolescents and presents primarily as a lymphoma, with predominant involvement of the lymphatic system. This lymphomatous type of ALL may present with mediastinal masses, marked lymphadenopathy and splenomegaly, and thymic involvement.
   Note: Because pre–B cells and pre–T cells can be difficult to distinguish morphologically, immunophenotyping based on cell surface markers is necessary to make a definitive diagnosis.

6. **How is diagnosis of acute lymphoblastic leukemia differentiated from acute myelogenous leukemia?**
   Although ALL and AML are both acute leukemias in which blast cells predominate, ALL occurs in children under the age of 15 years, and AML occurs in the age range of 15 to 59 years. Blood smears will show large lymphocyte precursors in ALL and myeloblasts (perhaps with Auer rods) in AML. ALL may spread to the central nervous system and testes—so-called sanctuary sites. These sites are generally spared in AML.

7. **If she is started on high-dose chemotherapy and suddenly develops marked hyperuricemia, hyperkalemia, hyperphosphatemia, and hypocalcemia, what has happened?**

    She has developed the tumor lysis syndrome, a metabolic emergency that is caused by massive destruction of tumor cells after initiation of high-dose chemotherapy. The death of large numbers of tumor cells results in the metabolism of large amounts of DNA. This produces excessive amounts of uric acid, which can precipitate in the renal tubules and cause renal damage. Intracellular ions such as potassium and phosphate are also released in large amounts by dying tumor cells. The released potassium can cause marked hyperkalemia, resulting potentially in fatal arrhythmias. The hyperphosphatemia can precipitate with calcium within tubules, further contributing to renal damage.

    Tumor lysis syndrome can be treated with hydration and allopurinol. Alkalization of urine to prevent uric acid precipitation is controversial because it may cause calcium precipitation.

SUMMARY BOX: ACUTE LYMPHOBLASTIC LEUKEMIA/ LYMPHOMA

- Acute lymphoblastic leukemia (ALL) classically presents in children. Symptoms include fatigue, night sweats, anorexia, and weight loss.

- Laboratory findings in ALL are notable for pancytopenia due to replacement of bone marrow by tumor. Note that the patient is deficient in *normal* white blood cells, while the actual white blood cell (WBC) count may be high owing to malfunctioning tumor cells.

- Tender lymphadenopathy typically indicates an infection. In contrast, painless lymphadenopathy may indicate a malignancy.

- Tumor lysis syndrome can develop after initiation of chemotherapy and is due to the release of large amounts of intracellular uric acid, potassium, and phosphate from dying tumor cells.

CASE 14-3

A 35-year-old woman complains of fatigue for the past 3 weeks and recurrent spontaneous nosebleeds. Physical examination is significant for nontender lymphadenopathy, hepatosplenomegaly, truncal petechiae, and multiple ecchymoses. A peripheral blood smear shows the presence of numerous myeloblasts, cytogenetic analysis of which shows a translocation between chromosomes 9 and 22. A CBC reveals a hematocrit of 25%, hemoglobin of 7.2 g/dL, WBC count of 22,000/μL, and platelet count of 30,000/μL.

1. **What is the likely diagnosis?**

    The presence of a translocation between chromosomes 9 and 22—the so-called Philadelphia chromosome—is highly suggestive of CML.

2. **What is the pathogenesis of this disorder?**

    CML is a myeloproliferative disorder in which a transformed hematopoietic progenitor cell causes an increased production of granulocytic cells (of the myeloid lineage) in the bone marrow, causing a myeloid leukocytosis (predominantly neutrophils). Bone marrow biopsy in these patients will reveal an abnormally increased myeloid-erythroid ratio of approximately 15:1 to 20:1. The Philadelphia chromosome, present in a majority of CML patients, involves a translocation between the *BCR* gene on chromosome 9 and the *ABL* gene on chromosome 22.

Note: Other myeloproliferative disorders include polycythemia vera and essential thrombocythemia.

3. **What is the blast crisis that may occur in chronic myelogenous leukemia?**
Blast crisis is an acute worsening of the disease, in which there is substantial medullary or extramedullary proliferation of blasts. Marrow blasts will often exceed 30% of marrow cells. This is an ominous prognostic sign.

4. **Compare and contrast chronic lymphocytic leukemia and chronic myelogenous leukemia.**
See Table 14-6 for this comparison.

TABLE 14-6.	CHRONIC LYMPHOCYTIC LEUKEMIA (CLL) AND CHRONIC MYELOGENOUS LEUKEMIA (CML)	
Feature	B-CLL/SLL	CML
Evolution	To prolymphocytic lymphoma or large B-cell lymphoma (both ominous events)	Blast crisis (ominous)
Immunophenotype and genetics	B-cell tumor that expresses B-cell antibodies and CD5 (an antibody unique to T cells); varied chromosomal abnormalities	9:22 translocation (Philadelphia chromosome); *BCR-ABL* fusion gene product
Peripheral blood smear	Smudge cells	Blasts, myelocytes
Typical age	Older adults	Young to middle-aged adults

SLL, small lymphocytic lymphoma.

SUMMARY BOX: CHRONIC MYELOGENOUS LEUKEMIA

- The Philadelphia chromosome is a translocation between chromosomes 9 and 22 and is associated with chronic myelogenous leukemia (CML).

- CML is a myeloproliferative disorder. Other myeloproliferative disorders include polycythemia vera and essential thrombocythemia.

- CML classically affects middle-aged adults, with symptoms of fatigue, spontaneous bleeding, lymphadenopathy, hepatosplenomegaly, and petechiae.

- CLL classically affects older adults and often is associated with "smudge cells" on a blood smear.

CASE 14-4

A 22-year-old male track athlete at the local university presents with a 3-month history of fatigue. Upon questioning he also admits to drenching night sweats and an unintentional 15-lb weight loss during this time. His past medical history is unremarkable.

1. **Is this history concerning for a serious disease?**
   These symptoms are very worrisome, especially for lymphoma. Lymphoma patients often present with so-called B symptoms, which include fever greater than 38° C, unintentional loss of >10% of body weight, and night sweats. This staging is used to distinguish symptomatic lymphoma patients from those without systemic symptoms.

2. **Other than malignancy, what else does the differential diagnosis include?**
   In a 22-year-old, you want to consider and search the question stem for the following clues:
   - Depression: Does the patient have a depressed mood, sleep disturbances, or loss of interest in normal activities?
   - Infection: Mononucleosis patients, for example, may also complain of a sore throat and have posterior cervical lymphadenopathy on examination. Also rule out human immunodeficiency virus (HIV).
     Note: In an older patient, you should also consider malignancies such as AML or CML, as well as diabetes (look for polydipsia/polyuria.)

CASE 14-4 continued:

On examination, nontender supraclavicular lymphadenopathy is noted as well as a feeling of fullness in the upper left abdominal quadrant. A computed tomography (CT) scan of the chest reveals a mediastinal mass, and he is referred to oncology for further evaluation.

3. **How does the location of the enlarged lymph nodes help in the differential diagnosis?**
   As mentioned earlier, mononucleosis or upper respiratory infections often are associated with enlarged cervical nodes, but cancer must always be ruled out in patients with enlarged supraclavicular nodes.

CASE 14-4 continued:

Biopsy of the enlarged supraclavicular node reveals the presence of large, binucleated cells amid normal-appearing lymphocytes, histiocytes, and granulocytes, as shown in Figure 14-4.

4. **Name these cells and describe their lineage of origin and relation to this patient's diagnosis.**
   This cellular description is classic for Reed-Sternberg cells, cluster designation (CD) 30$^+$ and CD15$^+$ monoclonal B cells, the presence of which indicates Hodgkin's lymphoma. Lymphoma can be categorized into Hodgkin's and NHL, with the basic distinction that Hodgkin's lymphoma has Reed-Sternberg cells.
   Note: This presentation was a classic description of Hodgkin's lymphoma (Table 14-7).

STEP 1 SECRET

Reed-Sternberg cells are commonly presented in image format on Step 1. You should be able to recognize these cells and distinguish them from the "owl's eye inclusion bodies" that are associated with cytomegalovirus (CMV).

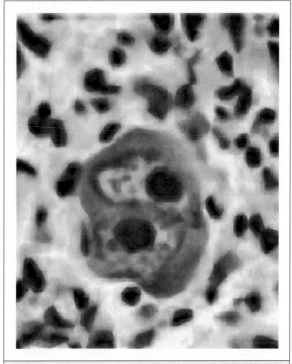

Figure 14-4. A Supraclavicular lymph node biopsy from patient in Case 14-4. (From Hoffman R, Benz EJ, Shattil SJ, et al: Hematology: Basic Principles and Practice, 4th ed. Philadelphia, Churchill Livingstone, 2005.)

TABLE 14-7. HODGKIN'S LYMPHOMA

Feature	Clinical Manifestations
Symptoms/ signs	Patients typically present with intermittent fevers, night sweats, unintentional weight loss, and fatigue.
Physical findings	Patients often have supraclavicular or cervical, nontender lymphadenopathy.
Imaging	The mediastinal mass is likely to represent lymphadenopathy, often seen in Hodgkin's lymphoma.
Epidemiology	Patients are predominantly male. Hodgkin's lymphoma shows a bimodal distribution, with one peak between 15 and 35 years of age and another after the age of 50. Patients with non-Hodgkin's lymphoma also are typically male, but the median age at diagnosis is around 65 years.

5. **What are the main variants of Hodgkin's lymphoma and how do they relate to the prognosis?**
   - Nodular sclerosis (60-80% of patients): Lacunar variant of Reed-Sternberg cell with fibrotic collagen bands that divide tumor into circumscribed nodules (excellent prognosis). Patients are predominantly young and female.
   - Mixed cellularity type (15-30%): Heterogeneous (mixed) cellular infiltrate of lymph nodes (good prognosis). These patients are usually older.
   - Lymphocytic predominance: Predominantly lymphocytic infiltrate of lymph nodes (excellent prognosis).
     Note: The lymphocytic depletion variant is controversial, so it is not addressed here.

6. **What is the value of distinguishing Hodgkin's lymphoma from non-Hodgkin's lymphoma?**
   Unlike other lymphomas, Hodgkin's lymphoma begins as a localized process and spreads in a consistent fashion to adjacent nodes, commonly only affecting a single set of axial nodes, and rarely has extranodal involvement. Consequently, this tumor is often susceptible to local cure. NHLs frequently involve multiple peripheral nodes and extranodal sites, so they are less likely to respond to purely localized therapy. Patients are classically 20 to 40 years old, are often HIV-positive or otherwise immunosuppressed, and do not have the hypergammaglobulinemia seen in multiple myeloma.

SUMMARY BOX: HODGKIN'S AND NON-HODGKIN'S LYMPHOMAS

- Lymphoma patients usually present with systemic (B) symptoms of fever, weight loss, and night sweats.

- Reed-Sternberg cells are large binucleated cells (owl's eyes) seen on node biopsy and are nearly pathognomonic for Hodgkin's disease.

- Hodgkin's lymphoma has many subcategories as listed here, each often with a unique genetic alteration and course.

CASE 14-5

A 62-year-old woman with an unremarkable medical history is evaluated for a 4-week history of headaches, dizziness, and generalized itching, particularly after taking hot showers. She also complains of bouts of sudden-onset intense burning in her hands and feet with accompanied bluish discoloration of the surrounding skin, though she has found through trial and error that aspirin brings rapid relief.

1. **What is the differential diagnosis?**
   The paresthesias and changes in skin color in her hands and feet might be seen with peripheral vascular disease, Raynaud's phenomenon, or diabetic neuropathy. The pruritus, particularly after warm showers, can sometimes be seen in myeloproliferative disorders such as polycythemia vera (PV) or essential thrombocytosis.

CASE 14-5 continued:

Physical examination is significant for elevated blood pressure and splenomegaly but is otherwise normal. Laboratory evaluation reveals the following:
Hemoglobin: 19.6 g/dL
Hematocrit: 60%
WBC count: 15,800
Platelets: 500,000

2. **What is the differential diagnosis of the erythrocytosis (elevated hematocrit)?**
Differential diagnosis includes dehydration, secondary polycythemia (due to hypoxemia, renal tumors, exogenous erythropoietin, Cushing syndrome, carboxyhemoglobinemia), and primary polycythemia (i.e., polycythemia vera [PV]), a myeloproliferative disorder.

CASE 14-5 continued:

Further blood work shows a low level of erythropoietin, normal oxygen saturation, and an elevated leukocyte alkaline phosphatase and uric acid. A peripheral smear is unremarkable, and a bone marrow aspirate shows hypercellularity with megakaryocytic hyperplasia and reduced iron stores

3. **What is the likely diagnosis?**
PV is likely. Patients with this disorder often complain of pruritus, which is due to increased basophils and consequently increased histamine production by mast cells. This is responsible for the generalized itching that occurs following hot showers, a clue often provided in the clinical history for PV on boards. The increased uric acid level is due to increased cell turnover associated with this condition. Patients also commonly present with a ruddy face, blurred vision, and headache secondary to vascular congestion.

4. **What is the pathophysiology of her symptoms of sudden-onset burning?**
This burning is a condition called erythromelalgia, and is caused by microvascular thrombi. It is seen in PV because this disorder also causes dysfunctioning platelets, resulting in increasing stickiness among the cells. Erythromelalgia is also seen in the myeloproliferative disorder essential thrombocytosis because the increased platelet count results in increasing clotting. Aspirin is the most effective treatment to reduce pain. Because of platelet dysfunction and markedly elevated blood viscosity and volume, patients are at an increased risk for other thrombotic events including myocardial infarction, deep venous thrombosis (DVT), stroke, and Budd-Chiari syndrome.

5. **What is the significance of low erythropoietin (epo) levels in diagnosing polycythemia vera?**
Erythropoietin (epo) is produced by the kidneys when the body senses low RBC volume. During states of RBC overproduction such as PV, epo levels are suppressed. This will be an important clinical clue in diagnosing PV versus other causes of polycythemia, which is a term used to describe an abnormally increased RBC count. Appropriate polycythemia occurs in hypoxemic states that reactively trigger RBC production such as high altitude, pulmonary disease, and certain forms of heart disease. In these cases, oxygen saturation is decreased and epo secretion is upregulated. A change in oxygen saturation does not occur in PV. In inappropriate absolute polycythemia, ectopic epo secretion is responsible for increased RBC mass. This most commonly occurs in renal cell carcinoma, pheochromocytoma, and

hepatocellular carcinoma. Oxygen saturation remains unaltered. The final form of polycythemia that you should know for boards is relative polycythemia, which is marked by decreased plasma volume secondary to dehydration. Because plasma volume is reduced, RBC count (number of cells/plasma volume) appears to be elevated, but RBC mass (absolute number of RBCs) remains unaltered. Blood oxygen levels are normal. You should know how to differentiate between these causes of polycythemia for Step 1, as this is another high-yield topic.

6. **What is the classic presentation for essential thrombocytosis?**
Patients with essential thrombocytosis present with many of the same symptoms seen in PV, such as erythromelalgia, bleeding, pruritus, and splenomegaly. They have "platelet counts greater" than 600,000/μL and may have associated increases in RBCs and granulocytes. A peripheral smear classically shows large, hypogranular platelets, and the bone marrow aspiration also shows megakaryocytic hyperplasia but normal iron stores.
   Note: A majority of PV cases and half of essential thrombocytosis cases occur secondary to mutations in *JAK2*, which is involved in hematopoietic growth factor signaling.

7. **What concerns would you have if her bone marrow cells revealed the Philadelphia chromosome?**
As discussed in a prior case, the presence of the Philadelphia chromosome would be concerning for CML. This patient would likely have increased neutrophils and metamyelocytes on peripheral smear, reduced serum LAP, and a bone marrow aspirate with a high myeloid-erythroid ratio.

SUMMARY BOX: MYELOPROLIFERATIVE DISORDERS

- Myeloproliferative disorders such as polycythemia vera and essential thrombocytosis often present with symptoms such as itching and burning as well as a marked proliferation in a single cell line.

- Secondary polycythemia is caused by hypoxemia, renal tumors, exogenous erythropoietin, Cushing syndrome, or carboxyhemoglobinemia.

CASE 14-6

A 75-year-old man is evaluated for worsening fatigue and persistent fever. On physical examination, you notice many bruises on his arms and legs, which he admits is a relatively new phenomenon that he has attributed to "getting old." No lymphadenopathy or hepatosplenomegaly is noted.

1. **What is the differential diagnosis for a combination of fatigue, easy bruising, and recurring fever or infection in an older man?**
The differential diagnosis is broad but for the most part comprises infection, malignancy, and vasculitis.

CASE 14-6 continued:

Blood work shows Hb 9.5 mg/dL, Hct 35%, platelet count 62,000, and WBC count 50,000 with 30% blast cells; a peripheral blood smear is shown in Figure 14-5.

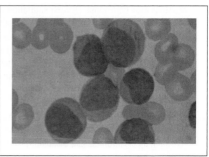

Figure 14-5. Peripheral blood smear from patient in Case 14-5. (From Goldman L, Ausiello D: Cecil Textbook of Medicine, 22nd ed. Philadelphia, WB Saunders, 2004.)

2. **What characteristics of the smear aid the diagnosis?**
   The smear in Figure 14-5 shows circulating granular leukocytes known as myeloblasts, with eosinophilic needle-like inclusions called Auer rods. Auer rods and peripheral blast cells are indicative of AML.

STEP 1 SECRET

You should be able to recognize Auer rods on a peripheral blood smear. This is a high-yield image for the USMLE.

3. **How do his laboratory values help to explain his presenting symptoms?**
   Anemia is the most likely cause of his complaint of fatigue, and thrombocytopenia explains his easy bruising. Although he has an excess of WBCs due to AML, these cells are nonfunctional, causing a clinical neutropenia with consequent fevers/infections.

4. **What cytochemistry tests are used to help diagnose acute myelogenous leukemia and to distinguish among acute myelogenous leukemia subtypes according to the French-American-British classification system?**
   Cluster designations (CDs), myeloperoxidase (MPO) and nonspecific esterase (NSE), periodic acid–Schiff (PAS), and Sudan black (SBB), as depicted in Table 14-8, should be performed.

CASE 14-6 continued:

Bone marrow biopsy showed a predominance of promyelocytes with strongly positive MPO and negative NSE. Fluorescence in situ hybridization (FISH) reveals a translocation between chromosomes 15 and 17 in the affected cells. The translocation involves the retinoic acid receptor-α gene on chromosome 15. The patient is diagnosed with acute promyelocytic leukemia (PML), French-American-British (FAB) classification of M3.

5. **What is the standard treatment for promyelocytic leukemia?**
   As mentioned earlier in the basic concepts section of this chapter, PML is unique in that induction therapy (usually anthracycline) is combined with all-trans-retinoic acid (ATRA), which binds to the mutated *RAR-α* gene and promotes differentiation and thus eventual cell death. Arsenic is used for refractory cases.

TABLE 14-8. CYTOCHEMISTRY TESTS USED TO DIAGNOSE ACUTE MYELOGENOUS LEUKEMIA AND DIFFERENTIATE ACUTE MYELOGENOUS LEUKEMIA SUBTYPES

FAB Subtype	Incidence	Morphology	Classical Characteristics	Diagnostic Features	Cytochemistry
M0	2%	Undifferentiated	Diploid	≥20% blasts of total nucleated cell, immunophenotyping CD33 and CD13	<3% reactive to MPO or SBB
M1	10-18%	Acute myeloblastic	Auer rods	≥20% blasts	>3% reactive to MPO or SBB
M2	27-29%	Acute myeloblastic	Auer rods	≥20% blasts, t(8:21) chromosome abnormality	MPO+, SBB+, NSE+
M3	5-10%	Acute promyelocytic	>30% promyelocytes, Auer rods	≥20% blasts and abnormal promyelocytes; intense MPO and SBB reactivity; t(15:17) cytogenetic abnormality	MPO+, SBB+, PAS−, NSE±
M4	16-25%	Myelomonocytic	Myelomonocytic blasts	Associated with inv(16) chromosome abnormality	PAS+, >20% NSE+
M5	13-22%	Monocytic	Monoblasts		NSE+
M6	1-3%	Erythroleukemia	Dysplastic	≥50% erythroid precursors	PAS+, MPO+
M7	1-3%	Megakaryocytic	Megakaryocytes	Infants <1 year old with t(1:22), myelofibrosis, Down syndrome	

CD, cluster designation; FAB, French-American British [classification]; MPO, myeloperoxidase; NSE, nonspecific esterase; PAS, periodic acid–Schiff; SBB, Sudan black B.
Modified from Hoffman R, Benz EJ Jr, Shattil SJ, et al: Hematology: Basic Principles and Practice, 4th ed., Philadelphia, Churchill Livingstone, 2005.

SUMMARY BOX: ACUTE MYELOGENOUS LEUKEMIA

- Auer rods on a peripheral blood smear are pathognomonic for acute myelogenous leukemia (AML).

- Cytochemistry tests and cell morphologic appearance are used to subclassify AML patients. Subclassifications often have different clinical courses and treatments.

- A t(15,17) involving the retinoic acid receptor-α gene on chromosome 15 is unique to acute promyelocytic leukemia (APML), French-American-British (FAB) classification of M3. Its treatment using all-trans-retinoic acid (ATRA) is equally unique.

CHAPTER 15

IMMUNOLOGY

Thomas A. Brown, MD, and Sonali J. Shah

INSIDER'S GUIDE TO IMMUNOLOGY FOR THE USMLE STEP 1

Immunology can be an intimidating subject for many medical students. Fortunately, immunology-related questions on the USMLE focus primarily on basic concepts that can be mastered by achieving a thorough understanding of the topics listed in First Aid and working through the questions and cases in this chapter. Pay close attention to the tables in this chapter. These topics are particularly high-yield for the USMLE Step 1 examination.

BASIC CONCEPTS

1. **Outline hematopoiesis, beginning with a pluripotent stem cell.**
   See Figure 15-1.

2. **What are the major primary and secondary organs that make up the human lymphoid system?**
   Primary lymphoid organs include bone marrow, thymus, and fetal liver and are the sites at which lymphocytes mature. Precursor B and T lymphocytes are produced in the bone marrow. In adults, B cells continue to mature in the bone marrow, but T cells leave the marrow to mature in the thymus. Maturation in these organs occurs in the absence of stimulating antigen and involves a stringent selection process that eliminates both poorly functioning and autoreactive lymphocytes. Secondary lymphoid organs include lymph nodes, spleen, and mucosa-associated lymphoid tissue (MALT). MALT ranges from poorly organized clusters of lymphoid cells to highly organized structures such as appendix, tonsils, and Peyer's patches. These secondary lymphoid organs provide a site for mature lymphocytes to respond to antigen presented on the surface of dendritic cells and other professional antigen presenting cells (APCs).

3. **What is the function of innate immune system?**
   The innate immune system forms the first line of defense against pathogens and toxic compounds. Cells of the innate immune system are activated non-specifically and contain various pattern recognition receptors (PRRs) that recognize a diverse group of pathogen-associated molecular patterns (PAMPs) shared by different classes of microbes (e.g., LPS and flagellin). The intensity of the innate immune response does not increase with repetitive exposure to identical antigens.
   The first component of innate immunity includes factors that prevent microbes from entering the body. Examples of this are intact epithelium, respiratory cilia, alveolar macrophages, lysozyme, cationic peptides (defensins), RNase (ribonuclease), and normal flora. The second component includes factors that destroy or limit the growth of microbes that have already entered the body. Examples of this are phagocytes, natural killer (NK) cells, complement, interferon (IFN), iron-sequestering proteins (e.g., lactoferrin), fever and the inflammatory response (i.e., release of

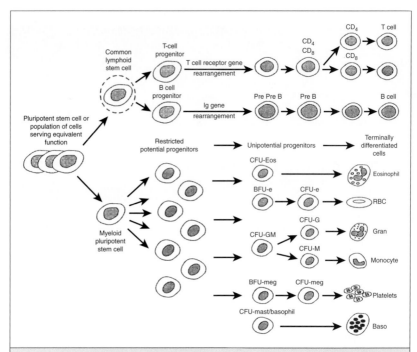

Figure 15-1. Stem cell–based model of hematopoiesis. (From Noble J: Textbook of Primary Care Medicine, 3rd ed. St. Louis, Mosby, 2001.)

interleukin 1 [IL-1], IL-6, and tumor necrosis factor [TNF]). Neutrophils form the most abundant type of phagocyte and are first to reach the site of infection. Here, they engulf and destroy microbes. Pus is a viscous exudate that is composed of dead neutrophils at the infection site.

4. **What is adaptive/acquired immunity?**
   Adaptive immunity involves the response of B and T cells following exposure to an antigen to which they are specific. It is characterized by memory, resulting in rapid, stronger, and more efficient elimination of the source of the offending antigen upon repeat exposure to said antigen (Table 15-1). It is very important to recognize that stimulation of the adaptive immune response depends on prior activation of the innate immune system. Dendritic cells are considered to form the bridge between the innate and adaptive immune systems, because they present antigen to naive T cells. Stimulation of dendritic cell PRRs results in antigen processing and presentation to naive T cells via major histocompatibility complex (MHC)-T-cell receptor (TCR) interactions.
   Note: The primary and secondary immune responses refer to the activity of the adaptive immune system. The primary response is the activity of this system after first exposure to the pathogen, whereas the secondary response occurs after immunologic memory has been generated from a previous exposure, so the secondary response is more rapid and powerful.

5. **What are the basic characteristics of cell-mediated and humoral immunity?**
   Cell-mediated immunity involves helper T (T_H) cells and is characterized by T_H cell–mediated defense against viruses, fungi, and mycobacteria. It is also responsible for type IV hypersensitivity reactions, tumor destruction, and graft rejection.
   Non-specific activation of dendritic cells and macrophages leads to secretion of IL-12, which stimulate naive T helper (T_H0) cells to differentiate into T_H1 cells. This T-cell subset secretes IL-2,

TABLE 15-1. CHARACTERISTICS OF INNATE AND ACQUIRED IMMUNITY

	Innate (Natural)	Acquired (Adaptive)
Effector cells	Neutrophils (polymorphonuclear neutrophils), macrophages, eosinophils, basophils, mast cells, natural killer (NK) cells	B cells and plasma cells, T helper cells (e.g., T_H1, T_H2 cells), cytotoxic T lymphocytes (CTLs)
Chemical mediators	Complement, lysosomal enzymes, cytokines, interferons, acute-phase proteins	Antibodies (immunoglobulins), cytokines, granzyme, perforin
Response characteristics	Rapid, nonspecific; same intensity against all antigens, no memory	Slow, antigen-specific; long-term memory and enhanced response generated after first exposure (e.g., more rapid and intense)

leading to propagation of the T_H cell response and activation/conversion of T_C cells to cytotoxic T lymphocytes (CTLs), which function to destroy tumors and virus-infected cells. Note that IL-2 secretion from T_H1 cells constitutes only part of the signal sequence necessary for CTL activation; CTLs also require TCR and CDB interaction with MHC class I on infected cells (see question 6, next). T_H1 cells also secrete interferon-γ (IFN-γ), which activates macrophages and stimulates intracellular microorganism destruction.

Humoral immunity is primarily mediated by B cell production of antibodies. Antibodies have a diverse set of roles, including neutralization of pathogens and toxins, opsonization of pathogens to facilitate phagocytosis, complement activation, stimulation of mast cell and basophil degranulation, and B cell activation. Antibodies are grouped into five different isotypes (IgM, IgD, IgA, IgE, IgG) according to their constant domains. Production of IgA, IgE, and IgG relies on B cell interaction with T cells in a process known as *class switching* (*see question 9*).

6. **Describe the difference between class I and class II major histocompatibility complex molecules.**
   T cells possess T-cell receptors (TCRs) that interact with MHC molecules. MHC class I molecules are found on the surface of all nucleated cells, thus excluding only mature erythrocytes, and interact with the TCR of CD8$^+$ T cells (i.e., cytotoxic T lymphocytes). The CD8 molecule is necessary to complete the interaction of the TCR and MHC class I. MHC class II lies on the plasma membrane of antigen-presenting cells (dendritic cells, macrophages, and memory B cells). It interacts with the TCR of CD4$^+$ T cells (i.e., T_H cells), with the CD4 molecule serving a necessary role for this interaction to occur. An easy way to remember which MHC molecule interacts with which T-cell type is to use the rule of 8:

$$\text{Class } 1 \times \text{CD}8 = 8$$
$$\text{Class } 2 \times \text{CD}4 = 8$$

For the purpose of boards, MHC class I displays nonself peptides that have been processed intracellularly (as might be seen in a cell infected with a virus), and MHC class II displays exogenous nonself peptides (obtained via phagocytosis or endocytosis). This is an important distinction to make. MHC class I, when displaying nonself peptides, marks the cell for destruction by the CTL with the TCR specific for that peptide. This destruction is mediated by Fas-Fas ligand binding (leading to apoptosis), granzymes (proteases), or perforins (creates a channel in the plasma membrane and mediates cytolysis), thus eliminating the infected cell. On the other hand, when MHC class II displays nonself peptides, it leads to activation of the T_H cell with the TCR specific for that peptide. This activation process upregulates T_H cytokine production, resulting in subsequent macrophage activation and proliferation of plasma cells with the appropriate specificity, thus catalyzing the elimination of the offending extracellular agent.

7. **How do antibodies eliminate extracellular pathogens?**
Extracellular pathogens (e.g., bacteria, free virions) commonly induce production of humoral antibodies. Extracellular pathogens that are coated with opsonizing antibodies (IgG) are efficiently phagocytized by macrophages and neutrophils. Following phagocytosis and processing of extracellular antigens, expression of antigenic peptides in association with MHC class II on the surface of antigen-presenting cells (APCs) stimulates T_H2 cells, which further enhances the humoral response. Keep in mind that IgG and IgM can activate complement that may lyse, neutralize, or opsonize extracellular pathogens.

8. **By what process can antibodies catalyze the elimination of intracellular pathogens?**
Antibody-dependent cellular cytotoxicity (ADCC) involves the binding of IgG (attached to antigens on the surface of the target cell) to $Fc\gamma$ receptors. This leads to destruction of the cell by phagocytic cells or NK cells possessing these receptors.

9. **What are the five classes (isotypes) of immunoglobulins? Describe their respective distributions in the body.**
See Table 15-2.
   Note: When B cells directly interact with CD4+ helper T cells, all classes of immunoglobulin can potentially be produced. The TCR interacts with MHC II on the B cell, and CD40L expressed on the activated T cell simultaneously binds to the constitutively expressed CD40 on the B cell. This interaction facilitates the production of various cytokines from the T cell that influence B cell class switching via VDJ recombination and production of IgG, IgE, and IgA. B cells capable of producing these antibodies are referred to as plasma cells.
   In contrast, the T cell–independent response consists almost exclusively of IgM. The T cell–independent response generally occurs when the primary antigen is a polysaccharide (e.g., bacterial capsule, lipopolysaccharide on the gram-negative outer membrane), because these molecules are not processed by APCs in the same manner as for peptide antigen. Therefore, T_H cells are not activated and isotype switching cannot occur. This means that only IgM will be produced and no secondary (memory) immune response will occur. Vaccines containing polysaccharide capsules (e.g., meningococcal vaccine, pneumovax, *Haemophilus influenzae* type B vaccine) are thus commonly conjugated to proteins in order to promote T_H cell activation, class switching and the formation of immunologic memory.

10. **Most humans can produce 10^6 to 10^9 unique immunoglobulin (Ig) molecules. However, the number of immunoglobulin genes is orders of magnitude less than this. How is this possible?**
This is primarily due to gene rearrangement. Note that each Ig molecule consists of two identical light chains (classified as λ or κ by the constant region) and two identical heavy chains (classified as α, δ, ε, γ, and μ according to the isotype, as determined by the constant region). Diversity is gained from "mixing and matching" these chains. However, each of these four chains also contains a variable region, which is created by gene rearrangement. In this process, various unique gene segments in groups named V, D (heavy chains only), and J are excised from the strand, reordered to create a unique code for the variable region, and reconnected by *RAG1* and *RAG2* (recombination-activating genes) to each other and to the constant region gene segments. This type of rearrangement is also seen in the α and β chains of the TCR to achieve diversity in these molecules as well.

TABLE 15-2. IMMUNOGLOBULIN ISOTYPES

Immunoglobulin Isotype	Location	Functions
IgA	Dimeric IgA, joined by a J chain, is found in secretions Monomeric IgA is found in the blood	Found in mucosal secretions (e.g., tears, saliva, colostrum, gastrointestinal secretions); mediates mucosal immunity Poor activator of complement
IgD	Surface of mature B cells; some found in the blood	Unclear
IgE	Bound to FcεR1 receptors on the surface of tissue mast cells and blood basophils	Mediates type 1 hypersensitivity Mediates parasitic killing via ADCC (eosinophils possessing Fcε receptors are the effector cells and induce damage with major basic protein)
IgG	Found in the blood; crosses placenta Has the longest half-life of all isotopes and is thus used for passive immunization	Ligand for Fc receptors Activates classical complement pathway Most abundant immunoglobulin in secondary immune response Highest affinity for antigen (greatest strength of interaction between antigen and antibody)
IgM	Found in the blood, often in pentamers (joined by J chains), on the surface of immature and mature B cells	Activates classical complement pathway Earliest antibody produced in any humoral response Most abundant immunoglobulin in primary immune response Highest avidity for antigen (greatest number of antigen-binding sites as a result of pentameric form)

ADCC, antibody-dependent cellular cytotoxicity.

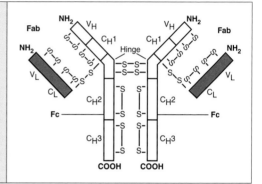

Figure 15-2. The structure of immunoglobulin (Ig) molecules. **Note:** The 12 complement-determining regions (CDRs) are the areas that most determine to which antigen the antibody will bind. (From Mason RJ, Murray JF, Broaddus VC, et al: Murray & Nadel's Textbook of Respiratory Medicine, 4th ed. Philadelphia, WB Saunders, 2005.)

11. **What are complement proteins and how do they function in an immune response?**

    Complement proteins comprise a network of soluble plasma proteins that become activated as a cascade by IgM and IgG (classical pathway) or by surface molecules of microorganisms (alternative and lectin pathways). The complement proteins have many important biologic activities. The membrane attack complex mediates cell lysis, whereas other components participate in opsonization, chemotaxis, neutralization of pathogens, and clearance of immune complexes (Fig. 15-3 and Table 15-3).

12. **Describe the ramifications of the most common complement protein deficiencies.**

    See Table 15-4.

    Note: Since complement represents a set of proteins produced by the liver, generalized complement deficiencies can be seen in liver failure or in dietary deficiencies of certain essential amino acids.

13. **Which complement components and cytokines are required for neutrophil chemotaxis?**

    Neutrophil migration is dependent on IL-8 C5a (complement component), and LTB_4 (a leukotriene). Leukotriene synthesis is dependent upon the enzyme lipoxygenase, which is inhibited by the drug zileuton.

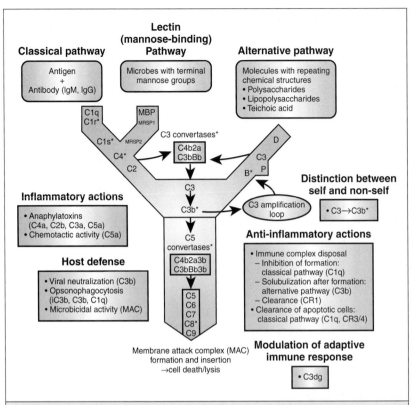

Figure 15-3. The complement cascade. (From Mandell GL, Bennett JE, Dolin R: Principles and Practice of Infectious Disease, 6th ed. Philadelphia, Churchill Livingstone, 2005.)

TABLE 15-3. COMPLEMENT PATHWAY COMPONENTS AND ACTIVITY

Biologic Activity	Complement Component(s)
Cell lysis	C5b-C9 (membrane attack complex [MAC])
Degranulation of mast cells and basophils	C3a, C4a, C5a (anaphylatoxins)
Opsonization of particulate antigens	C3b, C4b, iC3b (opsonins)
Chemotaxis of leukocytes (mainly polymorphonuclear neutrophils)	C5a, C3a, C5b67 (chemotactic factors)
Viral neutralization	C3b, C5b-9
Solubilization and clearance of immune complexes	C3b

14. **As a review, list the effector functions of the major leukocyte classes.**
    See Table 15-5.

TABLE 15-4. COMPLEMENT PROTEIN DEFICIENCIES

Complement Protein(s)	Deficiencies
C1 esterase inhibitor	Deficiency of C1 esterase inhibitor results in C1 esterase overactivity and overproduction of anaphylatoxins, leading to recurrent episodes of angioedema; this is also known as hereditary angioneurotic edema and is inherited in an autosomal dominant fashion. C1 esterase inhibitor also is inhibited directly by bradykinin, which explains the rare but life-threatening angioedema that may result as a side effect of ACE inhibitors (ACE is responsible for the degradation of bradykinin).
C2 or C4	These deficiencies often resemble autoimmune diseases (e.g., systemic lupus erythematosus, vasculitis) but frequently are asymptomatic. C2 deficiency is the most common complement deficiency and also may be associated with septicemia (typically due to *S. pneumoniae*).
C3	Reduced levels of C3b predispose patient to recurrent pyogenic infections as a consequence of decreased opsonization. Red blood cells also recognize antigen-antibody-C3b complexes in circulation and transport them to the liver or spleen for phagocytic degradation. Decreased C3b levels in serum thus predispose patients to type III hypersensitivity reactions due to decreased immune complex clearance from circulation.
C5-C8 or mannan-binding lectin (MBL), or mannose-binding protein	These greatly increase risk of *Neisseria* infections; of note, C5b-C9 forms the MAC, which can kill most unencapsulated gram-negative organisms.
Decay-accelerating factor (DAF) or CD55 and CD59	This protein is located on the surface of all human cells and destabilizes C3 convertase and C5 convertase, preventing MAC formation, thereby protecting human cells from lysis; deficiency is manifested as an increase in complement-mediated hemolysis, clinically apparent as paroxysmal nocturnal hemoglobinuria. DAF deficiency is diagnosed with the Ham test, which checks to see whether the fragility of red blood cells increases when placed in a mildly acidic solution.

ACE, angiotensin-converting enzyme; MAC, membrane attack complex.

TABLE 15-5. LEUKOCYTES AND THEIR EFFECTOR FUNCTIONS

Cell	General Description	Effector Mechanism
Monocyte	A phagocytic cell that constitutes 4-10% of the WBCs in peripheral blood. Several hours after release from the bone marrow, monocytes will die or migrate into the tissue and differentiate in macrophages or dendritic cells.	Phagocytosis
Macrophage	This is a highly phagocytic tissue-dwelling cell. Major functions include phagocytosis of particulate material, antigen presentation to T cells, and secretion of IL-1, TNF, IL-8, and IL-12.	Antimicrobicidal activity includes generation of both oxygen-dependent mediators (e.g., superoxide anion, hydrogen peroxide, hypoclorous acid) and oxygen-independent mediators (e.g., TNF-α, lysozyme, defensins, hydrolytic enzymes).
Dendritic cell	This potent antigen-presenting cell forms an extensive web in tissues for trapping antigen (e.g., Langerhan cells in the epidermis).	Phagocytosis
Neutrophil	This type of granulocyte makes up ~70% of WBCs in peripheral blood. Neutrophils are active phagocytes that are the first cell to arrive at sites of inflammation.	Like macrophages, neutrophils employ both oxygen-dependent and oxygen-independent pathways to generate antimicrobial substances.
Eosinophil	This type of granulocyte makes up 2-5% of the WBCs in peripheral blood. It is a phagocytic cell that migrates into the tissue spaces, where it plays a role in defense against parasitic organisms.	Exocytosis of granules contains extremely basic proteins.
Basophil	This nonphagocytic granulocyte makes up 0.5-1% of peripheral WBCs. Basophils play a major role in allergic responses.	Basophils release pharmacologically active substances from cytoplasmic granules (histamine and other vasoactive amines) on cross-linking of surface-bound IgE by allergen.
Mast cell	This tissue-dwelling cell plays a role in allergic responses similar to that of basophils. Mast cells have Fcϵ receptors (for IgE) and histamine-containing granules.	This cell releases pharmacologically active substances from cytoplasmic granules (histamine and other vasoactive amines) on cross-linking of surface-bound IgE by allergen.

Continued

TABLE 15-5. LEUKOCYTES AND THEIR EFFECTOR FUNCTIONS—continued

Cell	General Description	Effector Mechanism
Helper T cell	This CD4+ lymphocyte matures in the thymus and functions in cytokine production. Helper T cells play a central role in the immune response by regulating the function of cells such as CTLs, B cells, NK cells, and macrophages. Helper T cells are activated by foreign antigen in the context of MHC class II molecules.	T_H1 cells: IL-12 induces their differentiation (from T_H0 cells); secretes IFN-γ (activates macrophages), and IL-2 activates CTLs and propagates the response) T_H2 cells: IL-4 induces their differentiation; activate B cells to plasma cells with IL-4 and IL-5.
Cytotoxic T cell	This CD8+ lymphocyte matures in the thymus and functions in direct cell killing upon activation by foreign antigen presented by MHC class I molecules.	Perforins, granzymes, IFN-γ, TNF-β, FasL
B cell	This CD19+CD20+ lymphocyte has membrane-bound immunoglobulin. Upon activation by helper T cells, B cells may differentiate into plasma cells, which produce large volumes of antibodies. By presenting endocytosed antigen in the cleft of MHC class II, B cells also function as antigen-presenting cells in the activation of helper T cells.	Antibody
NK cell	This is a large granular lymphocyte that has no markers in common with B or T cells and is not MHC-restricted. NK cells act to lyse virally infected cells (via ADCC) and tumor cells with decreased levels of MHC class I.	Perforins, granzymes, IFN-γ, TNF-α

ADCC, antibody-dependent cellular cytotoxicity; CTLs, cytotoxic T lymphocytes; FasL, Fas ligand; IFN-γ, interferon-γ; IgE, immunoglobulin E; IL, interleukin; MHC, major histocompatibility complex; NK, natural killer; TNF, tumor necrosis factor; WBCs, white blood cells.

15. **List the functions of the major cytokines secreted by various classes of immune cells.**
Secreted by T cells:
- IL-3: Hematopoietic stem cell differentiation into myeloid progenitors

Secreted by T_H1 cells:
- IL-2: T-cell proliferation
- IL-12: T_H1 cell differentiation
- INF-γ: Activation of macrophages and T_H1 cells, suppression of T_H2 cells, killing of intracellular pathogens

Secreted by T_H2 cells:
- IL-4: T_H2 cell differentiation, promotes IgE and IgG class switch
- IL-5: Promotes eosinophil proliferation, aids in IgA class switch
- IL-10: Anti-inflammatory; activates T_H2 cells and inhibits T_H1 cells

Secreted by macrophages:
- TNF-α: Acute-phase cytokine that activates adhesion molecule expression on endothelium; promotes vascular leak; responsible for septic shock and cachexia
- IL-1: Acute-phase cytokine; activates adhesion molecule expression on endothelium and causes fever
- IL-6: Acute-phase cytokine; promotes fever
- IL-8: Neutrophil chemotaxis
- IL-12: T_H1 cell differentiation, NK cell activation

16. **List the major cell surface markers used to identify various classes of immune cells.**
See Table 15-6.

CASE 15-1

A 2-year-old boy becomes acutely short of breath, has audible wheezing, and develops pruritic hives. He also has a bout of nausea and diarrhea. His mother takes him to the emergency room, where he is found to be dangerously hypotensive, with marked tachycardia and tachypnea.

1. **What is the differential diagnosis for this presentation?**
Asthma, anaphylactic shock, bronchiolitis (inflammation of the small airways usually following a viral infection), foreign body aspiration, and toxin or allergen ingestion must be considered.

CASE 15-1 continued:

The mother is quickly questioned, and it is discovered that these symptoms developed shortly after the child took the first dose of a course of amoxicillin. The child is immediately given a subcutaneous injection of epinephrine, as well as intravenous (IV) diphenhydramine and methylprednisolone. It is explained to the mother that this acute episode was most likely due to the amoxicillin, but she seems confused because he had taken amoxicillin previously to treat an ear infection and had no problems with it.

2. **What is the most likely diagnosis?**
Acute systemic anaphylaxis (anaphylactic shock)—the combination of bronchospasm, urticaria, and hypotension makes this diagnosis much more likely than the others. It

TABLE 15-6. CELL SURFACE MARKERS USED TO IDENTIFY CLASSES OF IMMUNE CELLS

T Cells	B Cells	Macrophages	NK Cells	RBCs/WBCs/Platelets
CD2	Ig	CD14 (endotoxin receptor)	CD16	CD55 and CD59 (DAF; prevents complement-mediated damage)
CD3	CD19	CD16 (Fcγ receptor)	CD56	
CD4+ (helper T cells)	CD20	CD40	MHC class I	
CD8+ (CTLs)	CD21	B7		
CD28 (binds to B7)	CD40 (binds to CD40L)	MHC class I and II		
CD40L (binds to CD40)	B7 (binds to CD28)	CR1 (C3b receptor)		
TCR	MHC class I and II			

CD40L, CD40 ligand; CTLs, cytotoxic T lymphocytes; DAF, decay-accelerating factor; MHC, major histocompatibility complex; NK, natural killer; RBCs, red blood cells; TCR, T-cell receptor; WBCs, white blood cells.

should be noted that anaphylaxis is the most serious result of drug hypersensitivity. However, the most common type of drug hypersensitivity involves cutaneous symptoms, such as generalized flushing, urticaria (hives), or mild angioedema. Penicillins are the most common cause of medication-induced anaphylaxis, but this is still a very rare phenomenon with this class of antibiotics.

3. **Can free penicillin cause anaphylaxis?**
   No. Penicillin is only large enough to bind to one arm of an antibody (i.e., the variable regions of only one heavy chain and one light chain) and thus is referred to as univalent. Penicillin must be bound to a carrier protein to induce a response, and therefore it is a hapten. When penicillin is bound to its carrier protein, it can cross-link IgE (bind to one arm of two separate but identical antibodies and increase the propinquity of the corresponding Fc receptors on the mast cell surface), thus triggering the release of mediators.

4. **What type of hypersensitivity is anaphylaxis? What is its immunopathogenesis?**
   Anaphylaxis is the systemic form of the immediate hypersensitivity response (type I). Upon first exposure to antigen, the antigen binds to a B cell, which presents the antigen on MHC class II to a T_H2 cell. The T cell provides cytokines to induce IgE class switching. IgE binds to Fc receptors on the surface of mast cells and basophils, where it persists until the second exposure to antigen. This antigen then cross-links the IgE bound to mast cells and basophils,

triggering the release of pre-formed histamine (via cGMP, cAMP, and Ca^{2+}) and the de novo synthesis and release of lipid mediators (e.g., leukotrienes, prostaglandins, platelet-activating factor [PAF]). In the immediate phase (occurs within minutes; caused by degranulation of pre-formed mediators), histamine induces a widespread increase in vascular permeability and smooth muscle contraction. In the late phase (>6 hours later, as these mediators were synthesized at the time of exposure), leukotrienes elicit prolonged bronchoconstriction, mucus secretion, and an increase in vascular permeability, while prostaglandin D_2 and PAF cause leukocyte migration and activation. Eosinophilia occurs along with the late phase reaction due to release of eosinophil chemotactic factor. Eosinophils release cationic granule proteins intended to destroy parasites, but in the absence of parasites, tissue damage and remodeling occur.

5. **What is the pathophysiologic explanation for the wheezing and diarrhea that developed?**
   Release of mast cell mediators, such as histamine and leukotrienes, causes an increase in vascular permeability and contraction of certain smooth muscle types in multiple organ systems. In the airways, this leads to laryngeal edema, bronchoconstriction, and mucus hypersecretion, resulting in the clinical symptom of wheezing. In the gastrointestinal tract, the consequence of smooth muscle contraction and edema is nausea, vomiting, and diarrhea.

6. **How does anaphylaxis result in the urticaria observed in this patient?**
   The widespread vasodilation and increased vascular permeability that develop in anaphylaxis allow fluid to accumulate in the superficial dermis, producing small wheals with a pale center encircled by a red flare. This same mechanism is responsible for causing edema in the deep dermis (angioedema) and the laryngeal edema that can develop in anaphylaxis.

7. **Why did the child NOT have a reaction to amoxicillin when it was first administered for his previous ear infection?**
   He was not sensitized to the allergen at that time. Initial exposure to an allergen generates allergen-specific IgE antibodies after several days, which become bound to Fc receptors on the mast cell surface (sensitization). Re-exposure to the same allergen (challenge phase) cross-links the IgE-bound mast cells and stimulates degranulation (see question 4).

8. **What clinical testing can be performed to confirm that this immediate hypersensitivity reaction was caused by amoxicillin?**
   A few days following the attack, a skin test for amoxicillin and other common drug allergens can be performed. If the child is allergic, intradermal injections of amoxicillin will cause degranulation of local mast cells at the site of injection. The resultant release of histamine and other mediators will cause a large wheal and flare to develop within 30 minutes. The wheal is a central raised area reflecting leakage of plasma from venules (edema), and the flare is a surrounding red area caused by vasodilation (erythema).

9. **Why was the child immediately given epinephrine?**
   Epinephrine alleviates the symptoms of anaphylaxis through its positive adrenergic effects. By stimulating β_2-receptors, it relaxes bronchial smooth muscles to open the airways; by stimulating peripheral α_1-receptors, it constricts small blood vessels, thereby reducing vascular leakage and raising blood pressure.

10. **Why was the child given diphenhydramine and methylprednisolone?**
    Diphenhydramine (Benadryl) is an H_1 receptor antagonist and will ameliorate the histamine-mediated components of anaphylaxis.
    Methylprednisolone is a corticosteroid that acts synergistically with epinephrine by upregulating adrenergic receptors. It also blocks a portion of the late phase of the allergic response by demarginalizing neutrophils (preventing subsequent chemotaxis), reducing eosinophil counts,

and blocking phospholipase A_2 (the enzyme that produces arachidonic acid, which is eventually converted into prostaglandins and leukotrienes). Note that although corticosteroid administration decreases plasma counts of many leukocyte subtypes, it increases neutrophil count secondary to decreased adhesion molecule synthesis. This reduces adhesion of polymorphonuclear cells (PMNs) to the endothelial wall and thus allows more to enter the circulation.

RELATED QUESTIONS

11. **What was the motivation for developing the second-generation H_1 receptor antagonists such as fexofenadine (Allegra) and loratadine (Claritin)?**
These agents do not cross the blood-brain barrier like the first-generation H_1 receptor antagonists and do not cause as much drowsiness. They are generally used for allergic rhinitis, another (milder) type I hypersensitivity response.

12. **List the common classes of drugs that are used to treat type I hypersensitivity disorders and their general mode of action.**
See Table 15-7.

SUMMARY BOX: ANAPHYLACTIC SHOCK

- Anaphylactic shock has many potential manifestations, including bronchospasm, urticaria, hypotension, and gastrointestinal (GI) problems.

- Anaphylactic shock is a type I, IgE-mediated hypersensitivity reaction, with histamine and leukotrienes playing the major mediator roles.

- Epinephrine, diphenhydramine (an antihistamine), and corticosteroids are the most effective treatments for anaphylactic shock.

- See Table 15-8 for more information.

CASE 15-2

A 43-year-old man with uncomplicated pneumococcal pneumonia is prescribed a 10-day course of penicillin V. On the ninth day, he appears mildly jaundiced, and his hematocrit has dropped significantly from when he was first seen. He denies any hemoptysis, hematemesis, melena, or hematochezia.

1. **What is the differential diagnosis for this presentation?**
Hemolytic anemia, chronic liver disease (jaundice is common, as is a macrocytic anemia), occult hemorrhage, drug toxicity, tumor obstructing biliary tract (anemia is common in cancer, and biliary obstruction would lead to jaundice), and Gilbert syndrome (jaundice can occur if stressor—anemia in this case—is severe enough to induce markedly reduced uridine diphosphate (UDP) glucuronyl transferase activity) are all considered.

2. **What additional tests should be ordered to further analyze the anemia and jaundice?**
All patients with anemia should receive a complete blood count (CBC) with erythrocyte indices (mean corpuscular volume [MCV], mean corpuscular hemoglobin [MCH], mean corpuscular hemoglobin concentration [MCHC], red blood cell (RBC) distribution width, and a reticulocyte

TABLE 15-7. DRUGS USED TO TREAT TYPE I HYPERSENSITIVITY DISORDERS AND THEIR GENERAL MODE OF ACTION

Type of Drug	Mode of Action	Clinical Indication(s)	Comments
Antihistamines	Block histamine H_1 and H_2 receptors on target cells	Allergic rhinitis, atopic dermatitis, allergic conjunctivitis	Second-generation histamine receptor antagonists have fewer adverse side effects (e.g., they are nonsedating)
Mast cell stabilizers	Prophylactic inhibitors of mast cell mediator release	Allergic rhinitis and asthma	Include cromolyn sodium and nedocromil
Methylxanthines	Inhibition of phosphodiesterase, in addition to many other (debated) effects	Asthma, bronchospasm resistant to other modes of treatment	Include theophylline and aminophylline
Corticosteroids	Anti-inflammatory; block production of inflammatory cytokines; multiple effects on several types of leukocytes	Allergic asthma, atopic dermatitis	Include prednisone, beclamethasone, triamcinolone, flunisolide
Sympathomimetics	Adrenergic effects	Asthma; epinephrine in anaphylaxis	Epinephrine has both α- and β-adrenergic effects; albuterol, salmeterol, and metaproterenol are selective β-adrenergic bronchodilators
Monoclonal anti-IgE antibody	Binds to $Fc\varepsilon$ receptors, preventing IgE binding	Severe asthma, uncontrolled with corticosteroids	Includes omalizumab
Leukotriene pathway inhibitors	Prophylactic inhibitors of leukotriene synthesis or receptor antagonists	Asthma	Include cysteinyl leukotriene receptor antagonists (e.g., zafirlukast, montelukast) and 5-lipoxygenase inhibitors (e.g., zileuton)

IgE, immunoglobulin E.

count). The patient is also presenting with jaundice, necessitating liver function tests as well as direct (conjugated) and indirect (unconjugated) bilirubin levels.

CASE 15-2 continued:

The additional tests reveal a reticulocyte count of 7% (normal is <2.5%), an MCV of 90 fL (normal is 80-100 fL), and an elevated indirect bilirubin. With these results, you decide to immediately order one more test. The results of the direct Coombs' test are positive.

3. What is the most likely diagnosis?
   Drug-induced warm autoimmune hemolytic anemia (AIHA).

4. What is the significance of a positive direct Coombs' test and how does it support the diagnosis considered in this patient?
   A Coombs' test is an antiglobulin assay that detects both immunoglobulin that is attached to the surface of a patient's RBCs (direct test) and the presence of circulating immunoglobulin against RBCs (indirect test). A positive direct Coombs' test supports, but does not prove, the presence of an immune-mediated hemolytic process.
   Note: Distinguishing between direct and indirect Coombs' assays can be tricky, but it is important to understand the differences between the methodologies and uses for the two tests. In a direct Coombs' test, anti-Ig antibody is added to a patient's RBCs. If the RBCs are already bound to immunoglobulin present in the patient's own blood, the addition of anti-Ig antibody will cause agglutination. This test is used to detect the presence of immunoglobulins against a patient's *own* RBCs (e.g., hemolytic disease of the newborn, drug-induced AIHA, transfusion reactions). In contrast, an indirect Coombs' test requires addition of normal RBCs to a patient's serum. If immunoglobulins against the RBCs are present in the serum, agglutination will occur. Thus, an indirect test measures for immunoglobulins against *foreign blood products* that are not bound to the patient's own RBCs (e.g., screening for antibodies prior to blood transfusion, detecting Rh antibodies).

5. How do medications such as penicillin cause autoimmune hemolytic anemia?
   Certain antibiotics (e.g., penicillin, cephalosporins, streptomycin, tetracycline) and other small molecules may nonspecifically adsorb to proteins on RBC surfaces, forming a complex similar to a hapten-carrier complex. These drugs are generally too small to elicit an immune response by themselves; however, they can become immunogenic when combined with larger molecules such as membrane-associated proteins. In such individuals, this complex can induce the formation of antibodies, which then bind to the adsorbed drug on RBCs. It is the presence of these autoantibodies that is detected in the direct Coombs' test.

6. What type of hypersensitivity does autoimmune hemolytic anemia represent?
   This is an example of a type II hypersensitivity reaction, in which IgM or IgG antibodies bind to cell surface antigens. Other examples of type II hypersensitivity include blood transfusion reactions, hyperacute rejection of organ transplants, and hemolytic disease of the newborn.

7. What is the mechanism by which hemolysis occurs in drug-induced autoimmune hemolytic anemia?
   IgG damages RBCs by binding and activating effector cells carrying Fcγ receptors (e.g., neutrophils, macrophages, and NK cells). Note that both IgG and IgM can induce complement-mediated lysis of RBCs, but this mode of destruction is not common in this form of AIHA.

Note: In some individuals, the extended use of certain drugs, including methyldopa, levodopa, quinidine, and procainamide, can stimulate production of anti-RBC antibodies. The mechanism by which the autoantibodies are induced is unknown, and the antibodies do not cross-react with the drug that appears to elicit their production.

RELATED QUESTION

8. If this patient had had a *Mycoplasma pneumoniae* infection rather than a pneumococcal infection, what type of autoimmune hemolytic anemia would have been considered?
   Cold AIHA, in which anti-*M. pneumoniae* IgM cross-reacts with erythrocyte surface antigens. Optimal binding occurs at 0° to 5° C (compared with 37° C in warm AIHA), and IgM initiates complement-mediated hemolysis. This occurs intravascularly, whereas in warm AIHA, the site of sequestration and hemolysis is the spleen (extravascular hemolysis).

SUMMARY BOX: AUTOIMMUNE HEMOLYTIC ANEMIA

- Warm autoimmune hemolytic anemia (AIHA) involves antibodies against red blood cells (RBCs). Normocytic anemia with a high reticulocyte count is seen.

- Type II hypersensitivity is characterized by antibodies binding to cell surfaces and catalyzing cellular damage.

- Haptens are small molecules capable of inducing an immune response only when coupled to larger carrier proteins. Penicillin is a hapten.

- See Table 15-8 for more information.

CASE 15-3

A 12-year-old boy presents to the emergency department with puffy eyes, perioral swelling, a tight feeling in his throat, and widespread urticaria. A few hours after arrival, he develops a fever, swollen lymph nodes and spleen, and swollen and painful ankles. His mother reports that he stepped on a nail during vacation in Zimbabwe 1 week ago and was given horse antitetanus immune serum. His mother also notes that his urine appears foamy and discolored.

1. What is the differential diagnosis for this boy's presentation?
   Nephrotic syndrome, serum sickness, infectious mononucleosis, glomerulonephritis, anaphylaxis, juvenile rheumatoid arthritis (acute febrile type), and upper respiratory tract infection would be considered.

CASE 15-3 continued:

Laboratory tests of a blood sample from the boy reveal an elevated white blood cell (WBC) count in which a majority of the cells were lymphocytes. Plasma cells were detected in a peripheral blood smear. His total serum complement level and his C1q and C3 levels were decreased. Urinalysis revealed proteinuria and hematuria. The patient was started on prednisone, and all of his symptoms progressively improved.

2. What is the most likely diagnosis?
   Serum sickness.

3. **What is the pathogenesis of serum sickness?**

   Serum sickness is a type III hypersensitivity reaction caused by the formation of antibody-antigen (immune) complexes and their deposition in tissues, eventuating in the activation of the complement cascade. Immune complexes form when antigen and antibody bind together. In this case, the antibody is most likely the patient's IgG with specificity for the highly immunogenic horse serum proteins, most likely the Fc portion of the horse immunoglobulins. These complexes may deposit in tissues if large amounts of antigen and antibody are present, creating more immune complexes than the mononuclear phagocyte system can clear from the circulation. Additionally, some of the smaller immune complexes that are not cleared effectively by phagocytosis are taken up by endothelial cells in various parts of the body and deposited in tissues. Local activation of the complement system by these complexes provokes an inflammatory response.

4. **What is the reason for the delay from the serum administration to the onset of symptoms?**

   The presence of antigen (those in the horse antitetanus immune serum) alone is insufficient to produce the reaction seen in serum sickness. A time interval of 2 days to 2 weeks is generally necessary for the production of the responding antibody to reach a critical level at which the number of antibody-antigen complexes exceeds the threshold at which they could be effectively cleared. The resulting increasing serum concentration of antibody-antigen complexes leads to deposition in the tissues and the symptoms seen in this patient.

   Note: The number of antigens in the body will not increase in a one-time injection such as this one, so the symptoms will subside once the mononuclear phagocyte system "catches up" and is able to clear the antigens.

STEP 1 SECRET

Be sure to pay close attention to time intervals on the USMLE examination, as they can often provide significant clues to the type of hypersensitivity reaction taking place. Although serum sickness may cause urticaria similar to that associated with type I hypersensitivity, this reaction will occur days after antigen exposure in contrast with minutes after antigen exposure seen with type I reactions.

5. **What is the significance of decreased serum levels of complement?**

   This signifies consumption of complement secondary to the activation of the classical pathway by immune complexes. Note that only IgG- and IgM-containing complexes can fix complement, which, in the classical pathway, is accomplished by C1 binding to a site in the Fc region. Although only one IgM molecule is necessary to accomplish this, two cross-linked IgG molecules must be present if the classical pathway is to be initiated.

6. **What caused the hives and facial swelling in the patient?**

   Initiation of the complement cascade leads to the production of complement components C3a, C4a, and C5a (anaphylatoxins), which in turn elicit mediator release from mast cells. Histamine and leukotrienes cause vasodilation and increased vascular permeability that lead to localized and systemic edema.

7. **What is the significance of red blood cells and protein in the urine?**

   One potential site of immune complex deposition in type III hypersensitivity is the renal glomeruli. Inflammation at this site (glomerulonephritis) results in hematuria and mild proteinuria. Note that most cases of glomerulonephritis are also caused by a type III hypersensitivity reaction: poststreptococcal glomerulonephritis by complexes of IgG and *Streptococcus pyogenes* antigens and systemic lupus erythematosus (SLE) nephritis by complexes of IgG and nuclear components; the antigen involved in IgA nephropathy is unclear (but note that the mesangial deposition of IgA complexes and C3 suggests that this disease represents a rare instance of IgA fixing complement).

8. **What is the cause of this boy's joint pain?**
   Immune complex deposition in the synovial tissue (of the ankles in this case) results in inflammation and causes pain. This mechanism is identical to that for joint pain seen in rheumatoid arthritis, an autoimmune disease that is also classified as a type III hypersensitivity.

9. **Does a type III hypersensitivity reaction require previous exposure (sensitization) to antigen to occur?**
   No. If an exogenous antigen is given in large excess on first exposure, it can cause the formation of large numbers of immune complexes over time [see question 4] (during which sensitization is occurring), their subsequent deposition in tissue, and the activation of the complement cascade.

10. **Why has the increasing use of antibody therapy NOT led to a sharp increase in the incidence of immune complex–mediated illness?**
    Previously, therapeutic antibodies were typically synthesized in other species and thus were highly immunogenic in humans. However, recombinant technology has now allowed for the production of chimeric antibodies (Fab is nonhuman, Fc [the usual site of antigenicity] is human) that are much less immunogenic. Now that purely nonhuman serum/antibodies are rarely used, drugs are the most common cause of serum sickness.

SUMMARY BOX: SERUM SICKNESS/TYPE III HYPERSENSITIVITY

- Type III hypersensitivity involves immune complex (antigen bound to antibody) deposition at various sites.

- Immune complex deposition causes damage by activation of the complement cascade and resultant neutrophil attraction.

- Administration of nonhuman antibodies can lead to serum sickness, but by making the Fc antibody region nonantigenic (such as a chimeric antibody—Fab is nonhuman, Fc is human), this reaction can be avoided.

- See Table 15-8 for more information.

CASE 15-4

A 23-year-old woman comes to your office with a pruritic rash and no other symptoms. She is already wearing a gown when you enter the room, and you immediately notice large weepy, erythematous, crusted patches and plaques on her chest, face, and arms. As you move closer, you see within these areas clear and erythematous vesicles. She also has swollen eyelids.

1. **What is the differential diagnosis for this woman's rash?**
   Contact dermatitis (allergic type), contact dermatitis (irritant type), atopic dermatitis, varicella-zoster virus infection, and second-degree burn are considered.

2. **How can allergic type and irritant type contact dermatitis be differentiated?**
Allergic type contact dermatitis is a rash that develops from skin-substance contact, after the patient has been immunologically sensitized (as seen in poison ivy). Irritant type contact dermatitis is a rash that develops from repetitive skin irritation (as seen in repetitive body washing, often a manifestation of obsessive-compulsive disorder).

Additionally, atopic dermatitis and allergic type contact dermatitis can be differentiated by rash characteristics and by the time of onset. Atopic dermatitis tends to show lichenification from chronic scratching, and it appears on the flexural body regions, whereas contact dermatitis tends to be erythematous and weepy and it is sharply demarcated, as it only appears in the areas where direct contact occurred. Also, atopic dermatitis is a type I, IgE-mediated hypersensitivity reaction that tends to be chronic (and associated with asthma and allergic rhinitis), but when an acute exposure occurs, symptoms show up within minutes. Conversely, contact dermatitis is a type IV, delayed-type hypersensitivity reaction; thus, when an acute exposure occurs, symptoms show up 12 to 72 hours later (assuming the patient has already been exposed and sensitized).

STEP 1 SECRET

Both atopic and contact dermatitis are high-yield topics for the USMLE Step 1 examination.

CASE 15-4 continued:

You elicit the history from the patient and find that she recently began going to a tanning salon. About 1 week ago, she stayed in the light too long and acquired a sunburn covering her arms and upper chest. She used Solarcaine aerosol (benzocaine 20%, triclosam 0.13%) to relieve the pain of the sunburn. After 2 days, she had a rash covering both of her arms, her chest, and her face. She took diphenhydramine to control the itching, but the rash did not improve over the last week. She denies fever, fatigue, or any other associated symptoms.

3. **What is the diagnosis?**
She has contact dermatitis (allergic type).

4. **What is the causative agent and the mechanism by which it induced an immune response in the patient?**
Benzocaine and other ingredients in topical drugs constitute a major cause of contact dermatitis, a type IV or delayed type hypersensitivity (DTH) response. In this response, antigen-presenting cells in the skin (dendritic Langerhans cells) internalize self-proteins that have exogenous molecules bound to them (haptenated self-proteins), which renders these self-proteins immunogenic. These complexes are displayed on class II MHC molecules, which bind to T_H cell receptors (TCRs). This results in activation of sensitized T_H1 (T_{DTH}) cells, release of cytokines, and subsequent activation of tissue macrophages (via IFN-γ) and $CD8^+$ T cells (via IL-2). The release of lytic enzymes by the macrophages, as well as epidermal damage by CTLs, results in the erythema, weepiness, and vesicles that characterized this patient's reaction to benzocaine.

5. **Why did the patient have lesions in areas other than on her arms and upper chest (where she applied the spray)?**
The topical drug can be transferred from the initial point of contact to other areas of the skin by the fingernails after scratching the itchy lesions at the primary site. Therefore, unexpected sites can be affected (e.g., the eyelids and genitals). It is beneficial to cut fingernails short and thoroughly wash off the skin to remove the drug and prevent further spread.

6. **What is the treatment for allergic type contact dermatitis?**
   The patient should be given a corticosteroid-containing cream, and she can take oral diphenhydramine to control further itching. With this treatment, the rash should resolve in 1 to 2 weeks.

7. **Why is it important for the patient to avoid the use of benzocaine in the future?**
   Once an individual is sensitized, each subsequent exposure not only produces the hypersensitivity reaction but also generates more effector and memory T cells. Thus, the reaction becomes more severe with each subsequent exposure. Memory T cells can persist for the lifetime of an individual.
   Note: The first contact with an allergen does not typically result in a type IV allergic response (as is also the case in type I reactions). Accordingly, a contact hypersensitivity has a sensitization stage in which a clonal population of memory $CD4^+$ T cells is produced and an elicitation stage whereby the memory T cells become activated upon subsequent exposure to antigen. Additionally, an individual may be able to touch the material (allergen) for many years without suffering an adverse reaction (Table 15-8).

SUMMARY BOX: CONTACT DERMATITIS

- Type IV hypersensitivity is mediated by T_H1 cells, making it the only type of hypersensitivity that is not antibody-mediated.

- The direct causes of the damage in this type of hypersensitivity are activated macrophages and cytotoxic T lymphocytes (CTLs).

- Contact dermatitis appears only at sites of direct contact with the offending substance and can be treated most effectively with corticosteroids.

- See Table 15-8.

CASE 15-5

A 4-month-old baby boy is brought to your office by his parents for evaluation of a runny nose and a cough that have persisted for over a month. Examination reveals oral thrush, absence of tonsils and lymph nodes, and a fall from the 50th percentile in weight to the 10th percentile. A chest x-ray study is performed and demonstrates diffuse, symmetrical interstitial opacities. Laboratory tests reveal marked lymphopenia with normal numbers of $CD20^+$ cells (B lymphocytes) and an absence of $CD3^+$ cells (T lymphocytes).

1. **What is the differential diagnosis?**
   Severe combined immunodeficiency (SCID), human immunodeficiency virus (HIV) infection, bare lymphocyte syndrome, ataxia-telangiectasia, and atypical DiGeorge syndrome (thymic aplasia) are considered.

CASE 15-5 continued:

Further specialized testing revealed that blood lymphocytes were unresponsive to the B- and T-cell mitogen, pokeweed (PWM). A diagnosis of *Pneumocystis jirovecii* (formerly *Pneumocystis carinii*) pneumonia was made, and the baby responded well to intravenous trimethoprim-sulfamethoxazole (TMP-SMX). Although he was considered low-risk, testing to rule out HIV infection was performed and was negative.

TABLE 15-8. SUMMARY OF HYPERSENSITIVITY REACTIONS

Classification	Definition	Mediator	Mechanism of Destruction	Clinical Presentations	Detection
Type I	IgE-mediated immediate hypersensitivity	IgE	Mast cell degranulation induced by allergen–cross-linked IgE	Systemic anaphylaxis, allergic rhinitis, bronchial asthma, atopic dermatitis, food allergies	Skin testing, RIST, RAST
Type II	Antibody-mediated cytotoxic hypersensitivity	IgM, IgG	Antibodies directed against cell-bound antigens induce destruction of cells or tissues	Transfusion reactions, hemolytic disease of the newborn, autoimmune hemolytic anemia	Direct and indirect Coombs' test
Type III	Immune complex–mediated hypersensitivity	Usually IgG	Antibodies directed against soluble serum antigen form circulating complexes that deposit in tissue nonspecifically; damage is complement mediated	Serum sickness, glomerulonephritis, rheumatoid arthritis, SLE, hypersensitivity pneumonitis	WBC counts, total serum complement levels, serum C3 and C1q levels
Type IV	Cell-mediated delayed hypersensitivity	T_H1 cells	Antigen-specific T_H1 cells activate tissue macrophages and stimulate a local inflammatory response over 12-72 hours	Contact dermatitis, tuberculin-type hypersensitivity, granulomatous hypersensitivity, acute tissue graft rejection	Patch test

IgE, IgG, IgM, immunoglobulins E, G, M; RAST, radioallergosorbent test; RIST, radioimmunosorbent test; SLE, systemic lupus erythematosus; WBC, white blood cell.

2. **What is the most likely diagnosis in this infant, given the fact that specialized testing revealed defects in both cellular and humoral function?**
    SCID is most likely. This condition is invariably fatal in infants unless recognized and treated by bone marrow transplantation. Prior to this, SCID patients must avoid exposure to any microorganisms by residing in a plastic bubble. Typically, infants with SCID become ill within the first 3 months of life, suffering from recurrent respiratory infections, pneumonia, thrush, diarrhea, and failure to thrive. Opportunistic infections with intracellular pathogens such as *Candida albicans*, *Pneumocystis jirovecii*, *Cryptococcus neoformans*, cytomegalovirus, and mycobacteria are commonly observed in these infants.

3. **Why might a bone marrow transplant from an appropriate donor cure this boy?**
    The pathogenesis of SCID involves abnormal production and function of mature B and T cells. By transplanting normal lymphocyte precursors (no genetic defect) the infant's immune system will reconstitute with mature, functional B and T lymphocytes.

4. **What is the significance of the marked lymphopenia and complete lack of CD3⁺ cells?**
    SCID is a family of primary immune disorders that is characterized by low numbers of circulating lymphocytes while myeloid and erythroid cells appear normal in number and function. Within the lymphocyte population, T-cell numbers are typically low to absent, B-cell numbers can range from fairly normal to absent (although these B cells are typically nonfunctional), and NK cell numbers can be low to normal. Thus, there is failure to mount both humoral and cell-mediated immune responses, but the lack of cell-mediated immunity makes patients with SCID highly susceptible to opportunistic infections with intracellular organisms, the hallmark of this disease.

    Note: SCID may look very similar to DiGeorge syndrome, in which failure to develop the third and fourth pharyngeal pouches results in an absent thymus and complete lack of T cells. Both SCID and DiGeorge syndromes can produce an absent thymic shadow on chest x-ray films. However, DiGeorge syndrome does not affect B cells, is generally associated with congenital heart defects, and often produces symptoms of hypocalcemia due to absent parathyroid glands.

5. **Why are B-cell defects not evident in many babies when they are first diagnosed with severe combined immunodeficiency?**
    The infants have antibodies in their circulation that have been passively obtained from transplacental circulation (IgG) and from breast milk (IgA). As these antibodies are cleared over time and the infant becomes responsible for its own immunoglobulin synthesis, all levels will be low to absent.

6. **Mutations in the γ subunit of the IL-2 receptor are found in the most common, X-linked form of severe combined immunodeficiency (SCID). How can this explain the manifestations of the disease?**
    The γ common chain is encoded by the IL-2Rγ gene (located on the X chromosome) and is a protein shared by a large number of interleukin receptors involved in lymphocyte development. Thus, in addition to the IL-2 receptor, the γ subunit is associated with receptors for IL-4, IL-7, IL-9, and IL-15. Mutations in the IL-2Rγ gene result in an absence of these functional receptors and can lead to decreased growth and development (as well as decreased activation and proliferation) of both B and T cells. Interestingly, the lack of T cells results primarily from a nonfunctional IL-7 receptor. As discussed previously, the IL-2 receptor is also essential for T-cell development.

Note: Other genetic defects known to cause SCID include absence of class II MHC, dysfunctional ZAP-70 (T-cell signal transduction protein), defective *RAG1* or *RAG2* genes (TCR and Ig recombination), and absent adenosine deaminase or purine nucleoside phosphorylase (aids in purine breakdown). Adenosine deaminase deficiency is the second most common form of SCID and results in the buildup of dATP (deoxyadenosine triphosphate), which inhibits activity of ribonucleotide reductase. Decreased production of deoxyribonucleotides inhibits lymphocyte proliferation and thus results in immunosuppression.

RELATED QUESTIONS: B-CELL DISORDERS

7. **Which primary immunodeficiency should be suspected in a child with normal cell-mediated immunity but almost complete absence of plasma immunoglobulins?**
Bruton's agammaglobulinemia is an X-linked immunodeficiency syndrome. Affected boys have few B cells in their blood or lymphoid tissue, and their serum usually contains very low levels of all immunoglobulins. The defect involves Bruton's tyrosine kinase, which is crucial to the maturation of pre–B cells. Maternal immunoglobulin remains to protect the child until about 6 months of age.

STEP 1 SECRET

X-linked immunodeficiencies can be remembered using the mnemonic "Missing WBCs," which stands for hyper-Ig**M** syndrome, **W**iscott-Aldrich syndrome, **B**ruton's agammaglobulinemia, **C**hronic granulomatous disease, and **s**evere combined immunodeficiency (SCID) (most common type).

8. **Which B-cell disorder is associated with anaphylactic transfusion reactions?**
IgA deficiency (the most common immunodeficiency, ∼1:700) is due to a defect in heavy chain isotype switching, so affected patients cannot produce IgA (and sometimes IgG2 and IgG4 as well). Although many of these patients are asymptomatic, they may also present with recurrent sinus and pulmonary infections, persistent giardiasis, diarrhea, allergies, and asthma. The most serious complication of this condition is the production of specific IgE against the Fc portion of the IgA heavy chain, which can result in a life-threatening anaphylactic reaction to blood products that have not been purged of this immunoglobulin.

STEP 1 SECRET

The scenario of an anaphylactic reaction following blood transfusion is a favorite on the Step 1 examination. Consider this whenever a patient has an anaphylactic reaction after blood transfusion.

SUMMARY BOX: SEVERE COMBINED IMMUNODEFICIENCY

- Severe combined immunodeficiency (SCID) involves deficits in both T and B lymphocytes, leading to opportunistic infections.

- In infants before 6 months of age, most infections in SCID are by intracellular pathogens, evidence of deficient cell-mediated immunity. During this time, humoral immunity is kept intact by IgA-containing breast milk and IgG from transplacental circulation that has not yet been degraded.

- Bruton's agammaglobulinemia is a B-cell (and thus immunoglobulin) deficit. Severe (usually bacterial) infections appear after 6 months of age, when maternal immunoglobulin levels fall.

- See Table 15-10 for more information.

CASE 15-6

A 5-year-old boy presents to the emergency department with severe shortness of breath, a persistent cough, and chest pain. A chest x-ray film reveals the presence of multiple large, fuzzy opacities in both lung fields. Laboratory tests reveal a normal WBC with normal proportions of neutrophils, lymphocytes, and monocytes. A brief review of the boy's medical history shows multiple infections with organisms in the genera *Staphylococcus* and *Burkholderia*. Laboratory tests from 1 month ago showed a similar WBC profile, as well as serum antibody levels in the high normal range and normal levels of complement proteins.

1. **What is the differential diagnosis for this boy's apparent immunodeficiency?**
   Complement deficiencies and B-cell disorders can cause recurrent bacterial infections (although these generally involve encapsulated organisms [*Streptococcus pneumoniae*, *Haemophilus influenzae*, *Neisseria meningitidis*, *Salmonella* spp., etc.] rather than those seen in this patient), but these have been essentially ruled out with the results from 1 month ago. The presence of recurrent *Staphylococcus aureus* and *Burkholderia* (a genus of gram-negative rods quite similar to *Pseudomonas*) infections is strongly of suggestive of a phagocyte deficiency. The two WBC profiles make cyclic neutropenia and secondary neutropenia much less likely, thus leaving chronic granulomatous disease (CGD), Chédiak-Higashi syndrome (CHS), and leukocyte adhesion deficiency at the top of the differential diagnosis list.

CASE 15-6 continued:

In a WBC function test, the boy's monocytes and neutrophils failed to reduce nitroblue tetrazolium (NBT), a test of the adequacy of the oxidative respiratory burst. Sputum cultures return and are found to have grown *Aspergillus fumigatus*. He is promptly started on IV liposomal amphotericin B. He slowly improves over a 2-month period, but during this time in the hospital he contracts two bacterial respiratory infections. When he is discharged, he is started on treatment with injections of IFN-γ and daily prophylactic TMP-SMX.

2. **What is the diagnosis?**
   He has CGD.
   Note: It is important to understand the basis of the NBT test. The color of NBT is changed from yellow to deep blue in the presence of reactive oxygen species. Thus, absence of color change when NBT is added to a patient's WBCs indicates lack of functional nicotinamide adenine dinucleotide phosphate (NADPH) oxidase.

3. **What are the two mechanisms that a macrophage can employ to kill bacteria following phagocytosis?**
Destruction of internalized pathogens by macrophages (and neutrophils) involves both oxygen-dependent and oxygen-independent mechanisms. During phagocytosis, a metabolic process known as the respiratory burst occurs. This process is dependent upon the activity of NADPH oxidase, which catalyzes the production of superoxide (O^{2-}) from oxygen. Superoxide dismutase then converts superoxide to hydrogen peroxide (H_2O_2), which is converted to hypochlorite ($HOCl^-$, a very potent bactericidal oxidant, commonly known as bleach) by myeloperoxidase. The macrophage may also kill ingested pathogens using lysozyme, various hydrolytic enzymes, and cytotoxic peptides. The degradative activities of these factors do not require oxygen. Hydrogen peroxide that leaks out of the phagolysosome is potentially harmful to tissues and is thus neutralized to water by the enzyme catalase, which requires reduced glutathione for its action.

4. **What is the genetic basis of chronic granulomatous disease?**
All forms of CGD involve mutations in the gene encoding NADPH oxidase (65% of these are X-linked recessive and 35% are autosomal recessive). A deficiency in this enzyme results in an inability of phagocytes to kill many types of ingested pathogens. Therefore, these microorganisms persist, leading to the formation of granulomas in an attempt to "wall off" the invaders. Note that widespread granulomas are found in patients with CGD even in the absence of infection; this is presumably due to unopposed proinflammatory cytokine production.

5. **What are the contents of a granuloma and why is it formed?**
A granuloma is a collection of epithelioid and giant cells surrounded by a fibrous capsule. Generally, a granuloma forms to contain an intracellular pathogen that has been resistant to elimination (but sterile granulomas are common in CGD, as discussed previously). Note that epithelioid cells are modified macrophages, and giant cells are the result of the fusion of multiple macrophages (hence the supernumerary nuclei). These cells are maintained by continued secretion of IFN-γ by local T_H1 cells (Fig. 15-4).

STEP 1 SECRET

It is important to be able to recognize images of granulomas and their major constituents for the purpose of the USMLE.

6. **Patients with chronic granulomatous disease often experience recurrent staphylococcal infections, but streptococcal infections are rare. Why?**
Organisms in the genus *Streptococcus* are catalase-negative. As mentioned earlier, catalase catalyzes the degradation of hydrogen peroxide ($2H_2O_2 \rightarrow 2H_2O + O_2$). In the absence of catalase, hydrogen peroxide is not degraded and can be "stolen" by the phagocyte and converted to hypochlorite by myeloperoxidase. This allows for killing of the organism in the absence of functional NADPH oxidase.

Conversely, catalase-positive organisms quickly eliminate all hydrogen peroxide that they produce and thus cannot be killed via respiratory burst in hosts lacking functional NADPH oxidase. Therefore, common infecting organisms in CGD include *S. aureus*, *Serratia*, *Burkholderia cepacia*, *Aspergillus*, *Nocardia*, and *Candida*. Note that *Neisseria*, although catalase-positive, rarely causes infections in CGD because phagocytes have a propensity to kill this organism by oxygen-independent mechanisms (see question 3).

7. **What is the mechanism of action of amphotericin B?**
The polyene family, including amphotericin B and nystatin, acts by selectively binding to ergosterols (in the plasma membrane of fungal cells) and creating pores in the membrane. This

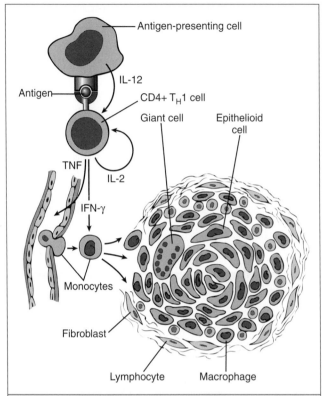

Figure 15-4. Schematic illustration of granuloma formation. (From Kumar V, Abbas AK, Fausto N: Robbins and Cotran Pathologic Basis of Disease, 7th ed. Philadelphia, WB Saunders, 2005.)

results in leakage of intracellular components, precipitating cell death. Amphotericin B possesses an extremely broad antifungal spectrum, but its undesirable side effect profile (chills, fever, nephrotoxicity, arrhythmias, hypotension) can be prohibitive. Nystatin is reserved for topical (diaper rash, vaginal candidiasis) and oral (oral candidiasis) use.

8. **How does liposomal amphotericin B differ from amphotericin B?**
The mechanism of action and the antifungal spectrum are identical, but liposomal amphotericin B causes significantly *fewer* side effects, most notably in the realm of renal toxicity. Note that amphotericin B's renal toxicity results from afferent arteriolar constriction and direct damage to distal tubular epithelium.

RELATED QUESTIONS: PHAGOCYTE DISORDERS

9. **How does Chédiak-Higashi syndrome differ from chronic granulomatous disease?**
CHS is also a primary immunodeficiency of the myeloid lineage. It is an autosomal recessive disorder that renders lysosomes of neutrophils incapable of fusing with phagosomes (membrane-bound pockets containing ingested microorganisms). CHS is thus characterized by

intracytoplasmic granules in PMNs and monocytes. Recurrent infections with *S. aureus*, as well as organisms of the *Streptococcus* and *Pseudomonas* genera, are seen. In addition to a failure of phagosome-lysosome fusion, defects affect melanocytes, nerve cells, and platelets. Common symptoms of CHS thus include neuropathy, partial albinism, and bleeding diathesis. In contrast with CGD, CHS yields a normal NBT or dichlorofluoroscein test because phagocytic NADPH oxidase is functional.

10. **Compare and contrast monocytes and macrophages with respect to origin, location, lifespan, and function.**
Both monocytes and macrophages are phagocytes derived from myeloid stem cells in the bone marrow. Monocytes circulate in the bloodstream for several hours, during which time many enlarge, migrate into various tissues, and differentiate into macrophages. Monocytes that remain in the blood will survive for 1 to 2 days, whereas those that become tissue-dwelling macrophages will have longer life spans of 4 to 15 days. Macrophages serve different functions in different tissues and are named according to their location (Table 15-9).

TABLE 15-9. MACROPHAGE TYPES WITH LOCATION AND FUNCTION

Macrophage Type	Tissue Location	Function(s)
Kupffer cells	Liver	Removal of senescent RBCs and debris
Splenic macrophages	Spleen	Removal of senescent RBCs and debris
Mesangial cells	Kidney	Phagocytosis, contraction, support
Microglial cells	CNS	Ingest degenerated myelin
Histiocytes	Connective tissue	Phagocytosis
Alveolar macrophages	Lung	Phagocytosis of inhaled particles

CNS, central nervous system; RBCs, red blood cells.

SUMMARY BOX: CHRONIC GRANULOMATOUS DISEASE

- Phagocytic cells can kill via oxygen-dependent (product is hypochlorite) and oxygen-independent (e.g., lysozyme, cytotoxic peptides) mechanisms.

- Chronic granulomatous disease (CGD) stems from defective nicotinamide adenine dinucleotide phosphate (NADPH) oxidase and results in recurrent infections with catalase-positive organisms.

- Chédiak-Higashi syndrome is a disorder of lysosomal fusion. Unlike in CGD, streptococcal (in addition to staphylococcal) infections are seen.

- See Table 15-10 for more information.

TABLE 15-10. SUMMARY OF PRIMARY IMMUNODEFICIENCIES

Classification	Example(s) of Immunodeficiency Syndromes	Immune Defect	Susceptibility
B cell deficiencies	Bruton's agammaglobulinemia (X-linked hypogammaglobulinemia)	Few to no B cells; only immunoglobulin found in serum is IgG (at very low levels)	Recurrent pyogenic infections appear after age of 6 months
	IgA deficiency	B cells fail to produce IgA and often IgG2 and IgG4	Recurrent sinus, respiratory, and gastrointestinal infections; anaphylactic transfusion reactions
	X-linked hyper-IgM syndrome	No B cell class switching from IgM to other isotypes (due to a defect in CD40 ligand)	Recurrent pyogenic infections, poor response to immunizations
	Common variable immunodeficiency	Late-onset (ages 20-35 years) agammaglobulinemia that has acquired and inherited characteristics; commonly follows viral infection	Recurrent pyogenic infections; increased risk of various autoimmune diseases and lymphoma
T-cell deficiencies	DiGeorge syndrome	T-cell deficit resulting from thymic aplasia (pharyngeal pouch maldevelopment)	Opportunistic infections: viral and fungal infections
	Chronic mucocutaneous candidiasis	T-cell dysfunction specific to *Candida albicans*	Recurrent skin and mucous membrane *C. albicans* infections
Combined	Severe combined immunodeficiency (SCID)	Deficit of both B and T cells	Opportunistic infections
	Ataxia-telangiectasia	11q22-23 (codes for DNA repair enzyme) deletion leads to T-cell deficit, IgA deficiency, cerebellar degeneration, and skin and conjunctiva telangiectasia	Recurrent infections, increased risk of lymphoma
	Wiskott-Aldrich syndrome	X-linked F-actin assembly defect in T cells and platelets; normal IgG, decreased IgM, and increased IgA and IgE	Infections with encapsulated bacteria; atopic dermatitis; thrombocytopenia
	Bare lymphocyte syndrome	Defective or absent class I and/or II MHC molecules	Recurrent infections, commonly viral

Continued

TABLE 15-10. SUMMARY OF PRIMARY IMMUNODEFICIENCIES—continued

Classification	Example(s) of Immunodeficiency Syndromes	Immune Defect	Susceptibility
Complement deficiencies	See Basic Concepts, question 12		
Phagocyte deficiencies	Chronic granulomatous disease (CGD)	Defective phagocytic respiratory burst, resulting from mutations in the NADPH oxidase gene	Increased susceptibility to certain bacteria and fungi; widespread granuloma formation
	Chédiak-Higashi syndrome	Defective neutrophil lysosomal fusion	Recurrent staphylococcal and streptococcal infections
	Leukocyte adhesion deficiency	Defective neutrophil integrin (LFA-1: mediates adhesion), resulting in defective migration	Recurrent severe pyogenic infections; delayed umbilical cord separation
	IL-12 receptor deficiency	Defective IL-12 receptor prevents the initiation of a T_H1 response	Disseminated, severe mycobacterial infections
	IFN-γ receptor deficiency	Defective IFN-γ receptor prevents macrophage activation (and the killing of intracellular pathogens)	Disseminated, severe mycobacterial infections
	Job's syndrome	Failure of helper T cells to produce IFN-γ, preventing macrophage activation and "tilting the balance" toward the T_H2 pathway; this leads to increased IgE and a level of histamine that inhibits neutrophil chemotaxis	Recurrent "cold" (i.e., the absence of inflammation) staphylococcal abscesses, atopic dermatitis
	Cyclic neutropenia	Autosomal dominant; irregular production of G-CSF leads to neutropenia for 3-6 days of a 21-day cycle	Severe bacterial infections during neutropenic phase only

G-CSF, granulocyte colony-stimulating factor; IFN-γ, interferon-γ; IgA, IgE, IgG, IgM, immunoglobulins A, E, G, M; IL, interleukin; LFA-1, lymphocyte function–associated antigen-1; MHC, major histocompatibility complex; NADPH, nicotinamide adenine dinucleotide phosphate [reduced].

CASE 15-7

A 5-day-old girl is brought to you by her mother for evaluation of "repeated muscle seizures" that began 3 days ago. She is afebrile. Physical examination reveals several facial abnormalities, including low-set ears, wide-set eyes (hypertelorism), and micrognathia. Laboratory tests are remarkable for hypocalcemia and lymphopenia. A chest x-ray film reveals a boot-shaped heart, decreased pulmonary vasculature markings, and the absence of a thymic shadow.

1. **What is the likely diagnosis in this infant and what is the pathophysiology of her disorder?**

   DiGeorge syndrome (thymic parathyroid aplasia). This genetic disorder is caused by microdeletions on the q arm of chromosome 22, resulting in dysmorphogenesis of the third and fourth pharyngeal pouches during embryologic development. Because the thymus (third pouch) and the parathyroids (inferior two from third pouch, superior two from fourth pouch) normally arise from this tissue, these structures may be absent in DiGeorge syndrome (Fig. 15-5). For similar embryologic reasons, the heart and aorta are often affected as well. DiGeorge syndrome is typically detected in the first week of life following evaluation of infants suffering from hypocalcemia (from hypoparathyroidism)-induced tetany, which, as seen in this infant, may resemble seizures.

   Note: The mechanism for hypocalcemia-induced tetany involves increased sodium influx into nerve terminals with decreased calcium concentrations.

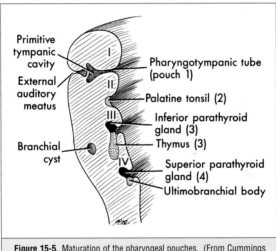

Figure 15-5. Maturation of the pharyngeal pouches. (From Cummings CW, Flint PW, Haughey BH: Otolaryngology: Head & Neck Surgery, 4th ed. Philadelphia, Mosby, 2005.)

2. **Joseph Heller might ask, "What tried and true medical school mnemonic can be used to remember the classic manifestations of DiGeorge syndrome?"**

   Congenital heart abnormalities (commonly truncus arteriosus or tetralogy of Fallot)
   Abnormal facial features
   Thymic aplasia
   Cleft palate
   Hypocalcemia from hypoparathyroidism
   22q deletion

3. **To what type of infections might this child be vulnerable, given that thymic development is abnormal?**

   The thymus is a primary lymphoid organ that is responsible for the maturation of progenitor T cells. When the thymus is underdeveloped or lacking, there is a dramatic decrease in all populations of T cells and a corresponding lack of cell-mediated immunity. Patients with DiGeorge syndrome who survive the immediate neonatal period are susceptible to recurrent or chronic fungal and viral infections that would normally be eradicated by CTLs. Additionally, because T_H cells and their cytokines (e.g., IL-2, IL-4, IL-5) are critical to the proliferation and differentiation of B cells, deterioration of humoral immunity will occur over time as maternal antibodies are degraded (by about 6 months of age). Thus, the patient will also become susceptible to infection with extracellular pathogens such as bacteria, which are normally warded off by the humoral system.

4. **What might a lymph node biopsy in this infant reveal?**
Thymic absence or hypoplasia in DiGeorge syndrome results in inadequate production of functionally mature T cells. Histologic analysis of lymph nodes would therefore reveal near complete absence of T cells in the normal T cell–dependent zones of lymph nodes, such as the paracortex (this lies between the nodular cortex and the medulla).

RELATED QUESTION

5. **What does the process of "thymic education" involve?**
The education of thymocytes involves both positive and negative selection and ensures that mature T cells will be MHC-restricted and self-tolerant, respectively. During positive selection, T cells able to recognize (bind) MHC molecules are selected to survive (others undergo apoptosis). Negative selection involves apoptosis of T cells that avidly bind self-peptide in association with MHC molecules (self-reactive T cells). Less than 5% of the thymocytes will survive these selection processes.
    A quick review of primary deficiencies is given in Table 15-10

SUMMARY BOX: DiGEORGE SYNDROME

- A 22q deletion results in DiGeorge syndrome (thymic parathyroid aplasia), in which the third and fourth pharyngeal pouches fail to develop properly.

  - The third pouch forms the thymus and the inferior two parathyroid glands.

  - The fourth pouch forms the superior two parathyroid glands.

  - Remember the mnemonic CATCH-22: **C**ongenital heart abnormalities (commonly truncus arteriosus or tetralogy of Fallot), **A**bnormal facial features, **T**hymic aplasia, **C**left palate, **H**ypocalcemia from hypoparathyroidism, **22**q deletion.

- See Table 15-10.

CASE 15-8

A 25-year-old man comes to your office, for the first time in many years, with complaints of general fatigue, a headache, muscle aches, and a mild fever. He states that this has persisted for "4 or 5 days" and that he "just wants to get my energy back." He takes no medications. He appears somewhat tired and shows mild psychomotor retardation. Physical examination is notable for scattered lymphadenopathy and a small patchy nonspecific rash on the neck.

1. **What is the differential diagnosis?**
Infectious mononucleosis, hypothyroidism, influenza, occult infection, anemia, depression, acute HIV infection, malnutrition, adrenal insufficiency, non-Hodgkin's lymphoma, and dermatomyositis should be considered.

CASE 15-8 continued:

You write orders for a battery of standard tests and give the patient directions to the laboratory. As you are about the leave the room, the patient stops you and asks, "A few months ago, I started using intravenous heroin. Do you think that might be related to these problems?"

2. **What must be suspected? What tests are used to diagnose this disease after the acute stage?**

HIV infection is now more likely. Detection of HIV antibodies is accomplished by enzyme-linked immunosorbent assay (ELISA), the preferred screening test (high-sensitivity test). If the ELISA is positive, the test must be confirmed by Western blot analysis (high-specificity test), which is positive if antibodies from the patient's serum are demonstrated to interact with HIV-1 proteins displayed on the acrylamide gel used in the test. A Western blot must be positive for antibodies to at least two important HIV antigens (e.g., gp120, gp41, p24). If only one antibody is positive, the result is indeterminate and the test must be repeated after a few months, or an HIV PCR assay must be done. HIV test results are often falsely positive in newborns born to HIV-infected mothers because these antibodies can cross the placenta, but are often falsely negative within the first few months of infection.

3. **Describe the enzyme-linked immunosorbent assay test.**

First, known antigens (HIV-1 proteins, in this instance) are fixed to the bottom of a well. Next, the patient's serum is added, and if he or she happens to possess the antibodies of interest, they will bind to the antigens in the well. Then, antibodies against human IgG with enzymes linked to their Fc region are added. If the originally mentioned antibodies are present (and they are IgG), the second antibody will bind, and when the substrate is added, the enzyme will induce a change in color. This activity can be detected using a spectrophotometer. The highest dilution of the original serum in which color change is detected represents the antibody titer.

CASE 15-8 continued:

The results of his HIV ELISA and Western blot test are positive. You continue to follow-up with him regularly, and 5 years later he comes for another regularly scheduled appointment with a few questions. You note in his chart that he has been on highly active antiretroviral therapy (HAART) for a few years now. He states that he has been reading about the HIV stages, and asks, "Which stage am I in?" Additionally, he said he heard about "something called *Pneumocystis carinii* pneumonia (PCP) that can happen when your CD4+ T-cell count gets below 200" and requests more information on this topic.

4. **What are the classes of drugs used in highly active antiretroviral therapy?**

The first class of antiretroviral drugs includes two types of reverse transcriptase inhibitors. Nucleoside analog reverse transcriptase inhibitors (nRTIs) are incorporated by reverse transcriptase into the transcribed DNA strand, where they block further extension of the strand and thereby inhibit viral replication. They require phosphorylation by thymidine kinase to become active. Non-nucleoside reverse transcriptase inhibitors (nnRTIs) inhibit the action of the reverse transcriptase enzyme but bind at a site other than the catalytic site and do not require activation by thymidine kinase. A second class of drugs called protease inhibitors (PIs) mimic peptides that HIV protease cleaves, but bind more tightly and specifically, thus inhibiting the protease. HAART refers only to combinations of two nRTIs plus either one nnRTI or one PI. Table 15-11 lists some anti-HIV drugs (common names) that are in clinical use.

STEP 1 SECRET

Learning the various human immunodeficiency virus (HIV) drugs can be a difficult task, as their names are somewhat complicated, but they are commonly tested on the USMLE. It is important to recognize both the mechanism of action and potential side effects for all HIV drugs mentioned in Table 15-11.

TABLE 15-11. DRUGS IN CLINICAL USE FOR TREATMENT OF HUMAN IMMUNODEFICIENCY VIRUS (HIV) INFECTION

Reverse Transcriptase Inhibitors		Protease Inhibitors*
Nucleoside Analogs	Non-nucleoside Analogs	
Bone marrow suppression and lactic acidosis	Bone marrow suppression and rash	Hyperglycemia, lipodystrophy (buffalo hump), and gastrointestinal intolerance
Zidovudine (azidothymidine [AZT]) *Megaloblastic anemia*	Delavirdine	Indinavir *Thrombocytopenia*
Lamivudine (3TC) *Fewer side effects*	Nevirapine	Ritonavir *Pancreatitis*
Stavudine (d4T) *Pancreatitis, peripheral neuropathy*	Efavirenz	Saquinavir
Didanosine (ddI) *Pancreatitis, peripheral neuropathy*		Nelfinavir
Zalcitabine (ddC) *Pancreatitis, peripheral neuropathy*		Amprenavir
Abacavir *Hypersensitivity reactions*		Lopinavir
Combivir (3TC and AZT)		Atazanavir

*Note that all of these agents end in "-navir."
Italic print indicates common side effects.
Other agents: tenofovir (nucleotide analog) and enfuvirtide (prevent HIV–T cell fusion; used only if multiple other drugs have failed).

5. **Suboptimal compliance with highly active antiretroviral therapy rapidly leads to resistance. Why?**
   Any allowance of continued viral replication (e.g., from missed doses) is dangerous, because the HIV reverse transcriptase enzyme is extraordinarily error-prone. Therefore, mutations arise quickly, and if one leads to drug resistance, it can proliferate rapidly. In general, nRTI resistance

occurs through mutations that prevent nucleoside analog incorporation or create a mechanism of ATP-mediated nucleoside analog removal. Resistance to nnRTIs and PIs usually occurs through mutations that alter the binding sites for these drugs.

6. **Briefly describe human immunodeficiency virus and its life cycle.**

HIV is an encapsulated retrovirus. Two viral envelope glycoproteins, gp120 and gp41, allow the virus to infect CD4$^+$ T cells (as well as some macrophages, dendritic cells, and microglial cells) that express an appropriate coreceptor (the chemokine receptors CXCR4 or CCR5). Note that macrophages and dendritic cells, once infected, display DC-SIGN (a C-type lectin receptor), which allows these cells to bind to and *directly infect* T cells. Upon entry into the cell, the virus efficiently copies its RNA genome into double-stranded DNA using the viral enzyme reverse transcriptase. The viral DNA copy is integrated into the host cell genome, aided by the viral enzyme integrase. This proviral form of the virus may remain latent in the cell until its expression is signaled. Expression of functional proteins by the virus involves a virally encoded protease that cleaves polyproteins into smaller functional proteins. When the provirus is expressed to form new virions, the host cells will often lyse (Fig. 15-6).

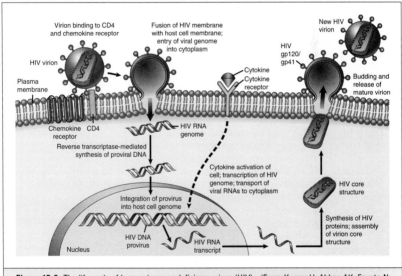

Figure 15-6. The life cycle of human immunodeficiency virus (HIV). (From Kumar V, Abbas AK, Fausto N: Robbins and Cotran Pathologic Basis of Disease, 7th ed. Philadelphia, WB Saunders, 2005.)

7. **What are the major mechanisms of CD4$^+$ T-cell depletion in human immunodeficiency virus infection?**

See Figure 15-7.

8. **Define the four major stages of human immunodeficiency virus infection.**

With *acute HIV infection*, the individual may remain asymptomatic or develop an acute illness that resembles influenza or infectious mononucleosis; symptoms usually develop within 2 to 6 weeks after infection (as seen in this patient). During this stage, antibodies to HIV are generally undetectable. Seroconversion usually occurs during *clinical latency*, an asymptomatic period that would last approximately 7 to 10 years in an untreated patient. Low-level (but persistent) replication of HIV causes a gradual decrease in CD4$^+$ T cells, and minor opportunistic infections may occur. During the *crisis* phase, escalation of viral replication leads to a more rapid T-cell

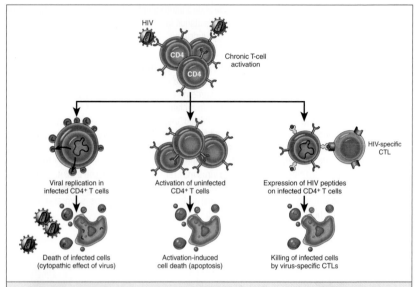

Figure 15-7. Mechanisms of CD4⁺ T-cell loss in human immunodeficiency virus (HIV) infection. CTLs, cytotoxic T lymphocytes. (From Kumar V, Abbas AK, Fausto N: Robbins and Cotran Pathologic Basis of Disease, 7th ed. Philadelphia, WB Saunders, 2005.)

decline (Fig. 15-8). This is clinically apparent as weight loss, fever, fatigue, and lymphadenopathy. Acquired immunodeficiency syndrome (AIDS) is the diagnosis for a person who is HIV-positive and has a T-cell count below 200 μL^{-1} or presents with one of the AIDS-defining opportunistic infections/malignancies.

9. **What are the most important determinants of the progression of human immunodeficiency virus infection?**

   CD4⁺T-cell count indicates the damage that has occurred to the immune system, and how close the patient is to progressing to AIDS (acquired immunodeficiency syndrome). A high count is ideal. Normal count ranges from 500 to 1500 μL^{-1}.

   Viral load is an indication of the pace at which the damage is occurring. A low viral load is ideal. Viral load serves as a marker for disease progression and drug therapy effectiveness by measuring the amount of actively dividing HIV virus.

10. **What is "PCP pneumonia" and what other opportunistic infections and malignancies might befall an AIDS patient?**

    PCP refers to *Pneumocystis carinii* pneumonia (the preferred name is now *Pneumocystis jirovecii* pneumonia). *P. jirovecii* (once considered a protozoan and now classified as a fungus) pneumonia is the most common significant opportunistic infection in HIV patients and typically occurs in patients with a CD4⁺ count of below 200. Patients with CD4⁺ counts below this level should be started on TMP-SMX prophylaxis. Other opportunistic pathogens and malignancies that are a major cause of death in AIDS are listed in Table 15-12.

    Common opportunistic infections at notable CD4⁺ counts: *Toxoplasma* encephalitis at <100, Cryptococcal meningitis at <100, *Mycobacterium avium* complex at <50, and cytomegalovirus retinitis at <50. CMV retinitis is treated with ganciclovir, a competitive guanosine analog. In the event that ganciclovir fails, foscarnet (viral DNA polymerase inhibitor) is used.

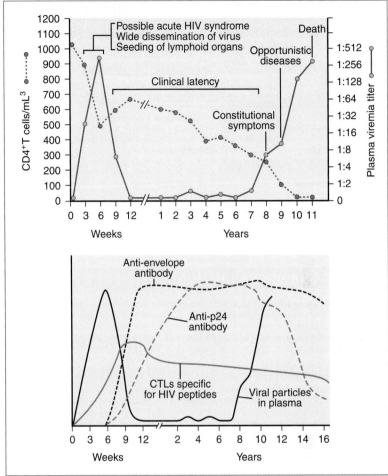

Figure 15-8. Typical course of human immunodeficiency virus (HIV) infection. CTLs, cytotoxic T lymphocytes. (From Kumar V, Abbas AK, Fausto N: Robbins and Cotran Pathologic Basis of Disease, 7th ed. Philadelphia, WB Saunders, 2005.)

11. **Explain why certain individuals remain infected with human immunodeficiency virus for longer than 10 years with no symptoms.**

    The clinical latency stage is variable and tends to run longer in patients whose viral load is low or who possess a mutant HIV strain with partially defective replication machinery. In these individuals, CTLs are able to control the virus (i.e., keep the viral load at low levels) without destroying very large numbers of CD4$^+$ T cells, thus delaying the onset of opportunistic infections. Additionally, certain genetic polymorphisms in the CXCR4 and CCR5 genes have been shown to delay disease progression. Homozygotes for CCR5 mutation have been shown to be resistant to HIV infection.

TABLE 15-12. OPPORTUNISTIC PATHOGENS AND MALIGNANCIES WITH MAJOR MORTALITY RISK IN ACQUIRED IMMUNODEFICIENCY SYNDROME

Parasites	Bacteria	Fungi	Viruses	Malignancies
Toxoplasma spp.	*Mycobacterium tuberculosis*	*Pneumocystis jirovecii*	Herpes simplex virus	Kaposi's sarcoma
Cryptosporidium spp.	*Mycobacterium avium* complex	*Cryptococcus neoformans*	Cytomegalovirus Varicella-zoster virus	Burkitt's lymphoma
Leishmania spp.		*Candida* spp.		
Microsporidium spp.	*Salmonella* spp.	*Histoplasma capsulatum*		Non-Hodgkin's lymphoma
		Coccidioides immitis		

SUMMARY BOX: HUMAN IMMUNODEFICIENCY VIRUS

- Acute human immunodeficiency virus (HIV) infection is characterized by many nonspecific symptoms and can resemble infectious mononucleosis.

- The HIV screening test is enzyme-linked immunosorbent assay (ELISA). Western blot is used as the confirmatory test.

- HIV, with gp120 and gp41, infects T cells that express CD4 and either CXCR4 or CCR5. HIV can also infect phagocytic cells (e.g., macrophages, dendritic cells, microglial cells). Microglia infected with HIV forms multinucleated giant cells in the central nervous system (CNS).

- HIV reverse transcriptase is very error-prone, and thus, suboptimal highly active antiretroviral therapy (HAART) compliance leads to rapid proliferation of resistant strains.

- HIV infection is said to have progressed to acquired immunodeficiency syndrome (AIDS) when the CD4$^+$ T cell count falls below 200 μL^{-1} or the patient presents with one of the AIDS-defining opportunistic infections/malignancies.

- *Pneumocystis jirovecii* pneumonia is the most common significant opportunistic infection in HIV patients and causes a diffuse symmetrical interstitial [lung] infiltrate. Trimethoprim-sulfamethoxazole (TMP-SMX) is the treatment (and prophylaxis) of choice.

CASE 15-9

A 55-year-old woman developed end-stage renal disease due to poorly controlled type 1 diabetes mellitus. She underwent hemodialysis twice a week for 6 months while waiting for a kidney transplant. Because she had no living blood relatives, she was in need of a cadaveric donor. A cadaveric kidney was found from a 28-year-old woman who was fatally injured in a car accident. The donor was blood type B, Rh-positive (matching "the patient's blood") with one matched HLA-A allele. Prior to the transplantation, a final crossmatch was performed in which the recipient was shown to be nonreactive. Immunosuppressive therapy following the transplant procedure consisted of azathioprine, cyclosporine, methylprednisolone, and antithymocyte globulin (ATG). Two weeks following the procedure, the patient was discharged from the hospital on azathioprine, cyclosporine, and prednisone. Her blood pressure and serum creatinine were normal.

She now presents to your office for her 2-week follow-up visit. She complains of decreased urine output, and her blood pressure is found to be 155/95 mm Hg. On physical examination, the region of the graft is enlarged and tender to the touch. You order standard laboratory tests, and the Chem-7 is notable for a serum creatinine of 4 mg/dL.

1. **What two diagnoses immediately rise to the top of your differential diagnosis list?**
    In view of her recent surgical history, transplant rejection (acute, given the timing of the progression of the variables in the case) must be considered. Additionally, note that the two most common adverse effects of cyclosporine are nephrotoxicity and hypertension, thus making cyclosporine toxicity quite likely as well.

2. **What is the mechanism of action of cyclosporine?**
    Cyclosporine binds to cyclophilin (one of the immunophilins), and this complex binds to and inhibits calcineurin. This prevents calcineurin from dephosphorylating the nuclear factor of activated T cells (NFAT). NFAT is a transcription factor, and dephosphorylation would allow it to enter the nucleus and induce transcription of the genes for IL-2 and the IL-2 receptor (essential for the clonal expansion and activation of T cells), as well as a number of other cytokines (Fig. 15-9).

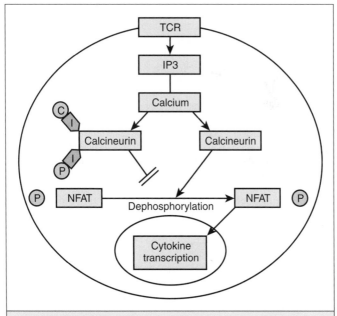

Figure 15-9. Mechanism of action of cyclosporine and tacrolimus. C, cyclosporine; T, tacrolimus; I, immunophilins. (From Adkinson NF Jr, Yunginger JW, Busse WW: Middleton's Allergy: Principles and Practice, 6th ed. Philadelphia, Mosby, 2003.)

CASE 15-9 continued:

A renal biopsy is undertaken and shows the presence of many lymphocytes in the transplant, indicating that the kidney is undergoing acute rejection. She is given high-dose methylprednisolone and OKT3. This immunosuppressive regimen proved successful, and within a year of the transplant, she is doing well. She continues to take low doses of azathioprine, prednisone, and cyclosporine.

3. **Discuss the genetics of the major histocompatibility complex molecules and the role of classes I and II in histocompatibility.**
   Every human has a set of MHC glycoproteins that are referred to as human leukocyte antigens (HLAs). Class I glycoproteins are known as HLA-A, -B, and -C antigens and appear on the surface of nearly all *nucleated* cells. Class II glycoproteins are known as HLA-DR, -DP, -DQ antigens and appear only on antigen-presenting cells (e.g., dendritic cells, B cells, macrophages, Langerhans cells). There are a large number of genes (multiple alleles) that code for each of the class I and class II glycoproteins. Each person receives one set of genes (a haplotype) encoding all six of these antigens from each parent. The HLAs are codominantly expressed on all cells and are antigenic among different individuals. Because of these molecular differences, transplanted tissues between genetically different members of the same species (allogeneic) are likely to be antigenically different and therefore stimulate an immune response.
   Note: Even when a tissue is transplanted between genetically different individuals with a perfect ABO blood group match and a perfect MHC match, rejection can occur because of differences at various minor histocompatibility loci. Although the rejection is usually less vigorous, successful transplantation between MHC-matched individuals still requires some immunosuppression.

4. **What types of rejection may occur in transplant recipients?**
   Hyperacute rejection is mediated by pre-formed serum antibodies in the recipient, usually against ABO antigens on graft endothelial surfaces. It generally occurs within minutes of transplantation, and often first appears as graft whitening (due to vascular thrombi) seen before the conclusion of the surgery. Hyperacute rejection is untreatable, so the organ should be removed.
   Acute rejection is mediated primarily by CTLs, which directly attack the parenchymal cells of the graft. HLA mismatches are the most common cause, and class II MHC mismatches are the most important determinants. As seen in this patient, it typically occurs 10 to 14 days after transplantation and is treatable with immunosuppressive drugs.
   Chronic rejection generally occurs several months to several years after transplantation. The major pathologic finding is graft vascular damage (atherosclerosis and fibrinoid necrosis), and it is thought that this is due to either antibody-mediated damage (resulting from minor histocompatibility antigen mismatches) or side effects of immunosuppressive drugs. Chronic rejection is untreatable.

5. **What is the significance of the patient's having no living blood relatives?**
   It is much easier to identify good HLA matches in blood relatives. Identical twins have the same histocompatibility type (HLA identical). The probability is approximately 0.25 that two siblings with the same parents are HLA identical at a given locus and approximately 0.50 that they are one-half HLA-matched (haploidentical) at a given locus. Furthermore, parents and children are almost always haploidentical across all loci. Because the patient had no living relatives, a cadaveric donor was her only option. A cadaveric donor that is blood group–compatible is often considered even with a poor MHC match.

6. **What does a nonreactive final crossmatch indicate?**
   It indicates that the recipient has no antibodies against the WBCs of the potential donor. Sensitizing events including blood transfusions, pregnancies, and previously failed

transplants may elicit the production of anti-HLA antibodies in the recipient. The presence of such pre-formed antibodies (as indicated by a positive crossmatch) is highly likely to cause hyperacute rejection (in this instance, with anti-HLA, rather than anti-ABO antibodies, as normally seen in this type of rejection) of the transplanted tissue.

Note: Hyperacute rejection of transplanted tissue is a type II hypersensitivity response.

7. **How does azathioprine work as an immunosuppressive agent? Antithymocyte globulin? OKT3? Methylprednisolone?**

Azathioprine, metabolized to 6-mercaptopurine, is a purine analog that interferes with purine synthesis/metabolism and can be incorporated into DNA to inhibit replication. It is most effective in interfering with rapidly dividing cells, such as activated lymphocytes.

Note: Mycophenolate mofetil is an IMP (inosine monophosphate) dehydrogenase inhibitor. This leads to a decrease in the synthesis of purines. Due to its increased specificity for lymphocytes (and thus, decreased side effects), it has replaced azathioprine in many protocols.

ATGs are antibodies against human lymphocytes that are produced in laboratory animals (heterologous antibodies). The antithymocyte (T cell) fraction is isolated and used in transplant recipients to decrease T cell numbers.

OKT3/muromonab is a murine monoclonal antibody that is specific for CD3 on the surface of T cells. It not only has the ability to inhibit T-cell recognition of alloantigen but also reduces T-cell counts. It is quite effective in management of acute rejection.

Methylprednisolone is a corticosteroid anti-inflammatory agent that functions to reduce the number of circulating lymphocytes as well as the ability of lymphocytes to activate and proliferate. It also causes decreased chemotaxis of cells so that fewer inflammatory cells are attracted to the site of activation (the graft) (Fig. 15-10 and Table 15-13).

SUMMARY BOX: TRANSPLANT REJECTION

- Cyclosporine inhibits calcineurin, preventing transcription of several important cytokines, such as interleukin 2 (and the IL-2 receptor). Its major side effects are nephrotoxicity and hypertension.

- Hyperacute rejection: Pre-formed anti-ABO antibodies occlude vessels of graft within minutes of transplantation.

- Acute rejection: T-cell–mediated destruction of graft parenchyma, usually due to human leukocyte antigen (HLA) mismatches, occurs within days to weeks and can be treated with immunosuppressive drugs.

- Chronic rejection: Graft vascular damage occurs months to years after transplantation (antibody-mediated vs. immunosuppressive drugs' adverse effects).

CASE 15-10

A 52-year-old man received a bone marrow transplant (from an HLA-matched brother) in an attempt to cure multiple myeloma. The patient was admitted to the hospital and given a course of busulfan and cyclophosphamide to eradicate his own lymphocytes. He was then intravenously administered bone marrow removed from the donor's iliac crest. His hospital recovery went smoothly and he was sent home, only to return 4 weeks after the transplant. He now presents to you with complaints of an itchy rash on his chest and upper extremities, as

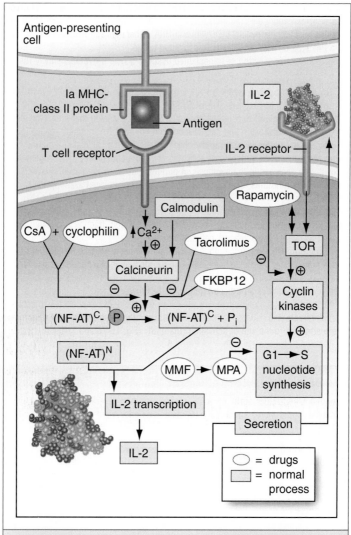

Figure 15-10. Mechanisms and sites of action of immunosuppressive drugs. CsA, cyclosporine; FKBP12, an immunophilin; IL, interleukin; MHC, major histocompatibility complex; MMF, mycophenolate mofetil; MPA, mycophenolic acid; (NF-AT)$^{C \rightarrow N}$, NFAT translocates from cytosol to nucleus; NFAT, nuclear factor of activated T cells; TOR, target of rapamycin. (From McPherson RA, Pincus MR: Henry's Clinical Diagnosis and Management by Laboratory Methods, 21st ed. Philadelphia, WB Saunders, 2006.)

well as severe diarrhea. Physical examination reveals a maculopapular rash with fine excoriations in the aforementioned distribution, mild jaundice, and mild hepatomegaly. The patient is then started on tacrolimus (FK506), methotrexate, and topical corticosteroids. Close follow-up over the next few weeks is recommended. The rash soon fades, but the intestinal symptoms persist. After initiation of weekly injections of a monoclonal antibody to CD2, the diarrhea finally resolves.

TABLE 15-13. TRANSPLANTATION-RELATED IMMUNOSUPPRESSIVE DRUGS

Agent(s)	Mode of Action	Comments
Cyclosporine and tacrolimus (FK-506)	Calcineurin inhibitors; block IL-2 synthesis, thereby preventing T-cell activation	Cyclosporine is nephrotoxic; FK-506 can be administered at lower doses and has fewer side effects than with cyclosporine
Rapamycin and sirolimus	TOR inhibitors, block IL-2–dependent activation of T cells	Rapamycin can be administered at lower doses and has fewer side effects than with cyclosporine
Cyclophosphamide	One metabolite is alkylating agent (cross-links DNA); suppresses B cells more than T cells	Acrolein (another metabolite) causes hemorrhagic cystitis (treated with mesna)
Azathioprine and mycophenolate mofetil (MMF)	Mitotic inhibitors (interfere with purine synthesis and metabolism), target proliferating lymphocytes	MMF has greater lymphocytic selectivity and therefore fewer side effects than those associated with its predecessors, azathioprine and cyclophosphamide
Corticosteroids	Block cytokine production by macrophages (TNF, IL-1); decrease number of circulating lymphocytes	Side effects include hypertension, osteoporosis, muscle wasting, acne, hyperglycemia, cataracts
Antilymphocyte globulin (ALG)/antithymocyte globulin (ATG)	Decrease lymphocyte numbers and T-cell numbers, respectively	Are heterologous sera (from another species), so adverse reactions include serum sickness, immune complex–induced glomerulonephritis, and anaphylactic reactions
OKT3/muromonab (anti-CD3)	Murine monoclonal antibody against CD3 that functions to eliminate T cells	Is a nonhuman antibody, so side effects in humans include serum sickness and immune complex–induced glomerulonephritis
Basiliximab and daclizumab (anti-CD25)	Monoclonal antibody against IL-2 receptor (CD25), blocks IL-2 binding, preventing T-cell activation	Chimeric murine-human monoclonal antibodies; thus, side effects less severe/frequent than with pure murine form

CTLS, cytotoxic T lymphocytes; IL-1, -2, interleukin 1, 2; TNF, tumor necrosis factor.
Note: The major goal of transplant-related immunosuppression is to decrease the generation and activation of helper T cells and CTLs, which mediate acute rejection.

1. **What caused the adverse reaction in this patient 4 weeks after transplantation?**
   Graft-versus-host (GVH) disease was acute, because the signs and symptoms began within 100 days of transplantation.

2. **What is the pathogenesis of graft-versus-host disease?**
   GVH disease is a reaction in which mature donor (graft) T cells in transplanted bone marrow act to attack cells in the immunosuppressed recipient (host). The reaction is initiated when immunocompetent T_H cells from the graft (allowed to survive because the host's leukocytes have already been eradicated in pretreatment) are activated by host proteins recognized as foreign. These cells produce high levels of cytokines that recruit and activate other T cells, macrophages, and NK cells to create the inflammation that is seen in GVH disease. However, note that the bulk of the damage is caused by graft CTLs and their unchecked destruction of host cells. These events lead to the classic GVH disease triad of skin rash, diarrhea, and hepatic dysfunction.

3. **Why did the donor's cells react against the recipient's when they were HLA-matched?**
   Individuals who are HLA-matched share the same MHC haplotypes. In other words, they have MHC class I and class II molecules that are genetically and antigenically identical. However, even in HLA-matched individuals, disparities in minor histocompatibility antigens exist. These allogeneic molecules, which are likely to vary in all donor-recipient pairs other than identical twins, have the potential to activate mature T cells of the donor.
   Note: Unlike MHC antigens, which are recognized directly by T cells, minor histocompatibility antigens are recognized only when presented by self-MHC molecules. Thus, tissue rejection due to minor histocompatibility differences takes longer to develop (several weeks) and is often less vigorous.

4. **Why are the skin and the intestinal tract the major sites of graft-versus-host disease?**
   Recall that the epidermal barriers of the skin and the gastrointestinal tract are two of the major portals of attempted entry for microorganisms. Therefore, the immunologic protection at these two sites is quite robust; this includes a high level of expression of histocompatibility antigens. In GVH disease, such expression would increase the probability (and severity) of attack at these two sites.

5. **How do monoclonal antibodies against CD2 help treat graft-versus-host disease?**
   CD2 is an antigen found on thymocytes and mature T cells. Antibody against CD2 is effective at decreasing T cell numbers by eliciting their clearance by the reticuloendothelial system (e.g., splenic macrophages). ATG would have a similar effect.

6. **What is the mechanism of action of busulfan?**
   Busulfan is an alkylating agent that causes DNA-DNA cross-linking and DNA-protein cross-linking. This leads to cytotoxicity, which is specific to myeloid cells and circulating lymphocytes at low doses and to hematopoietic stem cells at high doses. When given in combination with cyclophosphamide, high-dose busulfan can be used to eradicate a patient's leukocytes in preparation for bone marrow transplantation, as was seen in this patient. Common adverse effects include GI upset, pancytopenia, and hyperpigmentation. Pulmonary fibrosis is rare, but very serious.

7. **What is the mechanism of action of methotrexate?**
Methotrexate is a folic acid analog that inhibits dihydrofolate reductase. This leads to a lack of tetrahydrofolate (THF), causing a lack of multiple nucleotide precursors. This prevents DNA synthesis and, importantly for GVH disease, prevents lymphocyte proliferation. Notable adverse effects include myelosuppression, hepatotoxicity, interstitial lung disease, and a transient neurologic syndrome with protean manifestations.

8. **Performance of what laboratory test could have predicted that graft-versus-host disease would result in this patient?**
One-way mixed lymphocyte reaction (MLR) test measures proliferation (activation) of donor lymphocytes in response to irradiated (killed) recipient lymphocytes. Proliferation of these cells in vitro is a good predictor of GVH disease in vivo.

9. **How might the donor's marrow have been treated to prevent graft-versus-host disease?**
Partial T cell depletion of donor marrow before infusion can reduce the incidence of GVH disease. Monoclonal antibodies against T-cell antigens (e.g., OKT3, ATG, anti-CD2) are useful in the removal of T cells.

SUMMARY BOX: GRAFT-VERSUS-HOST DISEASE

- Graft-versus-host (GVH) disease is characterized by graft T cells attacking the cells of the [immunocompromised] host.

- The skin and gastrointestinal (GI) tract are two of the major sites of pathogen entry and therefore consist of cells with a very high major histocompatibility complex (MHC) expression density. GVH disease affects these two sites prominently because of this.

- Mismatches between donor and recipient occur not only from human leukocyte antigen (HLA) MHC mismatches but also from differences in minor histocompatibility antigens.

CASE 15-11

A 26-year-old man comes to your office with a chief complaint of new-onset pain in his right knee and left ankle after returning from a trip to northern New England 2 weeks ago. He also mentioned the onset of fatigue, a mild fever, and an "eye problem" to the medical assistant. Before seeing him, you briefly review his medical history and see only a history of psoriasis and a laboratory test result showing that he is HLA-B27–positive.

1. **His presentation, coupled with his HLA-B27 status, brings what three diagnoses into consideration?**
Ankylosing spondylitis, reactive arthritis (previously known as Reiter's syndrome), and psoriatic arthritis are possible.

2. **Complete the initial differential diagnosis.**
Trauma must be considered in a potentially active patient. Also, until the sexual history is known, gonococcal arthritis cannot be ruled out. Lyme disease should be considered as well, given his travel history, and the time course and symptoms would be suggestive of stage 2. Other possibilities, dependent on the pending detailed history, include rheumatoid arthritis, SLE, substance/drug-induced arthritis, septic arthritis, and viral arthritis.

CASE 15–11 continued:

You interview the patient and he recounts the following story about his joint pain: "First it was my right knee, then it was my left ankle, and now I think my right ankle might be hurting a little too." However, he also notes that he had multiple episodes of dysuria 2 weeks ago, and these have now returned. Upon further questioning, he admits to having had sexual intercourse with a partner he met for the first time on his trip. Physical examination reveals that the right knee and left ankle are tender and immobile, with moderate effusions. Ophthalmologic examination reveals anterior uveitis of the left eye. Examination of the genitals is unremarkable.

3. **What is the most likely cause of the patient's clinical picture?**
   Reactive arthritis is most likely.

4. **What organisms are most commonly associated with reactive arthritis?**
   Chlamydia trachomatis, *Campylobacter jejuni*, *Yersinia enterocolitica* and *Y. pseudotuberculosis*, *Salmonella enteritidis* and *S. typhimurium*, and *Shigella flexneri*.

5. **What should be done next?**
   Arthrocentesis should be performed to rule out infection. Owing to the high likelihood that his reactive arthritis is related to *Chlamydia*, he should have a urine test for this organism, as well as for *Neisseria gonorrhoeae*. Because he might not return to follow up on his results, it would be advisable to initiate presumptive treatment for *Chlamydia* (azithromycin or doxycycline) at this time. Additional testing for sexually transmitted infections, such as HIV and syphilis, should be considered. In terms of his reactive arthritis, the symptoms are best treated with nonsteroidal anti-inflammatory drugs (NSAIDs).

6. **Describe the pathogenesis of reactive arthritis.**
   Though still often debated, reactive arthritis likely results from bacterial antigen molecular mimicry. In short, this means that certain antigens (from *Chlamydia*, in this case) have a molecular composition that is similar to that of proteins in the joints, genitourinary tract, and the eye. Thus, when T and B cells initiate attack on the offending organism, these self proteins can be bound by TCR (if presented on MHC) or antibody, and damage ensues.

7. **The cardiac manifestations of rheumatic fever represent one of the best examples of molecular mimicry. Discuss the cross-reacting proteins.**
   The M protein of *Streptococcus pyogenes* is the organism's primary antiphagocytic factor. Certain types of the M protein very closely resemble myocardial myosin. If a *S. pyogenes* infection is not treated in less than 9 days, some patients will produce cross-reactive antibodies, leading to myocardial damage. Note that M protein molecular mimicry is thought to play a role in other symptoms of rheumatic fever (polyarthritis, cardiac valvular disease, skin nodules, skin rash, and Sydenham's chorea) as well.

8. **In addition to molecular mimicry, what are the two other proposed major mechanisms of autoimmunity?**
   Alteration of self proteins: A situation in which a substance binds to a normal self protein and causes it to appear foreign to the immune system. Examples are penicillin-induced AIHA (see Case 15-2) and drug-induced lupus. A similar scenario occurs when certain viruses infect a cell and alter select surface proteins.
   Compromise of immunologically privileged sites: Certain tissues are never exposed to the immune system, and thus tolerance toward them is never developed. Examples are the sperm (via the Sertoli cell barrier), the brain (via the blood-brain barrier), and certain parts of the eye. If damage to the tissue and the barrier occurs, proteins (now antigens) are released into

circulation, and immunologic attack on the source tissue ensues. Similarly, the immune system usually does not develop tolerance to intracellular proteins such as those associated with the nucleus (e.g., DNA, histones). Therefore, cellular damage and release of these antigens (as might be seen with a lytic virus) are thought to play a role in the development of autoimmune diseases such as SLE.

RELATED QUESTIONS: MECHANISMS OF TOLERANCE

9. **T-cell tolerance in the thymus (central tolerance) was discussed in Case 7, question 5. Discuss the important principles of peripheral T-cell tolerance.**
All T_H cells require two things to become activated: the interaction of the TCR and CD4 with MHC II plus antigen, and costimulatory signals. If the first interaction is present, but one of the vital costimulatory signals is absent, the T cell becomes anergic (nonreactive). The most commonly cited costimulatory signal is the binding of B7 from the APC to T cell CD28. The meeting of these two molecules can be prevented by downregulation of APC B7 expression or competition for B7 binding sites by CTLA-4 on the T cell. Cytokines are also important in T cell activation. A key player in peripheral tolerance is the suppressor T cell, a type of T_H cell. This cell strives to control self-reactive cells and to "put the brakes on" the immune response by secreting a myriad of inhibitory cytokines.

10. **Describe B-cell tolerance.**
B-cell tolerance is not as well characterized as T-cell tolerance. Central tolerance occurs in the bone marrow, but in contrast with thymic education, the approach is single-pronged: only self-reactive B cells are deleted (negative selection). Peripheral tolerance is also important and likely is directed to a large degree by suppressor T cells.

SUMMARY BOX: REACTIVE ARTHRITIS

- Molecular mimicry, one of the probable mechanisms of autoimmunity, describes a non-self molecule (often part of an infecting virion or bacterium) that resembles a self molecule. The resultant immune attack can cross-react and lead to damage of self tissues containing the mimicked molecule.

- Autoimmunity may also be due to virus/drug-induced alteration of self proteins and compromise of immunologically privileged sites.

- Helper T (T_H) cells require the interaction of the T-cell receptor (TCR) and CD4 with class II major histocompatibility complex (MHC) plus antigen AND a costimulatory signal to become activated. Absence of the costimulatory signal leads to T_H cell anergy.

  - Disruption of the CD28-B7 interaction (by CTLA-4, for example) is a common mechanism of costimulatory signal blockage and anergy induction.

- Reactive arthritis is a "reaction" to a bacterial infection, is associated with HLA-B27, and is seen clinically as asymmetrical arthritis, urethritis, anterior uveitis and/or conjunctivitis, rash, and fatigue.

CHAPTER 16

PSYCHOLOGY

Jaime Stevens, MD, MPH, Thomas A. Brown, MD, and Sonali J. Shah

INSIDER'S GUIDE TO PSYCHOLOGY FOR THE USMLE STEP 1

Psychology is a straightforward subject on the USMLE if studied for correctly. Focus on learning the diagnostic criteria for the diseases covered in First Aid. Popularly tested subjects include personality disorders, defense mechanisms, delirium versus dementia, eating disorders, panic disorder, drug abuse and withdrawal, and depression. Take time to learn the antipsychotic drugs and their side effects. They are commonly tested on Step 1.

CASE 16-1

A 20-year-old college student has been doing poorly for the past 8 months. He has become socially withdrawn and apathetic, and his grades, previously good, have been suffering. He complains to the campus physician that he has been hearing voices and that the TV news anchor has been giving him secret messages telling him to infiltrate the Russian KGB and thwart their assassination attempt of the President. He also wants to go into hiding because he believes that the CIA is after him. An extensive workup to identify organic causes of his symptoms (thyroid function tests, drug screening, head computed tomography [CT], and magnetic resonance imaging [MRI]) is negative.

1. **What is the most likely diagnosis?**
   Schizophrenia, a thought disorder that occurs in approximately 1% of the population, is most likely. However, the differential diagnosis includes schizoaffective disorder, mood disorder with psychotic features, and psychosis secondary to a general medical condition or substance abuse.
   Note: The typical age at onset of schizophrenia is 18 to 24 years in men and 26 to 45 years in women.

2. **According to the *Diagnostic and Statistical Manual of Mental Disorders* (DSM-IV), what criteria must be met in order to make the diagnosis of schizophrenia?**
   Two or more of the following active-phase symptoms must be present for a 1-month period (or less if successfully treated):
   1. Delusions (substantially irrational beliefs, e.g., a belief that you're the reincarnation of Fred Astaire)
   2. Hallucinations (e.g., hearing voices that only you can hear) (**Note:** The primary cause of auditory hallucinations in a psychotic patient is schizophrenia. You should make this association for the USMLE.)

3. Disorganized speech (e.g., incoherence)
4. Grossly disorganized or catatonic behavior
5. Negative symptoms (e.g., social withdrawal)

   In addition, the preceding symptoms must cause negative effects on major areas of functioning such as work, interpersonal relations, or self-care. The duration of the disturbance must persist for at least 6 months, including at least 1 month of active-phase symptoms listed here.

3. **What is the diagnosis if this man had suffered these symptoms for only the past 3 months rather than for 8 months (with a negative workup for other causes)?**
   Schizophreniform disorder, which is diagnosed in a patient displaying symptoms of schizophrenia for a period of more than 1 month and no longer than 6 months in duration.

STEP 1 SECRET

Many psychological disorders are associated with time intervals that are required to make a definitive diagnosis of the disease. The USMLE will expect you to know these time intervals (e.g., schizophreniform disorder and schizophrenia both present with the same symptoms, but schizophrenia is diagnosed only in patients who are symptomatic for at least 6 months).

4. **What is the likely diagnosis if this man presented with these symptoms and later developed depressive, manic, or mixed features?**
   Schizoaffective disorder is more likely because the "affect" is involved. There is also the usual laundry list of DSM-IV criteria to make this diagnosis, but you will not be required to know this for the Step 1 examination. Schizoaffective disorder differs from major depression with psychotic features in that the latter does not involve delusions and hallucinations in the absence of significant mood symptoms for more than 2 weeks (i.e., if longer than 2 weeks, it is schizoaffective disorder).

STEP 1 SECRET

You are responsible for learning about schizoaffective disorder for Step 1, but because it is such a nit-picky diagnosis to make, you are far more likely to be tested on schizophrenia and schizophreniform disorder than on schizoaffective disorder.

5. **What would your diagnosis be if this man had symptoms of schizophrenia following a severe stressor and these symptoms resolved within 2 weeks?**
   He would be suffering from a brief psychotic disorder; in this case, it would be a reactive psychosis, as it is associated with marked stressors. A brief psychotic disorder is a disorder that lasts a short period of time, less than a month, but at least 1 day. It cannot be due to a general medical condition, associated with a mood disorder, or caused by substance use. This disorder does not require that severe stressors be present. In women, it additionally may have postpartum onset (if within 4 weeks of delivery), in which case it would be called postpartum psychosis. If this had followed or had been attributed to a medical illness, it would be diagnosed as psychosis secondary to a general medical condition.

6. **What are the four primary types of schizophrenia?**
Catatonic schizophrenia is characterized by two or more of the following: cataplexy (define) or stupor, excessive motor activity, resistance to instructions or attempts of movement, peculiar movements or posturing and mannerisms or grimacing, and echolalia or echopraxia (mimicking of others' speech or movements).
   Disorganized schizophrenia includes disorganized speech and behavior and flat or inappropriate affect and does not meet criteria for catatonic schizophrenia.
   Paranoid schizophrenia is characterized by delusions of persecution and absence of disorganized speech, catatonic behavior, and flat or inappropriate affect. This patient's symptoms are most consistent with paranoid schizophrenia.
   Residual schizophrenia is characterized by absence of prominent delusions, hallucinations, or catatonia, and there is continuing evidence of the disease such as negative symptoms and odd beliefs.

STEP 1 SECRET

It is not hugely important to know the different types of schizophrenia for the USMLE. Read this section through once or twice, but do not worry about committing these facts to memory.

7. **What neurotransmitter abnormality is thought to play the primary role in this man's disorder?**
The current theory is that excess dopamine activity in certain regions of the brain is the cause of schizophrenia. There are several pieces of evidence in support of this theory. Some researchers have shown that positron emission tomography (PET) scans of schizophrenic patients' basal ganglia show an increased number of D_2 receptors when compared with unaffected control subjects. Patients with schizophrenia who are treated with dopamine receptor antagonists show a beneficial response. Additionally, drugs with dopaminergic effects will aggravate existing psychosis and, in some patients, can result in new-onset psychosis (see question 8).

8. **What are the differences between the positive and negative symptoms experienced by schizophrenics?**
Positive symptoms are symptoms whose *presence* is abnormal. They include thought disturbances, delusions, and auditory and visual hallucinations. These symptoms are mediated by increased levels of dopamine in the mesolimbic pathway and can be treated with typical antipsychotic drugs. Negative symptoms are those that indicate an *absence* of a habit, expression, or quality present in a majority of the general population. They can include social withdrawal and isolation, anhedonia, and apathy. Negative symptoms are the result of decreased activity of mesocortical dopaminergic projections. They can be exacerbated by use of typical antipsychotics.

9. **What is the relationship between schizophrenia and suicide?**
Unfortunately, people with schizophrenia are at greatly increased risk for attempting suicide, and between 10% and 15% of schizophrenics do successfully commit suicide.

10. **When initiating therapy for patients like this college student, it is important to keep potential side effects in mind and to educate the patient about them. What type of side effects are more commonly seen with high-potency antipsychotics such as haloperidol and fluphenazine than with other antipsychotics?**

Extrapyramidal side effects (EPS) such as acute dystonia, parkinsonism, akathesia, and tardive dyskinesia (TD) are more commonly seen. Acute dystonia results in excessive muscle tone and muscle spasms (e.g., torticollis, laryngospasm) after only short-term exposure (typically within 3-5 days) to antipsychotics. Parkinsonism is characterized by shuffling gait, cogwheel rigidity, bradykinesia, and resting tremor. Onset is usually not until after a couple of weeks of therapy. Akasthesia is a subjective sensation of inner restlessness or desire to move. Individuals with this condition may appear anxious or agitated and may move about and pace, as they are unable to sit still. TD presents with involuntary movements of the tongue, lips, face, trunk, and extremities (generally irreversible) and occurs in patients treated with long-term dopaminergic antagonist medications (months to years) of high-dose antipsychotics. The risk of developing TDs is about 3% per year with typical agents.

11. **What is the correct treatment for the previously mentioned extrapyramidal side effects?**

Both dystonia and drug-induced parkinsonian syndrome are best treated with an anticholinergic such as benztropine (note that this would be a good opportunity to review the role of acetylcholine in the basal ganglia pathways). In addition, if there is acute airway obstruction due to laryngeal spasms in acute dystonia, intravenous diphenhydramine should be used urgently. Akathesia frequently does not improve with anticholinergics; administration of a beta blocker is often the first step. Lowering the dose or switching medication may be necessary. If TDs appear, the offending drug should be discontinued immediately (hence the importance of the education). Unfortunately, TDs often do not improve or resolve despite discontinuation of the drug. All antipsychotics, with the exception of clozapine, may produce TD, but it is most commonly seen with the typical agents prescribed. The patient should therefore be switched to an atypical agent or to clozapine. Anticholinergics have no benefit in these patients and may actually worsen symptoms.

12. **How might this man develop the following symptoms if he is being treated with low-potency typical antipsychotics such as chlorpromazine or thioridazine?**

A. Urinary retention

The term *low-potency typical antipsychotics* refers to the fact that a greater dose is required to reach the same dopaminergic effect. The low-potency antipsychotics, in addition to blocking D_2 receptors, also block histaminic, α-adrenergic, and muscarinic receptors (i.e., the HAM receptors) to a much greater extent than the high-potency typical antipsychotics. Blockade of the muscarinic cholinergic receptors on the detrusor muscle of the bladder results in urinary retention.

Note: The muscarinic antagonism also causes the common anticholinergic side effects of dry mouth, loss of visual accommodation, and constipation.

B. Orthostatic hypotension

Orthostatic hypotension can be caused by α-blockade. As a result, higher doses are used, leading to increased antagonism of the α-receptor.

C. Sedation

H_1 blockade can produce a sedative effect. Administration of the drug at bedtime may reduce daytime sedation.

13. **Perhaps the most feared complication of antipsychotics is an idiosyncratic reaction characterized by severe muscle rigidity, myoglobinuria and elevated plasma creatine kinase, fever, autonomic instability, and altered mental status. What is the name of this lethal side effect and what is the treatment?**
Neuroleptic malignant syndrome (NMS) may occur with any antipsychotic, aside from clozapine, but more commonly is seen with the typical agents; the offending drug should be stopped immediately. In addition, NMS can be treated with dantrolene or dopamine agonists such as bromocriptine.

STEP 1 SECRET

Neuroleptic malignant syndrome (NMS) and side effects of high-potency and low-potency neuroleptics are frequently tested on Step 1. Be sure to know which drugs fall into which of these two categories.

14. **How do typical and atypical antipsychotics differ with respect to their mode of action and to their effect on positive and negative symptoms?**
Atypical antipsychotics (e.g., clozapine) are "atypical" in that they are more effective against the negative symptoms of schizophrenia and are much less likely to cause extrapyramidal side effects (e.g., acute dystonia, TD) than are the typical antipsychotics. In addition to dopamine receptor blockade, atypicals block the serotonin receptor of the $5-HT_2$ subtype; this is thought to offer some protection against EPS. The thought is that atypicals are effective in mesolimbic blockade of dopamine (hyperactive in schizophrenics) without significant blockade of the mesocortical circuit (hypoactive in schizophrenics). In addition, the atypicals have other dopamine receptor actions. For example, clozapine is a very effective D_4 antagonist, and aripiprazole is a dopamine autoreceptor agonist and a D_2 partial agonist.

15. **Which one of the four major dopamine pathways of the brain is responsible for the following symptoms in schizophrenia?**
A. Gynecomastia, galactorrhea, and menstrual dysfunction with antipsychotic use
   The tuberoinfundibular pathway involves projection of dopamine neurons in the arcuate nucleus to the median eminence (below the hypothalamus). Dopamine released at this site normally inhibits the secretion of prolactin from the anterior pituitary gland. Some antipsychotic drugs block dopamine in the tuberoinfundibular pathway, causing hyperprolactinemia. This may cause gynecomastia, galactorrhea, and menstrual dysfunction secondary to prolactin-mediated inhibition of gonadotropin-releasing hormone (GnRH).
B. Positive symptoms
   The mesolimbic pathway involves projection of dopamine neurons in the ventral tegmentum to the nucleus accumbens. Hyperactivity of this pathway is thought to be responsible for the positive symptoms such as hallucinations, delusions, and agitation.
C. Negative symptoms
   The mesocortical pathway involves projection of dopamine neurons in the ventral tegmentum to the frontal lobes. The idea is that hypoactivity of this pathway in schizophrenics may be responsible for the negative symptoms of social withdrawal and flat affect.
D. Parkinsonism with antipsychotic use
   The nigrostriatal pathway is a neural pathway that connects the substantia nigra with the striatum. Loss of neurons in this pathway is responsible for Parkinson's disease, so it is no wonder that blockade of dopamine will cause parkinsonism (bradykinesia, rigidity, masked facies, resting tremor, shuffling gait). Fortunately, these symptoms are reversible with discontinuation of the antipsychotics.

You should know the functions of each of the dopaminergic pathways and the symptoms involved with dysregulation of these pathways.

16. **Recent studies have suggested that there is no large difference in effectiveness and tolerability between the typical and atypical drugs, with the exception of clozapine. Although the typicals have significant side effects, the atypicals also come with their fair share of problems. Which atypicals are most strongly correlated with the following side effects?**

A. Gynecomastia, galactorrhea, and menstrual dysfunction

Risperidone is similar to typical antipsychotics in that it is a very potent blocker of the D_2 receptor. D_2 receptor blockade of the tuberoinfundibular pathway leads to hyperprolactinemia, which causes gynecomastia, galactorrhea, and menstrual dysfunction.

B. Hyperlipidemia and diabetes

Olanzapine and clozapine appear to carry the greatest risk, followed by risperidone and quetiapine. However, in 2003 the U.S. Food and Drug Administration (FDA) requested manufacturers of *all* atypical antipsychotics to include product label warnings about the potential for an increased risk of hyperglycemia and diabetes.

C. Increasing the QT interval

Of the atypical drugs, ziprasidone has the greatest effect on QT prolongation and should therefore be avoided in patients with increased QT intervals or known heart disease.

D. Increased mortality risk with treatment of dementia-related psychosis in the elderly

A placebo-controlled trial in which risperidone and olanzapine were studied found that for the treatment of dementia-related psychosis in the elderly, there was an associated higher death rate versus placebo. In April 2005, the FDA therefore required manufacturers of *all* atypical antipsychotics to include a boxed warning in their labeling noting this risk.

17. **Why is clozapine recommended for use only in schizophrenics whose symptoms are refractory to treatment with other antipsychotics?**

Clozapine is an atypical antipsychotic that often works in patients who have been refractory to other antipsychotics. The big drawback of using clozapine is that it can precipitate a fatal agranulocytosis (1% per year) and therefore necessitates weekly monitoring of blood levels for the first 6 months of therapy before the dose is reduced to a somewhat longer interval. Other drugs that can cause agranulocytosis include carbamazepine, colchicine, propylthiouracil, methimazole, and dapsone. The USMLE loves to ask questions on this concept!

SUMMARY BOX: PSYCHOTIC DISORDERS

■ Schizophrenia is defined as presence of two symptoms for 1 month (delusions, hallucinations, disorganized speech, disorganized or catatonic behavior, negative symptoms) AND signs of illness for at least 6 months.

■ Schizoaffective disorder meets criteria for schizophrenia and criteria for major depression, mixed disorder, or manic episode. It is accompanied by delusions and hallucinations for 2 weeks *without* mood symptoms.

■ Schizophreniform disorder meets criteria for schizophrenia, but duration is 1 to 6 months.

- Brief psychotic disorder is described as presence of schizophrenic symptoms lasting 1 day to 1 month.

- Delusional disorder consists of presence of *nonbizarre* delusions for at least 1 month AND no other symptoms of schizophrenia.

- Atypical antipsychotics are more effective against the negative symptoms of schizophrenia and are much less likely to cause extrapyramidal side effects.

- Low-potency typical agents have high incidence of anticholinergic side effects, sedation, and orthostatic hypotension.

- High-potency typical agents have high incidence of extrapyramidal side effects.

- There is no large difference in effectiveness and tolerability between the typical and atypical antipsychotics, with the exception of clozapine.

CASE 16-2

A 22-year-old college man nicknamed "Roller-coaster" by his friends complains of problems with his mood and is referred to a psychiatrist by the campus physician for further evaluation. He states that for the past week he has been incredibly productive because he has required very little sleep. During the interview, the physician notes pressured speech, distractibility, euphoric mood, and psychomotor hyperactivity. The patient denies any history of auditory or visual hallucinations or use of alcohol or other drugs. Just prior to this period, however, he experienced a 2-month period characterized by hypersomnia, anhedonia, decreased appetite, and psychomotor retardation. Physical examination is noncontributory, and laboratory tests indicate normal thyroid activity.

1. **What is the diagnosis?**
   He has bipolar disorder—specifically, bipolar I.
   Note: Bipolar I is characterized by manic episodes lasting at least 1 week, whereas the milder bipolar II requires only a hypomanic episode lasting at least 4 days for diagnosis. The major difference from a manic episode is the lack of social or occupational dysfunction.
   Manic episodes consist of abnormal mood with three or more of the following symptoms present for at least 1 week:
   - **B**efuddled/distracted
   - **I**deas upon ideas (racing thoughts)
   - **G**randiosity
   - **S**leep decrease
   - **H**ypersexuality
   - **I**rresponsible actions
   - **F**ocused activity
   - **T**alkative

STEP 1 SECRET

You can easily recall the symptoms of manic episodes by remembering that manic episodes cause a BIG SHIFT in mood.

2. **Was the previous depressive episode required to make the diagnosis of bipolar in "Roller-coaster"?**
   No, only a single manic episode is required. All patients who have experienced a manic episode are considered bipolar, regardless of whether they have additionally suffered a depressive episode or not. This can be confusing, as the term "bipolar" implies manic and depressive features. However, most patients with a history of manic episodes will ultimately develop a depressive disorder as well.

   Note: Unlike bipolar I, bipolar II *does* require at least one major depressive episode. There is also cyclothymia, which requires a period of at least 2 years during which there have been both periods of hypomania and depression, but the depressive episodes do not fulfill requirements for *major* depression and the patient has not been symptom-free for more than 2 months.

3. **The physician prescribes lithium and informs "Roller-coaster" that he needs to have his blood levels of lithium monitored regularly. Why is this necessary?**
   There is only a small difference between the therapeutic and toxic concentrations of lithium (i.e., its therapeutic index is low, which makes it a dangerous drug). Lithium toxicity presents with *coarse* tremor (fine tremor is a common side effect of lithium), stupor, ataxia, vomiting, diarrhea, and cardiac arrhythmias.

4. **After taking lithium for an extended period of time, "Roller-coaster" develops polyuria and polydipsia. The urine has a low osmolarity, and administration of antidiuretic hormone (vasopressin) does not have a significant effect on either the polyuria or the low urine osmolarity. What is happening?**
   A distinctive but rare side effect of lithium is nephrogenic diabetes insipidus. This occurs when the kidneys do not respond effectively to antidiuretic hormone (ADH) and so do not conserve water or concentrate the urine effectively—hence the polyuria and polydipsia.

5. **True or false: Treatment of this lithium-induced nephrogenic diabetes insipidus with loop diuretics may be effective in decreasing his symptoms of polyuria.**
   True. Although this effect is seemingly counterintuitive, loop diuretics and thiazide diuretics will actually decrease polyuria in nephrogenic diabetes insipidus because they promote proximal tubular reabsorption. However, extracellular fluid depletion can also increase the risk of lithium intoxication by enhancing lithium reabsorption at the proximal tubule, so careful monitoring is required to avoid lithium toxicity. Amiloride is perhaps the best choice of a diuretic because it is least likely to increase lithium levels.

6. **"Roller-coaster" also mentions that he has become rather depressed after being on the lithium for a while, is having memory problems, and seems to be cold all the time. Rather than just putting this patient on an antidepressant, the physician orders thyroid-stimulating hormone (TSH) and T_4 (thyroxine) levels first. Why?**
   Another side effect of lithium is hypothyroidism, which can cause the previously mentioned symptoms.

   Note: Although the issue is not pertinent to this patient, lithium can also lead to pregnancy problems. A well-established complication of lithium is Ebstein anomaly, which is a congenital malformation of the heart characterized by apical displacement of the tricuspid valve leaflets.

7. **Because "Roller-coaster" is not tolerating lithium well, his physician decides to substitute a drug that is effective not only for bipolar disorder but also for several seizure disorders. What is this drug and what regular monitoring should be done?**
   Because valproic acid has lower toxicity and fewer side effects than lithium, this drug has actually become the mood stabilizer of choice. Valproic acid is also effective for absence seizures, partial seizures, and generalized seizures. It is worth mentioning that valproic acid

is also more effective than lithium in rapid-cycling and mixed-state episode bipolar disorder. Very rare but potentially fatal side effects of valproic acid therapy include necrotizing hepatitis (children are at increased risk) and agranulocytosis. Periodic monitoring of liver enzymes and blood cells is therefore indicated in patients on long-term valproic acid therapy. Administration of valproic acid in pregnant women can also cause neural tube defects in the fetus.

8. **At his next visit, "Roller-coaster's" symptoms seem to be well controlled with valproic acid, but his liver enzymes are markedly elevated. The valproic acid is discontinued, and he is prescribed another anticonvulsant that may also cause a leukopenia or agranulocytosis but is not hepatotoxic. What drug was he likely given?**
   Carbamazepine, which is really only effective in acute manic episodes, is known to produce a persistent leukopenia. Therefore, regular monitoring of laboratory values would be required.

9. **Why should valproic acid be used with extreme caution in patients also taking phenobarbital?**
   Valproic acid inhibits the hepatic metabolism of phenobarbital and displaces phenobarbital from plasma proteins. These effects result in elevated levels of free plasma phenobarbital, putting the patient at risk for barbiturate-induced coma.

10. **In someone with a seizure disorder that is well controlled with phenytoin, why may the addition of carbamazepine cause seizures to occur again?**
    Carbamazepine induces hepatic enzymes, which increase the metabolism of phenytoin and can reduce its plasma level to subtherapeutic levels.

SUMMARY BOX: BIPOLAR DISORDER

- Bipolar I disorder is defined as one or more manic or mixed episodes (major depressive episode is not required).

- Bipolar II disorder consists of one or more major depressive episodes and at least one hypomanic episode.

- Cyclothymia describes many episodes of depression and hypomania occurring over a 2-year period.

- Lithium has a narrow therapeutic index.

- Side effects of lithium include nephrogenic diabetes insipidus and hypothyroidism.

- Valproic acid is now the mood stabilizer of choice due to side effect profile and lower toxicity.

- Valproic acid is more effective than lithium in rapid-cycling and mixed-state episode bipolar disorder.

CASE 16-3

A 48-year-old man complains of poor appetite, insomnia, decreased interest in activities that he used to enjoy, difficulty concentrating, and loss of energy for much of the past year. He has lost 20 lb in the past 6 months. He denies illicit drug use or alcohol abuse and is not taking any prescription medications. Physical examination is unremarkable. Laboratory evaluation reveals a normal TSH and T_4.

1. **What is the most likely diagnosis?**
   Major depressive disorder is most likely. However, the differential diagnosis for depression includes hypothyroidism, bipolar, schizophrenia, Parkinson's disease, chronic renal failure, anemia, dementia, substance withdrawal, and anxiety.

2. **According to the DSM-IV, what criteria must be met in order to make the diagnosis of major depressive disorder?**
   Major depressive disorder can be diagnosed when at least five of the following symptoms are present on an almost daily basis for at least the past 2 weeks, and when at least one of the symptoms is either depressed mood or loss of interest or pleasure in activities that were previously enjoyable (anhedonia):
   1. Depressed mood most of the day
   2. Anhedonia
   3. Significant change in weight or appetite
   4. Insomnia or hypersomnia nearly every day
   5. Psychomotor agitation or retardation nearly every day
   6. Fatigue or loss of energy nearly every day
   7. Feelings of worthlessness or excessive/inappropriate guilt
   8. Diminished ability to think or concentrate
   9. Recurrent thoughts of death, suicidal ideation with or without a plan, or a suicide attempt
   In addition, these symptoms must cause significant impairment in social, occupational, or other important areas of functioning. These symptoms cannot be better explained by a general medical condition (e.g., hypothyroidism), substance abuse, or loss of a loved one (bereavement).

3. **What does the monoamine deficiency theory propose with respect to the etiology of depression?**
   A deficiency in any one of the neurotransmitters norepinephrine, dopamine, or serotonin can result in depression. There is accumulating pharmacologic evidence in support of this theory because increasing central activity of serotonin, norepinephrine, and dopamine, either individually or in combination, has been shown to be beneficial in the treatment of depression.

STEP 1 SECRET

For Step 1 *and* for your clinical years, it will be important to remember which neurotransmitter levels are altered in various psychological and neurologic diseases because treatment is generally aimed at correcting these abnormalities. You can remember which neurotransmitters are affected in depression by considering our poor friend Ned. NeD'S DOWN because he has DEPRESSION. Ne = norepinephrine, D = dopamine, S = serotonin, and DOWN refers to decreased levels of all three of these neurotransmitters in depressed patients.

4. **Why does hypothyroidism have to be ruled out in this patient?**
   Hypothyroidism can produce symptoms similar to those of depression.

5. **What pharmacologic therapies are available to treat depression?**
   - Tricyclic antidepressants (TCAs)
   - Selective serotonin reuptake inhibitors (SSRIs) (e.g., fluoxetine, paroxetine, sertraline)
   - Monoamine oxidase inhibitors (MAOIs) (e.g., phenelzine, tranylcypromine)
   - Serotonin/norepinephrine reuptake inhibitors (SNRIs) (e.g., venlafaxine, duloxetine)
   - Mixed serotonin reuptake inhibitor–serotonin receptor antagonist (e.g., nefazodone, mirtazapine)

Note: Electroconvulsive therapy (ECT) and psychotheraphy are other options. ECT is a very safe and effective treatment for depression and is the therapy of choice when there is a high risk of suicide, the patient has been refractory to pharmacotherapy, or there is insufficient time for a trial of medication. ECT has a response rate of 90% compared with 70% for pharmacotherapy, the main side effect being anterograde amnesia. After ECT, combined pharmacotherapy and psychotherapy is the most effective treatment.

6. **On review of systems he expresses concern about a history of premature ejaculation. What class of antidepressant may help address this concern?**
   SSRIs commonly produce sexual dysfunction and delayed ejaculation in men. In a patient with premature ejaculation, however, the effects of delaying ejaculation would be desirable.

7. **Why have the selective serotonin reuptake inhibitors become first-line treatments for depression over the tricyclic antidepressants?**
   SSRIs have become a first-line treatment because of their more benign side effects and because they present less danger in overdose relative to the TCAs. TCAs cause anticholinergic, orthostatic hypotensive, and sedative side effects and in overdose can cause cardiac arrhythmias, convulsions, and even coma or death. Although SSRIs can cause sexual dysfunction (delayed orgasm or even anorgasmia), this is a relatively benign side effect compared with the side effect profile of the TCAs. When treating a severe depression with TCAs, one must also consider that they are quite lethal in overdose. A patient with a suicide plan may save up the medication and subsequently overdose on it. Their toxic potential makes this a very real potential, whereas SSRIs are quite safe, even if ingested in large quantities.

8. **Why might you want to avoid administering selective serotonin reuptake inhibitors and other antidepressants to this patient if his history was also significant for manic episodes?**
   He may have bipolar disorder, and antidepressants could precipitate a manic episode. This may happen in approximately 3% to 5% of bipolar patients.

9. **What class of antidepressant was this man likely started on if he experienced symptoms of dry mouth, blurred vision, constipation, orthostatic (postural) hypotension, urinary retention, and memory impairment?**
   TCAs have strong anticholinergic side effects (e.g., dry mouth, blurred vision, urinary retention) and antiadrenergic side effects (e.g., orthostatic hypotension). TCAs should be used with caution in elderly patients because the orthostatic effects may increase the risk for falling with the potential for a hip fracture. Nortriptylene and desipramine have the least sedative, orthostatic, and anticholinergic side effects of the TCAs.
   Note: The anticholinergic effects of the TCAs (urinary retention) make them effective for treating enuresis (bed wetting). Imipramine is usually used for this (in children and adolescents).

10. **Assume that this patient responded well to some form of antidepressant therapy but then presented to the emergency room 3 weeks later suffering from priapism. What antidepressant was he likely given?**
    Trazodone can cause this rare but rather serious complication in men. Trazodone and nefazodone are both mixed serotonin reuptake inhibitors–serotonin receptor antagonists; remember these two drugs as being in the *z-group* because they both have z's and the patient gets very sleepy (i.e., they are very sedating) from taking them.

11. **If this man is addicted to red wine with cheese, what class of antidepressant should be avoided and why?**
    MAOIs, such as phenelzine and tranylcypromine, should be avoided. The tyramine present in wine and cheese is ordinarily degraded by monoamine oxidase in the gastrointestinal (GI) tract.

Inhibition of MAO in the GI tract and liver can increase levels of tyramine in the blood. Massive displacement of norepinephrine by tyramine from adrenergic storage sites can then lead to hypertension.

When discontinuing MAOIs from a patient's treatment plan, it is recommended that the physician wait at least 2 weeks prior to administration of a new antidepressant medication to avoid hypertensive crisis that may occur with excess monoamine levels.

12. **How do monoamine oxidase inhibitors work and what are the two classes of monoamine oxidase inhibitors?**
MAOIs work by inhibiting the degradation of monoamines (dopamine, norepinephrine, and serotonin) in presynaptic neurons. Monoamine oxidase A inhibitors primarily reduce the breakdown of norepinephrine and serotonin and are therefore useful in treating depression.
Note: Monoamine oxidase B (e.g., selegiline) inhibitors primarily reduce the breakdown of dopamine and are therefore useful in treating Parkinson's disease.

13. **What is the main danger of prescribing both a selective serotonin reuptake inhibitor and a monoamine oxidase inhibitor?**
The combination of a MAOI and an SSRI or TCA can cause pathologically elevated levels of serotonin, resulting in the serotonin syndrome (SS). The SS is characterized by mental status changes, autonomic hyperactivity, and neuromuscular abnormalities. It can be very difficult to distinguish from neuroleptic malignant syndrome (NMS) if the patient has received both antipsychotics and drugs that can produce SS. Tachycardia, diaphoresis, fever, and agitation can be seen in both syndromes, but hyperreflexia and clonus (including horizontal ocular clonus) are more likely to occur in SS than in NMS. Symptoms can progress to hallucinations, hyperthermia, widespread rigidity, spontaneous clonus, rhabdomyolysis, delirium, and even death.
Note: The street drug MDMA ("ecstasy") is known for producing very severe cases of SS, even by itself. Amphetamines and cocaine can also contribute to SS, and it is important to keep in mind that any process that will elevate serotonin levels may contribute to the syndrome because they also cause increased serotonin release (increased synthesis from tyramine, decreased breakdown from MAOIs, and decreased serotonin reuptake from meperidine, TCAs, and SSRIs, as well as serotonin receptor agonism from lysergic acid diethylamide [LSD]).

14. **If this patient is suffering from depression and is additionally a smoker who is trying to quit, which drug might be effective?**
Buproprion would be an excellent choice for this patient. It has been shown to be effective in smoking cessation, especially when used with nicotine replacement therapy. Although its exact mechanism of action is not completely understood, it has been shown to inhibit the reuptake of both dopamine and norepinephrine, thereby enhancing both dopaminergic and noradrenergic transmission. Buproprion is a nice alternative to the SSRIs because it lacks their adverse sexual side effects.
Note: One major concern with this drug is that it lowers the threshold for seizure development, particularly in women with an underlying eating disorder such as anorexia nervosa.

15. **If this man experienced much milder symptoms of depression for longer than 2 years, what would be his probable diagnosis?**
Dysthymic disorder is likely.

16. **How might your diagnosis change if this man had been divorced 2 months ago and his symptoms of depression were milder?**
This man would be suffering from an *adjustment disorder* with depressed mood. The appearance of emotional or behavorial symptoms that are the response to an identifiable stressor within 3 months of the appearance of said stress is the hallmark of adjustment disorder.

These symptoms must either cause a person significant distress over what would be expected in that situation or cause significant social or occupational dysfunction to be considered an adjustment disorder. Upon removal of the stressor, the symptoms should resolve within 6 months. If the patient were experiencing loss of a loved one, then it would more appropriately be classified as bereavement. The adjustment disorder should be classified as chronic or acute and may be further classified as follows: with depressed mood, with anxiety, with mixed anxiety and depressed mood, with disturbance of conduct, with mixed disturbance of emotions and conduct, or unspecified.

17. **If this man's wife died 1 year ago and he was still experiencing these symptoms, what would his probable diagnosis be?**
    Major depressive disorder is more probable. Normal grieving, which can mimic depression, is largely resolved within 6 months.

SUMMARY BOX: DEPRESSION

- Major depressive disorder requires one or more major depressive episode(s).

- Dysthymic disorder is depressed mood for most of the day on more days than not for 2 years.

- Adjustment disorder with depressed mood: upon removal of the stressor, the symptoms should resolve within 6 months.

- Tricyclic antidepressants (TCAs) cause anticholinergic, orthostatic hypotensive, and sedative side effects and in overdose can cause cardiac arrhythmias, convulsions, and even coma or death.

- Electroconvulsive therapy (ECT) has a response rate of 90% compared with 70% for pharmacotherapy.

- The combination of a monoamine oxidase inhibitor (MAOI) and a selective serotonin reuptake inhibitor (SSRI) or TCA can cause pathologically elevated levels of serotonin, resulting in serotonin syndrome.

CASE 16-4

A 12-year-old boy's twin brother is killed in a car accident. The surviving twin suffers from depressed mood, feelings of guilt, and frequent emotional outbursts. He has begun to wear only his brother's clothing. He has been writing his thoughts in a diary since the accident. He also begins to treat his younger brother badly, talking to him harshly and even physically abusing him.

1. **Instead of speaking to his deceased brother, which he believes would be unacceptable, he begins to keep a diary, which he believes is a more acceptable outlet for his emotions. What is the defense mechanism employed by this boy?**
   Sublimation involves altering a socially objectionable aim or object into an acceptable one. By channeling the desire to communicate with his brother into writing his thoughts in a diary, the patient uses sublimation to express his inner thoughts and feelings.

2. **Why does this young man begin to wear his brother's clothing? What term is used to describe this type of activity?**
   Identification involves seeing oneself as like the other person. By wearing his deceased brother's clothing, he feels like part of his brother is still with him, and he does not have to face the loss of his brother.

3. **What term is used to describe him taking out his frustrations on his younger brother?**
   Acting out involves the expression of an impulse through action to avoid dealing with what the feelings mean. By abusing and showing anger toward his little brother, he does not have to be conscious of the anger he feels at having lost his older brother.

4. **What are the categories of defense mechanisms and what are some examples of each type?**
   - *Mature defenses* include altruism, humor, sublimation, and suppression.
   - *Neurotic defenses* include repression, intellectualization, identification, rationalization, displacement, and regression.
   - *Immature defenses* include acting out, fantasy, hypochondriasis, and projection.
   - *Psychotic defenses* include denial and distortion.

STEP 1 SECRET

There is some disagreement in the literature as to which ego defenses fall under which categories, so this is less important. However, the specific nature of each of the various defenses is a favorite topic on the boards, so spend sufficient time learning this.

CASE 16-5

A 42-year-old married businessman with six children is diagnosed with Huntington's disease after being seen by a specialist in movement disorders. The patient is told that there is no cure for his disease and that he will progressively decline both physically and mentally prior to death within 10 years. To make matters worse, he is told that several of his six children may have the disease. He comes home from his appointment and for the first time in his life is physically abusive to his wife.

1. **What are the five stages of grief this man will likely experience?**
   The stages of grief that one passes through are *denial, anger, bargaining, acceptance,* and *sadness.* The grieving person may not experience all of these stages and may pass through a stage quite rapidly, appearing not to pass through it at all.

2. **What term is used to describe alleviating his frustration by abusing his wife?**
   Acting out allows him to express anger without having to deal with the newfound knowledge of his diagnosis.

3. **What defense mechanism would he be employing if he ignored the doctor's visit and went on with his life without acknowledging his diagnosis?**
   Denial involves subconscious refusal to acknowledge that there is a problem. There is cognitive and emotional unawareness of the truth. The person does not believe what he has been told, and it does not register emotionally.

4. **What term would be used to describe his behavior if while hospitalized he begins crying for his mother and demanding that other people feed him and take care of things he is fully capable of?**

   Regression is an attempt to return to an earlier phase of functioning to avoid conflict. It is quite common in the medical setting and is a normal phenomenon.

5. **Cover the left column of Table 16-1 and attempt to name the defense mechanisms described in the middle column.**

TABLE 16-1. DEFENSE MECHANISMS

Defense Mechanism	Description	Example
Splitting	Categorization of things into good or bad ("everything is black or white," no gray); associated with borderline personality disorder	A patient describes you as "the best doctor," while her last physician is a "quack."
Altruism	The act of giving or serving, not for feeling of obligation or recognition, merely for the sake of doing good	A wealthy widow donates half of her husband's estate to benefit the local children's hospital.
Reaction formation	Turning a strong impulse that is unacceptable into the opposite, in order to "undo" the feeling	A boy is angry with his mother for grounding him and he wishes she would die. Feeling guilty, he runs downstairs, hugs her, and tells her how much he loves her.
Suppression	Consciously or semiconsciously postponing attention to a conscious impulse; discomfort is minimized, but still acknowledged	A woman tries to avoid thinking about her husband, who recently committed suicide, by removing his clothing from their shared closet.
Repression	Withholding an idea or feeling from consciousness; impulses are consciously inhibited to the point of losing, not just postponing, goals	A woman tries to avoid thinking about her husband, who recently committed suicide, by burning all his clothing and removing all his photos from the wall.

NOTE: All ego defenses are unconscious, with the exception of suppression.

SUMMARY BOX: EGO DEFENSES

- Sublimation involves altering a socially objectionable aim or object into an acceptable one.

- Identification involves seeing oneself as like the other person.

- Acting out involves the expression of an impulse through action to avoid dealing with what the feelings mean.

- Denial involves unconsciously refusing to acknowledge that there is a problem.

- Regression is attempting to return to an earlier phase of functioning to avoid conflict.

- See Table 16-1 for descriptions and examples of other ego defenses.

CASE 16-6

An 8-year-old boy is brought to the physician by his mother for behavioral problems. The mother says that for as long as she can remember he has been much more "difficult" than his other brothers and sisters. She is also concerned because he has been doing poorly in the first grade and his teacher has complained to her several times about his disruptive behaviors in class, which include excessive talking and leaving his seat in the classroom inappropriately. In the physician's office, he appears distracted and fidgety; when asked by the doctor to respond to five questions on a questionnaire, the boy answers only two of the questions. When addressed by the physician, he seems distracted and does not appear to be listening.

1. **What are the considerations in the differential diagnosis?**
   Attention-deficit/hyperactivity disorder (ADHD), oppositional defiant disorder (ODD), conduct disorder, and even normal behavior are all considered.
   The boy does not argue with adults, defy or refuse to comply with requests, or deliberately annoy people. He also does not display aggression to people and animals or destruction of property.

2. **What is this patient's likely diagnosis?**
   ADHD, a disorder characterized by a pattern of hyperactivity, impulsiveness, inattention, and distractibility, is likely. The diagnosis requires that the symptoms be present in at least two settings (i.e., school and at home), and the onset of these symptoms must occur before 7 years of age. Sometimes it can be difficult to exclude normal behavior, especially if the child behaves well in the office, and the doctor must rely on information from the parents and teachers; often rating scales are used for this purpose.
   Note: ODD involves a pattern of negative, hostile, and deviant behavior lasting at least 6 months. Affected patients show at least four of the following: they argue with adults, lose their temper, defy or refuse to comply with requests, deliberately annoy people, blame others for their mistakes, are angry and resentful, or are spiteful and vindictive.
   Conduct disorder is a pattern of behavior in which other peoples' basic rights are violated or societal rules or norms are broken, demonstrated by at least three of the following in the past 12 months, and at least one in the past 6 months: aggression to people and animals, destruction of property, deceitfulness and theft, or a serious violation of rules.

3. **Using the DSM-IV criteria, under what axis would ADHD be listed?**
   ADHD would be listed under axis I. By way of review, the five axes of diagnosis used in psychiatry are as follows:
   - Axis I: Psychiatric conditions (e.g., schizophrenia)
   - Axis II: Personality disorders, mental retardation (e.g., borderline personality disorder)
   - Axis III: Medical conditions (e.g., diabetes mellitus)
   - Axis IV: Social stressors (e.g., bad marriage)
   - Axis V: Global assessment of functioning (a numerical score of 0-100 that assesses the patient's emotional, social, and everyday functioning)

STEP 1 SECRET

Second-year medical students are not expected to know the *Diagnostic and Statistical Manual of Mental Disorders* (DSM-IV) axes for Step 1. Do not spend time learning these types of details for the examination. Instead, focus on the other material that we have marked as high-yield in this chapter.

4. **What class of drugs is the primary treatment for ADHD?**
   The first-line treatment of ADHD includes the use of amphetamine derivatives (e.g., methylphenidate, dextroamphetamine), which result in increased attention, decreased motor activity, and improvement in learning tasks.

5. **What psychiatric symptoms might be evident in an individual following an overdose of amphetamines?**
   Psychotic features may appear and are presumably related to increased dopamine, which may explain why a shot of haloperidol (an antipsychotic) will calm these patients down. This also illustrates the importance of ruling out substance abuse as a cause prior to making a diagnosis of schizophrenia in a patient.

SUMMARY BOX: CHILDHOOD DISORDERS

- Attention-deficit/hyperactivity disorder (ADHD): pattern of hyperactivity, impulsiveness, inattention, and distractibility; symptoms be present in at least two settings and must occur before 7 years of age

- Oppositional defiant disorder (ODD): a pattern of negative, hostile, and deviant behavior lasting at least 6 months

- Conduct disorder: peoples' basic rights are violated or societal rules or norms are broken, demonstrated by at least three of the following in the past 12 months, and at least one in the past 6 months: aggression to people and animals, destruction of property, deceitfulness and theft, or a serious violation of rules

CASE 16-7

A 4-year-old boy is brought to the pediatrician by his mother because he is having trouble "fitting in" with his peers at preschool. His teacher says he is a fine student academically but does not like to play with others during free time, only plays with the red blocks, and refuses to leave the room until all books are stacked perfectly. Yesterday, he showed no interest in show-and-tell. He can speak in four-word sentences, hop and skip, dress himself, and use a fork and a spoon. His mother says he has never been an emotional boy and has always been content spending time alone. In the office he does not make eye contact when spoken to, focusing instead on tapping his right thumb repetitively.

1. **What is the differential diagnosis?**
   Asperger's syndrome, autistic disorder, learning disorder, mental retardation, sensory impairment (such as difficulties with hearing or vision), and normal behavior should be considered.

2. **What are the criteria for Asperger's syndrome?**
   Impairment in social interaction and repetitive behavior without developmental delay in language, cognition, or self-help are features of Asperger's syndrome.

3. **What if the patient also repeated odd phrases and was unable to successfully engage in a conversation with his peers?**
   The likely diagnosis would be autistic disorder.

4. **How does autistic disorder differ from Asperger's syndrome?**
   Patients with autistic disorder must demonstrate not one but two deficits in social interaction (impairment in nonverbal behavior, peer relationships, sharing with others, or emotional reciprocity), they must also have impairment in communication, and onset must be prior to 3 years of age.

5. **What is known about the etiology of autism spectrum disorders?**
   Heritability estimates are around 92%, but no specific genes have been identified. There is no credible evidence that environmental factors contribute to the onset of autism, although some parents refuse vaccinations for their children because they believe vaccinations can contribute to autism risk.

6. **What if the patient was not doing well academically and these behaviors and social impairments were manifested only at school?**
   The diagnosis might be a learning disorder (reading disorder, mathematics disorder, disorder of written expression), as cognitive or academic difficulties are often associated with disruptive behavior in children.

7. **What should the workup include?**
   Intelligence quotient (IQ) testing and standardized tests for math, reading, and writing should be performed.

8. **What would be the diagnosis if the patient scored 70 or below on IQ testing?**
   Mental retardation (MR), a subtype of intellectual disability that presents prior to age 18, characterized by IQ below 70 and limitations in two behavioral areas including communication, activities of daily living (ADLs), problem solving, and interpersonal skills.
   MR is further classified by subtype depending upon the score on IQ testing:
   - 50 to 69: mild
   - 35 to 49: moderate
   - 20 to 34: severe
   - <20: profound

   IQ between 70 and 84 is considered borderline intellectual functioning, in which patients have trouble with abstraction.

SUMMARY BOX: CHILDHOOD DISORDERS

- Learning disorder: specific difficulty in mathematics, reading, or writing can present with disruptive behavior

- Mental retardation (MR): intellectual and multiple behavioral difficulties, intelligence quotient (IQ) <70

- Asperger's syndrome: repetitive behavior and impairment in social interaction

- Autism: multiple deficits in social interaction and impairment in communication

CASE 16-8

A 4-year-old boy is brought to see a psychiatrist by his parents. The mother reports three different episodes of walking into his room while he was masturbating, and she is worried that he has some kind of "problem."

1. **If the psychiatrist explains this boy's developmental maturation in terms of psychosexual development, what psychologist is he referring to and what are these stages of development?**
   Sigmund Freud identified five stages of psychosexual development:
   - *Oral stage*: birth to 18 months
   - *Anal stage*: 18 months to 3 years
   - *Phallic stage*: 3 to 6 years
   - *Latency stage*: 6 years to puberty
   - *Genital stage*: puberty to young adulthood

2. **Freud also discusses the id, ego, and superego. How do these concepts relate to this boy's problem?**
   The *id* represents the instinctual drives with which people are born. The id operates in the subconscience and lacks the ability to delay or change the drives with which one is born.
   The *ego* spans both the conscious and unconscious. Consciously, logical and abstract thinking and verbal expression are handled by the ego. Unconsciously, defense mechanisms are used by the ego. The ego uses external reality to harness instinctual drive of the id and substitutes realities for pleasure.
   The *superego* serves to monitor a person's behavior, thoughts, and feelings according to a strict set of morals and values internalized from that of the parents; it makes comparison to these standards and offers approval or disapproval. For example, the superego deems it inappropriate for the boy to keep masturbating and causes him to feel guilty about it. The id represents the pleasure he receives from masturbation. The ego processes the inputs from the id, the superego, and the external reality. The ego compromises by giving in sometimes and masturbating, but other times it substitutes other pleasurable activity, such as playing a board game, for masturbating.

3. **If the psychiatrist discusses the boy's development in terms of stages of cognitive development, what psychologist is he referring to and what are these stages of cognitive development?**
   Piaget identified four stages of cognitive development:
   Sensory-motor: Between the time of birth and about 2 years of age, babies begin to develop an understanding of object permanence. No longer do they fear that "mommy is gone" when she

covers her face with her hands. "Peek-a-boo" begins to lose its charm. They develop the ability to control movement and observe their surroundings via their developing senses.

Preoperational: As the child ages from about 2 to 7 years, he begins to associate events with external happenings, leading to a belief of phenomenalistic causality. For example, a negative thought directed toward someone who falls and breaks a leg causes the child to believe the fall was caused by the inappropriate thought. They also tend to operate in an egocentric fashion. These children are unable to process how their behavior or an outside event affects other people.

Concrete operational: From ages 7 to 11, children begin to understand conservation of objects. They develop the ability to understand that a small cup full of juice is "less" than a big cup that is half full, but still might have trouble understanding a nickel is less money than a dime ("it's bigger"), because they have not mastered abstract thought. Children in these stages may become strict rule followers; obsessive traits may begin to emerge.

Formal operations: From age 11 until the end of adolescence, teens begin to develop the ability to understand abstract thought and reason. They begin to be able to process ideas and concepts lacking a concrete basis.

4. **If the psychiatrist explains this boy's development in terms of development of the ego, what psychologist is he referring to and what are the stages of ego development?**
    Erikson theorized that a person must overcome certain basic conflicts in eight stages of life in the process of development. These stages are as follows:
    - Trust versus mistrust (birth–1 year): The child learns whether his basic needs will be met and if his care providers can be relied upon.
    - Autonomy versus shame (1–3 years): Toddlers begin to show mastery over excretory functions such as urination and defecation.
    - Initiative versus guilt (3–5 years): Children are allowed to initiate behavior and interests, their conscience is established,
    - Industry versus inferiority (6–11 years): Children learn they are able to master and complete tasks; inadequacy may develop if their social environment is unsupportive.
    - Identity versus role confusion (11–21 years): Young people develop a sense of who they are and where they are going.
    - Intimacy versus isolation (21–40 years): People establish sexual relationships, deep friendships, and deep associations, as long as there is no underlying identity confusion.
    - Generativity versus stagnation (40–65 years): People's main interest is in guiding and establishing future generations or improving society.
    - Integrity versus despair (over 65 years): Satisfaction is sensed if a person feels that his life has been productively lived.

    Failure to meet each of these conflicts result in stagnation of development, but successfully resolving each conflict allows the progression to the next stage of development.

SUMMARY BOX: PSYCHOLOGY

- Freud identified five stages of psychosexual development: oral, anal, phallic, latent, and genital.
- Freud's three structures of the mind are the id, ego, and superego.
- Piaget identified four stages of cognitive development: sensory-motor, preoperational, concrete operational, and formal operational.
- Erikson identified eight stages of life in the process of development:
    □ Trust versus mistrust (birth–1 year)

- Autonomy versus shame (1–3 years)

- Initiative versus guilt (3–5 years)

- Industry versus inferiority (6–11 years)

- Identity versus role confusion (11–21 years)

- Intimacy versus isolation (21–40 years)

- Generativity versus stagnation (40–65 years)

- Integrity versus despair (over 65 years)

CASE 16-9

A 75-year-old man presents to the emergency department complaining of severe midepigastric pain radiating to the back, malabsorption, steatorrhea, and polyuria. An abdominal x-ray film shows pancreatic calcifications.

1. **What is the most likely diagnosis?**
   Chronic pancreatitis is most likely.

2. **What is the most likely etiology?**
   Pancreatitis can be caused by alcohol abuse, gallstones, severe hypertriglyceridemia, hypercalcemia, scorpion bite, abdominal trauma, hereditary predisposition, embryologic malformation (e.g., annular pancreas), and numerous medications. However, by far the most common cause is alcohol abuse.
   The patient is promptly admitted to the medicine service. He denies a history of alcohol use until some "cute" nurse who seems interested in partying gets him to confess that his "wild and crazy days" are still alive and kicking. In fact, he had a fifth of vodka this morning with breakfast to put him in the mood for watching Jerry Springer.

3. **What concern does this man's alcohol abuse pose to the medicine team?**
   This man's pancreatitis is more than likely due to his alcohol problem, and if he is not treated appropriately for alcohol abuse, all that can be expected for his pancreatitis is symptomatic control of his periodic exacerbations. Additionally, patients who consume large quantities of alcohol (or have regular consumption of smaller quantities) are at risk for symptoms of withdrawal.

4. **What are the expected symptoms of withdrawal and how are they managed?**
   Withdrawal is displayed in two stages. Early on, symptoms of withdrawal might include tachycardia, tremors, nausea, vomiting, or hypertension. These initial symptoms are usually controlled with lorazepam, a benzodiazepine. The later, more life-threatening concern is the appearance of delirium tremens (DTs). Usually presenting after about 48 hours of abstinence, these severe tremors may be accompanied by hallucinations (generally these are tactile hallucinations, e.g., experiencing "bugs crawling on one's skin"), delirium, and mild fever. Often DTs are preceded by seizures, which rarely lead to status epilepticus. Seizures can be managed by intravenous benzodiazepines, or if there is a history of withdrawal seizures, prophylactic phenytoin may be started. The DTs can be managed with benzodiazepines and supportive care. The affected patient may need intensive care, especially in the case of autonomic instability. These symptoms typically last for around 3 days but may persist for weeks.

Note: Alcohol is one of few drugs that are cleared from the body through zero-order kinetics. In zero-order kinetics, a constant *amount* of the drug is cleared from the body per unit time, compared with first-order kinetics in which a constant *fraction* of the drug is cleared per unit time. Phenytoin, aspirin, and heparin are other examples of drugs with zero-order kinetics.

5. **What is the mechanism by which the administration of benzodiazepines is able to control the delirium tremens?**
   Management of a patient who ceases alcohol intake involves a taper, using benzodiazepines. Alcohol potentiates the γ-aminobutyric acid (GABA) receptor, as do the benzodiazepines. Gradual tapering, rather than abrupt termination, of this agonistic effect allows the central nervous system to acclimate to the increased stimulation experienced as alcohol is removed.

6. **Another class of drugs act as agonists of the GABA receptor at a different site. What is the name of this group of drugs and how do the pharmacokinetic effects differ from that of benzodiazepines?**
   Barbiturates also agonize the GABA receptor at a site distinct from that of the benzodiazepines. The benzodiazepines eventually reach a maximal effect, whereas barbiturates continue to increase their effect as dosage is increased. The result is that barbiturates are much more likely to cause a fatal respiratory depression than benzodiazepines (although this is still a concern).
   Note: Benzodiazepines work by increasing the frequency of chloride channel opening, and barbiturates increase the duration that the chloride channel is open.

7. **How are substance *abuse* and *dependence* differentiated?**
   A substance is being abused when *one* of the following has occurred over the past 12 months: the person experiences legal problems from the substance use, uses the substance in a situation in which that use is hazardous, continues to use the substance despite recurrent social problems due to the use of that substance, or shows a failure to fulfill major obligations at home, school, or work. The person meets the criteria for dependence when *three* of the following are present: tolerance, withdrawal symptoms, repetitive unintended excessive use, failure at cutting down, reduction in social/recreational/occupational functioning, excessive amount of time spent in pursuit of the substance, or continued use despite the knowledge that the substance is causing psychological difficulties.
   Note: Tolerance and withdrawal are neither necessary nor sufficient to meet criteria for substance dependence.

SUMMARY BOX: ALCOHOL

- Alcohol, benzodiazopines, and barbiturates all act at the γ-aminobutyric acid (GABA) receptor.

- Barbiturates are much more likely to cause a fatal respiratory depression than benzodiazepines.

- Substance abuse: one of the following in a 12-month period: legal problems from the substance use, use in situation where hazardous, continued use despite recurrent social problems due to the use of that substance, or a failure to fulfill major obligations at home, school, or work.

- Substance dependence: three of the following in a 12-month period: tolerance, withdrawal symptoms, repetitive unintended excessive use, failure at cutting down, reduction in social/recreational/occupational functioning, spending an excessive amount of time in pursuit of the substance, or continuing use despite the knowledge that the substance is causing psychological difficulties

- Tolerance and withdrawal symptoms are neither necessary nor sufficient to meet criteria for substance dependence.

CASE 16-10

Law enforcement officials bring a 27-year-old man to the emergency department. He is combative and disoriented and is screaming that bugs are crawling on his skin. His blood pressure, pulse, and respiratory rate are all elevated. He appears to be sweating profusely. On examination of the head, you notice some dried blood around one of his nostrils and see that his pupils are dilated. Once he settles down and begins talking with you, he complains that he feels light-headed and his chest hurts.

1. **Abuse involving what class of drugs should be expected in this man?**
   This patient is suffering from intoxication of a stimulant, in this case cocaine. Tactile hallucinations, impaired judgment, transient psychosis, and agitation are commonly seen in stimulant intoxication. Other characteristic symptoms include tachycardia or bradycardia, dilated pupils, hyper- or hypotension, chills or fever, nausea and emesis, and confusion. Amphetamine intoxication could present in a similar fashion.
   Note: Formication (bugs crawling on skin) is often called "cocaine bugs" because it so often is due to cocaine intoxication. However, it is also seen in DTs and in amphetamine psychosis.

2. **Would you be surprised if this man's electrocardiogram revealed myocardial ischemia?**
   It should not be surprising if this man's cardiac tissue has become ischemic. The cocaine he has been using can cause vasospasm, which can reduce cardiac perfusion leading to ischemia. Other drugs that can cause vasospasm include amphetamine and sumatriptan.

3. **What is the correct treatment for cocaine-induced coronary vasospasm?**
   Intravenous diazepam and aspirin are used in the treatment for cocaine-induced coronary vasospasm
   Note: If a patient has cocaine-induced chest pain and a normal cardiac enzyme profile, it is best to give a calcium channel blocker if one needs to control blood pressure and elevated heart rate. *Do not* give a beta blocker because that will lead to unopposed α-receptor stimulation by the cocaine causing further vasospasm.

4. **Why does this man have blood around his nostril?**
   The effect of cocaine on the nasal epithelium is vasoconstriction. This vasoconstriction can lead to infarction of the nasal septum and subsequent perforation. This is exacerbated by the sympathomimetic effects of cocaine, leading to increased blood pressure that increases the epistaxis.
   Note: Cerebral infarction is another all-too-common effect of cocaine intoxication.

5. **What are typical symptoms experienced by a person who is withdrawing from use of cocaine?**
   These patients experience severe psychological craving for the drug, extreme fatigue, hunger, headaches, cramps, and perspiration. These symptoms peak in 48 to 96 hours. These patients do not require inpatient management unless needed for the intense craving, as withdrawal is otherwise self-limited. Clonidine may be helpful in reducing the craving.

6. **A favorite on boards is to provide an emergency department presentation of somebody with a drug overdose and ask you to determine the drug responsible for the patient's symptoms. The question will provide enough information to narrow the choices down to a single drug and therefore will rely upon the use of trigger words. Try to memorize the trigger words in Table 16-2. Be sure to learn drug withdrawal symptoms as well. These symptoms are often opposite to those seen with drug toxicity.**

TABLE 16-2. DRUG INTOXICATIONS

Drug Intoxication	Trigger Words	Withdrawal
Opioids	Pupils constricted, ↓RR	"Flu-like" symptoms, rhinorrhea, anxiety, piloerection
Amphetamine	Pupils dilated, delusions, ↑HR, ↑BP	Hunger, hypersomnolence
PCP	Nystagmus, ataxia, ↑BP, clenching/grinding of the teeth (bruxism), random acts of violence and belligerence, hyperthermia	Depression
LSD	Flashbacks, pupillary dilation, depression, hallucinations	
Marijuana	Increased appetite, conjunctival irritation, paranoia, increased appetite, hallucinations	Irritability, depression, nausea, decreased appetite
MDMA ("ecstasy")	Hyperthermia, bruxism	
Anticholinergics—TCAs, pesticides*	Dry skin, flushing, fever, urinary retention, dilated pupils, delirium, cardiac conduction delays, thirst, ↑HR	
Benzodiazepines, barbiturates ("benzos," "barbs")	Anxiety, ataxia, somnolence, life-threatening ~~~~~~~~~~ with barbiturates	Anxiety, insomnia,
Cholinergic poisoning—organophosphates, anticholinesterases	Salivation, ↓HR, vomiting, urination, defecation, pupil constriction	

*You should know the antidotes for TCA and pesticide overdose: For TCA toxicity, administer sodium bicarbonate (NaHCO$_3$) to alkalize the serum. Organophosphate pesticides cause irreversible inhibition of acetylcholinesterase; overdose requires administration of atropine and pralidoxime (to regenerate acetylcholinesterase). Organophosphate poisoning is a commonly asked Step 1 concept.
BP, blood pressure; HR, heart rate; LSD, lysergic acid diethylamide; MDMA, 3,4-methylenedioxymethamphetamine; PCP, phencyclidine; RR, respiratory rate; TCA, tricyclic antidepressant.

STEP 1 SECRET

Drug-related causes of pupillary dilation and constriction are commonly tested on Step 1.

SUMMARY BOX: DRUG INTOXICATION

- Cocaine intoxication: dilated pupils, formication, transient psychosis, agitation, tachycardia or bradycardia, hyper- or hypotension; also risk of cerebral infarction and coronary vasospasm

- Know the signs of drug intoxication and withdrawal.

CASE 16-11

A 72-year-old woman with early-stage Alzheimer's disease is admitted to the hospital for extreme dyspnea and is diagnosed with pneumonia. Intravenous fluids and antibiotics are started. Upon admission, she is alert and oriented to person and time, but not to place. She is able to score 26/30 on a mini mental status examination administered to her shortly after her admission. The following morning she is found to be febrile. The attending physician believes feels that she is not responding as expected and changes her antibiotic. A few hours later, this woman has become confused and aggressive and believes that the hospital staff has been trying to kill her.

1. **Would this woman's current state be best described as dementia or delirium?**
    This is an important distinction that must be made when there are acute mental status changes. This woman is suffering from delirium. Although she may have an underlying dementia, she has clearly become acutely delirious.
    Note: One caveat applies if this patient has been misdiagnosed with Alzheimer's disease and in fact has Lewy body dementia (LBD), now thought to be the second most common cause of degenerative dementia. Along with dementia, the three core features of LBD are fluctuating cognition, visual hallucinations, and parkinsonism. Interestingly, one of the features of LBD is that it tends to worsen with neuroleptic agents.

2. **What is the most likely cause of this woman's delirium?**
    The two most common causes of a delirious state, especially in the elderly, are prescribed drugs and acute infections. This woman's pneumonia or the antibiotics being used to treat her pneumonia are most likely the cause of her delirious state. Other causes that should be investigated include drug or alcohol withdrawal, metabolic derangement, head trauma, epilepsy, and cerebral hypoperfusion.

3. **Distinguish dementia from delirium regarding onset, course, level of consciousness, and presence of delusions and hallucinations.**
    Dementia typically has a gradual, insidious onset. It often goes unnoticed by family members who see the person every day. The course tends to be a gradually progressive decline in cognitive function, especially in short-term memory, without any changes in level of consciousness. In early stages, patients can be quite oriented with a normal level of consciousness. Later stages involve behavioral alterations and impaired judgment. Delusions or hallucinations may or may not be seen in a patient with dementia.
    Delirium typically has an acute to subacute onset. It often has an abrupt onset, typically within hours to days. Electroencephalogram (EEG) results are abnormal. Short-term memory and poor attention span are common cognitive defects. It is a sudden impairment in the level of consciousness, and patients can rapidly fluctuate. Delusions are typically fleeting, often persecutory, and may be related to the disorientation. Hallucinations are common; visual hallucinations strongly suggest delirium.

STEP 1 SECRET

The USMLE often asks students to differentiate between delirium and dementia.

SUMMARY BOX: COGNITIVE DISORDERS

- Dementia: memory impairment plus one of the following: aphasia, apraxia, agnosia, or disturbance in executive functioning

- Delerium: disturbance in consciousness that develops over shorter period of time and fluctuates throughout the day

CASE 16-12

A 32-year-old previously healthy businesswoman presents to the emergency room with a recent onset of chest pain, shortness of breath, dizziness, and an intense fear that she is dying. Her symptoms came on "out of the blue" while she was working in her office on a presentation she was scheduled to give in a few days. She has a strong family history of cardiovascular disease and is convinced she is having a heart attack. An extensive workup including an electrocardiogram, chest x-ray, and serial cardiac enzymes is negative for a myocardial infarction. After a short while in the emergency room, her symptoms appear to resolve.

This woman most likely suffered a panic attack, which is frequently misinterpreted as a heart attack by patients. *Panic attacks* consist of a discrete period of intense fear or discomfort over which the symptoms develop abruptly and usually peak within 10 minutes. These symptoms often mimic those of a heart attack and can include perspiration, palpitations, chest pain, shaking, sensation of choking, nausea, dizziness, chills, fear of dying, fear of losing control, or a feeling of derealization. *Panic disorder* is characterized by recurrent, unexpected panic attacks. For at least 1 month, these people have had concerns about further attacks, fear the consequences of these attacks, or significantly altered their behaviors because of the panic attacks. Panic disorder has been associated with several other medical conditions including peptic ulcer disease and hypertension.

2. **If this woman subsequently developed a fear of leaving the house, what term should be used to describe this "phobia"?**
   Agoraphobia is intense anxiety felt about being in situations from which escape is difficult (or embarrassing) or where help may not be available in the event that a panic attack occurs. If the avoidance is limited to specific situations, specific phobias, social phobia, or obsessive-compulsive disorder (OCD) should be considered. Patients who suffer from panic disorder may or may not experience agoraphobia.

3. **What are the considerations in the differential diagnosis for panic disorder?**
   Generalized anxiety disorder, substance-induced anxiety disorder, and anxiety due to a general medical condition may resemble panic disorder.

4. **Why might the emergency department intern wish to check this woman's blood levels of thyroid hormone and urinary vanillylmandelic acid (VMA) and 5-hydroxyindoleacetic acid (5-HIAA)?**

   Multiple organic conditions can mimic a panic attack, including hyperthyroidism (or "thyroid storm"), pheochromocytoma (elevated VMA), and carcinoid syndrome (elevated 5-HIAA). These conditions can be ruled out by a laboratory workup.

5. **How can this woman's panic disorder be treated?**

   SSRIs are first-line drugs for the treatment of panic disorder. Additionally, benzodiazepines can be used to decrease the anxiety associated with panic attacks in the first few weeks of treatment with an SSRI or when other therapies have failed. Beta blockers can also be used to limit the physiologic effects of anxiety experienced in specific phobias, such as performance anxiety, when a person is certain to be exposed to that situation.

SUMMARY BOX: PANIC DISORDER

- Recurrent unexpected panic attacks followed by at least 1 month of persistent concern about having another, worry about the implications, or a significant change in behavior related to the attacks

- Can occur with or without agoraphobia

- Selective serotonin reuptake inhibitors (SSRIs) are first-line treatment

CASE 16-13

A 16-year-old girl is admitted to a tertiary psychiatric referral center. For several months she has been having severe emotional outbursts and fits of anger. She has had trouble falling asleep and has been having recurrent nightmares when she does sleep. She has a past history of sexual and physical abuse by her father at the age of 10 before he left the family. Her nightmares often revolve around these episodes of abuse.

1. **What is the most likely diagnosis in this girl?**

   She has posttraumatic stress disorder (PTSD), with delayed onset, as the symptoms appeared more than 1 month after the stressor and persist for at least 1 month.

   If symptoms last between 2 days and 1 month, the condition is termed "acute stress disorder."

2. **What are the requirements needed to make this diagnosis?**

   To make the diagnosis of PTSD, the patient has to have been exposed to, witnessed, or subjected to a traumatic event in which actual or threatened death or injury or a threat to the physical integrity of self or others has occurred. In addition, there must be a re-experiencing of the event, manifested either through distressing dreams, acting out, or intrusive recollections of the event. The person also avoids thoughts, feelings, and activities associated with the event; such patients may avoid activities, feel detached, and stop expressing their feelings. There is also an increase in arousal. The person may have trouble falling asleep, become irritable or have anger outbursts, have trouble concentrating, or show an exaggerated startle response. Once again, these symptoms must persist longer than 1 month. Recall that it is crucial to pay attention to time intervals on boards!

3. **Is this condition very disabling to patients and how is it best managed?**
PTSD can be very disabling to patients and can be a lifelong impairment. Group therapy has been very successfully used in the treatment of PTSD. In group therapy, patients are encouraged to talk about their trauma with other patients who have suffered from similar experiences. Pharmacologic therapy for PTSD involves use of the SSRIs. Typically, a combination of group therapy and SSRI is implemented for patients suffering from PTSD.

SUMMARY BOX: POSTTRAUMATIC STRESS DISORDER

- At least 1 month of the following after a traumatic event: persistent re-experiences, amnesia or emotional numbing, or increased arousal, causing impairment in social or occupational functioning

- If symptom duration is less than 1 month, then it is called acute stress disorder.

- Selective serotonin reuptake inhibitors (SSRIs) are first-line treatment

CASE 16-14

A thin, frail-looking 17-year-old girl comes into your office for a physical examination prior to joining the cheerleading team at school. When you ask her the date of her last menstrual period, she tells you she "can't remember but knows she hasn't bought tampons in months."

1. **What conditions are considered in the differential diagnosis for this patient?**
Anorexia nervosa, pregnancy, Turner syndrome, HPO axis abnormalities, Asherman's syndrome, stress, adrenal insufficiency, and thyroid disorder are all considered.
   Note: You must gather from this history that this girl has stopped having periods, making primary amenorrhea an unlikely cause. She is also thin, which makes obesity and polycystic ovary syndrome far less likely causes of her amenorrhea.

CASE 16-14 continued:

To confirm your suspicions of this patient's diagnosis, you look at the charts that the nurse has filled out and see that the patient is 5'4'' and weighs 98 lb (BMI = 16.8).

2. **What is this patient's likely diagnosis?**
Anorexia nervosa, which is an eating disorder associated with intense fear of weight gain and body weight that is <85% ideal body weight. A history of amenorrhea is required for diagnosis.

3. **Why does anorexia lead to amenorrhea?**
Anorexia nervosa is associated with a decrease in GnRH production by the hypothalamus, which decreases estrogen production, leading to a tertiary amenorrhea.

4. **What other conditions are associated with anorexia nervosa?**
   - *Depression:* Depression commonly coexists with anorexia but is not required for diagnosis. Contrary to what one might think, it is actually beneficial for an anorexic patient to have coexistent depression because it provides a possible route for therapy.
   - *Stress fractures* (particularly metatarsal stress fractures): Decrease in GnRH levels leads to decrease in estrogen levels, which reduces bone density and promotes bone fracture.

- *Lanugo* (fine, soft body hair)
- *Anemia*: Decreased food intake leads to inadequate levels of iron, vitamin B_{12}, and folate. If anorexia becomes severe, bone marrow will respond with pancytopenia.
- *Dental cavities*: Decreased food intake leads to inadequate salivary gland stimulation. Since saliva plays a role in the prevention of dental caries, this can be a common problem in anorexic patients. On similar lines, anorexic patients are also prone to halitosis.
- *Electrolyte disturbances and heart abnormalities*: Electrolyte disturbances are often secondary to vomiting, which induces metabolic alkalosis. The body responds to this by shifting potassium into cells in exchange for hydrogen out of cells (to restore blood pH). This results in a hypokalemic state, which can lead to ventricular arrhythmias. As mentioned in Chapter 5, Acid-Base Balance, metabolic alkalosis also results in a compensatory respiratory acidosis with increased CO_2 and decreased O_2 levels. Hypoxemia leads to hypoxia, which can induce arrhythmias such as ventricular fibrillation, and eventual death.

5. **Compare the diagnoses of anorexia nervosa and bulimia nervosa.**
A common misconception among students is that bulimia nervosa is marked by purging while anorexia is not. This, however, is not true. Both bulimics and anorexics exhibit purging behaviors, but neither disorder requires purging to make a diagnosis. The major difference between the two conditions is that bulimic patients maintain normal body weight while anorexic patients do not. Bulimia is also associated with a cyclic pattern of dieting and binge eating, while anorexia is marked by extreme starvation. Bulimia can lead to many of the same conditions as anorexia but is not generally associated with abnormal GnRH levels. It is, however, marked by conditions that arise from excessive vomiting, such as parotitis, enamel erosion, Mallory-Weiss syndrome, Boerhaave syndrome, and Russell's sign (calluses on the knuckles or back of the hand from repetitive induction of vomiting).

6. **How should this patient be managed?**
Unfortunately, anorexia nervosa is not an easy condition to manage. Treatment may involve antidepressants such as SSRIs and mirtazapine. Mirtazapine is especially beneficial for anorexic patients with depression because it has a side effect of weight gain. (Note that a skilled physician will try to use a drug's side effect profile to his or her advantage.) However, a majority of treatment programs for anorexia nervosa are geared toward weight stabilization and individual and family therapy. Treating this condition often requires extreme patience from health care providers.

SUMMARY BOX: ANOREXIA NERVOSA

- Anorexia nervosa is an eating disorder marked by fear of gaining weight and severe, self-inflicted starvation. The patient is <85% ideal body weight. Patients with bulimia nervosa are often of normal weight.

- History of amenorrhea is required for diagnosis of anorexia nervosa.

- Common symptoms of anorexia include depression, stress fractures, anemia, lanugo, dental cavities, electrolyte disturbances, and heart abnormalities.

- Anorexia is a difficult condition to manage clinically. Antidepressants may help in some cases, but treatment primarily involves weight stabilization and individual/family counseling.

CASE 16-15

A 35-year-old surgeon is 2 hours late for an appointment with his physician and is told by the secretary that he will need to reschedule his appointment. In a loud and argumentative voice he demands to be seen immediately by the physician and states that his time is just as important as this physician's, saying he is entitled be seen that day because he was held up in a very urgent procedure. While waiting to be worked in, he paces across the waiting room, muttering about how this university-affiliated clinic isn't good enough for the leading surgeon in his field. Finally, when seen by the physician, he challenges the doctor's understanding of his condition and argues against the recommended therapy.

1. What type of personality disorder is this man likely suffering from?
   Narcissistic personality disorder is most likely. These people have an exaggerated sense of self-importance, have a sense of entitlement, require excessive admiration from others, are arrogant, lack empathy, and take advantage of others to achieve their own ends.

CASE 16-16

A 22-year-old woman has a long history of unstable relationships with multiple suicide attempts and episodes of self-mutilation. After being seen by a particular physician for the first time, the woman tells the physician that she is the most amazing doctor she has ever seen. At the next appointment, he begins to discuss lifestyle changes to help her with her irregular sleep patterns. At this, she becomes enraged, yelling, "You are such a quack! I am going to see Dr. Jones. He knows how to treat insomnia!" She then storms out of the office.

1. What type of personality disorder is this woman likely suffering from?
   Borderline personality disorder is likely. These patients have unstable relationships, a poor self-image, labile affects, and poor impulse control and commonly employ splitting (see Table 16-1) as a defense mechanism. Psychotherapy, specifically dialectic behavioral therapy, is the treatment of choice.

CASE 16-17

A 42-year-old woman often appears preoccupied with herself, being inconsiderate and demanding of others. When seen by a male physician, she is flirtatious and makes inappropriate sexual comments. When the nurse enters the room, she feigns fainting just so the physician has to catch her. She has threatened suicide many times in the past, but her physician is convinced that these threats are not genuine and that the patient is manipulating him.

1. What type of personality disorder is this woman likely suffering from?
   Histrionic personality disorder is likely. These patients display excessive emotionality and are very attention-seeking.

CASE 16-18

A 28-year-old man has spent the last 5 years in prison after being convicted for assault and robbery. His behavior has always been characterized by utter disregard for the feelings of others. As a child, he was sexually abused by his father, and he frequently tortured animals for entertainment. He appears to have no conscience and lies whenever it is convenient. His father and grandfather are both alcoholics, and he has a long history of alcohol abuse.

1. **What type of personality disorder is this man likely suffering from?**
   He suffers from antisocial personality disorder, which can be diagnosed only in an individual 18 years of age or older.

2. **What type of psychiatric disorder did this man likely have as a child?**
   He had conduct disorder, which can be diagnosed only in children.

CASE 16-19

A physician frequently has calls from a 38-year-old female patient for very minor health concerns, such as common colds and minor cuts and scratches. When soliciting the physician's advice regarding her health care at regularly scheduled appointments, the woman invariably responds that she will do whatever he thinks is best and that her opinion doesn't matter in the slightest. At home, she defers almost all decision making to her husband, on whom she is very reliant.

1. **What type of personality disorder is this woman likely suffering from?**
   Dependent personality disorder is likely.

CASE 16-20

A 52-year-old man has worked in the same position in a large factory for 30 years. He is an excellent worker but has always turned down offers of promotion. He explains this by saying he loves his current job, but secretly he fears criticism of his job performance. He doesn't go out for dinner with his colleagues or attend the annual Christmas party because he becomes anxious in these situations.

1. **What type of personality disorder is this man likely suffering from?**
   He demonstrates avoidant personality disorder. Even though patients suffering from dependent personality disorder also crave acceptance and fear criticism, patients with avoidant personality disorder will not reach out to others and risk humiliation and rejection in order to get their needs met.

CASE 16-21

A 19-year-old female college student normally receives excellent grades in school, but sometimes her grades suffer because of handing in a "perfect" paper past the deadline. She is wonderfully reliable to her friends but causes them some frustration due to her insistence on maintaining a fixed rigid schedule and her moralistic and sometimes judgmental views. She pays excruciatingly close attention to minor details and is very sensitive to any criticism.

1. **What type of personality disorder is this young woman likely suffering from?**
   Obsessive-compulsive personality disorder (OCPD). Do not confuse this with OCD. Patients with OCPD *do not* have obsessions or compulsions that mark the diagnosis of OCD. Rather, they are preoccupied by perfectionism, order, control, and inability to change their routines. Patients with OCPD exhibit behaviors consistent with their own beliefs. This contrasts with patients who have OCD; these patients dislike performing their compulsive behaviors but exhibit little control over their actions.

CASE 16-22

A 32-year-old accountant is given new responsibilities at his job that he is not pleased with. Instead of discussing with his boss other ways to distribute this additional workload, he expresses his anger by sabotaging assignments, coming to work late, leaving early, and not achieving his usual quality of work.

1. What type of personality disorder is this man likely suffering from?
He demonstrates passive-aggressive personality disorder.

CASE 16-23

A 38-year-old woman has no close friends and "prefers to do things on my own." She has never had a boyfriend and is unperturbed by the frequent criticism of her parents regarding her unmarried status. Although she is a highly successful professional, she is indifferent to the praise of her coworkers and peers. She appears cold and unemotional but is not confrontational.

1. What type of personality disorder is this woman likely suffering from?
Schizoid personality disorder is demonstrated by a detachment from social relationships and restricted affect. Common manifestions include lack of desire to socialize or be part of groups or family, little interest in sexual relations or other pleasurable activities, detachment and emotional coldness, and indifference to the praise or criticism of others.

2. In addition to the previously mentioned personality characteristics, she states that she often sees her soul float away from her body and feels that after this happens she is able to predict the future. She adds that other people know of her abilities, and she feels they are "out to get her." What personality disorder might you diagnose in this woman?
Schizotypal personality disorder is a pattern of social and emotional deficits in addition to some cognitive or perceptual eccentricities. Persons who have schizotypal personalities often have odd beliefs, superstitions, or magical thinking. They may have inappropriate affect, odd speech patterns, and a paucity of close friends or confidants. Unlike those with schizoid personality disorder, patients with schizotypal personality disorder do not attempt to avoid people. It is others who generally avoid them!

3. What personality disorder would you diagnose if she were reclusive but really did yearn for social contact?
Avoidant personality disorder is seen in people who have fear of being ridiculed and view themselves as inept and inadequate. They desire social interaction, but the anxiety felt over being placed in social situations keeps them in the shadows. They are reluctant to take personal risks or engage in new activities for fear of being embarrassed.

SUMMARY BOX: PERSONALITY DISORDERS

- Personality disorders are lifelong by definition.
- Paranoid personality disorder: mistrust of others without justification
- Schizoid personality disorder: socially and emotionally detached individuals

- Schizotypal personality disorder: similar to schizoid but with ideas of reference, odd beliefs, or magical thinking

- Antisocial personality disorder: repetitive disregard for society at large and basic rights of others (narcissistic patients also lack empathy and use people to get what they want, but they are not as aggressive as antisocial patients)

- Borderline personality disorder: unstable relationships, poor self-image, labile affect, and poor impulse control

- Histrionic personality disorder: excessive emotionality and high need for attention

- Narcissistic personality disorder: requires constant admiration, displays envy, lack of empathy, and grandiose thinking

- Avoidant personality disorder: social inhibition, feelings of inadequacy, and fear of criticism

- Dependent personality disorder: excessive need to be taken care of

- Obsessive-compulsive personality disorder: orderliness, perfectionism and control without flexibility, and efficiency; no obsessions or compulsions

CHAPTER 17

NEUROLOGY

Thomas A. Brown, MD, and Sonali J. Shah

INSIDER'S GUIDE TO NEUROLOGY FOR THE USMLE STEP 1

Neurology is one of the toughest subjects on boards simply because of the broad range of information that you must learn for this topic area. Unfortunately, there is no way to comprehensively cover all of the information that you must know for neurology in this chapter or any single boards review book. The best-prepared students use a mix of review sources to study for neurology. You might consider having a proper neurology textbook nearby so that you can refer to some diagrams included in it as well.

High-yield neurology topics include degenerative disorders, Alzheimer's disease, spinal cord syndromes, and central nervous system (CNS) lesions that result from to neuronal damage (e.g., cranial nerve lesions, upper motor neuron [UMN] vs. lower motor neuron [LMN] signs) or arterial occlusions. When it comes to strokes and cranial nerve damage, simply knowing the general functional deficits that you would expect to find in the patient is not enough. Boards will expect you to predict the side of the body that will be affected based on the site of the lesion. Although this may seem like a simple task, be aware that it can be difficult to muster enough brain power to reason through this type of problem after sitting through such a long examination. Practice, practice, and practice while studying, and you will sharpen your intuition and minimize your efforts on test day.

We should mention that neuroanatomy is also high-yield for boards. You will be expected to recognize anatomic structures present at various levels of the brain or spinal cord and make clinical correlations to diseases that affect these structures. This will require you to know which section of the CNS you are looking at when presented with an image. First Aid will not adequately prepare you for this topic. We recommend using *High-Yield Neuroanatomy* of the High-Yield Series. Not only does this book cover the depth of information that you need to breeze through neuroanatomy on boards, but users also are quite impressed with its brevity.

BASIC CONCEPTS

1. **What is a motor unit? Will most α motor neurons innervate a few or many muscle fibers in a large muscle such as the gluteus maximus?**
   A motor unit is a group of muscle fibers that are all innervated by a single α motor neuron. In the large muscles, α motor neurons will innervate many muscle fibers, which is why fine control of muscle movement (contraction) is limited. On the other hand, in the smaller muscles (e.g., extraocular muscles or muscles of the hand), a given α motor neuron will innervate only a few muscle fibers, resulting in much finer control of movement. In both types of muscle, increasing the strength of muscle contraction occurs primarily by *recruitment* of additional motor units.

2. **How do upper motor neurons differ from lower motor neurons?**

Motor neurons, as the name implies, are neurons involved in stimulating movement. The axons of lower motor neurons (LMNs) (α and γ motor neurons) project directly to skeletal muscle fibers, while upper motor neurons (UMNs) originate in the motor region of the brainstem and cerebral cortex and have no direct contact with skeletal muscles (Fig. 17-1). The cell bodies of UMNs are supraspinal in location, and the axons of these neurons synapse either directly or indirectly, via interneurons, on LMNs located in the ventral horn of the spinal cord or brainstem motor nuclei (e.g., facial nerve motor nucleus).

UMN lesions produce a different set of symptoms than LMN lesions that you should recognize for boards. While LMN lesions result in flaccid paralysis and weakened reflexes due to decreased contractions from denervated muscles, UMN lesions result in a spastic paralysis and heightened reflexes due to loss of inhibition of γ motor neurons by UMNs. LMN lesions result in fasciculations (random twitches of denervated motor units) and muscle atrophy. UMN lesions are associated with a positive Babinski sign (toes extend upward with plantar stimulation), but LMN lesions are not. UMN and LMN symptoms are explored further in Case 17-1.

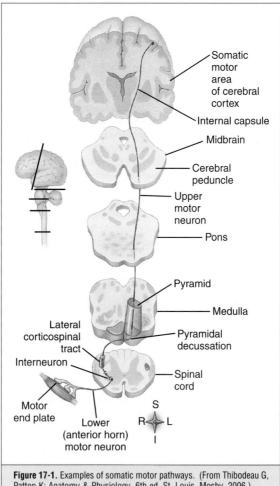

Figure 17-1. Examples of somatic motor pathways. (From Thibodeau G, Patton K: Anatomy & Physiology, 6th ed. St. Louis, Mosby, 2006.)

3. **What is the primary function of the cerebellum in movement?**
   The cerebellum fine-tunes movement. It does this by comparing commands sent by the motor cortex to the muscular system with proprioceptive feedback (via the spinocerebellar tracts) it receives about the movement that actually occurred. When differences in the planned movement and the actual movement occur, the cerebellum uses this feedback to correct errors and influence future output of the motor cortex.

4. **Why do cerebellar lesions classically produce ipsilateral symptoms?**
   The cerebellar hemispheres influence motor activity by their projections to the contralateral motor cortices (via the motor thalamus) and to the contralateral red nuclei. In turn, both the corticospinal tract and the rubrospinal tract arising from these structures cross back over en route to their target motor neurons, thereby producing symptoms on the same side of the body as the lesion.

5. **What are the two ascending sensory pathways and what information does each convey?**
   1. The *anterolateral system*, also referred to as the *spinothalamic tract*, conveys sensations of pain, temperature, and crude (nondiscriminative) touch.
   2. The *dorsal column–medial lemniscus pathway* conveys the sensations of fine touch, vibration, pressure, and conscious proprioception.
   Note: Unconscious proprioception is transmitted by the spinocerebellar pathways.

6. **What are the two anatomic divisions of the dorsal columns, and from which anatomic structures do these respective divisions relay sensory information?**
   1. The *fasciculus gracilis*, which relays information from the lower extremities and from the lower thorax (level T7 and below), is located most medially in the dorsal columns, just as the gracilis muscle is the most medial muscle of the thigh.
   2. The *fasciculus cuneatus,* which relays information from the upper thorax and the upper extremities (levels C2-T6; recall that the C1 spinal nerve provides motor innervation to the muscles of the occipital region) is immediately lateral to the fasciculus gracilis (Fig. 17-2).
   Note: Both fasciculi carry fibers that synapse on their respective nuclei in the medulla, the nucleus gracilis and nucleus cuneatus.

7. **At what neuroanatomic locations do projections in the corticospinal tract, dorsal columns, and anterolateral system (spinothalamic system) cross over?**
   The corticospinal tract crosses over (i.e., decussates) as it descends along the inferior aspect of the medulla through the medullary pyramids. The dorsal columns' (ascending) projections cross over between their nuclei in the brainstem and the thalamus, via the internal arcuate fibers of the medial lemniscus, which are located in the caudal medulla. The axons of the anterolateral system cross over almost immediately after their first-order neurons synapse in the dorsal horn of the spinal cord.

STEP 1 SECRET

You must know where common tracts such as the corticospinal tract, dorsal column–medial lemniscus pathway, and spinothalamic tract decussate because this will determine the side on which a patient experiences symptoms if one of the neurons in the aforementioned pathways is damaged. Remember, the USMLE is most interested in clinically relevant information! It will be far more valuable for you to practice pinpointing the site of a patient's lesion based on common sets of symptoms than to memorize a dozen different tracts.

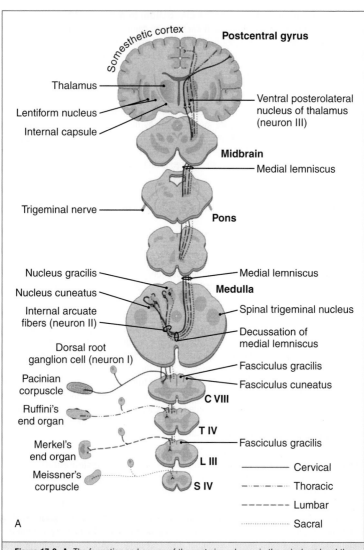

Figure 17-2. A, The formation and course of the posterior columns in the spinal cord and the medial lemniscus in the brainstem.

8. **Because you know where the major motor and sensory pathways cross over, identify and explain the neurologic deficits that occur in the Brown-Séquard syndrome.**

   Brown-Séquard syndrome is caused by a lateral hemisection of the spinal cord. The motor loss will be on the same side as that of the lesion, because the corticospinal tract has already crossed superior to the lesion (in the medulla), and in the spinal cord it innervates only motor neurons on the same side as it courses. Loss of LMNs in the anterior horn will result in ipsilateral symptoms of hyporeflexia and flaccid paralysis at the level of the lesion. However, ipsilateral UMN signs will also be present because UMNs synapse with LMNs at all levels of the spinal cord.

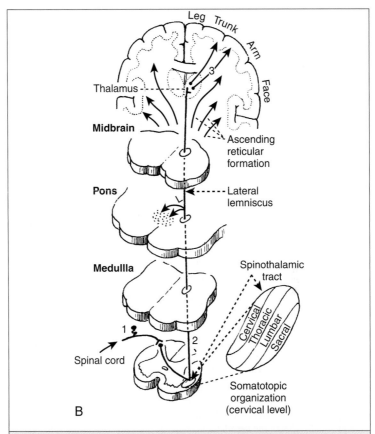

Figure 17-2.—Cont'd B, Divisions of the ascending sensory pathways. (**A** modified from Carpenter MB: Human Neuroanatomy. Baltimore, Williams & Wilkins, 1983. **B** from Lindsay KW, Bone I, Callander R: Neurology and Neurosurgery Illustrated, 3rd ed. Edinburgh, Churchill Livingstone, 2002.)

The loss of fine touch, vibration, and proprioception (modalities of the dorsal columns) will be on the same side as that of the lesion. This is because the sensory information of the dorsal columns does not cross over until a more superior location (between the brainstem nuclei and the thalamus). The loss of pain and temperature sensation (anterolateral system), however, will be contralateral to the side of the lesion, because the fibers of the anterolateral system ascend and cross over shortly after entering the spinal cord (Fig. 17-3).

Note: There may be some loss of all modalities at the level at which the lesion occurs.

9. **Where will the motor and sensory deficit manifest (below the head) if there is a lesion of the internal capsule?**
    The corticospinal tract, dorsal columns, and anterolateral system all travel to or from the cerebral cortex through the posterior limb of the internal capsule. Because all these tracts either originated from, or will eventually cross over to, the contralateral side, there will be a contralateral hemiplegia from effects on the corticospinal tract, along with a contralateral sensory loss from both ascending sensory systems.

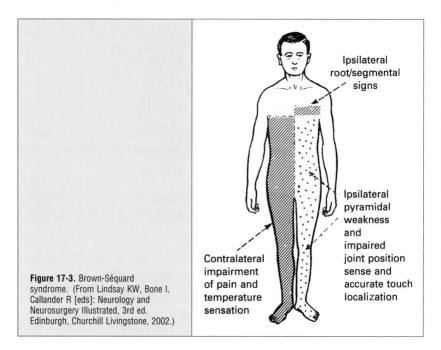

Ipsilateral root/segmental signs

Ipsilateral pyramidal weakness and impaired joint position sense and accurate touch localization

Contralateral impairment of pain and temperature sensation

Figure 17-3. Brown-Séquard syndrome. (From Lindsay KW, Bone I, Callander R [eds]: Neurology and Neurosurgery Illustrated, 3rd ed. Edinburgh, Churchill Livingstone, 2002.)

CASE 17-1

A 45-year-old man presents with a 6-month history of unexplained muscle weakness, dysphagia, and dysarthria. When reaching above his head to reshelve heavy board review books, he experiences arm weakness, accompanied by shoulder muscle cramps and neck cramps. His dysphagia and dysarthria manifest as difficulty swallowing both liquids and solids and a slow, strained speech pattern.

1. **How might we approach a case of suspected motor neuron disease?**
   Consider that the lesion might occur at the level of motor neurons, neuromuscular junctions, or muscles. For example, the differential diagnosis for muscle weakness, dysarthria, and dysphagia may include amyotrophic lateral sclerosis (a disease of motor neurons), myasthenia gravis (an autoimmune attack at the neuromuscular junction), or polymyositis (an inflammatory disease of muscle). Suspected motor neuron disease can then be investigated for UMN or LMN signs.

CASE 17-1 continued:

Physical examination of upper and lower extremities reveals a strange combination of flaccid and spastic paralysis, as well as hypo- and hyperreflexia. Diffuse muscle wasting and fasciculations are visible on the lateral aspects of the tongue. Sensation is intact to all modalities in all areas tested. A mini-mental status examination is within normal limits for the patient's age and cultural background, though he does have difficulty articulating.

2. **What upper motor neuron signs are present in this patient?**
   UMN lesion signs include spastic paralysis (the muscles have an increased resistance to passive movement or manipulation), hyperreflexia (hyperactivity of deep tendon reflexes [DTRs]),

and clonus (alternating contraction and relaxation of a muscle in rapid succession in response to sudden stretching of the muscle). Notice this patient has spastic paralysis and hyperreflexia.

3. **Why are the signs of hyperreflexia, spastic paralysis, and clonus seen with an upper motor neuron lesion?**
The most widely accepted theory is that UMNs are tonically inhibitory to LMNs, such that disruption of UMNs will *disinhibit* (i.e., allow activation of) LMNs. This makes the motor component of the DTRs more active and increases baseline muscle tone, which increases resistance to passive movement.

4. **What lower motor neuron signs are present in this patient?**
When an LMN is damaged, the muscle it innervates does not get stimulated, so the muscle atrophies and has less tone (*hypotonia*). The denervated muscle also has *flaccid paralysis* (the muscles have decreased resistance to passive movement or manipulation), and the efferent part of the DTRs is blunted, so the DTRs are weak or absent (*hyporeflexia*).
   Note: LMN involvement can be evaluated by electromyography (EMG) and nerve conduction studies.

CASE 17-1 continued:

Serum analysis is negative for antibodies to the acetylcholine (ACh) receptor. Cerebrospinal fluid (CSF) analysis is negative for oligoclonal bands (of immunoglobulins), elevated protein, or white blood cells (WBCs). Magnetic resonance imaging (MRI) of the brain and spinal cord appears normal. A muscle biopsy is shown in Figure 17-4.

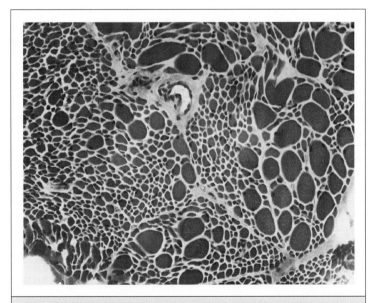

Figure 17-4. Muscle biopsy from a patient with spinal muscular atrophy type I demonstrating denervation atrophy with residual hypertrophic fibers (magnification × 300). (From Samuels MA, Feske SK: Office Practice of Neurology, 2nd ed. Philadelphia, Churchill Livingstone, 2003.)

5. **What process leads to the findings seen in this biopsy specimen stained with hematoxylin-eosin (H&E)?**
   The atrophied and angulated fibers reflect denervation due to the death of the innervating motor neurons. This death of an entire group of neighboring muscle fibers (of the same type, because they are innervated by the same motor neuron) is called *group atrophy*. It occurs with disease progression.

6. **What would myosin adenosine triphosphatase (ATPase) staining of this specimen show?**
   This histologic stain would distinguish type I (slow twitch) from type II (fast twitch) muscle fibers. Normally, these different types of muscle fibers will be intermingled in a checkerboard-like pattern, owing to the innervation of adjacent muscle fibers by different anterior horn motor neurons. However, when muscle fibers lose their motor innervation due to death of anterior horn cells, the axons that innervate neighboring muscle fibers will sprout new axons and take over the denervated fibers. This leads to *type grouping*, in which muscle fibers of the same type are grouped together, with loss of the checkerboard pattern.

7. **What is the most likely diagnosis?**
   Amyotrophic lateral sclerosis (ALS), or Lou Gehrig disease, is a chronic neurodegenerative disease of *both UMNs and LMNs* that results in muscle weakness, disability, and death typically within 3 to 5 years. Causes of death typically include respiratory failure, aspiration pneumonia resulting from respiratory muscle weakness, skin ulcers causing systemic infection, and deep vein thrombosis causing pulmonary thromboembolism.
   Note: Myotrophic means "muscle enlargement." *A*myotrophia means "muscle atrophy." Lateral sclerosis refers to palpable hardness of the lateral columns of the spinal cord at autopsy, due to sclerosis of the lateral corticospinal tracts.

8. **Why are the magnetic resonance imaging and cerebrospinal fluid findings notable?**
   The absence of periventricular plaques on MRI and oligoclonal bands in CSF makes the diagnosis of multiple sclerosis (MS) much less likely, as most MS patients have these findings. Another important distinction between MS and ALS is that ALS affects only the motor system, whereas MS affects both motor and sensory systems. The distinction between these diseases is important: Although both are incurable, ALS is relentlessly progressive, whereas MS has a more variable natural history.

9. **What are the principal pathologic findings in amyotrophic lateral sclerosis?**
   There is loss of pyramidal cells in the motor cortex, leading to fibrosis (which generally manifests in the central nervous system [CNS] as astrocytic gliosis) of the lateral corticospinal tracts. In addition, there is loss of ventral horn neurons throughout the length of the spinal cord, resulting in thinning of ventral (motor) nerve roots. The affected muscles show denervation atrophy with (muscle) fiber type grouping upon reinnervation. There usually is sparing of sensory tracts and cognitive function, which explains why this patient's mental status and sensory function are both completely normal. Extraocular muscles also are often spared, leaving some patients with severe disease progression no means of communication other than eye movements (Fig. 17-5).
   Note: Diffuse muscle atrophy with UMN lesions might occur secondary to muscle disuse but does not occur as a result of UMN loss. The group atrophy seen in ALS is secondary to muscle denervation due to LMN loss.

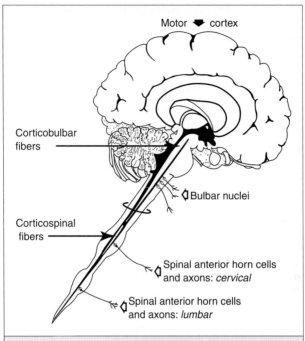

Figure 17-5. Sites of the lesions in amyotrophic lateral sclerosis (ALS). (From Pryse-Phillips WM, Murray TJ: Essential Neurology: A Concise Textbook. New York, Medical Examination Publishing, 1992.)

10. **What might you expect electromyography and nerve conduction studies to show in this patient?**
EMG could indicate LMN involvement by revealing signs of denervation (fibrillation potentials). *Fibrillations* are invisible contractions of single muscle fibers, seen on EMG only. *Fasciculations* are involuntary contractions of one or more muscle units (which are often visible) and may also be present in LMN lesions. Notice this patient had fasciculations, often visible in the tongue. Nerve conduction studies are typically normal (or close to normal).

11. **Is amyotrophic lateral sclerosis more commonly inherited or acquired?**
ALS is more commonly acquired than inherited. The precise etiology of the acquired form remains unknown. However, one of the familial forms has been associated with mutations in the zinc/copper superoxide dismutase 1 gene, which plays an important role in scavenging free radicals in metabolically active cells such as neurons.

12. **Why is amyotrophic lateral sclerosis often confused for syringomyelia and vice versa?**
Syringomyelia is a disease marked by enlargement of the central canal of the cervical spinal cord. This leads to destruction of the anterior horn cells in the upper levels of the spinal cord, resulting in atrophy of intrinsic hand muscles. Because atrophy and weakness of hand muscles are early signs of both ALS and syringomyelia, the disease presentations are often confused. However, enlargement of the central canal in syringomyelia also affects the decussating fibers of the anterolateral spinothalamic tract, resulting in bilateral loss of pain and temperature sensation in the upper extremities. ALS, on the other hand, has no sensory changes!

SUMMARY BOX: AMYOTROPHIC LATERAL SCLEROSIS

- Clinical presentation is one of chronic degeneration of upper and lower motor neurons, generally without sensory or cognitive involvement.

- Pathologic examination shows degeneration of pyramidal cells in the motor cortex and fibrosis of the lateral corticospinal tract. These areas are replaced with reactive astrogliosis.

- Muscle biopsy shows type grouping and group atrophy of muscle fibers.

- Most cases are acquired; one familial form is associated with superoxide dismutase 1 mutations.

- Amyotrophic lateral sclerosis (ALS) and syringomyelia both result in hand muscle atrophy. Syringomyelia also results in bilateral loss of pain and temperature sensation, while ALS is not associated with sensory changes.

CASE 17-2

A 70-year-old man presents with a tremor in one hand that causes him to appear to be rolling something between his fingers.

1. **With what actions is this tremor most likely to appear?**
   This patient's pill-rolling tremor is likely a resting tremor, most prominent when the arms are relaxed and the patient is not paying attention to his position or action.

2. **Differentiate among resting tremor, intention tremor, and postural tremor.**
   Resting tremor occurs when the patient is not moving (*resting*) and typically decreases with voluntary activity. Intention tremor, which typically has cerebellar origins, appears as the patient moves a limb toward a target, and is often irregular in amplitude and trajectory. Postural tremor, the most common cause of which is essential tremor, appears as the patient actively holds the limbs in a position against gravity.

CASE 17-2 continued:

During the interview, you note that the tremor appears at rest and disappears when the patient either extends his arms parallel to the floor or reaches for a pen. However, he has difficulty initiating movement to reach for a pen (akinesia), finally doing so successfully, albeit slowly (bradykinesia). You also note an expressionless face, decreased spontaneous blink rate, and forward stooped posture. On physical examination, the patient maintains this posture and walks with a slow, narrow-based, festinating gait. Motor examination shows that his muscles demonstrate a cogwheel rigidity, in which muscle rigidity gives way to passive stretching in series of successive jerks.

3. **In light of these signs, what is the most likely diagnosis for the tremor?**
   This is a classic presentation for Parkinson's disease, which is the most common cause of resting tremor. Parkinson's disease frequently presents with a triad of resting tremor, bradykinesia, and cogwheel rigidity. This patient has the triad, as well as characteristic masked facies, stooped posture, and festinating gait.

4. **How does a festinating gait differ from an ataxic gait?**
   A festinating gain is due to lesions of the substantia nigra pars compacta, a member of the basal ganglia, and manifests as an unsteady, shuffling gait consisting of narrow-based steps. When directed to turn around, patients often do so "en bloc," by taking many small steps without twisting the torso. An ataxic gait is due to lesions of midline cerebellar structures and manifests as unsteady wide-based steps, with staggering side to side. A subtly ataxic gait can be detected with heel-to-toe gait testing.

5. **Why should we determine whether this patient is taking medications such as haloperidol or metoclopramide?**
   The pathophysiology of Parkinson's disease is related to insufficient dopaminergic activity within the brain, because the substantia nigra pars compacta serves as the site of dopamine production. Certain antipsychotic and antiemetic agents that act as central dopamine receptor antagonists may cause or exacerbate parkinsonian symptoms such as rigidity, bradykinesia, and resting tremor. When making the diagnosis, it is critical for physicians to distinguish Parkinson's disease from parkinsonism, which can present with a similar symptomatology and may be drug-induced, postencephalitic, or neurodegenerative but with different anatomic lesions from those in Parkinson's disease.

6. **What cerebral structures are affected in Parkinson's disease, and how does this play into the bradykinesia and akinesia observed?**
   In Parkinson's disease, the dopaminergic, neuromelanin-containing neurons in the substantia nigra selectively degenerate over time. These neurons normally project to the basal ganglia via the nigrostriatal tract. The basal ganglia then influence execution of learned motor plans by modulating signals between the thalamus and motor cortex. Within the basal ganglia, there are two pathways leading to output to the thalamus: the direct and indirect pathways. Activation of the direct pathway facilitates desired movement by stimulating the thalamus via inhibition of the globus pallidus internus and substantia nigra pars reticularis (both of which normally inhibit the thalamus), whereas activation of the indirect pathway inhibits unwanted movement by inhibiting the thalamus. Nigrostriatal dopaminergic inputs activate the direct pathway and inhibit the indirect pathway, thus stimulating motion. Decreased dopamine levels in Parkinson's disease manifest with a net decrease in motor activity. However, this model does not yet account for the patient's tremor. Because dopamine decreases release of ACh, a decrease in dopamine levels leads to a relative excess of striatal ACh in patients with Parkinson's disease. ACh opposes the actions of dopamine and activates the indirect pathway, which disinhibits suppression of unwanted movements and results in the pill-rolling tremor that is characteristic of the disease. It is important that you understand the imbalance of dopamine and ACh levels in Parkinson's patients because dopamine agonists and anticholinergics are useful in treating this disease (Fig. 17-6).

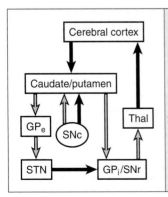

Figure 17-6. Schema of anatomic nuclei and pathways involving the basal ganglia. Black arrows represent excitation, and speckled arrows represent inhibition. GP$_e$, globus pallidus, external segment; GP$_i$, globus pallidus, internal segment; SNc, pars compacta of the substantia nigra; SNr, pars reticularis of the substantia nigra; STN, subthalamic nucleus; thal, thalamus. (From Goetz CG: Textbook of Clinical Neurology, 2nd ed. Philadelphia, WB Saunders, 2003.)

Note: The striatum consists of the caudate nucleus and putamen, both of which are part of the basal ganglia. You should be able to identify the basal ganglia on an anatomic section. The caudate and thalamus lie medial to the internal capsule, and the globus pallidus and putamen lie lateral.

CASE 17–2 continued:

When you see the patient in clinic 6 months later, you note marked improvement of his bradykinesia and resting tremor. You attribute this success to the patient's current treatment course.

7. **What medication did you start the patient on, and why is it, rather than dopamine, used to treat Parkinson's disease?**
   Dopamine cannot cross the blood-brain barrier. However, levodopa (L-dopa), a lipid-soluble precursor to dopamine, can cross the blood-brain barrier and increases CNS dopamine levels once converted by dopa decarboxylase. In fact, parkinsonian syndromes are often initially misdiagnosed as Parkinson's disease, and the diagnosis later corrected when the patient does not respond to L-dopa.

8. **Why is levodopa typically administered along with carbidopa?**
   Carbidopa is a dopa decarboxylase inhibitor that cannot cross the blood-brain barrier, so it inhibits the peripheral metabolism of L-dopa to dopamine. This both increases the delivery of L-dopa to the brain and minimizes the side effects of peripheral L-dopa/dopamine. These side effects include autonomic symptoms such as orthostatic hypotension, nausea/vomiting, confusion, hallucinations, and infrequently, arrhythmias. Long-term side effects include dyskinesia, particularly choreoathetosis of the face and distal extremities. CNS symptoms (confusion and hallucinations) are last to disappear.

9. **Drugs such as bromocriptine and pergolide are also used to treat Parkinson's disease. How do they exert their effects?**
   These drugs are dopamine receptor agonists and increase central dopaminergic activity without increasing dopamine levels, which of course is beneficial in Parkinson's disease.

10. **What is the mechanism of action of selegiline, a drug used in treating Parkinson's disease?**
    Selegiline selectively inhibits monoamine oxidase B (MAO-B), an enzyme that degrades dopamine. Selegiline can cross the blood-brain barrier, so it can be used without L-dopa.

11. **Why is it preferable to selectively inhibit monoamine oxidase B, rather than both monoamine oxidase A and monoamine oxidase B, in Parkinson's disease?**
    Monoamine oxidase A (MAO-A) principally degrades norepinephrine and serotonin, whereas MAO-B is more selective for dopamine degradation. Because MAO-A inhibitors increase serotonin and norepinephrine levels, they have been used for treating depression, but they are not expected to be as effective in treating the motor symptoms of Parkinson's disease.

12. **What is benztropine and why is it useful in Parkinson's disease?**
    Benztropine is an anticholinergic drug (like atropine) that crosses the blood-brain barrier. Recall that there is a *relative* excess of striatal ACh in Parkinson's disease because of the deficiency of dopamine. Thus, anticholinergics that can enter the CNS are also useful in treating the bradykinesia and akinesia of Parkinson's disease.

13. **Which antiviral medication is also effective in treating Parkinson's disease?**
    Amantadine, which is effective against influenza A, was incidentally discovered to be effective in Parkinson's disease. Though its mechanism is not fully understood, amantadine has anticholinergic and antiglutamatergic effects and also acts by increasing dopamine output from intact nerve terminals.

14. **How does the drug MPTP (1-methyl-4-phenyl-1,2,3,6-tetrahydropyridine) cause parkinsonism, and is this a reversible process?**
    MPTP is an analog of the opioid meperidine and is occasionally present as a contaminant in certain illicit drugs. It causes irreversible parkinsonism by selectively destroying neurons in the substantia nigra. In fact, the clinical and pathologic consequences of MPTP toxicity mimic those of Parkinson's disease so well that MPTP is often used in animal models to study Parkinson's disease.

15. **Why should you be suspicious of a diagnosis of Parkinson's disease in a patient being treated for schizophrenia?**
    Antipsychotic drugs that block dopamine receptors in the mesolimbic system to achieve their effect can also block dopaminergic activity in the nigrostriatal tract and cause symptoms similar to those of Parkinson's disease (pseudoparkinsonism, which is often reversible with discontinuation of the antipsychotics). However, the choreoathetoid motor disorders that develop after prolonged use of antipsychotics (e.g., tardive dyskinesia) may prove to be irreversible.

16. **What would a pathologist look for to establish the diagnosis of Parkinson's disease in evaluation of the brain at autopsy?**
    - Bilateral depigmentation of the midbrain substantia nigra, due to loss of dopaminergic, neuromelanin-containing neurons (Fig. 17-7A [normal] and B [Parkinson's])
    - The presence of neuronal Lewy bodies in degenerated substantia nigra neurons (eosinophilic, cytoplasmic inclusions containing α-synuclein and ubiquitin) (Fig. 17-7C)

SUMMARY BOX: PARKINSON'S DISEASE

- This hypokinetic movement disorder classically presents with pill-rolling tremor, bradykinesia, akinesia, festinating gait, stooped posture, and masked facies.

- Pathophysiologically, think of an imbalance between acetylcholine (too much) and dopamine (too little) in the basal ganglia.

- Pathologic examination shows degeneration of neuromelanin-containing dopaminergic cells in the substantia nigra.

- Pharmacologic treatment is targeted at increasing levels of dopamine in the brain, as well as decreasing acetylcholine activity in the central nervous system.

CASE 17-3

A 40-year-old man has become notably demented and has developed involuntary movements, such as facial grimaces and a dance-like gait in which his legs move in sudden, rapid, jerky movements. During the interview, you note that the patient makes continuous jerky movements with his arm, which he seems to complete as purposeful movements to smooth his hair. The patient also complains that his mind does not feel as sharp as it used to be.

1. **What term describes the patient's movements, and what conditions may cause these movements?**
   Chorea describes involuntary, sudden, rapid movements of a body part. Choreic movements often appear on a spectrum with athetosis, which are involuntary movements of the trunk and extremities that may give a writhing, snakelike, or dancing appearance to the gait.

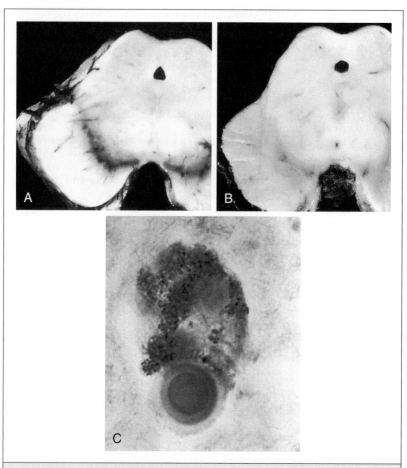

Figure 17-7. Parkinson's disease (PD). **A,** Normal substantia nigra. **B,** Depigmented substantia nigra in idiopathic PD. **C,** Lewy bodies in a substantia nigra neuron stain bright pink. (From Kumar V, Abbas AK, Fausto N: Robbins and Cotran Pathologic Basis of Disease, 7th ed. Philadelphia, WB Saunders, 2005.) (C courtesy of Dr. R. Kim, VA Medical Center, Long Beach, CA.)

The differential diagnosis of chorea is broad, but includes Huntington's disease, Sydenham's chorea (poststreptococcal autoimmune–mediated, and often accompanied by rheumatic fever), Wilson's disease (abnormal copper accumulation), cerebrovascular causes, and senile-related chorea.

2. **Why might medications such as haloperidol and L-dopa cause chorea?**
   Neuroleptics such as haloperidol block dopamine receptors. Although the goal of drugs such as haloperidol is to block dopamine receptors in the mesolimbic-mesocortical pathway and reduce psychotic behavior, long-term antagonism of dopamine receptors in the nigrostriatal pathway can cause choreoathetoid movements. This side effect is called tardive dyskinesia, which as the name implies, develops slowly after medication is started and may persist after the medication is discontinued.

   A variety of dyskinesias are often seen in patients who have been taking L-dopa for long periods of time. The most common presentation is choreoathetosis of the face and distal extremities.

CASE 17-3 continued:

While talking with the patient and his wife, the wife tells you that the patient saw a psychiatrist a few years ago due to some gradual changes in his mood.

3. **What sort of psychiatric changes might the patient's wife be referring to?**
    She might describe a gradual development of emotional lability, increased aggression and irritability, hypersexuality, or depression. Such behavioral changes are often initially misdiagnosed as psychiatric disease.

4. **If a mini-mental status examination shows the patient to be mildly demented, with deficits in organization, concentration, and short-term memory, what is the most likely diagnosis?**
    The classic clinical triad of dementia, behavioral changes such as aggression and depression, and chorea points toward Huntington's disease. This diagnosis is often supported by the family history, as this is a genetic disorder characterized by trinucleotide repeats.

5. **What pathologic lesion would be visible on imaging?**
    MRI of the head is notable for significant atrophy of the basal ganglia, especially the caudate nucleus. In fact, Huntington's disease is caused by degeneration of γ-aminobutyric acid (GABA) neurons belonging to the indirect pathway in the caudate nucleus. This is significant because the striatal nuclei are the main inhibitors of undesirable movement. The ventricular enlargement that is often apparent on autopsy (Fig. 17-8, right) is due to loss of neurons in the basal ganglia.

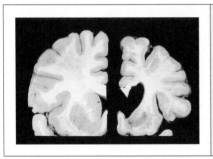

Figure 17-8. Huntington's disease (HD). Normal hemisphere on the left compared with the HD hemisphere on the right showing atrophy of the striatum and ventricular dilation. (Courtesy of Dr. J.P. Vonsattel, Columbia University, New York, NY.)

CASE 17-3 continued:

After discussions of your initial diagnosis, the patient reveals that he has known for a while that this was going to happen to him because he had tested positive for the gene that caused his father to have similar problems. However, the patient is upset because the disease has developed several years earlier in his life than in his father's.

6. **What is the mode of inheritance?**
    Huntington's disease is inherited in an autosomal dominant manner.

7. **What neurotransmitter is reduced in the basal ganglia in Huntington's disease and how does this relate to the hyperkinetic motor abnormalities seen in Huntington's disease?**
    GABA, the major inhibitory neurotransmitter of the CNS, is reduced. In Huntington's disease, loss of inhibitory signals within the basal ganglia results in *disinhibition* of the motor

thalamus, explaining the hyperkinetic motor abnormalities seen in this disease. Note that the deficiency of GABA within the basal ganglia has the opposite effect (i.e., hyperkinesia) from that seen with the deficiency of dopamine associated with Parkinson's disease (i.e., hypokinesia).

8. **What does the term "penetrance" imply with respect to genetic diseases, and is the penetrance of Huntington's disease high or low?**
   Penetrance is the frequency with which a pathologic phenotype is observed in the presence of the disease genotype. In Huntington's disease, which has a penetrance of 100%, every individual with the gene defect will eventually develop the disease. This is why this patient knew he was going to get the disease. Fortunately, most genetic diseases have incomplete penetrance.

9. **What is the meaning of anticipation with respect to genetic diseases and what is the cause of anticipation in Huntington's disease?**
   Anticipation is the expression of a hereditary disease at an earlier age and in a more severe form throughout succeeding generations. In Huntington's disease, anticipation is caused by an increase in the number of trinucleotide repeats within the gene responsible for the disease.

10. **What type of gene mutation gives rise to Huntington's disease?**
    A trinucleotide repeat (CAG) expansion, located in the huntingtin gene on chromosome 4, translates into insertion of a polyglutamine tract in the huntingtin protein. It is not known whether Huntington's disease results from a loss of function (such as neuroprotection) or a gain of function (such as neurotoxicity) of the gene product.

11. **How is it possible for someone with a negative family history of Huntington's disease to develop the disease?**
    There is a set range of the number of CAG repeats in the huntingtin gene that is considered to be normal. It is possible that the first case of Huntington's disease in a family represents the instance in which the number of repeats has increased beyond the normal range such that it manifests in disease symptoms.

12. **Why might it make sense to measure levels of serum ceruloplasmin in patients who present with similar motor abnormalities and a similar family history?**
    Serum ceruloplasmin is a screening test for Wilson's disease (hepatolenticular degeneration), which is also hereditary and causes movement abnormalities. In this disease, serum levels of copper are abnormally high and serum levels of ceruloplasmin, a serum protein that transports copper, are abnormally low. Copper deposition in the lenticular nuclei (globus pallidus and putamen) results in motor abnormalities.

SUMMARY BOX: HUNTINGTON'S DISEASE

- Classic clinical triad consists of dementia, behavioral changes, and choreoathetosis.

- The diseae is inherited in autosomal dominant manner, with 100% penetrance.

- This disease is caused by expansion of CAG repeats in the huntingtin gene in chromosome 4.

- The disease typically presents in middle-aged patients, but because of genetic anticipation in which the number of CAG repeats increases, it presents at younger ages with successive generations.

CASE 17-4

A 30-year-old woman complains of a long history of double vision (diplopia) and some difficulty swallowing solid foods (dysphagia). Her physical appearance is remarkable only for ptosis and slight atrophy of facial muscles. While thinking about whether her motor symptoms reflect abnormality of motor neurons, the neuromuscular junction, or muscle, you perform a cranial nerve examination.

1. **Given her diplopia, which cranial nerves should you examine particularly carefully?**
   Diplopia may reflect asymmetrical pathology of the extraocular muscles (EOMs), which would be detected during the test of cranial nerves CN IV (innervating superior oblique), CN VI (innervating lateral rectus), and CN III (innervating all other EOMs). Diplopia may also be due to lesions of the medial longitudinal fasciculus (MLF), a midbrain circuit that coordinates the EOMs of the left and right eyes in order to move both eyes in a given direction, or of the optic nerves, both of which can be affected in MS. Diplopia may reflect pathology of the globes (e.g., trauma, Graves' disease) or brain (e.g., stroke). Finally, diplopia can occur from ischemic damage to one of the cranial nerves controlling eye movement (mononeuropathy), as can occasionally be seen in diabetes.
   Note: Diplopia and other ocular pathologic conditions are discussed in further detail in Chapter 18.

CASE 17-4 continued:

After a complete physical examination, you notice that her ptosis seems more pronounced than it was 30 minutes ago. When asked to look upward for 1 minute without closing her eyes, she closes her eyes after only 15 seconds due to muscle weakness. She then admits that she has been feeling fatigued lately; after mild exercise, her arms and legs feel weak, though not painful. All these symptoms seem worse in the evening.

2. **Why would an edrophonium chloride (Tensilon) test help determine whether the symptoms are of nerve, neuromuscular junction, or muscle origin?**
   The Tensilon test involves the administration of edrophonium, a short-acting cholinesterase inhibitor. The function of cholinesterase is to degrade synaptic acetylcholine (ACh). By antagonizing cholinesterase, edrophonium increases the concentration of ACh in the synaptic cleft. This helps to overcome a deficiency of available ACh receptors by activating a higher percentage of the ACh receptors that are present. Thus, a positive test (one where muscle strength improves in response to edrophonium) reflects deficiency of ACh action at the neuromuscular junction, possibly due to reduced availability of ACh receptors. This occurs in myasthenia gravis, in which the serum of affected patients contains autoantibodies to postsynaptic ACh receptors.

3. **If computed tomography and magnetic resonance imaging scans of the chest were ordered, what diagnosis would be supported by finding a thymoma?**
   Myasthenia gravis is often associated with thymoma or thymic hyperplasia, and a thymectomy frequently helps reverse the symptoms.

STEP 1 SECRET

You may be expected to identify a thymoma on chest x-ray study and use this finding to aid your diagnosis of myasthenia gravis on Step 1.

4. **What is the pathophysiology of the motor weakness in myasthenia gravis?**

   As mentioned previously, myasthenia gravis is an autoimmune disorder characterized by the production of autoantibodies to proteins involved in signaling at the neuromuscular junction. The antibodies are most commonly directed against postsynaptic nicotinic ACh receptors present on skeletal muscle fibers. These antibodies reduce the number of ACh receptors on the motor end plate, making the motor end plate less responsive to ACh. Less frequently, autoantibodies are directed against a muscle-specific tyrosine kinase involved in ACh receptor clustering.

   Reduced binding of ACh to its receptor at the neuromuscular junction results in striated muscle weakness, particularly of muscles involved in eye movement. Common initial findings in patients with myasthenia gravis include diplopia, ptosis, dysphagia to solids and liquids (due to esophageal striated muscle weakness), and proximal muscle weakness.

5. **What is the normal mechanism by which an action potential is generated in skeletal muscle cells?**

   Recall that nicotinic ACh receptors are ligand-gated sodium channels, and that binding of ACh to ACh receptors produces an end plate potential in skeletal muscle cells. This end plate potential has to be above a certain threshold value for activation of fast voltage-gated sodium channels and generation of an action potential, which causes muscle contraction by triggering release of calcium from the sarcoplasmic reticulum. In myasthenia gravis, there are not enough ACh receptors to respond to the synaptic ACh and depolarize the cell to reach the threshold for action potential formation.

6. **Why is edrophonium not used to treat myasthenia gravis, and what are other treatment options?**

   Edrophonium is a *short-acting* cholinesterase inhibitor. For long-term management of myasthenia gravis, the long-acting cholinesterase inhibitors pyridostigmine and neostigmine are used.

7. **If someone being treated for myasthenia gravis overdosed on one of the cholinesterase inhibitors, what side effects might occur?**

   A side effect profile with an overdose of cholinesterase inhibitors would mimic excessive stimulation of the parasympathetic nervous system (i.e., excessive cholinergic activity), resulting in diarrhea, miosis, bronchospasm, excessive urination, bradycardia, salivation, and lacrimation. Additionally, because the sympathetic nervous system stimulates sweating via the release of ACh from postganglionic sympathetic fibers, excessive sweating may also occur. All these side effects occur due to ACh activity at *muscarinic* ACh receptors at end organs. *Nicotinic* ACh receptors exist at the neuromuscular junction and at sympathetic ganglia.

   Note: If someone is poisoned with organophosphates (e.g., parathion), which are *irreversible* cholinesterase inhibitors, treatment is aimed at reducing total cholinergic activity. This is accomplished with pralidoxime, which regenerates active cholinesterase, and also with the anticholinergic atropine.

STEP 1 SECRET

Autonomic nervous system (ANS) pharmacology is one of the highest-yield topics to know for boards. This topic will be further explored in Chapter 23.

8. **What is the mechanism of action of the nondepolarizing neuromuscular blockers and why are these drugs particularly dangerous in patients with myasthenia gravis?**

   These agents are analogs or derivates of curare (e.g., pancuronium, tubocurarine), and work by antagonizing the nicotinic ACh receptor at the neuromuscular junction. They are often used as an adjunct in surgical anesthesia to achieve muscle relaxation. Obviously, these drugs will exacerbate muscle weakness in myasthenia gravis and may even produce respiratory failure from diaphragmatic dysfunction.

9. **Myasthenia gravis and Lambert-Eaton syndrome can have very similar clinical presentations. How is Lambert-Eaton syndrome similar and what is this disease due to?**
    Lambert-Eaton syndrome is an autoimmune disease caused by the abnormal production of self-reactive antibodies to voltage-gated calcium channels located in the terminal bouton of presynaptic neurons, which results in insufficient neurotransmitter (ACh) release. Thus, muscle strength increases with continued effort (contraction) and buildup of released ACh. This distinguishes Lambert-Eaton syndrome from myasthenia gravis, in which continued effort at contraction causes decreased strength and increased muscle fatigue, as seen in our patient.
    Note: Lambert-Eaton syndrome is often associated with paraneoplastic syndromes, particularly small cell carcinoma of the lung.

SUMMARY BOX: MYASTHENIA GRAVIS

- Autoimmune attack on neuromuscular junction; antibodies usually are directed against acetylcholine (ACh) receptors.

- Causes motor weakness, often of extraocular, bulbar, and facial muscles; weakness and fatigue increase with increased use of muscles.

- Diagnose with edrophonium (short-acting cholinesterase inhibitor).

- Treat with pyridostigmine and neostigmine (long-acting cholinesterase inhibitors).

- Contrast with Lambert-Eaton syndrome: autoimmune attack on presynaptic calcium channels, often paraneoplastic, increased strength with increased effort.

CASE 17-5

A 35-year-old man presents with bilateral loss of pain and temperature sensation in the arms and upper thorax, as well as several painless ulcers on his fingers from burning his hands repeatedly while cooking. Fine touch, vibration, and proprioception remain intact in all areas, although pain and temperature sensation are severely compromised in both arms and the upper thorax. MRI reveals a fluid-filled cavity within the spinal cord (Fig. 17-9).

1. **What is the diagnosis and which ascending sensory system is affected in this man?**
    This patient has syringomyelia, which is caused by an expanded fluid-filled cavity (a syrinx) in the central canal of the spinal cord. The anterolateral system is affected due to compression from the syrinx on the anterior white commissure, which is located just ventral to the central canal and contains the decussating fibers of second-order neurons in the spinothalamic system. The anterolateral system, also called the spinothalamic system, conveys modalities of pain, temperature, and crude touch. Thus, the sensory deficit will occur in areas supplied by fibers that decussate at the level of the fluid-filled cavity. Recall that tactile information (which includes fine touch, pressure, and vibration) and proprioception are conveyed by the dorsal column–medial lemniscus pathway.
    Note: Syringobulbia is a variant of syringomyelia in which fluid-filled, slit-like cavities are located in the medulla. Remember, myelo = spinal cord and bulbar = brainstem.

2. **At what general level in the cord is syringomyelia most commonly found?**
    Syringomyelia most commonly occurs in the cervical spinal cord, as shown in the MRI in Figure 17-9. In the image shown, the syrinx extends into the thoracic spinal cord as well.

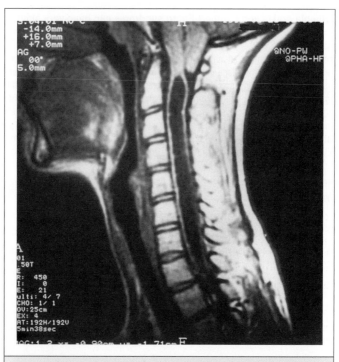

Figure 17-9. Magnetic resonance image demonstrates a large syringomyelic cavity in the cervical cord. (From Bradley WG, Daroff RB, Fenichel GM, et al: Neurology in Clinical Practice, 4th ed. Philadelphia, Butterworth-Heinemann, 2004.)

3. **If the patient also had the cerebellar anomaly shown in Figure 17-9, what diagnosis should be suspected?**
    Figure 17-9 shows herniation of the cerebellar tonsils into the foramen magnum. This anatomic anomaly in association with syringomyelia is typical of type II Arnold-Chiari malformations.

4. **Why is the sensory loss caused by syringomyelia typically called "suspended-dissociated" loss?**
    The loss of pain and temperature sensation caused by syringomyelia is generally limited to the dermatomes innervated by the spinal nerves affected by the spinal level of the syrinx. Sensation above and below the syrinx is expected to be intact. Thus, the body area of sensory loss is "suspended" between two areas of normal sensation. The sensory loss is said to be "dissociated" because only the modalities of pain and temperature (and crude touch) are affected; tactile and proprioceptive sense are intact, because the dorsal column–medial lemniscal pathway is not affected (Fig. 17-10).

5. **How can this disease progress to cause atrophy of the muscles of the hands and hypoactive reflexes of the upper extremities?**
    The syrinx can expand to compress the ventral horns of the spinal cord, thereby producing the LMN signs of muscle atrophy and hyporeflexia.

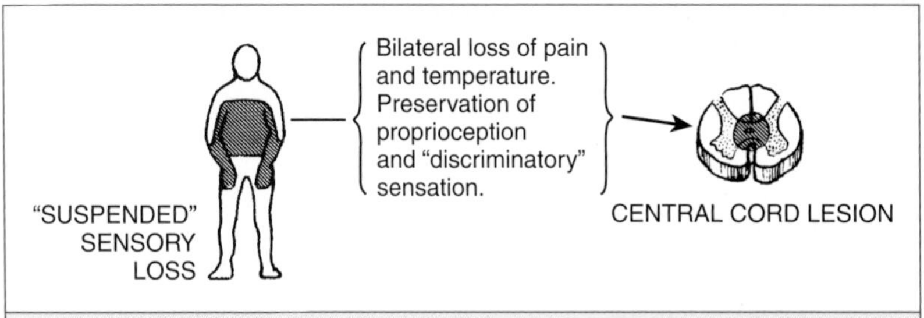

Bilateral loss of pain
and temperature.
Preservation of
proprioception
and "discriminatory"
sensation.

"SUSPENDED"
SENSORY
LOSS

CENTRAL CORD LESION

Figure 17-10. Syringomyelia. (From Lindsay KW, Bone I, Callander R [eds]: Neurology and Neurosurgery Illustrated, 3rd ed. Edinburgh, Churchill Livingstone, 2002.)

Note: If the interossei and lumbrical muscles of the hand were primarily affected, suspect involvement of the C8-T1 segments.

6. **From what area of the body does pain and temperature sensation travel to the cerebral cortex via the medial lemniscus?**
Recall that the anterolateral system carries pain and temperature sensation for most of the body, with the exception of the areas innervated by the trigeminal nerve. Though we generally think of the trigeminal nerve as innervating the face, remember that it does not innervate the angle of the jaw and does not stop at the anterior hairline. The trigeminal nerve can more accurately be thought of as innervating the anterior two thirds of the head. This innervation includes the modalities of fine touch, pressure, vibration, proprioception (for the muscles of mastication), pain, temperature, and crude touch. In this trigeminal mechanosensory pathway, pseudounipolar neurons in the trigeminal ganglion synapse with second-order neurons in one of three nuclei in the trigeminal brainstem complex. The axons of these second-order neurons decussate in the pons before ascending in the medial lemniscus on their way to the ventral posteromedial nucleus of the thalamus.

SUMMARY BOX: SYRINGOMYELIA

■ Syringomyelia refers to a fluid-filled expansion of the central canal of the spinal cord. A similar syrinx can occur in the brainstem and is called syringobulbia.

■ This often occurs in the cervical spinal cord but can extend into the thoracic spinal cord.

■ Compression of the anterior white commissure of the anterolateral (spinothalamic) system causes suspended-dissociated loss of pain and temperature sensation.

■ Compression of the ventral horn motor neurons can cause atrophy of muscles innervated by the spinal nerves arising from the level of the syrinx.

CASE 17-6

A 65-year-old woman complains of intermittent episodes of lancinating pain in her right lower jaw. She is occasionally wakened at night from this pain. She mentions that she read about something called trigeminal neuralgia on the Internet and wonders if this might be related. An extensive workup does not reveal any dental disease, and an MRI does not reveal any mass lesions in the posterior fossa.

1. **In following up on her suggestion of trigeminal neuralgia, what aspects of history should you inquire about?**
   Trigeminal neuralgia (tic douloureux) is diagnosed on the basis of the medical history. Classic presentation includes pain of a sudden, shooting quality that involves one or more branches of the trigeminal nerve unilaterally and lasts seconds to minutes. The pain may be accompanied by brief facial spasms or tics.

2. **What is the value of imaging the posterior fossa for any masses in this woman?**
   The trigeminal nerve courses from its nuclei in the pons through the posterior fossa, and exits the cranium via the superior orbital fissure (V_1), foramen rotundum (V_2), or foramen ovale (V_3). Compression or meningeal inflammation anywhere along this pathway may cause similar symptoms.

3. **In thinking about associated neurologic problems, what disorder might trigeminal neuralgia be associated with in a younger patient?**
   Trigeminal neuralgia in a young patient might suggest MS. Trigeminal neuralgia in an older patient is more often idiopathic.

4. **Which division of the trigeminal nerve is affected in this woman? What is the anatomic distribution of the other divisions?**
   In this woman it is the mandibular division (or V_3), which innervates the lower jaw *but does not extend to the angle of the jaw*. The maxillary division (V_2) innervates the upper jaw and cheek, and the ophthalmic division (V_1) innervates the region of the nose, eyes, and forehead, *extending posterior to the hairline* (Fig. 17-11).

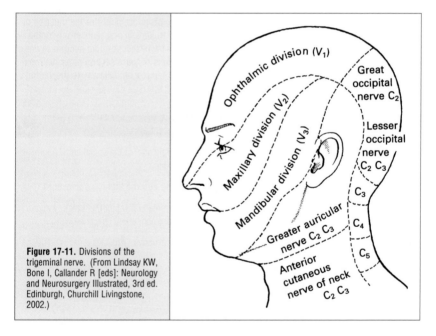

Figure 17-11. Divisions of the trigeminal nerve. (From Lindsay KW, Bone I, Callander R [eds]: Neurology and Neurosurgery Illustrated, 3rd ed. Edinburgh, Churchill Livingstone, 2002.)

5. **If surgical sectioning of the involved branch were performed in this woman, what modalities of sensation would we expect to be impaired?**
   All modalities of sensation would be lost in the distribution of the mandibular division in this woman because the trigeminal nerve conveys all sensory information from the face (i.e., pain, temperature, fine touch, vibration, and proprioception). These trigeminal nerve afferents then synapse in

the appropriate subdivision of the trigeminal brainstem complex: the principal sensory nucleus for tactile sensation, the spinal nucleus for pain and temperature, and the mesencephalic nucleus for proprioceptive information from the muscles of mastication. (The trigeminal brainstem complex is extensive, spanning from the midbrain to upper cervical spinal cord.)

6. **Why might therapy with carbamazepine (Tegretol) make sense for this woman?**
   Carbamazepine is an anticonvulsant medication that is also used for trigeminal neuralgia and is prescribed for treating neuropathic pain of almost any etiology. It acts by reducing the rate of nerve transmission by inhibiting voltage-gated sodium channels in neurons.

SUMMARY BOX: TRIGEMINAL NEURALGIA

- Diagnose by history: Attacks of sharp pain, often unilaterally, involve one division of the trigeminal nerve and are accompanied by facial spasm or tic.

- Trigeminal nerve anatomy: Pseudounipolar neurons in the trigeminal ganglion provide motor innervation to muscles of mastication and sensory innervation to the anterior two thirds of the head. Three sensory divisions exit the cranium through different foramina.

- First-line therapy for trigeminal neuralgia is with carbamazepine, an anticonvulsant that inhibits voltage-gated sodium channels.

CASE 17-7

A woman who had been previously diagnosed with a megaloblastic anemia and put on folic acid supplements presents complaining of confusion, difficulty remembering things, depression, and a feeling of pins and needles in her extremities for the past few months. Physical examination is notable for the absence of papillae over much of the surface of the tongue (atrophic glossitis), positive Romberg sign, and bilateral Babinski signs. Laboratory tests reveal an elevated methylmalonic acid and a normal fasting plasma glucose. An MRI of the brain appears normal.

1. **What should you reflexively think of when you see "megaloblastic anemia" on boards?**
   Try to make a quick association with vitamin B_{12} or folate deficiency. There are a number of ways to become deficient in vitamin B_{12} or folate, such as malnutrition, chronic alcoholism, or malabsorption, but the initial association will help you focus. Because we know the patient is taking folic acid, vitamin B_{12} deficiency seems likely.

2. **What findings might you see on a peripheral blood smear from a patient deficient in folate or vitamin B_{12}?**
   If you are given a blood smear, you likely will see large, immature, oval red blood cells (RBCs) (remember, you can use a lymphocyte as a scale for judging RBC size) and hypersegmented (five or more visible segments of the nucleus) polymorphonuclear neutrophils (PMNs).

3. **Why would both vitamin B_{12} and folate deficiency cause a preponderance of large, immature red blood cells (macro-ovalocytes) on a blood smear?**
   Vitamin B_{12} and folate are needed for production of the nucleotide precursors of deoxyribonucleic acid (DNA), specifically, the conversion of dUMP $\rightarrow$ dTMP (deoxyuridine monophosphate to thymidine monophosphate) and of homocysteine $\rightarrow$ methionine. When DNA synthesis is

impaired by vitamin B_{12} or folate deficiency, cell division is blocked while ribonucleic acid (RNA) and protein synthesis continue. The expanding cytoplasmic volume and prevention of mitosis lead to large, immature RBCs.

4. **How is a positive Romberg sign elicited on examination? Why might vitamin B_{12} deficiency give rise to a positive Romberg sign?**
To elicit the sign, ask the patient to stand with her feet close together. If she is steady and not swaying when her eyes are open, but sways or falls when you ask her to close her eyes, this is a positive Romberg sign. A positive sign indicates proprioceptive sensory loss that can be compensated for by visual input but becomes apparent when visual input is removed. In this case, the proprioceptive loss is due to demyelination of the dorsal columns. Recall that vitamin B_{12} deficiency leads to a buildup of propionyl coenzyme A (CoA), which prevents normal myelination from occurring.
Note: It is a common misconception that a positive Romberg sign indicates cerebellar dysfunction, but this is not the case.

5. **Given the atrophic glossitis and neurologic symptoms, what is the likely diagnosis?**
This patient most likely has a vitamin B_{12} deficiency neuropathy (subacute combined degeneration). Vitamin B_{12} deficiency can cause a megaloblastic anemia, which can be corrected with folic acid supplementation. However, folic acid supplementation does not prevent the neurologic manifestations of vitamin B_{12} deficiency. Therefore, in a patient with megaloblastic anemia, both serum folate and vitamin B_{12} levels should be tested, and both vitamins should be supplemented. Should the patient become pregnant, adequate folate supplementation also helps prevent neural tube defects in the fetus. However, note that *folate deficiency does not cause neurologic dysfunction*.

6. **What is a positive Babinski sign and what does it indicate?**
As was mentioned in the Basic Concepts section of this chapter, a positive Babinski sign refers to spontaneous dorsiflexion of the big toe upon stroking the lateral plantar surface of the foot from the heel toward the big toe. It indicates an upper motor neuron lesion and likely represents demyelination of the corticospinal tracts in this patient.
Note: Positive Babinski signs are normal in infants (up to 12 months) because of inadequate myelination at this time in life. Suppression of the Babinski reflex by higher brain centers is a prerequisite for learning to walk.

7. **What is the value of obtaining a fasting plasma glucose level in this patient?**
Diabetic neuropathy has paresthesias and sensory loss similar to that seen with vitamin B_{12} deficiency, and generally presents in a "stocking and glove" pattern (meaning that the symptoms commonly appear initially in the feet and lower legs and then in the hands, both bilaterally).

8. **What is the value of obtaining a methylmalonic acid level?**

$$\text{Propionyl CoA} \rightarrow \text{Methylmalonyl CoA} \rightarrow \text{Succinyl CoA}$$

In the fatty acid metabolic pathway shown here, vitamin B_{12} is a cofactor for the conversion of methymalonyl CoA to succinyl CoA. Thus, vitamin B_{12} deficiency causes a buildup in propionyl CoA and methylmalonyl CoA. A serum methylmalonic acid level is the *most sensitive test* for vitamin B_{12} deficiency.
As an aside, propionyl CoA replaces acetyl CoA in neurons, possibly accounting for the neurologic symptoms that occur with vitamin B_{12} deficiency. However, the lack of methionine and *S*-adenylmethionine might also contribute to the neurologic dysfunction (do not worry about this for Step 1).

9. **Given the paresthesias, and positive Romberg and Babinski signs, where is the anatomic lesion?**

Vitamin B$_{12}$ neuropathy, also called *subacute "combined" degeneration*, can cause degeneration of both the lateral corticospinal tract and the dorsal columns. Lesions of the latter lead to paresthesias; upper motor neuron loss in the corticospinal tract leads to a positive Babinski sign and spasticity. Lesions of the dorsal columns lead to proprioceptive dysfunction. Tabes dorsalis (tertiary syphilis) also results in degeneration of the dorsal columns, leading to a positive Romberg sign and sensory ataxia. Tabes dorsalis is associated with an Argyll Robertson pupil (a pupil that can accommodate but does not react to light).

Vitamin B$_{12}$ deficiency is commonly seen in pernicious anemia (autoimmune gastritis) and in patients who have had surgical resection of the terminal ileum (e.g., patients with Crohn's disease).

SUMMARY BOX: VITAMIN B$_{12}$ (COBALAMIN) DEFICIENCY

- This deficiency can present as some combination of paresthesias, proprioceptive dysfunction, cognitive changes, and corticospinal tract dysfunction.

- Vitamin B$_{12}$ is important for DNA synthesis. Its deficiency can cause megaloblastic anemia, with macro-ovalocytes and hypersegmented polymorphonuclear neutrophils (PMNs) (as can folate deficiency).

- Folate acid supplementation will treat the anemia but *not* the neurologic symptoms.

- An increased serum methylmalonic acid level is highly sensitive for vitamin B$_{12}$ deficiency.

CASE 17-8

A 32-year-old woman presents complaining of a recent episode of visual impairment in which she was temporarily unable to see out of her right eye and felt extremely dizzy and nauseated. Upon examination, her funduscopic and neurologic examinations are normal. She asks you whether she might have MS.

1. **Why is it impossible to make a definite diagnosis of multiple sclerosis at this time?**

A hallmark of MS is its variability over time. To make a definite diagnosis of this disease, one needs to see a larger picture of recurrent attacks of neurologic dysfunction. One episode, especially one that presents as classically as it does here (and as it will on boards)—a young adult woman with optic neuritis and vertigo—may raise a suspicion of MS, but it is insufficient to make a diagnosis.

STEP 1 SECRET

The USMLE loves to test students on multiple sclerosis. Be sure to pay close attention to the details of this case.

CASE 17-8 continued:

The patient returns 1 year later and describes episodes of sudden-onset clumsiness, due to weakness of her left leg, slight tremor with movement, frequent bladder incontinence, and numbness and tingling sensations in her right arm. The episodes were occasionally accompanied by double vision. She has experienced three such episodes over the past year, each lasting about 2 weeks. Ocular examination demonstrates intact convergence. However, when she is asked to look left, her left eye abducts while her right eye stays at midline, and when she is asked to look right, her right eye abducts while her left eye stays at midline. There is also bilateral nystagmus of the abducting eye.

2. **Where is the lesion underlying her oculomotor abnormalities?**
   The lesion is likely in the medial longitudinal fasciculus (MLF). The MLF is a white matter tract in the brainstem that connects the abducens cranial nerve (CN VI) nucleus with the contralateral oculomotor (CN III) nucleus, allowing for conjugate gaze. Lesions of the MLF can cause *internuclear ophthalmoplegia* that manifests as diplopia, as seen here. The pathology of MLF syndrome is further described in Chapter 18.
   Note: Bilateral internuclear ophthalmoplegia is pathognomonic for MS.

CASE 17-8 continued:

Given the constellation of episodes and symptoms, you order some studies. MRI reveals periventricular plaques in the brain. CSF analysis reveals the presence of oligoclonal immunoglobulin bands (absent in the serum), elevated immunoglobulin G (IgG), and myelin basic protein.

3. **What is the diagnosis at this time?**
   The patient's time course of symptoms, MRI, and CSF findings are definitive for diagnosis of MS, an autoimmune disease that involves demyelination of various white matter areas of the CNS. This occurs secondary to T-cell recognition of myelin basic protein as an antigen, which results in T-cell activation, cytokine production, and subsequent activation of macrophages and B cells. This sequence of events further destroys myelin sheaths and oligodendrocytes (myelin-producing cells of the CNS) in a type IV hypersensitivity reaction. In addition, MS may involve production of autoantibodies against the myelin sheath and oligodendrocytes.
   MS can have a relapsing and remitting course (as in this patient) or a chronically progressive course. The various neurologic manifestations that develop are due to inflammation and demyelination at different sites within the CNS.
   MRI classically shows multiple plaques in different areas of white matter, most notably in the periventricular areas. Oligoclonal immunoglobulin bands on electrophoresis of CSF are a sign of demyelination.

4. **What cell type is attacked and destroyed in multiple sclerosis?**
   As mentioned in the preceding discussion, oligodendrocytes are attacked by $CD8^+$ T cells. In contrast, Schwann cells, which provide myelination in the peripheral nervous system, are spared in MS. However, Schwann cells are attacked in Guillain-Barré syndrome.
   Note: One oligodendrocyte can myelinate many neurons, but one Schwann cell can myelinate only one neuron.

5. **Is there any reason to consider the diagnosis of Guillain-Barré syndrome in this patient?**
   No. This patient's symptoms are not consistent with Guillain-Barré syndrome, which classically presents as an ascending muscle paralysis that begins in the distal lower extremities. It typically follows an acute infectious process, and is most commonly associated with *Campylobacter*

jejuni infection due to autoimmune attack of peripheral myelin, which resembles *Campylobacter* proteins (molecular mimicry). Although Guillain-Barré is similar to MS in being an *inflammatory demyelinating disease*, it does not involve alterations in the CNS (e.g., demyelinated plaques in the brain). Rather, it is due to demyelination of the peripheral nerves. Laboratory findings include increased protein in the CSF and a normal cell count. Papilledema may result secondary to increased CSF oncotic pressure. In addition, patients may present with severe irregularities in autonomic system function. Finally, you should remember that Guillain-Barré is an acute illness and thus does not relapse and remit as MS does.

6. **Would electromyography reveal slow, fast, or normal peripheral nerve conduction velocity in this woman?**
   Myelinated nerve fibers conduct impulses faster than unmyelinated nerve fibers, but because the peripheral nerves are not subject to demyelination in MS, the conduction speed of peripheral nerves would not be altered in this patient. However, in Guillain-Barré syndrome, there may be a reduction in nerve conduction velocity due to peripheral nerve demyelination.

7. **Would you expect patients with multiple sclerosis to show signs of upper or lower motor neuron lesions when the motor system is involved?**
   They will show UMN signs, because MS involves white matter in the brain and spinal cord and does not affect LMNs.

8. **Given the inflammatory basis of the disease, what treatment might be considered?**
   Interferon-β is considered first-line therapy and has been shown to decrease the rate of relapse. Immunosuppressive drugs are also given to decrease the progression of MS. However, there is no known effective treatment to decrease the severity of attacks once they occur.

SUMMARY BOX: MULTIPLE SCLEROSIS

- The classic patient is a young woman presenting with multiple episodes of neurologic dysfunction, such as limb paresthesias, motor weakness, and visual impairment due to optic neuritis or internuclear ophthalmoplegia. Other symptoms of multiple sclerosis (MS) include bladder/bowel incontinence, intention temor, and sensory deficits on one side of the body.

- The pathogenesis involves an autoimmune attack on oligodendrocytes, leading to inflammation and demyelination in the central nervous system (CNS) (*not* the peripheral nervous system).

- Laboratory findings include elevated IgG level and myelin basic protein in cerebrospinal fluid (CSF) and oligoclonal bands on CSF electrophoresis. Brain MRI classically reveals diffuse periventricular white matter plaques.

- Gross findings are demyelinating plaques in brain and spinal cord white matter, especially in periventricular regions.

CASE 17-9

A 70-year-old man presents with acute-onset paralysis and loss of sensation in his left leg, with slight weakness in the left arm. His past medical history is notable for hypertension, hyperlipidemia, and a 40-pack-year history of cigarette smoking.

1. **What is the most likely diagnosis?**
   The patient's age and symptom severity should raise immediate suspicion for a stroke. There are two major classifications of stroke: ischemic and hemorrhagic. In the absence of other information, you should reason that ischemic stroke is more likely than hemorrhagic stroke, simply because ischemic stroke is the more common of the two types of stroke. Note that transient ischemic attack (TIA) should also be considered, particularly if his symptoms resolved quickly, and no lesions were found on imaging.

   CASE 17-9 continued:

   An emergent non-contrast computed tomography (CT) scan of the brain is performed and does not reveal any intracranial bleeding. MRI is subsequently performed, and the site of arterial occlusion is identified. The patient is examined and questioned for contraindications to treatment with tissue plasminogen activator (tPA) (e.g., severe hypertension, recent gastrointestinal [GI] bleeding, intracranial bleeding, recent surgery) and is cleared for thrombolytic therapy.

2. **Why is the lack of intracranial bleeding on computed tomography important?**
   Prior to administering tPA, it is important to rule out intracranial hemorrhage using CT, because any thrombolytic therapy could exacerbate active or recent bleeding. This is why thrombolytic therapy is contraindicated in hemorrhagic stroke.

3. **What are some possible causes of intracranial hemorrhage?**
   There are four main categories of intracranial hemorrhage that you must know for boards. Epidural hemorrhage is due to rupture of the middle meningeal artery, which is most commonly attributed to temporoparietal bone fracture (e.g., blow to the head). This type of hemorrhage presents with a lucid interval in which the patient briefly loses consciousness, appears asymptomatic for a bit, and then deteriorates again. Look for the presence of a biconvex disk that does not cross suture lines on CT scan.
   Subdural hemorrhage is attributed to rupture of the bridging veins that extend between the dura and the arachnoid layers. This is generally due to blunt/generalized trauma or anticoagulation. The elderly are particularly susceptible to subdural hemorrhage because the stretched bridging veins, due to brain atrophy, are more susceptible to injury. Shaken baby syndrome also predisposes to subdural hemorrhage. Look for the presence of a crescent sign that is capable of crossing suture lines on CT scan.
   Subarachnoid hemorrhage (SAH) is generally attributed to arteriovenous malformation or a ruptured aneurysm. Suspect aneurysm rupture in patients with connective tissue disorders or adult polycystic kidney disease. Look for a star-shaped area of hemorrhage on CT scan.
   The fourth type of intracranial hemorrhage to know for boards is parenchymal hematoma, which results from vessel rupture secondary to hypertension or amyloid angiopathy. Note that hypertension is a risk factor for both hemorrhagic and ischemic stroke.

STEP 1 SECRET

You should expect to have at least one question on causes of intracranial hemorrhage. We will consider this topic in greater detail later in the chapter.

4. **Why is the patient's history of hypertension, hyperlipidemia, and smoking important to the etiology of ischemic stroke?**
   Ischemic strokes result predominantly from atherosclerosis and subsequent thromboembolic phenomena either intra- or extracranially. Hypertension, hyperlipidemia, and smoking all increase the risk of ischemic stroke by contributing to a state of vascular endothelial damage, hypercoagulability, and inflammation.

5. **How does atrial fibrillation predispose to stroke?**
    Atrial fibrillation makes it easier for blood to pool and clot within the atria, and the clots can then embolize to the brain. This is why patients with atrial fibrillation are routinely put on the anticoagulant warfarin.

6. **How does myocardial infarction predispose to stroke?**
    Similar in concept to atrial fibrillation, inefficient ventricular ejection after myocardial infarction can lead to clotting and subsequent embolus. For this reason, patients who have akinesis or severe hypokinesis of the left ventricle following a myocardial infarction are often placed on the anticoagulant warfarin (Coumadin).

7. **Where does intracerebral vessel rupture due to hypertension occur most often?**
    Branches of the lenticulostriate vessels, which supply the basal ganglia, often develop aneurysms that may rupture. These are referred to as Charcot-Bouchard microaneurysms and most commonly affect the thalamus and basal ganglia. Note that these regions of the brain are especially prone to ischemia.

8. **Given the patient's loss of sensation in his left leg, what artery was probably occluded in this patient?**
    The right anterior cerebral artery or branches thereof were likely occluded because this artery serves the motor and sensory cortex that is devoted to the contralateral (left) leg (Fig. 17-12).

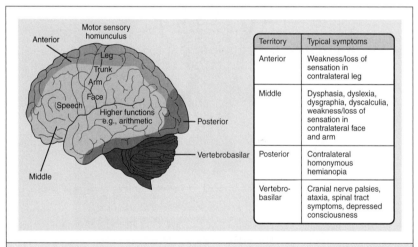

Territory	Typical symptoms
Anterior	Weakness/loss of sensation in contralateral leg
Middle	Dysphasia, dyslexia, dysgraphia, dyscalculia, weakness/loss of sensation in contralateral face and arm
Posterior	Contralateral homonymous hemianopia
Vertebro-basilar	Cranial nerve palsies, ataxia, spinal tract symptoms, depressed consciousness

Figure 17-12. Cerebral artery territories and symptoms of strokes in those areas. (From Mihailoff GA: Crash Course: Nervous System. Philadelphia, Mosby, 2005.)

9. **What motor and sensory abnormalities might develop from occlusion of the middle cerebral artery or its branches?**
    The middle cerebral artery supplies the motor and sensory cortex for the contralateral upper extremity, head, neck, and face, so occlusion can cause abnormalities in this distribution.

10. **If someone suddenly developed difficulty understanding or articulating speech due to an ischemic stroke, branches of which major cerebral artery are most likely occluded?**
    The middle cerebral artery on the dominant (typically the left) side of the brain, which controls speech, is likely occluded. Difficulty understanding speech (*receptive aphasia*) results from

lesions in Wernicke's area of the *temporal lobe* and is called *Wernicke's aphasia*. Although people with this lesion can articulate, their speech is devoid of logical structure and often amounts to what is called a "word salad." Difficulty articulating speech (*expressive aphasia*), without impaired comprehension, is due to a lesion in Broca's area of the *frontal lobe* and is called *Broca's aphasia*. Global aphasia impairs both Wernicke's and Broca's areas, such that patients have difficulty articulating words and have impaired comprehension. On the other hand, conduction aphasia, which affects the arcuate fasciculus that connects Broca's and Wernicke's areas, impairs neither speech nor comprehension (Fig. 17-13). These patients have trouble with speech repetition.

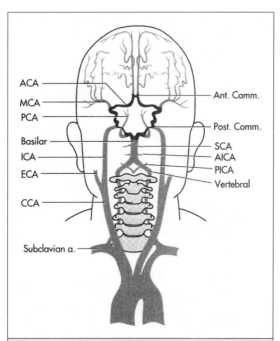

Figure 17-13. Coronal view of the extracranial and intracranial arterial supply to the brain. ACA, anterior cerebral artery; AICA, anterior inferior cerebellar artery; Ant. Comm., anterior communicating artery; CCA, common carotid artery; ECA, external carotid artery; ICA, internal carotid artery; MCA, middle cerebral artery; PCA, posterior cerebral artery; PICA, posterior inferior cerebellar artery; Post. Comm., posterior communicating artery; SCA, superior cerebellar artery. (From Andreoli TE: Cecil Essentials of Medicine, 5th ed. Philadelphia, WB Saunders, 2001.)

11. **How might occlusion of the right posterior cerebral artery or its branches cause loss of the left visual field of each eye (left homonymous hemianopia)?**
   - The posterior cerebral artery supplies the visual cortex in the occipital lobe. The visual cortex on the right receives sensory input from the nasal retina of the left eye and the temporal retina of the right eye, each of which receives sensory information from the left visual field.
   - A branch of each posterior cerebral artery also supplies the lateral geniculate nucleus on the same side, which is the major relay center from the optic tract to the visual cortex.

12. **Why does occlusion of the most proximal segment of the anterior cerebral artery typically not result in stroke symptoms?**
    If the occlusion is proximal to the anterior communicating artery, collateral blood flow from the contralateral anterior cerebral artery through the communicating artery can prevent a perfusion deficit.

STEP 1 SECRET

It is important to know the arrangement of blood vessels that supply the brain and spinal cord. The USMLE will commonly ask second- or third-order questions for which the answer depends on the student's ability to correctly identify cerebral blood vessels on an angiogram.

13. **In a sudden hypotensive episode, what regions of cerebral circulation are particularly susceptible to infarction and why?**
    Watershed areas, or the bordering zones between regions of the brain that are supplied exclusively by an artery such as the anterior or middle cerebral artery, for example, are particularly susceptible.

14. **What mechanism exists to protect the brain tissue from inadequate perfusion during systemic hypotension?**
    The cerebral circulation is "autoregulated." With activation of either vasodilation or vasoconstriction, cerebral blood flow remains constant over a mean arterial pressure range of 60 mm Hg to 140 mm Hg. This autoregulatory mechanism also protects the brain from *excessive* arterial pressure, which can cause vascular rupture and hemorrhage.

15. **Describe the gross pathologic findings in stroke.**
    Classic findings include a wedge-shaped area of pale (in ischemic stroke) or hemorrhagic infarction that develops first at the periphery of the cerebral cortex. The brain undergoes liquefactive necrosis with potentially dangerous swelling. Then, myelin will break down, causing loss of demarcation between the gray and white matter. Astrocytes will proliferate near the infarct as a reaction to injury, and microglia cells (macrophage-like cells for the brain, derived from mesenchymal lineage) will remove debris from liquefactive necrosis. After many days to weeks, cystic areas may develop.

SUMMARY BOX: CEREBROVASCULAR ACCIDENTS

- The two types of cerebrovascular accidents, or strokes, are ischemic and hemorrhagic. Hemorrhagic strokes must be ruled out with a computed tomography (CT) scan to determine whether the patient is eligible for thrombolytic therapy.

- Major risk factors are hypertension, smoking, hyperlipidemia, and atherosclerosis.

- Recent surgery, recent gastrointestinal (GI) bleeding, intracranial bleeding, and severe hypertension are contraindications to thrombolytic therapy.

CASE 17-10

A 37-year-old man presents to the emergency room (ER) complaining of the "worst headache of his life." On questioning, he also complains of nausea, vomiting, and discomfort to bright lights (photophobia). On physical examination, he has a stiff neck (nuchal rigidity).

1. **What is the classic cause of the "worst headache of one's life," especially in association with the other symptoms presented here?**
   This presentation is classic for SAH. Though atypical presentations are common clinically, Step 1 boards will use a classic presentation.

2. **If the patient presented with hematuria, bitemporal hemianopia, and impaired renal function, why would subarachnoid hemorrhage be more strongly suspected?**
   This patient may have polycystic kidney disease, which is associated with berry (also known as saccular) aneurysms, which occur most commonly at the bifurcation of the anterior communicating artery. Berry aneurysms of the anterior communicating artery can compress the optic chiasm and cause visual deficits.

3. **What is the first step that should be taken to diagnose this patient?**
   A CT scan should be performed first, as it can be done quickly and is reasonably sensitive for the detection of SAH.

CASE 17-10 continued:

A CT scan is performed and shows blood in the basal cisterns (areas of expansion of the subarachnoid space, located rostral to the pons and between the temporal lobes). Subsequently, cerebral angiography is performed and localizes the site of bleeding.

4. **If a computed tomography scan did not reveal any characteristic bleeding into the subarachnoid space, what other diagnostic test can be done to establish the diagnosis of subarachnoid hemorrhage?**
   A lumbar puncture should be performed if the CT scan is negative or equivocal. Blood found in the CSF, which is sampled from the subarachnoid space, supports a diagnosis of SAH.
   Note: Because the spinal cord terminates at the level of L1-L2 in adults, lumbar punctures are performed at the level of the L3-L4 or L4-L5 interspace. An external landmark to use to locate the L4 spinous process is the iliac crest.

5. **Why does subarachnoid hemorrhage cause headache, nuchal rigidity, photophobia, and nausea/vomiting?**
   The headache, photophobia, and nuchal rigidity are caused by meningeal irritation; blood is very irritating to the meninges. Nausea and vomiting are due to increased intracranial pressure and meningeal irritation.

6. **What are some common causes of subarachnoid hemorrhage?**
   As was mentioned in Case 17-9, common causes of SAH include ruptured berry aneurysm, ruptured arteriovenous malformation, and head trauma. Ruptured aneurysm is the most common cause of SAH, though head trauma is also a common cause of SAH. Berry aneurysms can be congenital or acquired.

7. **What are some major risk factors for acquired berry aneurysms?**
   Hypertension and cigarette smoking are major modifiable risk factors. Family history and connective tissues disorders are also risk factors for SAH.

8. **Where do berry aneurysm typically develop and why?**
They often develop in the circle of Willis, at the junction of communicating arteries with main cerebral arteries. This is because these junctions lack an internal elastic lamina and have an attenuated tunica media. The most common site is the junction containing the anterior cerebral artery (Fig. 17-14).

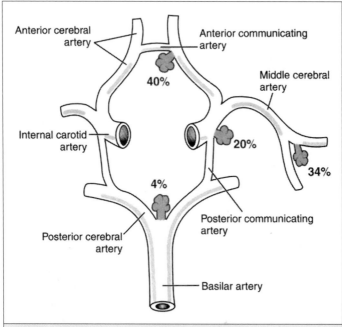

Figure 17-14. Frequency of aneurysmal sites. (From Cotran RS, Kumar V, Collins T: Robbins Pathologic Basis of Disease, 6th ed. Philadelphia, WB Saunders, 1999.)

SUMMARY BOX: SUBARACHNOID HEMORRHAGE

- Subarachnoid hemorrhage (SAH) classically presents with severe ("the worst of my life") headache, photophobia, meningeal irritation, and nausea/vomiting.

- Diagnostic studies include computed tomography (CT), followed by lumbar puncture.

- The most frequent cause is ruptured aneurysm.

- Hypertension, such as in the setting of polycystic kidney disease, predisposes one to develop berry aneurysms.

- Berry aneurysms frequently occur at the junctional points of the circle of Willis, especially in the anterior circulation.

CASE 17-11

The patient in the previous vignette managed to survive the SAH after some heroic neurosurgical procedures. However, several months later, he develops severe headaches and difficulty walking. Additionally, his wife now complains that his memory has become very poor and that he has difficulty paying attention to anything.

1. **What are some potential complications of subarachnoid hemorrhage?**
    The most worrisome acute complication is rebleeding, for which the risk is highest within a few days after the SAH presents. Later complications include hydrocephalus and delayed ischemia due to vasospasm at the site of a subarachnoid blood clot.

CASE 17-11 continued:

Ophthalmic examination shows papilledema, and a CT scan of the brain is as shown in Figure 17-15.

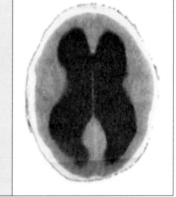

Figure 17-15. Massively dilated lateral ventricles. (From Lindsay KW, Bone I, Callander R: Neurology and Neurosurgery Illustrated, 3rd ed. Edinburgh, Churchill Livingstone, 2002.)

2. **What is the diagnosis?**
    He has hydrocephalus, most likely secondary to his SAH.
    Note: About a third of hydrocephalus cases in adults are idiopathic, and the remaining two thirds develop following meningitis, SAH, intracranial surgery, head injury, intracranial tumor, or congenital aqueductal stenosis. For example, an ependymoma is a tumor derived from the cells that line walls of the ventricular system, so its growth can easily obstruct CSF flow by compressing the cerebral aqueduct.

3. **How is cerebrospinal fluid produced and what is its function?**
    CSF is produced via an active secretory process (rather than mere filtration of plasma) by the choroid plexus of the lateral ventricles, third ventricle, and fourth ventricle. Its function is to cushion and suspend the brain and spinal cord, protecting these soft tissues from the compressing forces of gravity and their own weight.

4. **What is the pathway of cerebrospinal fluid flow?**
   CSF flows from the lateral ventricles into the third ventricle via the (intraventricular) foramen of Monro. From the third ventricle, it flows through the cerebral aqueduct (of Sylvius) into the fourth ventricle. From the fourth ventricle it then flows into the subarachnoid space via the *lateral* foramina of Luschka and the *medial* foramen of Magendie (Fig. 17-16).

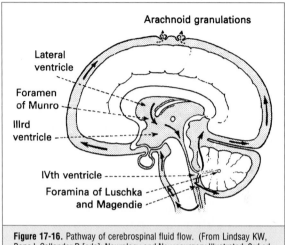

Figure 17-16. Pathway of cerebrospinal fluid flow. (From Lindsay KW, Bone I, Callander R [eds]: Neurology and Neurosurgery Illustrated, 3rd ed. Edinburgh, Churchill Livingstone, 2002.)

5. **How is cerebrospinal fluid reabsorbed?**
   CSF empties from the subarachnoid space into the dural venous sinuses via the arachnoid granulations. To be more specific, arachnoid granulations protrude into the superior sagittal sinus, which eventually drains into the internal jugular vein.

6. **What happens if the cerebral aqueduct is blocked?**
   This creates a backup of CSF in the ventricles, thereby enlarging the ventricles, compressing the brain, and possibly leading to headache and neurologic dysfunction. This type of hydrocephalus is called "noncommunicating" because the communication between the ventricular system and subarachnoid space is blocked. On CT scan or MRI study, the lateral and third ventricles are enlarged, but the fourth ventricle is normal in size because its outflow is not obstructed.

7. **In contrast with noncommunicating hydrocephalus, what is communicating hydrocephalus?**
   In communicating hydrocephalus, the communication between the ventricular system and subarachnoid space is preserved. In this case, hydrocephalus may be caused by excess production of CSF (which is rare) or by defective absorption of CSF (more common; may be caused by scarring of the arachnoid layer after meningitis). The overall increase in CSF leads to elevated intracranial pressure, which can result in bilateral papilledema and herniation. If not properly managed, papilledema can result in vision loss.

8. **What type of hydrocephalus does our patient, status post subarachnoid hemorrhage, likely have?**

   SAH and subsequent clotting of blood can cause fibrosis of the arachnoid granulations. This prevents effective outflow of CSF from the subarachnoid space, though the communication between the ventricular system and the subarachnoid space is preserved. Thus, this type of hydrocephalus is called obstructive communicating hydrocephalus.

SUMMARY BOX: HYDROCEPHALUS

- Cerebrospinal fluid (CSF) is secreted by the choroid plexus lining the ventricular system. CSF flow: lateral ventricles → foramen of Monro → third ventricle → cerebral aqueduct → fourth ventricle → foramina of Luschka and Magendie → subarachnoid space → arachnoid granulations → dural venous sinuses.

- Excess volume of CSF can cause expansion of the ventricular system and compression of the brain.

- Symptoms include headaches, ataxia, and neurologic deficits such as dementia. Nausea/vomiting, incontinence, and visual disturbances are also possible.

- Hydrocephalus can be communicating or noncommunicating, depending on whether communication between the ventricular system and subarachnoid space is open.

- Obstructive communicating type is a potential complication of subarachnoid hemorrhage.

CASE 17-12

A boy playing baseball gets hit on the left side of his head by a pitch and falls unconscious.

1. **What types of bleeds can result from blunt trauma to the head?**

   The major types of bleeds resulting from trauma to the head are epidural (extradural) or subdural in location. Epidural and subdural hemorrhage differ in the vessels involved and in clinical presentation. However, both can cause increased intracranial pressure, leading to herniation and death.

CASE 17-12 continued:

The boy quickly recovers consciousness and refuses to be taken to the hospital but agrees to sit out the rest of the game. After a few minutes he appears to act confused, lethargic, and disoriented, and an ambulance is called to take him to the hospital. Examination at the hospital shows a dilated left pupil. CT scan shows the presence of a rapidly expanding biconcave disk-shaped mass between the dura and the skull.

2. **What type of injury did this boy most likely sustain?**

   This is likely an epidural hematoma, which is the result of intracranial bleeding that dissects the periosteal layer of dura away from the cranium. The *lucid interval* (a period of clear consciousness between the initial blow and later changes in consciousness) seen here is classic for epidural hematoma.

3. **What are the three different layers of the meninges?**
The outermost layer is the dura mater ("dura" means tough or "durable") and is made of a fibrous connective tissue. The next layer is the arachnoid layer, which contains the subarachnoid space that CSF flows through and that blood vessels course through. The innermost layer is the pia mater, which is attached directly to the brain parenchyma.
   Note: Recall that the dura mater comprises two layers: a periosteal layer, adherent to bone, and a meningeal layer, continuous with the arachnoid mater. Because these two layers are normally also adherent to each other, no true space exists on either side of the dura under normal circumstances.

4. **What vascular structures are typically involved in an epidural hematoma?**
An epidural hematoma occurs when there is a rupture of a blood vessel, usually an artery, between the outermost membrane covering of the brain (the dura mater) and the skull. The middle meningeal artery is most commonly involved, and the rupture is associated with fracture of the temporoparietal bone overlying it.

5. **What vascular structures are typically involved in a subdural hematoma?**
The bridging veins that connect the subarachnoid space and the dural venous sinuses are severed. Subdural hematomas are more common in elderly people whose brains have atrophied. Because the atrophied brain can move around more in the skull, mild trauma such as a fall can tear these bridging veins more easily (Fig. 17-17).

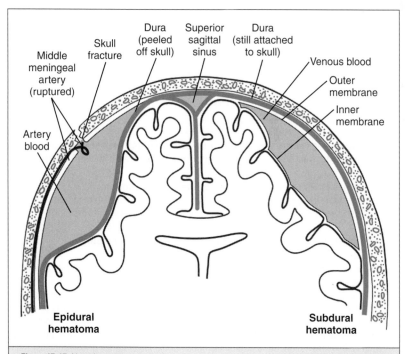

Figure 17-17. Vascular structures typically involved in a subdural hematoma. (From Kumar V, Abbas AK, Fausto N: Robbins and Cotran Pathologic Basis of Disease, 7th ed. Philadelphia, WB Saunders, 2005.)

6. **Why do the symptoms of subdural hematomas typically develop slowly?**
   Because these hematomas result from tearing of the low-pressure bridging veins, it takes more time for blood to accumulate and cause compressive symptoms.

7. **How does the radiographic appearance of a subdural hematoma differ from the biconcave disk shape of an epidural hematoma?**
   A subdural hematoma is crescent-shaped, following the contours of the skull, because flow of the hemorrhaged blood is not limited by the strong attachment points of the dura mater to the cranium at the cranial suture lines.

8. **Would cerebrospinal fluid analysis in this patient show multiple red blood cells?**
   No. Blood from an epidural bleed does not reach the subarachnoid space, where the CSF is located.

SUMMARY BOX: EPIDURAL AND SUBDURAL HEMATOMAS

- Epidural bleeding results from rupture of a high-pressure artery, most often the middle meningeal artery after temporal bone fracture.

- Epidural hematoma is associated with lucid intervals.

- Subdural hematomas are more common in the elderly and result from rupture of low-pressure bridging veins. The slow oozing of blood here implies that symptoms develop slowly.

- Epidural hematoma is a biconcave disk limited by suture lines. Subdural hematoma is crescent-shaped and not limited by suture lines.

- Both hematomas can eventually cause an altered level of consciousness, herniation, and death.

CASE 17-13

Upon awakening one morning, a 50-year-old neurologist realizes she cannot smile or grimace on her right side. Her initial worry is that she may have suffered a small stroke.

1. **Lesion of what cranial nerve might cause these symptoms?**
   Damage to the facial nerve (CN VII), which provides motor innervation to muscles of facial expression such as the orbicularis oris and platysma, can cause such symptoms.

2. **Assuming a stroke has caused these symptoms, where would the lesion be located?**
   She would have a lesion of the contralateral facial area of the motor cortex or its associated corticobulbar tract (i.e., an upper motor neuron lesion). The upper motor neurons of the facial motor cortex send fibers through the corticobulbar tract down to the facial motor nucleus. For upper motor neurons controlling the *upper face* (muscles such as orbicularis oculi and frontalis, necessary for blinking and frowning, respectively), there is *bilateral innervation* from both cerebral hemispheres. For upper motor neurons controlling the *lower face*, there is only *contralateral* innervation. So, unilateral disruption of the motor cortex or corticobulbar tract will cause paralysis of the lower face, but the other hemisphere can still provide adequate innervation and motor control to the upper face.

CASE 17-13 continued:

This neurologist then realizes that she cannot blink her right eye. While talking with her husband, she realizes that his voice seems louder than usual and is somewhat painful to listen to (hyperacusis). Her husband then takes her to the emergency room, where the examining physician detects an absent corneal reflex on the right and a lack of taste sensation in the anterior two thirds of the right side of her tongue.

3. **Given these findings, what is the likely diagnosis?**
   This patient likely has Bell's palsy (facial paralysis) caused by paralysis of the facial nerve (generally due to inflammation within the facial canal).

4. **What is causing the hyperacusis in this patient?**
   This is due to paralysis of the stapedius muscle, which functions to dampen the oscillations of the stapes footplate against the oval window. The facial nerve innervates the stapedius.

5. **Why is the corneal reflex absent in this woman?**
   The corneal reflex causes blinking of the eye when the cornea is touched. Touch sensation from the cornea is carried by the ophthalmic division (V_1) of the trigeminal nerve (afferent loop of the reflex). The efferent part of the reflex is carried by the facial nerve and causes contraction of orbicularis oculi. Because the facial nerve is paralyzed in this patient, the efferent part of the reflex is defective.

6. **Why is taste sensation absent from the anterior two thirds of the right side of this woman's tongue?**
   A branch of the facial nerve called the chorda tympani joins the lingual nerve (a division of the mandibular part of the trigeminal nerve). This path allows the chorda tympani to provide taste sensation to this part of the tongue.

STEP 1 SECRET

Innervation of the tongue is rather complicated, and it may be for that reason that the USMLE loves to ask questions about it. Touch sensation from the anterior two thirds of the tongue is mediated by CN V, while taste from the anterior two thirds of the tongue is mediated by CN VII. Touch and taste sensation of the posterior one third of the tongue is innervated by CN IX. The muscles of the tongue are innervated by CN XII.

7. **Why do the following produce symptoms similar to those seen in Bell's palsy?**
   - *Mumps infection:* The parotid gland, through which the facial nerve travels, becomes inflamed (parotitis) in mumps. Note that other viral infections such as herpes simplex virus (HSV) 1 and varicella zoster are also potential causative agents.
   - *Acoustic neuroma (schwannoma):* Acoustic neuromas (tumors of the Schwann cells of the eighth cranial nerve) commonly arise adjacent to where the facial nerve exits the pons. These tumors can compress the facial nerve at this location and should be suspected if a patient also presents with hearing loss or difficulties with balance.

8. **If this patient reported the recent development of palpitations, as well as a long-time passion for hiking, what diagnosis should be suspected?**
Bell's palsy and arrhythmias can represent the neurologic and cardiac manifestations of stage 2 Lyme disease. Recall that Lyme disease is caused by the spirochete *Borrelia burgdorferi* and transmitted by the *Ixodes* tick. Stage 2 Lyme disease occurs many weeks to months after transmission, so a recent episode of outdoor exposure need not have occurred.

SUMMARY BOX: BELL'S PALSY

- Paralysis of the facial nerve causes paralysis of the muscles of facial expression, loss of innervation to the stapedius, and loss of taste sensation in the anterior two thirds of the tongue.

- Potential causes include viral infections, acoustic neuroma, and Lyme disease.

- Upper motor neurons in the facial nerve nucleus provide bilateral cortical innervation for upper facial muscles and contralateral (unilateral) cortical innervation for lower facial muscles.

- Facial nerve paralysis can be distinguished from stroke by whether there is paralysis of upper facial muscles.

CASE 17-14

Steven is an 8-year-old boy who is brought to the neurologist by his concerned mother. His mother tells the neurologist that Steven occasionally experiences episodes during which he appears to lose consciousness and wets his pants. In addition, his whole body seems to become rigid. After a minute, his seemingly rigid body undergoes rhythmic jerks, and he simultaneously begins frothing at the mouth. After he stops seizing, his mother notes that Steven appears to be confused and lethargic for about an hour (postictal state).

1. **What kind of seizure does Steven seem to experience?**
A generalized tonic-clonic seizure (previously referred to as grand mal seizures) is likely. Patients who undergo this type of seizure typically experience loss of consciousness and whole body rigidity (tonic phase) followed by whole body jerks (clonic phase).

2. **If whole body rigidity is described as tonic, what happens in an atonic seizure?**
Atonic seizures, or "drop" seizures, are associated with sudden loss of muscle tone.

3. **What is the principal difference between a partial and a generalized seizure?**
A partial seizure begins focally within one cerebral hemisphere (although it may secondarily become generalized, it begins in one hemisphere). In contrast, a generalized seizure has its focus of onset diffusely throughout both hemispheres.

4. **What is the difference between a simple and a complex seizure?**
In a simple seizure, there is no alteration in consciousness. A complex seizure, by definition, implies alteration in consciousness.

5. Differentiate the seizure types listed in Table 17-1 in terms of their origin in the brain and any alteration in consciousness.
See Table 17-1 for these comparisons.

TABLE 17-1. SEIZURE TYPES

Seizure Type	Seizure Origin	Alteration in Consciousness
Partial	Focal (one cerebral hemisphere)	Yes *or* No
Simple partial	Focal	No
Complex partial	Focal	Yes
Generalized	Diffuse (both hemispheres)	Yes
Absence seizure	Diffuse	Yes
Tonic-clonic	Diffuse	Yes

6. What effects do most anticonvulsants have on neuronal firing?
They decrease the frequency of neuronal firing by increasing the threshold required for neuronal depolarization (i.e., they stabilize neuronal membranes). For most anticonvulsants, this is achieved by blocking sodium or calcium channels, but the benzodiazepines (e.g., diazepam) and barbiturates (e.g., phenobarbital) facilitate the inhibitory action of GABA by increasing chloride channel activity.

7. In Table 17-2, cover the right column and, looking at the side effects listed on the left, name the anticonvulsants best known for causing them.
Note: *Ethosuximide* is first-line therapy for *absence* seizures and blocks calcium channels. *Valproic acid* is first-line therapy for *tonic-clonic* seizures, with phenytoin and carbamazepine as good second-line options. Benzodiazepines are used as first-line agents for acute status epilepticus, in which the brain undergoes a state of persistent seizure. As this generally lasts for greater than 30 minutes, it can result in widespread neuronal death and be extremely damaging to the brain. Phenytoin is used as a first-line agent for prevention of status epilepticus.

TABLE 17-2. ANTICONVULSANTS AND THEIR SIDE EFFECTS

Side Effect(s)	Seizure Medication(s)
Agranulocytosis	Carbamazepine
Gingival hyperplasia, nystagmus, ataxia, cytochrome P-450 induction	Phenytoin
Hepatotoxicity	Valproic acid
Respiratory depression	Phenobarbital, diazepam
Stevens-Johnson syndrome	Lamotrigine, ethosuximide
Tremor	Gabapentin

STEP 1 SECRET

You should know key mechanisms and side effects for the anticonvulsant drugs, as well as which drugs are first-line agents for various seizure types.

8. **If this was the first seizure that Steven experienced, can he be diagnosed with epilepsy?**
   No. Epilepsy describes the presence of *recurrent, unprovoked seizures*. Unprovoked seizures are seizures that occur spontaneously, such that they are not secondary to infection (meningitis), toxic conditions (uremia), drug withdrawal (delirium tremors), fever (febrile seizures), head trauma, hyperventilation, or sleep deprivation. A diagnosis of epilepsy can be made only after a patient experiences another seizure and all possible other causes of seizure have been ruled out.

SUMMARY BOX: EPILEPSY

- Seizures can be accompanied by prodromal periods, autonomic dysfunction, and a postictal state of confusion or no memory of the event.

- Recurrent seizures must be documented and not provoked by an underlying medical condition to make the diagnosis.

- Seizures can be partial or generalized, depending on whether one or more than one area of the brain is involved.

- Seizures can be simple or complex, depending on whether consciousness is altered.

CASE 17-15

An 80-year-old woman has become increasingly demented over the past 10 years. She has difficulty remembering recent things (like where she put her keys) and recent conversations, but has a good memory of her earlier years. Her son, who accompanies her on her visit to the office, says that when relating events that have happened to her recently, she makes things up to fill in gaps in her memory but seems unaware that she is doing so (confabulation). Past medical history is negative for stroke, and there are no focal neurologic deficits on physical examination. A mini-mental status examination reveals that she is moderately demented.

1. **Assuming this woman is victim to the most common cause of dementia, what specific pathologic microscopic findings are characteristic of this disease at autopsy?**
   Neurofibrillary tangles and neuritic senile plaques are characteristic of Alzheimer's disease, the most common cause of dementia in the elderly. The plaques are extracellular aggregates of β-amyloid protein (a cleavage product of amyloid precursor protein), and the neurofibrillary tangles are cytoplasmic tangles of hyperphosphorylated tau protein. These changes are toxic to neurons.

2. **Why might this patient be at higher risk for intracerebral hemorrhage?**
   Deposition of β-amyloid protein in intracranial vessels (amyloid angiopathy) causes weakening of the vessel walls and may lead to intracranial hemorrhage.

3. **What is the second most common cause of dementia in the elderly and how does it arise?**
Multi-infarct (vascular) dementia occurs because of the cumulative effect of multiple small or large infarcts. It often presents with focal neurologic deficits because of the infarcts, which helps to differentiate it from Alzheimer's disease clinically.

4. **How would the pattern of cortical atrophy differ if this woman had Pick's disease rather than Alzheimer's disease?**
Pick's disease is characterized by selective atrophy of the frontal and temporal lobes, as opposed to the diffuse cerebral atrophy of Alzheimer's disease. In addition to dementia, symptoms of Pick's disease include parkinsonian aspects and personality changes. Intracellular tau protein aggregates called Pick bodies can be found at autopsy.

5. **What is the pathophysiologic rationale for treating Alzheimer's disease patients with cholinesterase inhibitors?**
In Alzheimer's disease, there is a selective destruction of cholinergic neurons (though other transmitter systems are variably affected). Cholinesterase inhibitors are believed to compensate for this to some degree by increasing the concentration and prolonging the action of acetylcholine in the synaptic cleft.
Note: Donepezil is a relatively new anticholinesterase used in Alzheimer's disease that does not have the hepatotoxic effects that tacrine does.

6. **If this woman also suffered from depression, as many Alzheimer's disease patients do, why should we avoid prescribing tricyclic antidepressants?**
Tricyclic antidepressants have powerful anticholinergic side effects that could exacerbate her cognitive decline due to Alzheimer's disease. The newer selective serotonin reuptake inhibitors (SSRIs) would therefore be a better choice for treating her depression.

7. **Based on what you know about the brain regions that are selectively destroyed in Alzheimer's disease, why would you expect long-term potentiation to be affected in these patients?**
Long-term potentiation, which occurs in the hippocampus (among other locations), is currently believed to be the mechanism by which neurons form "memories" of previous synaptic inputs of importance. The hippocampus is an early site of degeneration in Alzheimer's disease and this degeneration is believed to be one of the causes of the memory loss in these patients.

8. **Our patient's son worries that if his mother in fact does have Alzheimer's disease, he and his siblings might also get Alzheimer's disease. Is this likely to happen?**
No. Most cases of Alzheimer's disease are sporadic. About 10% of cases have a known genetic basis, usually associated with genes on chromosome 1, 14, 19, or 21.

9. **What important gene related to Alzheimer's is on chromosome 21? On chromosome 19?**
The gene encoding amyloid precursor protein (APP) is located on chromosome 21. APP is cleaved into Aβ-amyloid by β/γ-secretases. Extracellular Aβ-amyloid protein is responsible for the formation of senile plaques. Because Down syndrome patients have three copies of this chromosome and thus increased levels of APP, they are at high risk for early-onset (before age 40) Alzheimer's disease.
Chromosome 19 contains the apolipoprotein E gene. The E4 allele confers increased risk for late-onset Alzheimer's disease and thus accounts for some familial forms.
Note: Phosphorylated tau protein (insoluble cytoskeletal components) form the neurofibrillary tangles that are also seen in Alzheimer's patients. These tangles accumulate intracellularly and correlate directly with the degree of dementia that the patient has.

SUMMARY BOX: ALZHEIMER'S DISEASE

- Alzheimer's disease is the most common cause of dementia in the elderly; the second most common cause is multi-infarct (vascular) dementia.

- Alzheimer's disease is clinically distinguished by the presence/absence of focal neurologic deficits.

- Pathology involves defective degradation of amyloid precursor protein, leading to β-amyloid plaques, and hyperphosphorylated tau protein, leading to neurofibrillary tangles.

- Cholinesterase inhibitors are a potential treatment.

- This differs from Pick's disease in frontotemporal versus diffuse cortical atrophy.

- Amyloid can deposit in and weaken vessel walls, causing hemorrhage.

- Most forms are sporadic. Amyloid precursor protein (*APP*) and apolipoprotein E4 (*APOE4*) genes are important in familial forms.

- Down syndrome patients are at high risk for early-onset Alzheimer's disease.

CASE 17-16

A homeless alcoholic tries to gain admission to the hospital in order to get something to eat. He enters the ER and uses his usual trick of complaining about "pain all over." However, he also honestly admits that his memory is getting increasingly worse, and he has difficulty standing up when sober. After sitting in the ER for a few hours, he appears to be confused and irritable and complains of a headache. A quick blood glucose test reveals hypoglycemia.

1. **This patient was given intravenous (IV) glucose to relieve his hypoglycemic condition. Why should thiamine be administered just before administering glucose to this patient?**
   Thiamine (vitamin B_1) deficiency is commonly observed in alcoholics. Thiamine is a necessary cofactor for pyruvate dehydrogenase, which catalyzes the conversion of pyruvate (from glucose breakdown) to acetyl CoA. In the absence of thiamine, pyruvate (from glucose metabolism) is converted to lactic acid by lactate dehydrogenase, causing lactic acidosis within the CNS, which is detrimental to neuronal cells.

2. **What syndrome is most often caused by thiamine deficiency? What does each part of the syndrome's name mean?**
   Wernicke-Korsakoff syndrome is often found in chronic alcohol abuse. Acute CNS changes due to thiamine deficiency are called *Wernicke's encephalopathy*. These findings of confusion, ataxia, nystagmus, and ophthalmoplegia are *reversible*. However, chronic, *irreversible* CNS changes due to thiamine deficiency such as retrograde (as this patient complains of) and anterograde memory impairment, as well as confabulation, are called *Korsakoff's psychosis*.

3. **What brain regions are typically affected in Wernicke-Korsakoff syndrome?**
   Petechial hemorrhage and infarction often are seen in the mammillary bodies, thalamus, and periaqueductal gray matter (Fig. 17-18). The limbic system is also affected in Korsakoff psychosis.

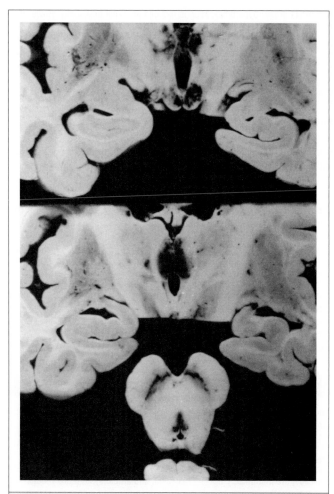

Figure 17-18. Wernicke's encephalopathy. Gross appearance of the brain characterized by petechial hemorrhages in the typical locations. (Reprinted with permission from Okazaki H: Fundamentals of Neuropathology, 2nd ed. New York, Igaku Shoin, 1989.)

4. **While our malingering alcoholic patient is in the hospital, he becomes agitated and develops anxiety, muscle cramps, tremors, delusions, and hallucinations. What is happening and what drugs could have been used to prevent/relieve these symptoms?**
He is going through alcohol withdrawal, the most severe manifestations of which are termed the delirium tremens. He could have been given long-acting benzodiazepines or barbiturates to prevent this.

5. **Explain why benzodiazepines and barbiturates are useful in treating alcoholic withdrawal.**
Alcohol, benzodiazepines, and barbiturates all bind to and activate the same receptor type, GABA$_A$. When activated, this receptor opens a chloride channel, resulting in hyperpolarization.

The net effect of this hyperpolarization is reduced neuronal excitability. However, if given for prolonged times or in large doses, any of these pharmacologic agents can cause downregulation of the GABAergic system. If these substances are then acutely withdrawn, the CNS loses inhibitory signals and becomes hyperexcitable. This causes manifestations similar to what this patient experienced. Consequently, the benzodiazepines and barbiturates are effective in treating withdrawal because they are essentially "alcohol substitutes."

Note: The longer-acting benzodiazepines and barbiturates cause significantly milder withdrawal symptoms than the short-acting agents. The benzodiazepine competitive antagonist flumazenil can be used for overdoses of benzodiazepines.

6. **How do the mechanisms of action of benzodiazepines and barbiturates differ?**
Benzodiazepines increase the *frequency* of chloride channel opening, whereas barbiturates increase the *duration* of chloride channel opening.

7. **Why do alcoholics often require a larger dose of benzodiazepines than healthy nonalcoholics in order to achieve the same pharmacologic effect?**
Alcoholics can develop *cross-tolerance* to other $GABA_A$ agonists. Alcohol consumption causes downregulation of the $GABA_A$ receptor, which makes $GABA_A$ agonists such as the benzodiazepines and barbiturates less effective.

8. **Why is it dangerous to discharge this alcoholic with a benzodiazepine or barbiturate prescription?**
Because this person is expected to resume alcohol abuse, the interactions of the benzodiazepines or barbiturates with alcohol can lead to respiratory depression and possibly even respiratory failure. Both drug classes also have a potential for dependence.

SUMMARY BOX: ALCOHOL AND RELATED DRUGS

- Thiamine (vitamin B_1) is an important cofactor for the production of adenosine triphosphate (ATP) from glucose.

- Thiamine deficiency, as seen in alcoholics, can cause Wernicke-Korsakoff syndrome, characterized by confusion, ataxia, ophthalmoplegia, and memory loss.

- Pathologically, the mammillary bodies, thalamus, and limbic system are affected in Wernicke-Korsakoff syndrome.

- Alcohol withdrawal can be treated with benzodiazepines or barbiturates, which act as $GABA_A$ agonists and affect chloride channels.

CASE 17-17

A 48-year-old woman presents complaining of a new-onset headache that is worse in the morning. She additionally complains of being nauseated and has vomited several times in the past few weeks. Funduscopic examination reveals papilledema.

1. **What does the clinical finding of papilledema in this woman represent?**
It represents edema of the optic disk, which is most commonly due to increased intracranial pressure, malignant hypertension, or central retinal vein occlusion.

2. **Why might a brain tumor present with these symptoms?**
Brain tumors often present with mass effects, meaning that the symptoms are related to the effect of a mass compressing the brain and raising the pressure within the restricted space of the skull. Mass effects include hydrocephalus, papilledema, nausea/vomiting, headache, and mental status changes. Tumors may also present with seizures, focal neurologic signs, or dementia.

3. **Given that our patient is an adult, what is the most likely location of a primary brain tumor? What about in a pediatric patient?**
Adult: Supratentorial, meaning that the tumor is located above the tentorium cerebelli (where the dura mater folds on itself, between the cerebrum and cerebellum
Child: Infratentorial, meaning that the tumor is located below the tentorium cerebelli

CASE 17-17 continued:

The neurologic examination reveals focal deficits with strength and sensory loss in her left arm. An MRI reveals a brain mass in the right cerebral hemisphere. An extensive workup does not reveal any primary tumor outside the CNS. A biopsy is then performed and reveals the diagnosis of astrocytoma.

4. **Prior to biopsy, why is a presumptive diagnosis of astrocytoma reasonable?**
Astrocytoma is the most common *primary* brain tumor in adults, although metastases are the most common sources of brain tumor *overall*. Biopsy must be done to distinguish between these two possibilities.

5. **What is the most unfortunate type of astrocytoma this patient could have?**
Glioblastoma multiforme carries the worst prognosis, with life expectancy under a year. Other lower grades of astrocytoma, such as juvenile pilocytic astrocytoma or anaplastic astrocytoma, may evolve into a glioblastoma multiforme.
Note: Glioblastoma multiforme has a characteristic *pseudopalisading arrangement* of tumor cells under the microscope and often crosses over into both hemispheres.

STEP 1 SECRET

When studying primary brain tumors, it will be helpful to focus on unique histologic characteristics of the tumor cells themselves.

6. **If our patient's computed tomography scan had shown calcifications in the intracranial mass, what tumor types might we suspect?**
Meningioma and oligodendrogliomas can both calcify and both often arise in the frontal lobe. Microscopically, meningiomas have a whorled pattern with psammoma bodies; oligodendrogliomas have a "fried egg" appearance.

7. **What is the second most common primary brain tumor in adults? In children?**
Adults: Meningioma, a benign tumor of arachnoid cells of the meninges. Because meningiomas are external to the brain, they can typically be resected easily during surgery.
Children: Medulloblastoma, a malignant tumor of the cerebellum. (Most common type in children is astrocytoma.)

8. **What pharmacologic property of drugs such as lomustine and carmustine make them more suitable for treatment of brain tumors?**
These drugs belong to a class of alkylating agents called nitrosoureas and can effectively penetrate the blood-brain barrier.

9. **What biophysical properties allow a drug to cross the blood-brain barrier?**
Generally, small, lipid-soluble, nonpolar molecules cross most easily.

SUMMARY BOX: BRAIN TUMORS

- Tumors in the brain often present with mass effects, seizures, focal neurologic signs, or dementia.

- Most brain malignancies metastasize from tumors in other organs, rather than from primary brain tumors.

- Most primary brain tumors are located above the tentorium in adults and below the tentorium in children.

- The most common type of brain tumor is astrocytoma.

- The second most common type of brain tumor is meningioma in adults and medulloblastoma in children.

- Drugs that are small, nonpolar, and lipid-soluble penetrate the blood-brain barrier most easily.

CASE 17-18

You are examining a 6-year-old child with a history of epilepsy, mental retardation, and cardiac murmur that was initially present at birth but resolved shortly there after. On physical examination, you note the presence of multiple, ovate, hypopigmented macules and a rough skin patch on the lower back.

1. **What is the most likely diagnosis in this child?**
Tuberous sclerosis, which is a rare, autosomal dominant neurocutaneous disorder that is marked by the presence of epileptogenic subependymal tubers. Patients with tuberous sclerosis commonly experience seizures and some degree of mental retardation. The dermatologic findings in this patient (hypopigmented ash-leaf spots and the shagreen patch on his back) strengthen our confidence in this the diagnosis.

2. **Patients with neurocutaneous disorders are generally at risk for several different types of tumors. What tumors are most commonly associated with tuberous sclerosis?**
Renal angiomyolipoma, cardiac rhabdomyoma, CNS hamartomas (including retinal glial hamartomas), and subependymal giant cell astrocytomas are associated with tuberous sclerosis. The history of cardiac murmur at birth that eventually resolved is good evidence that this child most likely had a cardiac rhabdomyoma, which often regresses spontaneously in these patients. Patients with tuberous sclerosis should be monitored regularly for evidence of these tumor types.

3. **If the patient in this case presented with hyperpigmented macules, pigmented nodules on the iris, and multiple neurofibromas covering the skin, what neurocutaneous disorder would you expect?**
This is a classic description of neurofibromatosis type I, which is characterized by café au lait spots, Lisch nodules, and multiple neurofibromas. It is an autosomal dominant disorder that results from a mutation on chromosome 17. In contrast, neurofibromatosis type II results from a mutation on chromosome 22 and presents with tinnitus and sensorineural deafness due to the presence of bilateral schwannomas (this tumor type often localizes to and impinges on CN VIII).

SUMMARY BOX: NEUROCUTANEOUS DISORDERS

- Symptoms of tuberous sclerosis result from the presence of subependymal tumors and include epilepsy, mental retardation, ash-leaf spots, and shagreen patches. Associated tumors include cardiac rhabdomyoma, renal angiomyolipoma, central nervous systems (CNS) hamartomas, and giant cell astrocytoma.

- Neurofibromatosis I presents with neurofibromas, café au lait spots, and Lisch nodules on the iris.

- Neurofibromatosis II presents with tinnitus and sensorineural deafness due to the formation of bilateral schwannomas that impinge on CN VIII.

CHAPTER 18

OPHTHALMOLOGY

Edmund Tsui, Thomas A. Brown, MD, and Sonali J. Shah

INSIDER'S GUIDE TO OPHTHALMOLOGY FOR THE USMLE STEP 1

All in all, ophthalmology is a fairly low-yield subject on boards, but there are specific topics that are known to appear quite frequently, particularly within the context of neurology. First Aid lists quite a bit of information under its ophthalmology section. This chapter points out which of that information is worth your time to study. As a general rule of thumb, you should know the pathways and lesions associated with visual perception, pupillary constriction, horizontal gaze, and extraocular eye muscle movement. We will highlight these for you within this chapter. The USMLE is far less focused on pathology of the eye, but you should at least have a general understanding of cataracts, glaucoma, and age-related macular degeneration (AMD).

We understand that visual pathways are quite confusing in the beginning, but we are here to help you simplify them. The best advice we can give you with regard to ophthalmology is to *actively* learn as much of this material as possible by diagramming the pathways as they appear throughout the chapter. This will make it much easier to reason through the deficits that occur when specific components of these pathways are lesioned. Assuming that you can understand all of this material by reading it without trying to actively test yourself may land you in an unfortunate spot on test day.

BASIC CONCEPTS

1. **Describe the course of visual information arriving from the left and right visual fields.**

   Light from the *left* visual field encounters the *right* half of each retina, temporally in the right eye and nasally in the left. Fibers from the temporal retina of the right eye travel in the right optic nerve and pass on the outside of the optic chiasm without any crossing. Fibers from the nasal retina of the left eye travel in the left optic nerve to the optic chiasm, where they cross to the other side and join the temporal fibers from the right eye to form the right optic tract. The *right* optic tract, which compromises the nasal fibers from the left eye (*left* visual field) and temporal fibers from the right eye (*left* visual field), synapses primarily in the right lateral geniculate nucleus (LGN) and in the Edinger-Westphal nucleus for pupillary reactions. Projections from the right LGN will then divide so that the left upper visual field information will travel through the temporal lobe and left lower visual field information will travel through the parietal lobe. These optic projections synapse in the right visual cortex within the occipital lobe. The visual information coming from the *right* visual field follows the same concepts as described for the left visual field but encounters the *left* half of each retina. The input from the two eyes is combined at the chiasm and travels to the left side of the brain (Figs. 18-1 and 18-2).

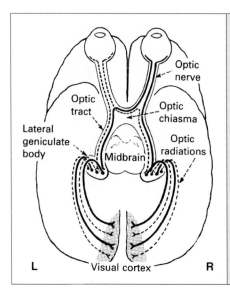

Figure 18-1. The left side (*L*) shows the course of sensory information from the left visual field. The right side (*R*) shows the course of sensory information from the right visual field. (From Lindsay KW, Bone I, Callander R: Neurology and Neurosurgery Illustrated, 3rd ed. Edinburgh, Churchill Livingstone, 2002.)

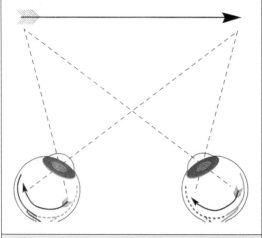

Figure 18-2. The temporal visual field information is received by the nasal retina, and the nasal visual field is received by the temporal retina. (From Nolte J: The Human Brain, 4th ed. St. Louis, Mosby, 1999.)

2. **What visual field defect results from midline sectioning of the optic chiasm? Explain.**

   Bitemporal hemianopia is a loss of the temporal (lateral) fields of vision in both eyes, resulting in "tunnel vision." Fibers from the nasal retina, which receive visual input from the contralateral temporal visual field, cross over in the optic chiasm and would be severed by a midline section of this structure or by a pituitary tumor. Figure 18-3 shows the visual field deficits resulting from lesions at various points in optic pathways.

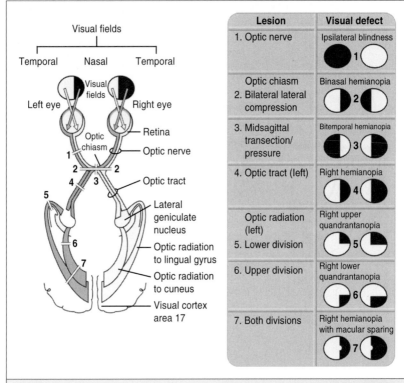

Lesion	Visual defect
1. Optic nerve	Ipsilateral blindness
Optic chiasm 2. Bilateral lateral compression	Binasal hemianopia
3. Midsagittal transection/ pressure	Bitemporal hemianopia
4. Optic tract (left)	Right hemianopia
Optic radiation (left) 5. Lower division	Right upper quadrantanopia
6. Upper division	Right lower quadrantanopia
7. Both divisions	Right hemianopia with macular sparing

Figure 18-3. The visual pathways, showing the consequences of lesions at various points. (From Brown TA: Rapid Review Physiology. Philadelphia, Mosby, 2007.)

STEP 1 SECRET

Boards may not openly make the diagnosis of bitemporal hemianopia for you when, for instance, describing a patient with a pituitary tumor. You will often have to arrive at this conclusion for yourself in the context of patient history. Be on the lookout for clues such as a patient's inability to see traffic on the left and the right (i.e., peripheral vision defect) when driving.

3. **What visual field deficit will occur with sectioning of the left optic tract and why?**
    Right homonymous hemianopia results from the loss of the right field of vision in both eyes. The left optic tract receives input from the right nasal retina and left temporal retina, both of which receive information from the right visual space (see Figs. 18-1 and 18-2).

4. **What visual field deficit is likely with a tumor in the right temporal lobe?**
    Left superior homonymous quadrantopia, loss of left upper quadrant of the visual field in both eyes ("pie in the sky"), would result. Temporal radiations from the right LGN travel through the temporal lobe on their way to the visual cortex. A tumor in this area will damage these fibers, causing loss of the contralateral superior quarter of the visual field from each eye. These patients might also experience seizures or olfactory hallucinations.

STEP 1 SECRET ✓

Visual field defects that result from damage to the optic nerve, optic chiasm, optic tract, lateral geniculate body, or occipital cortex are favorites on boards. Be sure to pay special attention to the side on which the damage occurs (left or right). Do not hesitate to diagram these pathways on your markerboard if you encounter one of these problems on test day.

5. **A physician shines a light into a patient's right eye and notes bilateral constriction of both pupils (normal response). Describe the pupillary light reflex.**
   When light is shone into the right eye, the photosensitive retinal ganglion cells of the right eye convey this information to the right optic nerve, which connects to the right pretectal nucleus of the upper midbrain. Axons then connect from the pretectal nucleus to the neurons in the right Edinger-Westphal nucleus, whose axons run along both right and left oculomotor nerves. The oculomotor nerves synapse on the ciliary ganglion neurons of each respective eye, which innervate the constrictor muscles of the irises. This stimulates bilateral pupillary constriction (Fig. 18-4).

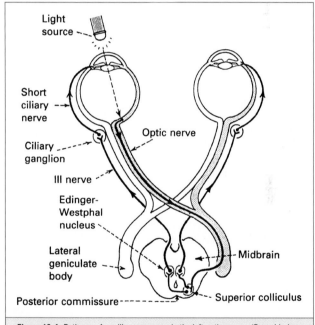

Figure 18-4. Pathway of pupillary response in the left optic nerve. (From Lindsay KW, Bone I, Callander R: Neurology and Neurosurgery Illustrated, 3rd ed. Edinburgh, Churchill Livingstone, 2002.)

6. **If there is a lesion in the left optic nerve, what would be the pupillary response if a light is shone into the right eye versus the left eye?**
   A. Right eye
      There will be pupillary constriction of both eyes, because the signal is transmitted from the right optic nerve to bilateral Edinger-Westphal nuclei. These nuclei then transmit the signal to the efferent part of the reflex arc (left and right oculomotor nerves), which is intact for both eyes. Oculomotor nerves signal to both pupillary constrictor muscles via the ciliary ganglia.

B. Left eye

There will be no pupillary response in either eye, because no signal is transmitted by the damaged left optic nerve to activate the reflex arc (Fig. 18-4).

7. **What will the pupillary response be to shining a light in either eye if there is a lesion in the left oculomotor nerve?**

Because both optic nerves and tracts and all the remainder of the afferent pathways are intact, regardless of which eye is getting the light, the right pupil will constrict, but because of the damaged left oculomotor nerve, the left pupil will not constrict. However, since the left oculomotor nerve conducts the efferent response to the left eye when light is shone in either the left or right eye, the left pupil will not constrict. (see Fig. 18-4).

8. **What is an Argyll Robertson pupil?**

An Argyll Robertson pupil demonstrates a normal near reflex (accommodation), but there is no reaction to light (pupil that "accommodates but does not react"). This is seen in patients with neurosyphilis damaging the Edinger-Westphal nucleus.

9. **If the oculomotor nerve is paralyzed on one side, why is the eyeball on that side rotated laterally and inferiorly ("down and out")?**

The oculomotor nerve innervates all the extraocular muscles other than the lateral rectus and superior oblique, which are innervated by the abducens nerve (CN VI) and the trochlear nerve (CN IV), respectively (remember the mnemonic LR_6SO_4). The lateral rectus moves the eyeball laterally, and the superior oblique rotates it inferiorly, giving the "down and out" position in oculomotor nerve palsy. Note that the pupil is also dilated, as would be expected in oculomotor nerve palsy.

STEP 1 SECRET

The pupillary light reflex and functions of the eye muscles are routinely tested on boards. You should know what happens with lesions of specific cranial nerves (e.g., damage to cranial nerve [CN] VI prevents lateral rectus action and leaves the medial rectus unopposed, such that the eye is permanently adducted). The functions of the extraocular muscles are listed for you in Table 18-1:

TABLE 18-1. FUNCTIONS OF EXTRAOCULAR MUSCLES

Extraocular Muscle	Innervation	Function(s)
Inferior rectus	CN III	Depression
		Extorsion
Superior rectus	CN III	Elevation
		Intorsion
Lateral rectus	CN VI	Abduction
Medial rectus	CN III	Adduction
Superior oblique	CN IV	Intorsion
		Depression
Inferior oblique	CN III	Extorsion
		Elevation
Levator palpebrae superioris	CN III	Elevates eyelid

10. **Describe the function of the medial longitudinal fasciculus.**

The medial longitudinal fasciculus (MLF) allows both eyes to move in the same direction in an attempt to track an object when one eye is stimulated. The horizontal gaze center, also called the paramedian pontine reticular formation (PPRF), is activated by the contralateral superior colliculus and frontal eye field. When the PPRF is activated, it sends a signal to the lower motor neurons of the ipsilateral abducens nucleus, which causes abduction of the ispilateral eye. The PPRF also stimulates the activity of internuclear neurons, which project via the MLF to the contralateral oculomotor nucleus. This activates the lower motor neurons of the oculomotor nucleus to cause adduction of the contralateral eye. Without the MLF, the contralateral eye would not be able to move in the same direction as for the ipsilateral (abducting) eye, a conjugate movement. Lesions of the MLF thus result in internuclear ophthalmoplegia, which leads to nystagmus of the abducting eye and complete lack of movement in the adducting eye. Internuclear ophthalmoplegia is associated with multiple sclerosis, which is discussed further in Chapter 17, Neurology.

Note: The MLF does not affect convergence, which is the simultaneous inward movement of both eyes toward one another (adduction) and is a disconjugate movement. Convergence is part of a triad that allows us to see nearby objects. The other two components of this triad are accommodation and pupillary constriction (Fig. 18-5).

11. **What is pathologic nystagmus?**

Pathologic nystagmus refers to an involuntary smooth pursuit movement of the eye in one direction followed by a saccadic movement in the opposing direction. It can occur with damage to the vestibular system, including the semicircular canals, and the vestibulocerebellum.

SUMMARY BOX: OPTIC PATHWAYS, VISUAL DEFICITS, PUPILLARY REFLEX

- Fibers from the nasal retina of each eye cross in the optic chiasm before merging with fibers in the contralateral optic tract, ultimately destined for the visual cortex of the contralateral occipital lobe.

- Visual hemifield information from both eyes is ultimately projected to the contralateral brain.

- Compression of the optic chiasm, as with an expanding pituitary tumor, can result in a bitemporal hemianopia.

- Sectioning of the optic tract results in a contralateral homonymous (same on both sides) hemianopia (half of visual field lost).

- A tumor in the temporal lobe can lead to contralateral homonymous superior quadrantopia ("pie in the sky"), seizures, and olfactory hallucinations.

- The pupillary (light) reflex arc consists of an afferent arm (the optic nerve), a central nervous system (CNS) integrator (Edinger-Westphal nucleus), and an efferent arm (parasympathetic fibers of oculomotor nerve). The normal light reflex is constriction of both pupils in response to light shined in either eye. Lesions in the optic and oculomotor nerves will affect the reflex in predictable ways.

- An oculomotor nerve palsy results in a "down and out" eyeball due to continued function of the lateral rectus (abducens) and the superior oblique (trochlear).

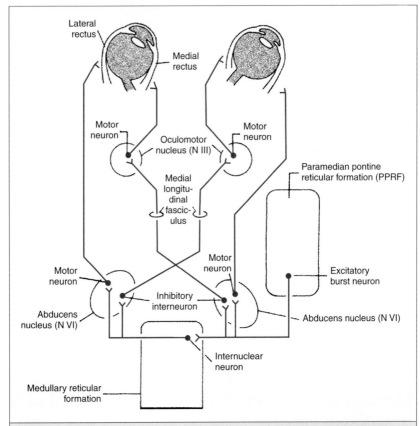

Figure 18-5. Neural circuit by which the horizontal gaze center elicits conjugate eye movements. Excitation of burst neurons of the right horizontal gaze center causes activation of abducens motor neurons on the right and medial rectus motor neurons on the left. The ascending pathway to the oculomotor nucleus is through the medial longitudinal fasciculus. The left horizontal gaze center is simultaneously inhibited by way of the reticular formation. (From Berne RM, Levy MN, Koeppen BM, Stanton BA: Physiology, 5th ed. Philadelphia, Mosby, 2003.)

CASE 18-1

A hyperopic ("farsighted") man presents with acutely decreased vision, redness, and pain in one eye. Funduscopic examination reveals cupping of the optic nerve, and a tonometer measurement indicates a significant elevation of the intraocular pressure.

1. **What is the most likely diagnosis?**
   Glaucoma, which describes a group of diseases associated with elevated intraocular pressure, is likely.

2. **What is the difference between open-angle glaucoma and closed-angle glaucoma?**
   The "angle" refers to the junction of cornea and iris, where the aqueous humor drains through the trabecular meshwork into the canal of Schlemm. In open-angle glaucoma, the angle is clinically open but drainage is still chronically compromised, leading to chronic elevation of pressure without pain and gradual damage to the optic nerve.

In closed-angle glaucoma, the angle is acutely closed by the peripheral iris. This leads to a sudden obstruction of outflow, pain, and severe elevation of intraocular pressure. If not treated immediately, closed-angle glaucoma can lead to severe loss of vision.

3. **What is the mechanism by which beta blockers reduce intraocular pressure in glaucoma?**
   Beta blockers inhibit the secretion of aqueous humor, thereby lowering the intraocular pressure. Because of some systemic absorption, these drugs should be avoided in severe asthmatics.

4. **What is the mechanism of action by which topical and oral carbonic anhydrase agents (e.g., acetazolamide) could be used to treat this man's glaucoma?**
   Like beta blockers, Carbonic anhydrase inhibitors also inhibit the production of aqueous humor, thereby lowering intraocular pressure.

RELATED QUESTIONS

5. **Why are cholinomimetics like pilocarpine and carbachol useful for closed-angle glaucoma?**
   One of the mechanisms causing angle closure is iris dilation by the peripheral iris tissue. Angle closure caused by peripheral iris dilation can be relieved by stimulating constriction of sphincter pupillae via parasympathetic cholinergic nerves. Cholinomimetics such as pilocarpine will constrict the pupil, pulling the iris from the angle and allowing it to open and improve drainage.

6. **Why should epinephrine be avoided in closed-angle glaucoma?**
   Although epinephrine is useful in open-angle glaucoma by preventing aqueous humor synthesis, it also causes mydriasis by stimulating the pupillary dilator muscle. Mydriasis will increase the obstruction between iris and lens in closed-angle glaucoma.

STEP 1 SECRET

The drugs used to treat glaucoma and their mechanisms of action are far more important for boards than the anatomy or pathophysiology of the disease (though you should know the basics!).

SUMMARY BOX: GLAUCOMA

- Glaucoma is a group of diseases associated with elevated intraocular pressures.

- In open-angle glaucoma, drainage of aqueous humor is *chronically* impaired despite a *normal-appearing* angle and trabecular meshwork. Pain is very unusual.

- In closed-angle glaucoma, drainage of aqueous humor is impaired *acutely* due to an obstructed angle. Pain is very common. This condition is an ophthalmologic emergency.

- Beta blockers and carbonic anhydrase inhibitors lower intraocular pressure by reducing aqueous humor secretion. α-Agonists and prostaglandin analogs can also decrease the pressure by affecting aqueous production and drainage.

- In closed-angle glaucoma, cholinomimetics constrict the pupil, pulling the iris from the angle and allowing for better drainage.

CASE 18-2

A 70-year-old man presents with central vision loss, complaining that straight lines appear wavy. Funduscopic examination reveals abnormal blood vessel growth and bleeding in the macula.

1. **What is the most likely diagnosis?**
   Age-related macular degeneration (AMD) with choroidal neovascularization ("wet" AMD) is most likely.

2. **What is the difference between "dry" and "wet" age-related macular degeneration?**
   "Dry" AMD is the most common form of AMD and occurs because of a breakdown of the photoreceptor cells. Drusen, which are yellow-white deposits, can form in the macula and are associated with vision loss. Dry AMD can progress to wet AMD, in which there is an abnormal growth of blood vessels in the choroid. Rupturing of these blood vessels can cause blood to leak into the retina and damage the macula.

3. **Where is the macula and what is its function?**
   The macula is a yellow spot near the central part of the retina. The fovea is located in the macula. The fovea has the highest concentration of cone photoreceptor cells, allowing us to see at the highest visual acuity.

4. **What is the mechanism of action for the intravitreal injection of ranibizumab that will be used to treat this man's age-related macular degeneration?**
   Ranibizumab is an antibody fragment that can bind to and inactivate vascular endothelial growth factor A (VEGF-A), a potent angiogenic factor. Inhibition of VEGF-A can prevent the growth of new vessels, potentially improving vision.

5. **What simple diagnostic test can be carried out to detect age-related macular degeneration?**
   In patients with AMD, straight lines may start appearing wavy. An Amsler grid, which is a grid made up of vertical and horizontal lines, can be used to quickly assess a patient's vision.

SUMMARY BOX: AGE-RELATED MACULAR DEGENERATION

- Age-related macular degeneration (AMD) causes a loss of central vision, and straight lines start appearing wavy.

- Dry AMD causes a blurring of central vision, and drusen deposits can be found near the macula. Dry AMD can progress to wet AMD.

- Wet AMD "is characterized by" abnormal blood vessel growth and "leakage of blood," leading to severe vision loss.

- The macula contains the fovea, which is the region of highest visual acuity.

- An intravitreal injection of ranibizumab is a common treatment for wet AMD: It inhibits vascular endothelial growth factor A (VEGF-A), stopping the growth of new blood vessels.

- Use of the Amsler grid is a simple and rapid method to assess a patient for AMD.

CHAPTER 19

RHEUMATOLOGY

Thomas A. Brown, MD, and Sonali J. Shah

INSIDER'S GUIDE TO RHEUMATOLOGY FOR THE USMLE STEP 1

When it comes to rheumatology on the USMLE, practice makes perfect. You are highly likely to encounter "textbook" presentations of the rheumatologic and bone conditions you must learn for Step 1, so the more cases you read before your examination, the better you will get at spotting the unique features that distinguish one disease from another. We have specifically designed this chapter to include high-yield cases that closely resemble the clinical presentations you should expect to see on boards. As you go through these cases, pay special attention to buzzwords and laboratory values (including autoantibodies) that will clue you into the correct diagnosis.

BASIC CONCEPTS

1. **What is a "diarthrodial" joint?**
   A diarthrodial joint is a joint in which bones meet in cartilage-covered surfaces. They are designed for mobility, such as that seen in the shoulder, hip, and interphalangeal joints, where substantial degrees of movement are possible. The diarthrodial joint is the most common type of joint found in the body.

2. **What are the components of a diarthrodial joint and which sites within a diarthrodial joint are vulnerable to disease?**
   These joints are composed of articulating bones covered by cartilage (usually hyaline cartilage). A fibrous capsule surrounds and protects the joint. The diarthrodial joint cavity is lined with a synovial membrane, which produces synovial fluid to lubricate the joint space. Ligamentous connections provide support and typically allow for a large amount of movement. Each of these components of the joint may be involved in disease processes (Fig. 19-1).

3. **What are synarthrodial and amphiarthrodial joints?**
   Synarthrodial joints exist where bones meet by fibrous connections without a joint space. These joints prevent motion between bones. The suture lines in the skull are an example of synarthroses. Amphiarthrodial joints consist of bones bound by fibrocartilage, which allows some limited degree of movement. The joints between vertebrae and the pubic symphysis are examples of amphiarthroses.

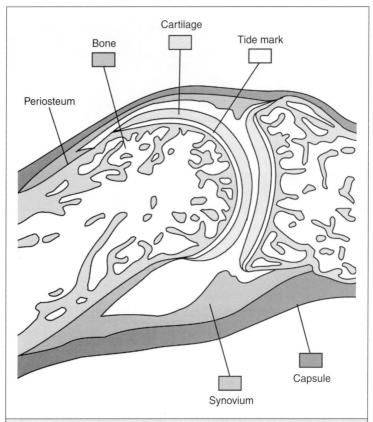

Figure 19-1. Normal interphalangeal joint, in sagittal section, as an example of a synovial, or diarthrodial, joint. (From Sokoloff L, Bland JH: The Musculoskeletal System. Baltimore, Williams & Wilkins, 1975.)

SUMMARY BOX: BASIC CONCEPTS

- Diarthrodial joints are the most common sort of joint and allow a large degree of motion between bones (examples: knees, hips).

- The diarthrodial joint is made up of bone, cartilage, a joint space lined with synovium, synovial fluid, a surrounding capsule, and ligamentous insertions.

- Synarthrodial joints consist of bones bound together by fibrous tissue and are nearly immobile (example: sutures in skull).

- Amphiarthrodial joints consist of bones bound together by cartilage and are slightly more mobile than synarthrodial joints (example: pubic symphysis).

CASE 19-1

A 55-year-old obese woman presents with several months of bilateral knee pain of several months' duration. The pain is exacerbated by activity and decreases with rest. She experiences approximately 10 to 15 minutes of morning stiffness each day but otherwise denies constitutional complaints such as fever, anorexia, weight loss, or fatigue.

1. What is the differential diagnosis?
   The differential diagnosis for symmetrical joint pain is broad and includes osteoarthritis, rheumatoid arthritis, and spondyloarthropathies such as ankylosing spondylitis or psoriasis, crystal arthropathy such as gout or pseudogout, and septic arthritis. In a middle-aged obese woman with involvement of weight-bearing joints, osteoarthritis seems likely.

CASE 19-1 continued:

The patient is moderately obese. None of her joints are warm, swollen, or tender. Aside from some crepitus with passive movement, examination of her knees is normal. The proximal and distal interphalangeal joints in both hands are enlarged but nontender. Plain film of the right knee shows narrowing of the medial compartment joint space (Fig. 19-2).

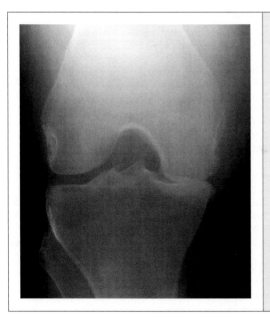

Figure 19-2. Plain film of the knee for patient in Case 19-1. (From Harris ED, Budd RC, Genovese MC, et al: Kelley's Textbook of Rheumatology, 7th ed. Philadelphia, WB Saunders, 2005.)

2. What is the likely diagnosis?
   Osteoarthritis (also known as OA, osteoarthrosis, degenerative joint disease, hypertrophic arthritis) is likely and is the most common joint disease worldwide. OA is characterized by loss of articular cartilage, which results in damage to the underlying bone. This process results primarily in pain (especially in weight-bearing joints), as well as stiffness and loss of joint mobility. The process is noninflammatory, so there is no ankylosis (fusion) of the joint.

Loss of the smooth articulating surface accounts for the finding of crepitus when the joint is moved. Pain is typically worse with use of the joint and decreases with rest. Reactive bone formation resulting in osteophytes (bone spurs) also occurs at the joint margins and may cause slight elevations in serum alkaline phosphatase. Joints typically affected include the proximal and distal interphalangeal joints (Bouchard's and Heberden's nodes, respectively), knees, and hips. Figure 19-3 shows both Heberden's and Bouchard's nodes. Recall that rheumatoid arthritis typically does *not* affect the distal interphalangeal joints.

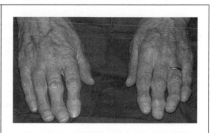

Figure 19-3. Typical hand deformities in osteoarthritis. Heberden's nodes are seen on the distal interphalangeal joints, and Bouchard's nodes are seen at the proximal interphalangeal joints. (From Forbes CD, Jackson WF: Color Atlas and Text of Clinical Medicine, 3rd ed. London, Mosby, 2003.)

3. **Is the pathogenesis of this condition primarily related to degeneration of bone, cartilage, or synovial membrane?**
Osteoarthritis is characterized by degeneration of articular cartilage and is often associated with "overuse" or trauma to the joint. Chondrocytes produce the type II cartilage that makes up the articular cartilage, and altered chondrocyte function has been demonstrated to occur in osteoarthritis. When articular cartilage is not maintained properly, the bones in the diarthrodial joint may come into direct contact with one another. The wear and tear that bones experience in this situation leads to abnormal bone proliferation, with the formation of osteophytes (bone spurs).
Rheumatoid arthritis differs in that the primary site of damage is the synovium, via an autoimmune mechanism. Unlike rheumatoid arthritis, osteoarthritis is not characterized by systemic inflammation or autoimmune phenomena. Rheumatoid joints often appear red and swollen (synovitis), whereas joints affected by osteoarthritis typically do not.

4. **What is the anatomic source of the joint pain in osteoarthritis?**
Although cartilage is the primary site of injury in this disease, there is no neural input to cartilage and therefore no pain transmission from it. The pain of osteoarthritis actually comes from the periosteum (dense fibrous tissue) surrounding the bone. The periosteum is highly innervated and is damaged when the cartilage has worn away to the point that bone is rubbing on bone.
Note: Joint cartilage is also completely avascular, which explains why injured cartilage will not heal.

5. **What are some risk factors associated with developing osteoarthritis?**
Obesity, occupation (repetitive motions), intense physical activity, joint trauma, and muscle weakness (likely from joint instability) play a role. Notice that all of these factors increase the mechanical forces to which the joint cartilage is exposed.
Gender, hormones, and genetics are involved as well. Women are more likely to suffer from osteoarthritis than men, and elderly populations are affected by this disease much more often than young people. There are certain forms of osteoarthritis that appear to be heritable.
Obesity is the strongest modifiable risk factor.
Note: Osteoarthritis can be classified as primary (idiopathic), the most common, or secondary, with an underlying cause (e.g., trauma, obesity, Paget disease, metabolic disorders). Diseases that involve the systemic deposition of certain compounds, such as hemochromatosis (iron), Wilson's disease (copper), and the crystal arthropathies, may be causes of secondary osteoarthritis.

6. **Would you expect the erythrocyte sedimentation rate (ESR) or C-reactive protein (CRP) to be elevated in this patient?**

No. An elevated ESR or CRP is a nonspecific indicator of a systemic inflammatory process. Because osteoarthritis is a local degenerative disease, these measurements would probably not be elevated in this patient (note that unlike rheumatoid arthritis, osteoarthritis does not result in systemic symptoms). In addition, although severe joint degeneration caused by OA may lead to inflammation, this inflammatory response would be confined to the joint space.

Note: Although osteoarthritis is classically considered a noninflammatory disease, it is interesting to note that pharmacologic treatment frequently involves the use of nonsteroidal anti-inflammatory drugs (NSAIDs) and intra-articular injections of steroids, which clearly act by reducing inflammation.

7. **How do the findings on x-ray studies generally differ between osteoarthritis and rheumatoid arthritis?**

The characteristic radiologic finding in osteoarthritis is joint space narrowing, as in this patient, due to the loss of cartilage between the bones. There may also be evidence of bony proliferation, such as increased density of the bones abutting the joint (subchondral sclerosis or eburnation) and presence of osteophytes. Chondrocalcinosis (calcium in the articular cartilage) and subchondral cysts may also be evident.

In rheumatoid arthritis, on the other hand, there are often marginal erosions of bone and osteoporotic changes (demineralization), and the joint space is typically normal. However, if the rheumatoid arthritis is severe enough, the inflammatory process may eventually destroy articular cartilage also and narrow the joint space.

Figure 19-4A demonstrates nearly complete loss of the lateral and medial joint spaces in rheumatoid arthritis, whereas Figure 19-4B demonstrates loss of only the medial joint space with subchondral sclerosis (increased density) of the underlying bone in OA.

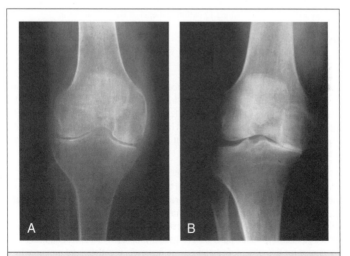

Figure 19-4. Radiographs of the knees in the two most common forms of arthritis: rheumatoid arthritis and osteoarthritis. **A,** Severe involvement in rheumatoid arthritis, with almost complete symmetrical loss of joint space in both the medial and lateral compartments, with little subchondral sclerosis or osteophyte formation. **B,** Typical osteoarthritis, with severe, near-total loss of joint space of one compartment and a normal or actually increased joint space of the other compartment. (From Goldman L, Ausiello D: Cecil Textbook of Medicine, 22nd ed. Philadelphia, WB Saunders, 2004.)

8. **Nonsteroidal anti-inflammatory drugs and cyclooxygenase-2 inhibitors are both possible treatments for this patient. What is similar about their mechanisms of action, and what is different?**

Regarding similarities, both classes of drug inhibit prostaglandin synthesis by inhibiting cyclooxygenase (COX), and by doing so cause relief of pain. All NSAIDs reversibly inhibit COX, except aspirin, which irreversibly inhibits COX. The COX-2 inhibitors (rofecoxib, celecoxib) selectively inhibit a form of COX that is induced in inflammatory cells, but not the constitutively expressed COX-1 that is produced for various normal body functions.

9. **What is the principal therapeutic advantage of the cyclooxygenase-2 inhibitors? What can be given to this patient with a nonsteroidal anti-inflammatory drug to prevent their principal side effect?**

By not inhibiting gastrointestinal (GI) prostaglandin synthesis, COX-2 inhibitors are supposed to cause less gastric ulceration, a very common problem with the NSAIDs. Drugs such as misoprostol, a synthetic prostaglandin analog, can be given orally with NSAIDs to reduce the risk of gastric ulceration and bleeding. However, more commonly proton pump inhibitors such as omeprazole are given to reduce the GI side effects of NSAIDs.

Note: NSAID use can also precipitate renal failure in patients with borderline renal function due to reduced synthesis of vasodilatory prostaglandins that help maintain renal perfusion.

10. **Why are cyclooxygenase-2 inhibitors considered dangerous in some patients?**

COX-2 inhibitors *do not* inhibit COX-1 in platelets. They therefore leave platelets capable of aggregating and forming thrombi. Additionally, COX-2 inhibitors *do* inhibit the production of prostaglandins in endothelial cells, potentially creating a prothrombotic state and promoting vasoconstriction. It is therefore believed that COX-2 inhibitors may pose a cardiovascular threat to certain patients at risk for stroke or myocardial infarction (MI), which is why Vioxx (rofecoxib) was withdrawn from the market in 2004.

11. **Is acetaminophen a reasonable option for treating joint pain in this patient?**

Yes. Actually, acetaminophen should be first-line therapy. Acetaminophen primarily works in the central nervous system (CNS) by raising the pain threshold. Its primary use is therefore as an analgesic. Because acetaminophen is not an NSAID and does not inhibit peripheral prostaglandin synthesis to a significant extent, it does not have the potential GI or renal side effects of the NSAIDs.

12. **What sort of analgesic would you prescribe for a patient with preexisting renal disease? Or liver disease? Or pregnancy?**

NSAIDs are renally excreted, and they decrease perfusion to the kidneys. They would therefore be relatively contraindicated in a patient with kidney disease, and acetaminophen is a better choice for this patient. Acetaminophen, however, is metabolized primarily by the liver (remember that patients who overdose on acetaminophen develop liver failure). A patient with cirrhosis or other liver disease would be better served by an NSAID than by large doses of acetaminophen. In a pregnant patient, NSAIDs should be avoided, particularly in the third trimester. The fetal ductus arteriosus is kept open by prostaglandins, and NSAIDs cause it to close prematurely in utero. However, in the case of a patent ductus arteriosus that persists after birth, indomethacin can be given to promote closure.

13. Quick review: Look only at the left column in Table 19-1 and try to list the class of drug, mechanism of action, and major side effects for each drug listed.

TABLE 19-1. TYPES OF ANALGESICS			
Drug	Class of Drug	Mechanism of Action	Side Effect(s)
Celecoxib (Celebrex)	COX-2 inhibitor	Inhibition of prostaglandin synthesis by inflammatory cells	Renal toxicity, increased cardiovascular disease risk
Indomethacin, naproxen, ibuprofen, etodolac, ketorolac (Toradol)	NSAID	Reversible COX-1/ COX-2 inhibition	GI ulcers and bleeding, renal damage
Aspirin	NSAID	Irreversible COX-1/ COX-2 inhibition	GI ulcers and bleeding, renal damage
Acetaminophen	No class	"Raises pain threshold"	Hepatotoxicity

COX, cyclooxygenase; GI, gastrointestinal; NSAID, nonsteroidal anti-inflammatory drug.

SUMMARY BOX: OSTEOARTHRITIS

- Osteoarthritis is the most common joint disease worldwide.

- Although there may be local joint inflammation, it is considered a noninflammatory condition without systemic (constitutional) symptoms.

- The disease process is centered in the cartilage and leads to destruction of bone.

- Pain is typically worse with activity.

- Obesity, gender, age, and trauma all contribute to its development.

- Radiographs show joint space narrowing, subchondral sclerosis, and osteophytes.

- Acetaminophen, cyclooxygenase (COX)-2 inhibitors, and nonsteroidal anti-inflammatory drugs (NSAIDs) are the mainstay of pharmacotherapy.

CASE 19-2

A 52-year-old woman presents with a chief complaint of polyarticular joint pain for several months. Her pain is worst in the morning and lessens with activity over the course of the day. She typically experiences 1 hour of stiffness after she wakes up. She also reports malaise, anorexia, night sweats, and a persistent low-grade fever. Her symptoms seem to come and go at will.

1. **What is the differential diagnosis?**

   The differential diagnosis for polyarticular arthritis includes osteoarthritis, rheumatoid arthritis, septic arthritis (e.g., disseminated gonococcal infection), reactive arthritis (e.g., in response to infections, previously known as Reiter's syndrome), systemic lupus erythematosus (SLE), hepatitis, and paraneoplastic syndromes. Although the differential here is broad, her morning stiffness and constitutional complaints are suggestive of an inflammatory arthropathy such as rheumatoid arthritis.

CASE 19-2 continued:

Upon examination, she has symmetrical involvement of the metacarpophalangeal (MCP) and proximal interphalangeal joints, with sparing of the distal interphalangeals (Fig. 19-5). Involved joints in her hands are swollen, warm, and tender to palpation. She has moderate-sized bilateral knee effusions. Laboratory tests show elevated ESR and CRP and positive rheumatoid factor (RF). She is diagnosed with a chronic autoimmune disease and prescribed methotrexate, an NSAID, and prednisone.

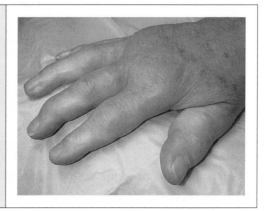

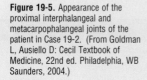

Figure 19-5. Appearance of the proximal interphalangeal and metacarpophalangeal joints of the patient in Case 19-2. (From Goldman L, Ausiello D: Cecil Textbook of Medicine, 22nd ed. Philadelphia, WB Saunders, 2004.)

2. **What is the diagnosis?**

   This patient presents with classic signs of rheumatoid arthritis, which is an autoimmune disease of synovial joints. The principal pathologic process in rheumatoid arthritis is synovitis—inflammation of the synovial membrane—which leads to destruction of the joint. Because rheumatoid arthritis is a systemic inflammatory condition, patients often present with constitutional symptoms such as fever, weight loss, and fatigue as well as joint pain. Note that joint involvement in rheumatoid arthritis is usually symmetrical.

3. **What are the criteria for the diagnosis of rheumatoid arthritis?**

   Four of the following seven criteria must be met for the diagnosis to be made:
   1. Morning stiffness lasting at least 1 hour
   2. Arthritis of three or more joints
   3. Arthritis of hand joints
   4. Symmetrical joint involvement
   5. Rheumatoid nodules
   6. Serum RF
   7. Radiographic changes

This patient has morning stiffness, symmetrical arthritis of more than three joints including the hand, and positive RF. She therefore meets the criteria for the definitive diagnosis of rheumatoid arthritis.

4. **What sort of damage occurs in the joints of patients with rheumatoid arthritis?**
The initial site of damage is the synovium lining the joint space, which becomes the center of an inflammatory process that will involve the entire joint. Lymphocytes, macrophages, osteoclasts, and fibroblasts are all involved and ultimately lead to destruction of the cartilage and bone of the joint. Pannus formation occurs as synovial tissue is aberrantly stimulated to proliferate, and bony erosions develop as the inflammatory process continues. Joints will be painful, show signs of inflammation, and eventually lose normal architecture and mobility.

5. **What is the significance of rheumatoid factor in this disease?**
RF is an autoantibody (IgM) directed against the Fc region of IgG. This autoantibody forms immune complexes (type III hypersensitivity reaction), which deposit throughout the body and are implicated in the extra-articular manifestations of rheumatoid arthritis. RF is present in roughly 80% of rheumatoid arthritis patients, but it is not highly specific for the condition; RF can also appear in lupus, tuberculosis, Sjögren's syndrome, and other disorders. It is therefore not necessary for the diagnosis of rheumatoid arthritis, but it is useful for determining prognosis. Virtually 100% of patients with extra-articular manifestations have a positive RF.
   Note: The current best serologic test for the diagnosis of rheumatoid arthritis is the anti-CCP (citrullinated cyclic peptide) antibody. Its sensitivity is the same as that for RF, but it is more specific for rheumatoid arthritis and is a better predictor of disease progression.

6. **What is the epidemiology of rheumatoid arthritis?**
As is the case with most autoimmune conditions, rheumatoid arthritis affects women more often than men, and its prevalence increases with age. However, there is no ethnic background or geographic distribution associated with the disease. Genetic susceptibility has been demonstrated, as the disease is associated with certain major histocompatibility complex (MHC) class II proteins expressed by antigen-presenting cells. The HLA-DR4 haplotype confers risk for rheumatoid arthritis, and a specific HLA-DR epitope is shared by many people with rheumatoid arthritis. However, these HLA genes do not tell the whole story, and many genes are likely to be responsible for the development of the disease.

7. **What is the typical treatment for rheumatoid arthritis?**
Three classes of medications are used to manage rheumatoid arthritis: analgesics to treat pain, corticosteroids to suppress inflammation, and disease-modifying antirheumatic drugs (DMARDs) to limit progression of the disease. NSAIDs are commonly used as analgesics and have the added benefit of dampening inflammation. Corticosteroids can be injected directly into affected joints and may be used to manage acute flares of rheumatoid arthritis. DMARDs include a variety of drugs such as methotrexate, sulfasalazine, gold, and tumor necrosis factor (TNF) inhibitors. Early use of DMARDs is desirable, as these drugs halt progression of irreversible joint damage.

8. **What would be learned from aspiration of this patient's knee?**
Probably not much would be revealed by aspiration. The synovial fluid should have an inflammatory composition with 2000 to 50,000 white blood cells (WBCs)/mm^3, with the cells being predominantly polymorphocnuclear neutrophils (PMNs). If crystals or bacteria were present, or the WBC count was not in this range, one would need to consider other diagnoses on the differential.
   Note: Rheumatoid arthritis may also show decreased C3 protein in the synovium but increased C3 levels in the serum.

CASE 19-2 continued:

Your rheumatoid arthritis patient is lost to follow-up but then returns to your office years later. She complains of diffuse arthralgias, weight loss, and shortness of breath. Her hands appear as shown in Figure 19-6, and subcutaneous nodules are present at the olecranon bilaterally. She has decreased breath sounds at the lung bases, and chest x-ray film shows bilateral pleural effusions and several pulmonary nodules.

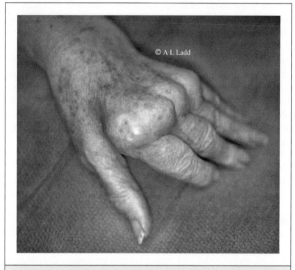

© A L Ladd

Figure 19-6. Left hand of the patient in Case 19-2. (Copyright A.L. Ladd.)

9. **What are the characteristic deformities in the hands in advanced rheumatoid arthritis?**
   Destruction of the metacarpophalangeal joints leads to ulnar deviation (shown in Fig. 19-6) as the distal portions of the digits shift toward the ulna. Boutonnière and swan-neck deformities consist of contractions of the fingers at the proximal interphalangeal and distal interphalangeal joints. Remember that the distal interphalangeal joints are not typically involved with rheumatoid arthritis, though they may be forced into flexion/extension due to involvement of the proximal interphalangeal joints and the tendons of the hand.

STEP 1 SECRET

Symmetrical joint involvement, sparing of the distal interphalangeal joints, and morning stiffness that resolves with joint use are unique characteristics of rheumatoid arthritis. Be on the lookout for mention of these clues if you suspect a diagnosis of rheumatoid arthritis.

10. **What are the extra-articular manifestations of rheumatoid arthritis?**
Because rheumatoid arthritis is a systemic inflammatory disease, it is not limited to the joints; immune complexes deposit in the vasculature and may affect nearly any organ system. Rheumatoid nodules typically form in the subcutaneous tissue or along tendon sheaths. Pericarditis, pulmonary nodules, interstitial fibrosis, episcleritis, and effusions in the pleural and pericardial space may all be seen in rheumatoid patients. Carpal tunnel syndrome can result from median nerve compression. A normocytic normochromic anemia (anemia of chronic disease) is also common.
    Note: Felty's syndrome is the combination of seropositive (RF+) rheumatoid arthritis, granulocytopenia, and splenomegaly.

SUMMARY BOX: RHEUMATOID ARTHRITIS

- Rheumatoid arthritis is a systemic inflammatory disease caused in part by immune complex deposition in the joints and potentially various other tissues.

- Gender, age, and human leukocyte antigens (HLAs) have been associated.

- The disease process is centered in the synovium of the joint.

- Joints are typically warm, erythematous, swollen, and tender (synovitis).

- Distal interphalangeal joints are typically spared.

- Pain is worse in the morning, classically lasting more than an hour.

- Rheumatoid factor is an autoantibody, the presence of which confers a poor prognosis.

- Extra-articular manifestations include rheumatoid nodules, pericarditis, pleural effusions, pulmonary nodules, pulmonary fibrosis, carpal tunnel syndrome, ocular manifestations, and anemia of chronic disease.

- Treatment includes nonsteroidal anti-inflammatory drugs (NSAIDs), glucocorticoids, and disease-modifying antirheumatic drugs (DMARDs). In recent years there has been a strong push to start DMARDs at the time of initial diagnosis.

CASE 19-3

A 47-year-old man presents with excruciatingly pain in the right knee that began 24 hours earlier. He had been to a banquet the night before and woke up with a red, swollen knee. He tried taking aspirin, but his pain only worsened. He has a history of hypertension treated with hydrochlorothiazide, and his body mass index (BMI) is 32.

1. **What is your differential diagnosis?**
The differential diagnosis for an acutely inflamed joint includes septic arthritis, cellulitis, gout, pseudogout, and osteomyelitis.

2. **How can crystal and septic arthritis be differentiated?**
Examination of joint fluid is of paramount importance. Both conditions will cause a high WBC and PMN percentage in the fluid, but Gram stain and culture must be done to look for infectious causes. Septic arthritis may cause more systemic illness, with symptoms such as fever, malaise, lymphadenopathy, and skin lesions. Organisms responsible for septic arthritis include *Staphylococcus aureus*, *Streptococcus* species, and *Neisseria gonorrhoeae*. Rapid diagnosis and treatment are crucial in septic arthritis.

CASE 19-3 continued:

On examination, the right knee is warm, erythematous, swollen, and tender to touch. The patient is afebrile, and the remainder of his examination in unremarkable. You aspirate cloudy yellow fluid from the joint and find 24,000 WBCs, 70% PMNs, and needle-shaped crystals that are strongly negatively birefringent under polarized light (Fig. 19-7).

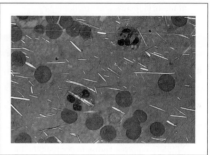

Figure 19-7. Microscopic appearance of synovial fluid under polarized light aspirated from patient in Case 19-3. (From McPherson RA, Pincus MR: Henry's Clinical Diagnosis and Management by Laboratory Methods, 21st ed. Philadelphia, WB Saunders, 2006.)

3. **What is the likely diagnosis?**
   Gout is an inflammatory arthritis caused by the intra-articular deposition of uric acid crystals. Although this patient's presentation is consistent with the other diseases listed for the differential diagnosis, the crystals seen here are pathognomonic for gout.
   The term to associate with gout is negative birefringence, which means that when the crystals are examined under polarized light, they appear yellow when oriented parallel to the direction of slow light vibration, and blue when oriented perpendicularly.

4. **What is the pathophysiology of this condition?**
   Uric acid is the end product of purine nucleotide metabolism and is excreted from the body by the kidneys. High levels of serum uric acid may occur with either overproduction or underexcretion of uric acid. The vast majority of the time (>90% of cases), gout is caused by underexcretion. In either situation, uric acid is deposited in synovial fluid in the form of monosodium urate crystals, which are phagocytosed and induce a local inflammatory response. Free uric acid crystals also activate synovial cells, leukocytes, and complement proteins including C5a, which recruits large numbers of PMNs into the joint space.

5. **Do most people with hyperuricemia develop gout?**
   No. Most people with hyperuricemia do not have gout, and many gout patients do not have high serum levels of urate. The risk of developing gout becomes substantial only with quite high levels of uric acid (>9 mg/dL vs. normal level of ~5 mg/dL). Other risk factors for gout are a purine-rich diet (e.g., seafood, certain meats), male gender age (fifth decade), obesity, hypertension, alcohol intake, renal disease, family history of gout, use of certain drugs, and certain genetic conditions.

6. **What is Lesch-Nyhan syndrome and why might it predispose to gout?**
   Lesch-Nyhan syndrome consists of mental retardation, spasticity, choreoathetosis, aggressive behavior, and self-mutilation, as well as gouty arthritis. It is due to an X-linked defect in hypoxanthine phosphoribosyltransferase (HGPRT), an enzyme involved in the purine salvage pathway. Absence of HGPRT leads to overproduction of uric acid with resultant hyperuricemia.

7. **Are there any complications of gout besides the monoarticular inflammatory arthritis?**
   The classic location for gouty arthritis is in the metatarsophalangeal joint of the great toe, which is known as podagra. In patients with chronic gout, monosodium urate crystals can also deposit in subcutaneous tissues, forming nodules called tophi. Tophi are often found in the helix of the ear and over the elbow. Figure 19-8 shows olecranon bursitis in chronic tophaceous gout.
   Uric acid calculi may form in the renal pelvis or ureters, leading to obstruction of the urinary tract. Crystals may also cause damage to the renal interstitial tissue, a condition termed gouty interstitial nephropathy.

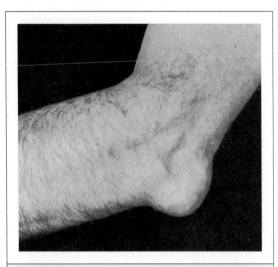

Figure 19-8. Olecranon bursitis in a patient with tophaceous gout. (From Polley HF, Hunder GG: Rheumatologic Interviewing and Physical Examination of the Joints, 2nd ed. Philadelphia, WB Saunders, 1978.)

8. **Are there any medications that can precipitate attacks of gout?**
   Drugs that decrease the renal excretion of uric acid may contribute to gout. Such offenders include low-dose salicylates, thiazide diuretics, and furosemide. Our patient may have been predisposed to developing gout because of his hydrochlorothiazide use, and the aspirin he took decreased his renal excretion of uric acid even further. Other precipitants include alcoholic beverages and purine-rich foods (meats and seafood).
   Note: Although low-dose aspirin (<2 g/day) decreases renal excretion of uric acid, high-dose aspirin actually increases renal clearance.

CASE 19-3 continued:

He is given colchicine and experiences rapid improvement.

9. **What other treatment options exist for an acute gout attack?**
   Acute attacks can be managed with NSAIDs (typically indomethacin), glucocorticoids, and colchicine, all of which dampen the inflammatory response and inhibit the continued phagocytosis of monosodium urate crystals.

Note: Colchicine works by binding to the molecule tubulin and inhibiting the polymerization of microtubules, thereby inhibiting mitosis in inflammatory cells. By inhibiting microtubule function, it also serves to limit the mobility of inflammatory cells. A worrisome side effect of colchicine is bone marrow suppression. It also commonly causes intestinal upset and diarrhea.

10. **Who needs chronic treatment for gout, and what does this treatment consist of?**
    Patients with recurrent bouts of gouty arthritis, radiographic evidence of joint damage, and extra-articular manifestations such as tophi and urate kidney stones merit chronic treatment. Note that asymptomatic hyperuricemia is *not* reason for treatment. Probenecid is used for most chronic gout patients (underexcretors), as it serves to increase renal excretion of uric acid. Allopurinol, an inhibitor of the uric acid-synthesizing enzyme xanthine oxidase, can be used to treat overproducers. For boards, patients are designated underexcretors or overproducers using a 24-hour urinary uric acid excretion test, although in clinical practice this is rarely done.
    Note: Patients undergoing treatment for hematologic malignancies are at risk for tumor lysis syndrome. As malignant cells are killed, their DNA is degraded into purine and pyrimidine nucleotides. Allopurinol is often given before radiation therapy or chemotherapy to prevent the production of uric acid through purine catabolism.
    Note: At the time of this writing, febuxostat (Uloric) has recently been approved as an alternative to allopurinol. While febuxostat has been shown to be more effective than allopurinol at lowering serum urate concentration, it has not been shown to be more clinically efficacious at preventing gouty flares.

11. **What is pseudogout?**
    Pseudogout is a crystal arthropathy caused by calcium pyrophosphate dihydrate (CPPD) deposition. Synovial fluid shows rhomboid, weakly positively birefringent crystals that are blue when parallel to light and yellow when perpendicular (versus the needle-shaped, strongly negatively birefringent crystals of gout). This condition usually affects larger joints such as knees and occurs in women more often than in men. Radiographs might show chondrocalcinosis-CPPD deposition within cartilage. Hemochromatosis and hyperparathyroidism are two metabolic disorders that predispose to pseudogout.

STEP 1 SECRET

Be sure that you understand the concepts of positive and negative birefringence and their associations with pseudogout and gout, respectively.

ONE LAST CRYSTAL . . .

A 78-year-old woman with a history of osteoarthritis presents with increasing left shoulder pain during the past few months. On examination, her shoulder is warm and an effusion is present. Her range of motion is severely limited by pain, and you note obvious crepitance. Aspiration reveals blood but no crystals in the synovial fluid. You order an x-ray study and compare it with one from 3 months ago, and find that the head of her humerus has been severely eroded during this short time.

12. **What is going on here?**
    This condition, termed "Milwaukee shoulder syndrome," is caused by deposition of hydroxyapatite crystals. It typically affects elderly women and causes rapid destruction of the shoulder. These crystals are visible only with electron microscopy.

SUMMARY BOX: GOUT, PSEUDOGOUT, AND MILWAUKEE SHOULDER

- Gout is an inflammatory typically monoarticular arthritis caused by the intra-articular deposition of urate crystals.

- Uric acid is a product of purine nucleotide catabolism.

- Uric acid crystals are needle-shaped and demonstrate strongly negative birefringence.

- Hyperuricemia is neither necessary nor sufficient for the development of gout.

- Risk factors for gout include a purine-rich diet, male gender, age (fifth decade), obesity, hypertension, alcohol intake, diuretic use, renal disease, and family history.

- Although this has little clinical relevance, for boards you should know that most gout patients are underexcretors of uric acid.

- Lesch-Nyhan syndrome is an X-linked defect in hypoxanthine phosphoribosyltransferase (HGPRT) associated with cognitive and behavioral symptoms including aggression and self-mutilation.

- Subcutaneous tophi, renal calculi, and interstitial nephropathy may occur in gout.

- Acute gout treatment includes nonsteroidal anti-inflammatory drugs (NSAIDs), steroids, and colchicine.

- Chronic gout treatment includes probenecid for underexcretors and allopurinol for overproducers of uric acid, although this distinction is rarely made clinically.

- Pseudogout is caused by calcium pyrophosphate dihydrate (CPPD) crystals.

- CPPD crystals are rhomboid and demonstrate weakly positive birefringence.

- Milwaukee shoulder is caused by deposition of hydroxyapatite crystals.

CASE 19-4

A 42-year-old woman presents with the complaint of "feeling sore all over" with constant aching pain. She complains of persistent fatigue as well. She has felt this way for years and has been to see several physicians without receiving a definitive diagnosis.

1. **What is your differential diagnosis for diffuse musculoskeletal pain and fatigue?**
This is a truly broad differential diagnosis. Hypothyroidism, chronic viral hepatitis, Lyme disease, sleep apnea, anemia, and many rheumatologic conditions can cause pain and fatigue. Certain medications may cause musculoskeletal pain, particularly the lipid-lowering HMG-CoA (3-hydroxy-3-methylglutaryl coenzyme A) reductase inhibitors (statins). Any number of malignancies could be responsible for this presentation as well.

CASE 19-4 continued:

Your patient states that along with the pain and fatigue, she has alternating episodes of constipation and diarrhea. She has a history of migraine headaches and takes fluoxetine (Prozac) for depression. Physical examination is remarkable only for tenderness to palpation at many points across her body. Laboratory tests show a normal complete blood count (CBC), ESR, CRP, and creatinine phosphokinase. Muscle biopsy and electromyography findings are normal.

2. **What is the likely diagnosis?**

   Fibromyalgia, a condition characterized by diffuse musculoskeletal pain, is likely. A diagnosis of fibromyalgia requires the presence of pain in all four quadrants of the body for at least 3 months, and in at least 11 of 18 anatomically specific tender points (Fig. 19-9).

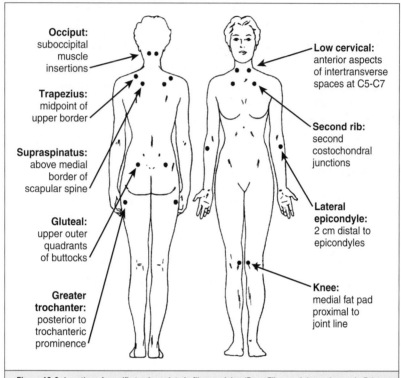

Occiput: suboccipital muscle insertions

Trapezius: midpoint of upper border

Supraspinatus: above medial border of scapular spine

Gluteal: upper outer quadrants of buttocks

Greater trochanter: posterior to trochanteric prominence

Low cervical: anterior aspects of intertransverse spaces at C5-C7

Second rib: second costochondral junctions

Lateral epicondyle: 2 cm distal to epicondyles

Knee: medial fat pad proximal to joint line

Figure 19-9. Location of specific tender points in fibromyalgia. (From Fibromyalgia syndrome. In Primer on Rheumatic Diseases. Atlanta, Arthritis Foundation, 1993.)

3. **What causes fibromyalgia?**

   The pathophysiology of this syndrome is poorly understood. Most believe that it is due to abnormalities in the CNS, leading to a heightened sensitivity to painful stimuli. Fibromyalgia patients have been shown to have lower-than-normal levels of serotonin and elevated levels of substance P (a neuropeptide that mediates the transmission of pain signals from the peripheral nervous system to the CNS).

4. **Are steroids indicated?**

   No. This is not an inflammatory disorder, as evidenced by the lack of laboratory abnormalities. Steroids should not be used in this situation. Sleep medications, NSAIDs, antidepressants, and muscle relaxants may be of some help. Physical therapy, cognitive-behavioral therapy, and aerobic exercise may be useful as well.

5. **Who is prone to developing fibromyalgia?**

   This disorder is seen predominantly in women (affecting four to seven times more often than men). Fibromyalgia is often seen alongside mood disorders such as depression and anxiety, sleep disorders, headaches, and irritable bowel syndrome.

CASE 19-5

The next patient is a 57-year-old woman who presents for evaluation of a 4-week history of diffuse aching pain of abrupt onset in her shoulders, hips, and low back. She has lost 8 lb and reports occasional low-grade fever. On examination, she is tender to palpation in many proximal muscles and large joints but shows no signs of muscle atrophy, muscle weakness, or sensory losses. Laboratory tests show an ESR of 84 mm/hour, hematocrit of 35%, mean corpuscular volume (MCV) of 93 fL, and an elevated ferritin level. Serum creatinine phosphokinase is not elevated, and electromyography and muscle biopsy findings are normal as well.

1. **What is the diagnosis in this patient?**
   This woman has polymyalgia rheumatica (PMR), another rheumatologic condition that presents primarily with diffuse myalgias. Unlike fibromyalgia, PMR is a systemic inflammatory disorder. Proximal muscles of the neck, shoulders, back, and thighs are typically involved. Fever, weight loss, and fatigue may be in the history, and a normochromic, normocytic anemia occurs in 50% of cases. PMR usually has an abrupt onset.
   Note: Ferritin is one of the acute-phase reactants—a group of proteins synthesized by the liver in response to inflammation. To attribute the high ferritin level to an acute response (versus iron overload, as in hemochromatosis), one should look for other signs of inflammation, such as an elevated ESR or CRP.

2. **How is this condition treated?**
   PMR is highly sensitive to corticosteroid administration, which is the mainstay of therapy for this disease. It typically responds within days to relatively low dose prednisone (10–20 mg/day). If symptoms do not rapidly improve, other conditions should be considered.

3. **What else should be looked for in patients with suspected polymyalgia rheumatica?**
   PMR is often associated with giant cell (temporal) arteritis, one of the vasculitides, and patients with polymyalgia should be evaluated for giant cell arteritis. Signs of arteritis include claudication involving the arms and legs, arterial bruits, and asymmetrical blood pressures in the extremities. Involvement of the temporal artery may cause jaw pain and unilateral headaches and, if left untreated, may lead to blindness.

SUMMARY BOX: FIBROMYALGIA AND POLYMYALGIA RHEUMATICA

- Fibromyalgia is a syndrome of diffuse musculoskeletal pain.

- While the etiology remains unclear, fibromyalgia is likely causes in part by heightened sensitivity to pain in the central nervous system (CNS).

- It is NOT an inflammatory disorder.

- Pharmacotherapy includes nonsteroidal anti-inflammatory drugs (NSAIDs) and antidepressants.

- Polymyalgia rheumatica (PMR) is an inflammatory disorder that causes musculoskeletal pain.

- PMR is treated with relatively low-dose corticosteroids.

- PMR is often associated with giant cell (temporal) arteritis.

CASE 19-6

A 37-year-old man presents with a several-month history of burning pain in his hands. His wife notices that he often wakes from sleep because of this pain and paces around their bedroom, shaking his hands to relieve the pain. He works for a moving company and spends much of the time lifting furniture. He finds that the pain sometimes shoots up from his wrists into his forearms, and he is beginning to notice hand weakness.

1. What is your differential diagnosis?
   This presentation is consistent with a tendonitis, enthesopathy, or a neuropathy.
   Note: Pathology at the site of insertion of tendons, ligaments, muscle, and joint capsule into bone is referred to as an enthesopathy.

CASE 19-6 continued:

On examination, you note bilateral thenar atrophy, and evoke positive Phalen and Tinel signs.

2. What is the Phalen sign? What is the Tinel sign?
   The Phalen test (Fig. 19-10) consists of having patients flex their wrists and hold their hands together for 60 seconds, which will cause numbness and tingling in the distribution of the median nerve if carpal tunnel syndrome is present. The Tinel sign is positive if similar paresthesias are evoked by simply tapping the wrist over the transverse carpal ligament in the area of the median nerve.
   Note: A 2002 study evaluating these tests in carpal tunnel syndrome confirmed patients and healthy controls showed a sensitivity and specificity of 85% and 89%, respectively, for the Phalen test and 66% and 67%, respectively, for the percussion test.

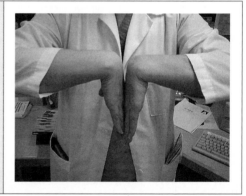

Figure 19-10. Phalen test. (From Marx JA, Hochberger RS, Walls RM, Adams JG: Rosen's Emergency Medicine: Concepts and Clinical Practice, 6th ed. Philadelphia, Mosby, 2006.)

3. What is your diagnosis?
   This man has carpal tunnel syndrome, which is a compressive or entrapment neuropathy of the median nerve at the wrist.

4. What causes carpal tunnel syndrome?
   The median nerve passes into the hand via the carpal tunnel. This space is bounded by carpal bones and the transverse carpal ligament (flexor retinaculum). Compression of the nerve in this location leads to carpal tunnel syndrome, which is characterized by neuropathic pain in the distribution of the median nerve. Repetitive wrist flexion may lead to irritation and inflammation within the carpal tunnel, making carpal tunnel syndrome a common work-related injury. Several medical conditions may also be responsible, including pregnancy, obesity, hypothyroidism, and amyloidosis.

5. **What structures pass through the carpal tunnel?**
   Ten anatomic structures reside within this space: four tendons of the flexor digitorum profundus, four tendons of the flexor digitorum superficialis, the tendon of the flexor pollicis longus, and the median nerve.

   Note: The flexor carpi radialis tendon passes through the wrist just lateral to these 10 structures but is *not* found within the flexor retinaculum.

6. **What does the median nerve innervate in the hand?**
   The median nerve originates in spinal roots C6-T1 and supplies the muscles of the anterior forearm. In the hand, it provides sensory innervation to the palmar surface of the first three and a half digits, as well as the distal dorsal portion of these fingers. The median nerve also supplies motor innervation to the thenar (thumb) muscles and the first two lumbrical muscles (Fig. 19-11).

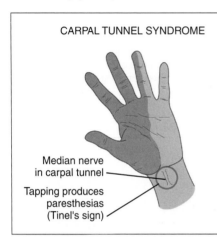

CARPAL TUNNEL SYNDROME

Median nerve in carpal tunnel

Tapping produces paresthesias (Tinel's sign)

Figure 19-11. Distribution of pain and paresthesias (*dark-shaded area*) when the median nerve is compressed by swelling in the wrist (carpal tunnel). (From Arnett FC: Rheumatoid arthritis. In Andreoli TE [ed]: Cecil Essentials of Medicine, 4th ed. Philadelphia, WB Saunders, 1997.)

7. **What are treatment options for carpal tunnel syndrome?**
   Conservative measures include splinting and limitation of aggravating factors. Steroid injections may be helpful. Surgical treatment involves releasing the transverse carpal ligament to reduce pressure in the canal. Although this has traditionally been an open surgery, it is now routinely performed laparoscopically.

SUMMARY BOX: CARPAL TUNNEL SYNDROME

- Carpal tunnel syndrome is a compressive (entrapment) neuropathy of the median nerve at the wrist.

- Symptoms include pain and paresthesias (numbness/tingling) in the distribution of the median nerve.

- The median nerve supplies cutaneous innervation to the first three and a half fingers and motor supply to the thumb.

- Phalen and Tinel tests may reproduce the symptoms of the entrapment neuropathy, with considerably better diagnostic value of the Phalen test relative to the percussion test.

CASE 19-7.1

A 26-year-old man presents with a 9-month history of low back pain and stiffness that is worse in the morning and generally subsides after a few hours of activity. On examination, you find tenderness to palpation of the sacroiliac joints, reduced flexibility of the lumbar spine, and limited expansion of the chest. Ten years later, x-ray films of the lumbar spine are obtained and shown in Figure 19-12.

1. **What is the diagnosis?**
   This man suffers from ankylosing spondylitis, one of the seronegative arthropathies. This disease generally occurs in young men and involves the axial skeleton. The x-ray films show the classic "bamboo spine" (Fig. 19-12B), which is caused in part by syndesmophytes (see white arrowheads), curvilinear calcifications linking one vertebral body to another.
   Note: The seronegative spondyloarthropathies are "seronegative" in that patients are typically negative for RF. These diseases all seem to occur most frequently in people who share a certain MHC I antigen, the HLA-B27 allele. Not all people with this allele will develop one of the spondyloarthropathies, but most patients with these diseases do have the HLA-B27 allele. This relationship is not fully understood, but the spondyloarthropathies obviously share a strong genetic component. They tend to affect the axial skeleton, along with the eyes, skin, genitalia, and GI tract.

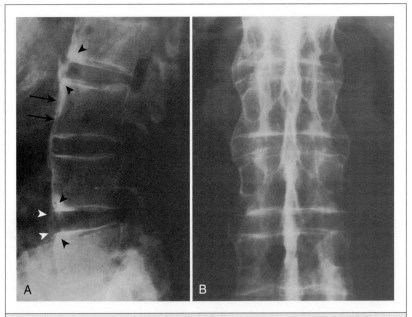

Figure 19-12. A, Early manifestations of this condition in the lumbar spine include the development of an osteitis (*black arrowheads*) at the corners of vertebral body end plates that results in sclerosis and bone resorption. Early syndesmophytes (*white arrowheads*) are gracile, curvilinear calcifications extending from corner to corner. Mineralization of the anterior longitudinal ligament (*black arrows*) may contribute to the squared appearance of a vertebral body. **B,** Gracile syndesmophytes at all levels create the "bamboo spine" appearance. (From Grainger RG, Allison D, Adam A, et al: Grainger & Allison's Diagnostic Radiology: A Textbook of Medical Imaging, 4th ed. Philadelphia, Churchill Livingstone, 2001.)

2. **What is the bamboo spine?**
As the inflammatory process unfolds in the spine, fibrous and cartilaginous structures are replaced with bone. This leads to diminished flexibility and eventual fusion of the vertebrae, giving the spine the appearance of bamboo on plain x-ray films.

CASE 19–7.2

A 32-year-old man presents with a 2-week history of pain in multiple joints, painful red eyes, and burning with urination. He has had several sexual partners in the past few months. Polymerase chain reaction (PCR) assay is positive for *Chlamydia trachomatis* and negative for *N. gonorrhoeae*. You note a few ulcerated lesions of the oral mucosa on examination.

1. **What is the likely diagnosis?**
This is reactive arthritis, also known as Reiter's syndrome. The classic triad of arthritis, conjunctivitis/uveitis, and urethritis makes up the clinical presentation in many cases of this seronegative arthropathy.

2. **What triggers this condition?**
Reactive arthritis occurs in response to an infection in patients with the HLA-B27 allele. Common agents include *Shigella*, *Yersinia*, *Chlamydia*, and *Salmonella*. Reactive arthritis is a systemic inflammatory response to these bacterial antigens; it is *not* a septic arthritis, and these bacteria will not be found in any affected joint. This differs from gonococcal arthritis, which typically involves bacterial seeding of affected joints.

CASE 19–7.3

A 40-year-old man presents with a 3-month history of pain and stiffness in his back, neck, and hands. You note large erythematous scaly plaques over the extensor surfaces of his elbows and knees, which he states he has had for years. There is tenderness to palpation of the left sacroiliac joint, and the distal interphalangeal joints are warm and swollen. You note that the first finger on his left hand is extensively red and swollen all along its length. You examine his feet and find that the toenails have extensive pitting.

1. **What is the diagnosis here?**
This man has psoriatic arthritis, another member of the group of seronegative spondyloarthropathies. This entity is associated with the dermatologic condition psoriasis, which is characterized by large red plaques covered with silvery white scales over extensor surfaces (Fig. 19-13).

STEP 1 SECRET

The USMLE loves to include pictures of common dermatologic lesions on the exam. Psoriasis is a particular favorite, but you should make a point of looking at as many images of skin lesions as possible as you encounter them throughout your studies.

2. **What joints are affected by psoriatic arthritis?**
Commonly the joints of the hands and feet (including the distal interphalangeal joints) are involved, but the axial skeleton can also be affected. The nails can show characteristic deformities in psoriatic arthritis, including pits, horizontal ridges, or abnormal coloration. Dactylitis, or inflammation of the soft tissue of an entire digit, is seen as well; this is known colloquially as a "sausage digit" (Fig. 19-14).

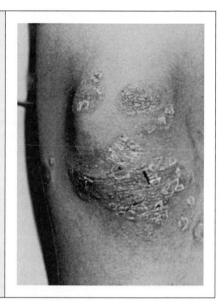

Figure 19-13. Chronic psoriatic plaques on the knee. (From Behrman RE: Nelson Textbook of Pediatrics, 16th ed. Philadelphia, WB Saunders, 2000.)

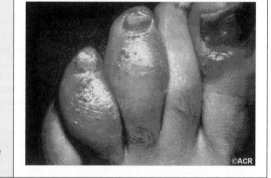

Figure 19-14. Sausage toes, or dactylitis, in a patient with psoriasis. (From American College of Rheumatology: Clinical Slide Collection on the Rheumatic Diseases. Atlanta, American College of Rheumatology, 1998.)

SUMMARY BOX: SERONEGATIVE SPONDYLOARTHROPATHIES ✔

- The seronegative spondyloarthropathies are associated with the HLA-B27 allele.

- These conditions are inflammatory arthritides not associated with rheumatoid factor.

- Involvement of the axial skeleton and extra-articular manifestations are common.

- Ankylosing spondylitis affects the spine and leads to fusion of vertebrae.

- Reiter's syndrome is a reactive arthritis that occurs in response to an infection.

- Psoriatic arthritis is associated with the dermatologic condition psoriasis.

CASE 19-8

A 33-year-old African-American woman presents with an odd complaint. She states that when she goes outside in the cold, her finger tips turn white, then blue, then red. The condition is painful and has been occurring for several months. She also complains of swelling and puffiness of her fingers, hands, and forearms, which has been persistent for the last few weeks.

1. **What do you think is going on here?**
   This condition of painful fingers that change color in cold is known as Raynaud's phenomenon (Fig. 19-15). It is caused by vasospasm of small vessels and can affect the hands, feet, nose, and ears. Cold, vibration, and emotional stress may provoke this condition. It is termed Raynaud's disease when it occurs idiopathically and Raynaud's syndrome when there is an underlying cause (such as a rheumatologic disorder).

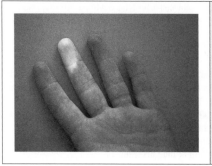

Figure 19-15. Raynaud's phenomenon in the acute phase, with severe blanching of the tip of one finger. (From Forbes CD, Jackson WF: Color Atlas and Text of Clinical Medicine, 3rd ed. London, Mosby, 2003.)

CASE 19-8 continued:

You educate your patient about Raynaud's disease and advise her on ways to avoid the painful episodes. For the puffiness in her hands and feet, you come up with a differential diagnosis that includes thyroid disorder, nephrotic syndrome, venous thrombi, heart failure, and vena cava syndrome. You find no protein in her urine, and her thyroid-stimulating hormone (TSH) is normal. You realize that the other conditions on your differential diagnosis are highly unlikely in a healthy 25-year-old woman, so you decide to see her back in a few weeks.

Your patient returns several months, rather than weeks, later. Her puffiness is gone, but she feels that the skin over her hands and feet has become thickened. She is now having frequent symptoms of gastric reflux, including burning in her chest after meals and when she lies down. She complains of diffuse arthralgias and also of dry mouth. You are beginning to think you may know what is going on here, so you order a few antibody tests. The results follow:

ANA: positive
Anticentromere: negative
Antitopoisomerase (Scl-70): positive

2. **What is your diagnosis?**
   This woman has systemic sclerosis, also known as scleroderma, which is a rheumatologic disease characterized by abnormal proliferation of connective tissue. Scleroderma is seen in several varieties: limited cutaneous, diffuse cutaneous, and localized.

3. **What is the pathogenesis of scleroderma?**

In this autoimmune disease fibroblasts are pathologically stimulated to deposit collagen and other extracellular matrix proteins. The cause of this disease is unknown. Like other autoimmune disease, theories posit that infectious agents, environmental factors, and genetics all play a role.

4. **Which sort of scleroderma does this patient have?**

So far your patient has skin and GI involvement, which may occur with either limited or diffuse systemic sclerosis. The antibody findings, however, point to a diagnosis of diffuse scleroderma. The anticentromere antibody is relatively specific for limited disease, but the antitopoisomerase antibody is associated with diffuse disease. Diffuse systemic scleroderma is associated with a higher mortality rate and more rapid progression than the other forms. It is more common and often has a worse prognosis in African Americans, particularly in younger women.

5. **What is the reason for the reflux?**

With systemic disease, the esophagus may become infiltrated with collagen, and motility is impaired. Reflux occurs as the lower esophageal sphincter loses tone. Gastroparesis may also occur with involvement of the stomach. Any portion of the GI tract may be affected by systemic sclerosis.

CASE 19-8 continued:

You see your patient again several years later. She now has extensive thickening and tightening of the skin of her extremities and face. The skin on her hands appears thickened and shiny, with several of the fingers contracted (Fig. 19-16). She reports frequent dyspnea. Her blood pressure is 165/98 mm Hg, and her weight is down 12 pounds from last year. You note bilateral basilar rales on pulmonary examination. CBC shows a normocytic anemia consistent with chronic inflammatory disease, and her creatinine is 1.6 mg/dL. You order pulmonary function tests, which show a restrictive pattern of lung disease.

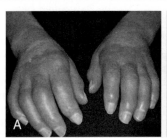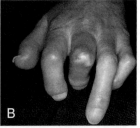

Figure 19-16. Scleroderma involving the hands. **A,** Edematous phase with diffuse swelling of the fingers. **B,** Atrophic phase with contracture and thickening sclerodactyly (thick skin over the fingers). (From Goldman L, Ausiello D: Cecil Textbook of Medicine, 22nd ed. Philadelphia, WB Saunders, 2004.)

6. **What are the renal manifestations of diffuse scleroderma?**

The renal vasculature may be compromised by collagen deposition, limiting blood flow to the kidneys. This leads to activation of the renin-angiotensin system, with a resultant rise in blood pressure. Patients with scleroderma may develop malignant hypertension and ultimately renal failure. Before the advent of angiotensin-converting enzyme (ACE) inhibitors, renal failure was the leading cause of death in scleroderma patients.

7. **What is the current leading cause of death for these patients?**

Pulmonary involvement now poses the biggest threat. The lung parenchyma and the pulmonary vasculature can be infiltrated with fibrotic material, leading to both interstitial fibrosis and pulmonary hypertension. Interstitial fibrosis reduces the compliance of the lungs and also limits the diffusing capacity. The increase in pressure in the pulmonary arteries places an afterload burden on the right ventricle, which can lead to heart failure.

8. **What is the CREST syndrome?**

CREST syndrome is another name for *limited* diffuse scleroderma, and stands for the following:

C: Calcinosis
R: Raynaud's syndrome
E: Esophageal dysmotility
S: Sclerodactyly
T: Telangiectasias

Calcium deposits may occur in subcutaneous tissue, tendons, or ligaments. Raynaud's syndrome is seen in nearly 100% of scleroderma patients. Esophageal dysmotility leads to dysphagia and reflux, as mentioned previously. Sclerodactyly is the condition of contracted, hardened skin and soft tissues of the hands. Patients with CREST syndrome tend to have skin involvement only of the distal extremities, with sparing of the trunk. Telangiectasias are groups of dilated superficial blood vessels visible on the skin.

9. **What is localized scleroderma?**

This form of scleroderma affects only the skin and subcutaneous tissue, not the internal organs. It is sometimes referred to as morphea and includes several specific subtypes. Figure 19-17 shows an example of *en coup de sabre* ("stroke of a sword"), which is a form of localized scleroderma that affects the face and scalp.

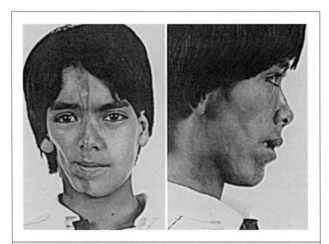

Figure 19-17. Linear scleroderma of the face (en coup de sabre) in a 13-year-old boy who had the disease for 8 years. (From Harris ED, Budd RC, Genovese MC, et al: Kelley's Textbook of Rheumatology, 7th ed. Philadelphia, WB Saunders, 2005.)

10. **How is scleroderma treated?**

Unlike most other rheumatologic diseases, systemic sclerosis does not respond well to immunosuppressant agents such as steroids. However, a majority of patients do respond to therapy with D-penicillamine. Although its precise mechanism of action remains unclear, D-penicillamine appears to inhibit cytokines such as interleukin 1 (IL-1), which stimulates fibroblast proliferation and collagen deposition, and retard the maturation of newly synthesized collagen. Other drugs used in treatment of scleroderma include ACE inhibitors to prevent the progression of renal disease, calcium channel blockers to alleviate the symptoms of Raynaud's phenomenon, and H_2 blockers or proton pump inhibitors to prevent gastric reflux. As mentioned earlier, pulmonary disease is the least treatable complication of scleroderma at this point. Cyclophosphamide is currently being evaluated for treatment of interstitial fibrosis, and prostacyclins and nitric oxide may be helpful in treating pulmonary hypertension.

11. Quick review: Cover columns 2, 3, and 4 in Table 19-2 and describe the various characteristics of diffuse, limited, and localized scleroderma.

TABLE 19-2. TYPES OF SCLERODERMA

	Diffuse Cutaneous Scleroderma	Limited Cutaneous Scleroderma (CREST)	Localized Scleroderma (Morphea)
Organ involvement	Extensive and diffuse skin involvement; significant visceral involvement (pulmonary, renal, gastrointestinal, cardiac, other)	Skin involvement, primarily of extremities; little visceral involvement; may evolve to diffuse scleroderma	Limited skin involvement with *no* visceral involvement
Antibodies	+ Antitopoisomerase (Scl-70)	+ Anticentromere	None/variable
Prognosis	Poor	Better	Good

CREST, *c*alcinosis, *R*aynaud's syndrome, *e*sophageal dysmotility, *s*clerodactyly, *t*elangiectasias.

SUMMARY BOX: SCLERODERMA

- Scleroderma is a disease characterized by abnormal collagen deposition.

- The skin and internal organs are involved to varying extents.

- Diffuse systemic sclerosis affects the entire body, including the kidneys and lungs.

- Pulmonary complications are the current leading cause of death in systemic disease.

- Limited sclerosis is expressed as the CREST syndrome: calcinosis, Raynaud's syndrome, esophageal dysmotility, sclerodactyly, and telangiectasias.

- Morphea or localized scleroderma affects only the skin.

- Treatments include D-penicillamine, angiotensin-converting enzyme (ACE) inhibitors, calcium channel blockers, H_2 blockers, and proton pump inhibitors.

CASE 19-9

A 22-year-old woman presents for evaluation of a painless facial rash that has been present for the past 3 weeks. She otherwise feels well, and is taking no medications. She can think of no precipitating factors other than sun exposure, as she is recently back from vacation. On examination, the rash involves both cheeks and the bridge of the nose but spares the nasolabial folds. The lesions appear as erythematous patches with scaling and a crusty appearance, similar in appearance to the facial rash shown in Figure 19-18.

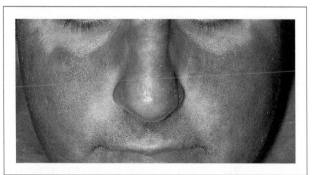

Figure 19-18. Classic appearance of a malar (butterfly) rash. (From Habif TP: Clinical Dermatology, 4th ed. Philadelphia, Mosby, 2004.)

1. **What is the likely diagnosis in this patient?**
   In the absence of other symptoms, the differential diagnosis for a malar rash includes rosacea, pellagra, psoriasis, dermatomyositis, and discoid lupus, a poorly understood autoimmune disease. If symptoms were present we would suspect SLE.

2. **How can a diagnosis of discoid lupus be confirmed?**
   Skin biopsy is the method of definitive diagnosis.

3. **What treatment options exist for discoid lupus?**
   Topical corticosteroids and antimalarial agents such as hydroxychloroquine can be used. Patients should be advised of the importance of sun protection as well.

CASE 19-9 continued:

Your patient's skin improves with the topical steroids, and she remains well for 10 years. She then returns to you with worsening facial rash, as well as diffuse arthralgias and fatigue. She complains of constant dryness of her mouth and eyes. Further history reveals that she has had several early miscarriages, and she was diagnosed with syphilis 3 years ago in the absence of clear symptoms or risk factors.

On physical examination, you find an erythematous facial rash in the malar distribution. Her metacarpophalangeal and proximal interphalangeal joints are tender, swollen, and erythematous bilaterally. Her mucous membranes appear dry, and you note the presence of aphthous ulcers (canker sores) and fissures in her lips. You draw several laboratory tests and find a mild anemia, protein in the urine, and the following serum autoantibodies:
   Antinuclear antibody: positive
   Anti-Smith: positive
   Antihistone: negative

4. **What is the likely diagnosis?**
This patient has SLE, an autoimmune disease that damages multiple organ systems primarily via pathological immune complex deposition.

5. **What is the pathogenesis of systemic lupus erythematosus?**
The primary immune phenomenon in lupus is the generation of autoantibodies directed against cellular components, a process that forms immune complexes. Note that SLE is a type III hypersensitivity reaction. Although the exact mechanism is not fully understood, there is evidence that immune cells become hyperreactive, leading to a sustained pathologic immune response. It is important to realize that SLE is truly a systemic disease and may manifest in the dermatologic, renal, cardiac, pulmonary, musculoskeletal, hematologic, GI, vascular, and nervous systems.

6. **What causes lupus?**
As with most autoimmune diseases, a combination of genetic and environmental factors is thought to be responsible. Lupus tends to occur most frequently in women aged 15 to 40, and African Americans are at highest risk. However, men and women of any age or race are capable of developing the disease.

7. **What are the criteria for diagnosing systemic lupus erythematosus?**
SLE is diagnosed on the basis of a combination of clinical and laboratory findings. If four or more of the following criteria are present at *any time* in the patient's history, the diagnosis can be made with 95% specificity.
    1. Malar rash
    2. Discoid rash
    3. Photosensitivity
    4. Oral ulcers
    5. Arthritis
    6. Serositis (pleurisy, pericarditis)
    7. Renal dysfunction +/− proteinuria/cellular casts
    8. Neurologic disorder (unexplained seizures or psychosis)
    9. Hematologic disorder (hemolytic anemia, leukopenia, lymphopenia, thrombocytopenia)
    10. Anti–double-stranded DNA (dsDNA), anti-Smith, or antiphospholipid antibodies
    11. Antinuclear antibodies

8. **What are "antinuclear antibodies," and are they sensitive or specific for systemic lupus erythematosus?**
The antinuclear antibodies are a diverse group of autoantibodies, all of which bind antigenic targets within the cellular nucleus. Because they are sensitive for SLE (>95% of patients with SLE have them), they are a good screening test for the disease. However, they are not specific, because they are present in many other autoimmune diseases and are often present in the healthy elderly. Anti-dsDNA and anti-Smith antibodies are very specific for SLE and are useful for confirming the diagnosis. Anti-dsDNA antibodies, in particular, are associated with SLE-induced renal disease and indicate poorer prognosis. Antihistone antibodies are found in drug-induced lupus.

9. **What is causing this patient's dry mouth and dry eyes?**
The complaint of dry mouth (xerostomia) and dry eyes (xerophthalmia) together constitutes sicca complex, also known as Sjögren's syndrome. This is an autoimmune disorder of the exocrine glands that can occur either on its own (primary Sjögren's) or alongside another autoimmune

disease (secondary) such as lupus, scleroderma, or rheumatoid arthritis. The anti-Ro and anti-La antibodies are often found in Sjögren's syndrome. Anti-Ro is capable of crossing the placenta and causing third-degree heart block in neonates born to mothers positive for this antibody.

10. **What is the reason for the proteinuria?**
Immune complexes are deposited in the renal glomeruli, leading to a type III hypersensitivity reaction. This entity is termed lupus nephritis and may progress to varying degrees in different patients with SLE. Renal biopsy is often needed to accurately determine prognosis and therapy. Other type III reactions seen in lupus include pericarditis, pleuritis, endocarditis, and the malar rash.
   Note: Libman-Sacks endocarditis is a nonbacterial form of endocarditis seen in SLE. Fibrinous vegetations are formed on valve leaflets in response to immune complex deposition. The mitral valve is most often involved.

11. **What is the reason for this woman's anemia?**
Lupus is a chronic inflammatory disorder, and as such, it is capable of causing anemia of chronic disease. This sort of anemia is often normochromic and normocytic, but it may be hypochromic and microcytic in some cases. Although anemia of chronic disease is the most frequent hematologic manifestation of lupus, other potential complications include autoimmune hemolytic anemia, leukopenia, lymphopenia, and thrombocytopenia.

12. **Why did this patient have a positive Venereal Disease Research Laboratory (VDRL) test?**
Some lupus patients produce the inaptly named "lupus anticoagulant," which is an antibody directed against certain phospholipid molecules. While this antibody delays in vitro coagulation assays, it actually predisposes to thrombus formation in vivo. This accounts for the increased incidence of venous and arterial thrombi, fetal loss, and thrombocytopenia in lupus patients. The lupus anticoagulant happens to bind the phospholipid used in the VDRL assay, which is the reason for the false positive result when testing for syphilis.

STEP 1 SECRET

The correlation between systemic lupus erythematosus (SLE) and positive Venereal Disease Research Laboratory (VDRL) test results is a high-yield fact to know for boards.

13. **What are the treatment options for systemic lupus erythematosus?**
The mainstay of treatment is systemic glucocorticoids. High doses are used for short periods of active disease, and low doses can be used to prevent flares. The side effects of glucocorticoids are frequently encountered in lupus patients, who may take these medications for years. The cytotoxic drug cyclophosphamide is also useful in the treatment of lupus nephritis.
   Note: Side effects of glucocorticoids include hypertension, hyperglycemia, osteoporosis, central obesity, and increased rates of infection.

14. **What medications are responsible for drug-induced lupus?**
Procainamide, quinidine, hydralazine, isoniazid, sulfonamides, methyldopa, and chlorpromazine have all been shown to cause a disease syndrome that mimics SLE. Drug-induced lupus typically resolves once the offending agent is withdrawn.

15. Quick review: Cover the right column in Table 19-3 and give the primary disease(s) associated with the autoantibodies listed in the left column.

TABLE 19-3. AUTOANTIBODY SUMMARY	
Autoantibody	**Primary Disease**
Antiacetylcholine receptor	Myasthenia gravis
Anticentromere	Limited cutaneous scleroderma (CREST syndrome)
Anti-dsDNA	SLE (specific)
Anti–glomerular basement membrane	Goodpasture's syndrome
Antihistone	Drug-induced SLE
Anti-IgG (RF)	Rheumatoid arthritis
Anti–islet cell	Type 1 diabetes mellitus
Anti-La (SS-B)	Sjögren's syndrome
Antimicrosomal	Hashimoto's thyroiditis
Antimitochondrial	Primary biliary cirrhosis
Antineutrophil (c-ANCA)	Wegner's granulomatosis
Antineutrophil (p-ANCA)	Microscopic polyangiitis
Antinuclear	SLE, scleroderma, dermatomyositis
Antiphospholipid	SLE
Anti-Ro (SS-A)	Sjögren's syndrome
Anti-Smith	SLE (specific)
Anti–smooth muscle	Chronic autoimmune hepatitis
Anti–tissue transglutaminase	Celiac
Antitopoisomerase (Scl-70)	Diffuse cutaneous scleroderma

c-ANCA, cytoplasmic antineutrophil cytoplasmic antibodies; CREST, *c*alcinosis, *R*aynaud phenomenon, *e*sophageal dysmotility, *s*clerodactyly, *t*elangiectasia; ds, double-stranded; IgG, immunoglobulin G; p-ANCA, perinuclear antineutrophil cytoplasmic antibodies; RF, rheumatoid factor; SLE, systemic lupus erythematosus.

SUMMARY BOX: SYSTEMIC LUPUS ERYTHEMATOSUS

- Lupus is an autoimmune disease that primarily occurs in young women.

- The disease is caused by autoantibodies directed against nuclear antigens and can affect all organs.

- Discoid lupus is primarily a skin disease but may progress to lupus.

- Antinuclear antibodies are highly sensitive, but not specific, for SLE.

- Anti-Smith and anti-dsDNA antibodies are highly specific, but not specific, for SLE.

- The lupus anticoagulant is an autoantibody that causes thrombosis, early miscarriages, thrombocytopenia, and false positive results on Venereal Disease Research Laboratory (VDRL) assays.

- Lupus nephritis is a type III hypersensitivity reaction associated with high morbidity and mortality rates.

- Lupus is primarily treated with steroids; lupus nephritis is typically treated with cyclophosphamide.

- Procainamide, quinidine, hydralazine, isoniazid, methyldopa, and chlorpromazine can cause drug-induced lupus.

- Sjögren's syndrome is an autoimmune disease of the exocrine glands that causes dry eyes and mouth and is often found along with other autoimmune diseases.

CASE 19-10

A 58-year-old woman presents to your office for evaluation of a several-month history of progressively worsening muscle weakness. She has had difficulty getting into and out of chairs, climbing the stairs, and lifting things over her head. She also reports recently developing a violet-colored rash around her eyes (Fig. 19-19). Review of systems is positive for fatigue, joint stiffness, and an unintentional 10-lb weight loss over the past 6 months. She takes no medications.

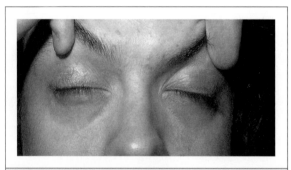

Figure 19-19. Periorbital rash from patient in case 19-10. (From Habif TP: Clinical Dermatology, 4th ed. Philadelphia, Mosby, 2004.)

1. **What is your differential diagnosis?**
   This patient has several symptoms of systemic disease (weakness, fatigue, weight loss) as well as a rash and joint pain. One could entertain diagnoses of a thyroid disorder, rheumatic arthritis, myasthenia gravis, polymyalgia rheumatica, Cushing disease, paraneoplastic syndrome or other malignancy, or various myopathies (e.g., muscular dystrophy, dermatomyositis, polymyositis).

CASE 19-10 continued:

You order several laboratory tests and find an elevated levels of creatinine kinase (CK), aldolase and aspartate transaminase (AST). Electromyographic studies are suggestive of myopathy, and a muscle biopsy shows an infiltration of lymphocytes and muscle atrophy.

2. **What is the diagnosis?**
   This patient has dermatomyositis, one of the idiopathic inflammatory myopathies. This autoimmune disease causes inflammatory damage to muscle fibers, with resultant proximal muscle weakness and elevated muscle enzymes (CK).

3. **What causes this disease?**
   Although the exact cause is unknown, a substantial fraction of patients with dermatomyositis have an underlying malignancy. It is therefore important to consider the presence of a neoplastic process in a patient who presents with dermatomyositis.

4. **What is the treatment?**
   As this is an inflammatory disorder, immunosuppressant drugs are the mainstay. Prednisone is first-line therapy, and methotrexate can be used if corticosteroids are unsuccessful.

5. **What are the other "idiopathic inflammatory myopathies"?**
   Dermatomyositis and polymyositis are both inflammatory myopathies characterized by symmetrical proximal muscle weakness, elevated serum muscle enzymes, and evidence of myopathy on electromyography. Dermatomyositis often presents with skin findings, such as the heliotrope rash, Gottron's sign (see Figure 19-20), and the shawl sign; polymyositis does not have these dermatologic manifestations. Dermatomyositis and polymyositis appear distinct on muscle biopsy, with dermatomyositis showing immune complex deposition, and polymyositis revealing predominantly T-cell invasion of muscle fibers. Inclusion body myositis is another inflammatory myopathy, which presents with both proximal and distal muscle weakness and normal or mildly elevated muscle enzymes and is associated with distinctive changes on electromyogram (EMG) and biopsy. Figure 19-20 shows Gottron's papules on the hands in dermatomyositis.

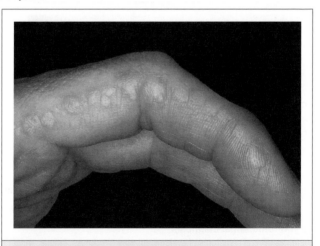

Figure 19-20. Gottron's papules, a pathognomonic sign of dermatomyositis, are round, smooth, flat-topped papules that occur over the knuckles and along the sides of the fingers. (From Habif TP: Clinical Dermatology, 4th ed. Philadelphia, Mosby, 2004.)

6. **What disease that is transmitted by pork can cause similar muscular symptoms?**
   Trichinosis is caused by eating raw or undercooked meats that contain the viable larvae of the roundworm *Trichinella spiralis*. Although most infections are subclinical, exposure to a heavy inoculum of larvae can result in trichinosis, which may present manifest clinically with diarrhea, myositis, fever, and periorbital edema. Laboratory evaluation will typically reveal hypereosinophilia as well.

SUMMARY BOX: INFLAMMATORY MYOPATHIES

- Dermatomyositis, polymyositis, and inclusion body myositis are idiopathic inflammatory myopathies.

- Dermatomyositis is characterized by proximal muscle weakness, elevated serum muscle enzymes, electromyogram (EMG) abnormalities, dermatologic manifestations, and characteristic muscle pathologic changes.

- Polymyositis is a similar myopathic process with distinct muscle disease but without skin involvement.

- Inclusion body myositis causes both proximal and distal muscle weakness without markedly raised serum muscle enzymes.

- The inflammatory myopathies are treated with steroids.

- Trichinosis is a parasitic disease that may cause myopathy.

CASE 19-11

The parents of a 3-year-old boy are concerned that he is not walking as well as other boys his age. Both parents are healthy, and there is no family history of neuromuscular disease. He has three older brothers who are healthy. On physical examination, he has large calf muscles and lower extremity proximal muscle weakness, as demonstrated by the need to use his arms and hands to assist in standing from a seated position. Examination is otherwise unremarkable.

1. **What is your differential diagnosis?**
   This child with muscle weakness may be suffering from a myopathy such as juvenile dermatomyositis, an inflammatory disease such as juvenile rheumatoid arthritis, an inherited muscular dystrophy, a neurologic disorder such as Guillain-Barré syndrome, or an infection such as Lyme disease or trichinosis.

CASE 19-11 continued:

Laboratory tests are significant only for a markedly elevated CK. A skeletal muscle biopsy reveals complete absence of dystrophin staining.

2. **What is the most likely diagnosis?**
   Duchenne's muscular dystrophy is most likely.

3. **Is this condition more commonly acquired or inherited?**
   About two thirds of cases of Duchenne's muscular dystrophy are inherited in an X-linked recessive manner. However, approximately one third of the cases are secondary to spontaneous mutations within the dystrophin gene. The dystrophin gene is subject to a high rate of spontaneous mutations because of its enormous size ($>2 \times 10^6$ bases). Because his parents were unaffected and he has three healthy older brothers, this condition was likely acquired in this boy following a spontaneous mutation in the dystrophin gene.

STEP 1 SECRET

Boards will often relate its genetics questions to pedigrees, which means that you should know the inheritance patterns of the genetic diseases that you study. X-linked recessive diseases are a particular USMLE favorite. These include **G**6PD deficiency, **O**cular albinism, **L**esch-Nyhan syndrome, **D**uchenne's muscular dystrophy, **W**iskott-Aldrich syndrome, **B**ruton's agammaglobulinemia, **C**hronic granulomatous disease, **H**unter's syndrome, **F**abry's disease, and **H**emophilia (A and B).

You can use this mnemonic to remember the X-linked recessive diseases: "**Good OLD WBCs Hunt and Fight Heroically**."

4. **What is the function of dystrophin?**
   Dystrophin is a cytoskeletal membrane protein that plays an important structural role in skeletal muscle cells. It is absent in Duchenne's muscular dystrophy.

5. **How do the manifestations of Becker's muscular dystrophy differ?**
   This disease is also due to mutations in the dystrophin gene, but there is some level of protein present rather than a complete absence, so the clinical manifestations are not as severe as in Duchenne's muscular dystrophy.

6. **Why does this boy have such large calf muscles on examination? What term is used to describe this finding in Duchenne's muscular dystrophy patients?**
   Patients with Duchenne's muscular dystrophy ironically have the appearance of enlarged calf muscles, referred to as pseudohypertrophy of the calf muscles (Fig. 19-21). This hypertrophy occurs initially in response to hypertrophy of muscle fibers but secondarily in response to fatty infiltration of the muscle and abnormal proliferation of connective tissue within the muscle.

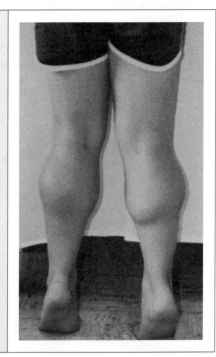

Figure 19-21. Enlarged calf muscles in a patient with Duchenne's muscular dystrophy. (From Fenichel GM: Clinical Pediatric Neurology. Philadelphia, WB Saunders, 1997.)

7. **How is a Gowers' sign elicited on examination and what does it indicate?**
    A Gowers' sign can be elicited by asking the child to stand from a sitting position. Children with muscular dystrophy and other disorders involving muscle wasting will not have the muscle strength to simply stand. They may instead first roll over into a prone position, push themselves onto all fours, and then "walk" their hands up their thighs to a standing position (i.e., positive Gowers' sign). The presence of a Gowers' sign indicates marked proximal muscle weakness (Fig. 19-22).

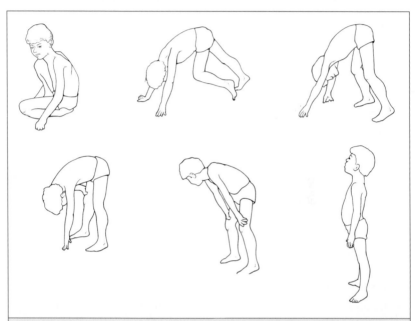

Figure 19-22. Gowers' sign. (Redrawn from Siegel IM: Clinical management of muscle disease. In Canale STS: Campbell's Operative Orthopedics, 5th ed. London, William Heinemann, 1977.)

A FEW MORE MUSCULAR DYSTROPHIES . . .

A patient complains of a long history of generalized muscle weakness. On examination, his facial muscles show marked atrophy, and when you ask him to shake your hand, he appears unable to relax his grip for an extended period.

8. **What diagnosis might you suspect?**
    You might suspect myotonic dystrophy, which is the most common adult dystrophy. The term myotonia refers to a sustained involuntary contraction of muscles, which this man is exhibiting by not being able to release his grip.

    Other symptoms of myotonic dystrophy include facial muscle weakness, frontal balding, testicular atrophy, cataracts, cardiac conduction defects, and glucose intolerance.

9. **What is the mechanism of inheritance of myotonic dystrophy?**
    Myotonic dystrophy results from impaired expression of the myotonin protein kinase gene. The mechanism causing impaired expression involves expansion of a trinucleotide repeat sequence located in the 3′ untranslated region of the myotonin protein kinase gene. This disorder

is inherited as an autosomal dominant disease, and because this mechanism involves expansion of trinucleotide repeat sequences (CTG), the phenomenon of amplification is seen (i.e., family members get the disease at earlier and earlier ages throughout the generations).

Note: Other trinucleotide repeat disorders include Huntington's disease (CAG), fragile X syndrome (CGG), and Friedreich's ataxia (GAA).

An adult patient with a long history of muscle weakness has maintained a slow, steady course of declining function and is now wheelchair-bound. His weakness is most prominent in proximal muscles, with complete sparing of facial and extraocular musculature. A muscle biopsy shows normal dystrophin expression. The patient's father and grandfather had similar courses.

10. **What is the diagnosis?**
    This is limb-girdle muscular dystrophy, which is actually a group of myopathies that affect the shoulder and pelvic girdles. Limb-girdle dystrophies can be inherited in both autosomal dominant and recessive fashion and may display a heterogeneous phenotype. The recessive form of the disease tends to have an earlier onset and progresses more quickly, whereas the dominant form follows a slower and more variable course. Several different genes have been implicated in this disease.

SUMMARY BOX: THE MUSCULAR DYSTROPHIES

- Duchenne's muscular dystrophy is an inherited loss of the dystrophin protein, which is a structural component of skeletal muscle cells.

- Duchenne's muscular dystrophy is inherited in a recessive X-linked fashion, or may be an acquired spontaneous mutation.

- Becker's muscular dystrophy is an inherited defect in dystrophin that results in partial loss of the dystrophin protein.

- Myotonic muscular dystrophy is a trinucleotide repeat disorder.

- Limb-girdle muscular dystrophy is a heterogeneous group of heritable defects in proteins that result in proximal muscle weakness and atrophy.

- Gowers' sign indicates proximal muscle weakness.

CASE 19-12

Dr. Rheumatoid is a specialist widely known for his interest and skill in treating rare disorders of the musculoskeletal system. His particular expertise is in diagnosing and treating metabolic and developmental disorders of bone. A third-year medical student working with him one afternoon is delighted to encounter one "zebra" after another in clinic.

CASE 19-12.1

The first patient was referred to Dr. Rheumatoid with complaints of bone pain and a diagnosis by a hematologist of myelophthisic anemia. A bone scan reveals abnormally thick and dense bones with an "Erlenmeyer flask" deformity (Fig. 19-23).

1. **What is your diagnosis?**
   Osteopetrosis (also known as marble bone disease).

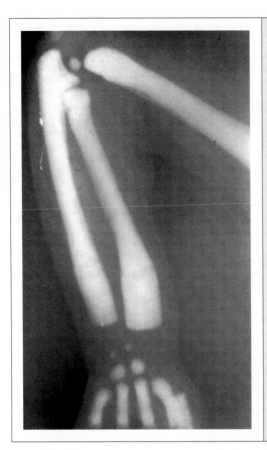

Figure 19-23. Radiograph of the upper extremity in a patient with this condition (see text for discussion). (From Kumar V, Abbas AK, Fausto N: Robbins and Cotran Pathologic Basis of Disease, 7th ed. Philadelphia, WB Saunders, 2005.)

2. **What causes the bones to be dense and thick in this patient?**

   In osteopetrosis, osteoclasts are less active than normal (or inactive entirely) and therefore do not resorb bone effectively during bone remodeling. This generally is the result of failure of the osteoclasts to acidify the resorption pit (e.g., due to carbonic anhydrase or chloride channel gene mutations). Additionally, the process whereby woven (immature) bone is converted to compact (mature) bone is disrupted in osteopetrosis. This combination of reduced remodeling of bone and inadequate bone "maturation" results in thick and brittle bones.

3. **Why might you see anemia in osteopetrosis and why is it referred to as a myelophthisic anemia?**

   The term myelophthisis describes the replacement of hematopoietic tissue in the bone marrow with abnormal tissue. Myelophthisic anemia is therefore caused by the replacement of bone marrow by abnormal tissue. In the case of osteopetrosis, the failure of osteoclasts to remodel existing bone allows newly formed bone to encroach on the space of the bone marrow, making hematopoiesis less effective and resulting in pancytopenia (anemia, thrombocytopenia, leukopenia).

4. **Should you observe any laboratory value abnormalities in a patient who has osteopetrosis?**

   No. Serum calcium, phosphate, alkaline phosphatase, and parathyroid hormone (PTH) levels are normal in osteopetrosis.

STEP 1 SECRET

Laboratory value abnormalities associated with various bone disorders are high-yield for Step 1. When studying this topic, you should classify these disorders according to their unique clinical and radiographic features as well as their expected laboratory values (i.e., calcium, phosphate, alkaline phosphatase, parathyroid hormone [PTH]). **Note:** You do not need to know exact laboratory value ranges, but you should be able to compare them with normal values using relative terms (increased, decreased, normal).

CASE 19-12.2

A 13-year-old boy with sickle cell anemia is referred for persistent right hip pain and intermittent fevers, although he cannot recall any specific trauma to the hip. An x-ray of the hips suggests avascular necrosis of the femoral heads.

5. **Infection with what organisms should be suspected?**
    Although *S. aureus* is the most common organism responsible for osteomyelitis, patients with sickle cell anemia are uniquely susceptible to *Salmonella* bacteremia and osteomyelitis. This susceptibility stems from the impaired splenic and mononuclear cell function associated with sickle cell anemia, as *Salmonella* is an encapsulated organism.

CASE 19-12.3

A 42-year-old woman with end-stage renal failure is referred to Dr. Rheumatoid because recent bone scans revealed marked osteopenia throughout her body.

6. **What most likely explains this?**
    The most likely explanation is osteomalacia caused by vitamin D deficiency secondary to renal failure. Recall that an important endocrine function of the kidneys is the production of 1,25-dihydroxycholecalciferol, the active form of vitamin D. Because vitamin D is necessary for bone mineralization, and because bone is constantly being remodeled, impaired mineralization results in an imbalance between mineralization and degradation, causing marked osteopenia (Fig. 19-24).
    Note: Additional causes of renal osteodystrophy include bone buffering of excess acid and hypocalcemia from calcium phosphate precipitation in hyperphosphatemia.

CASE 19-12.4

A 6-year-old boy is brought to the clinic by his mother because he has suffered multiple bone fractures throughout his short life. These fractures were all unexpected, as they invariably occurred in response to very minor accidents. Additionally, the boy has been doing poorly in school recently because he is having trouble hearing the teacher. The examination is remarkable only for slightly blue sclerae. X-ray of the lower extremity shows marked bowing of the bones (Fig. 19-25).

7. **What is your diagnosis and what is the etiology of this condition?**
    Osteogenesis imperfecta is due to genetic defects that result in structural or quantitative abnormalities of type I collagen, which is the primary component of the extracellular matrix of bones, including the middle ear bone (explaining the hearing loss seen in this child). Type I collagen is also found in corneal tissues. A defect in type I collagen results in translucency of the connective tissue over the vascular choroid layer of the eye, such that the veins impart a blue appearance to the sclerae.

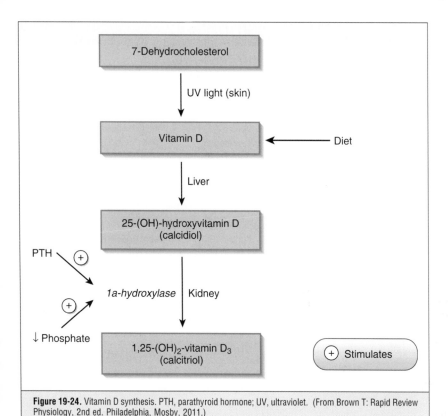

Figure 19-24. Vitamin D synthesis. PTH, parathyroid hormone; UV, ultraviolet. (From Brown T: Rapid Review Physiology, 2nd ed. Philadelphia, Mosby, 2011.)

Note: A wide spectrum of genotypes and phenotypes is associated with osteogenesis imperfecta, ranging from fairly minor to very severe.

8. **Quick review: Cover the right column in Table 19-4 and list the pathophysiologic abnormality associated with each of the rheumatologic disorders listed in the left column.**

SUMMARY BOX: OSTEOPETROSIS, SICKLE CELL AVASCULAR NECROSIS, OSTEOGENESIS IMPERFECTA

- Osteopetrosis is a disorder of osteoclasts that results in thick, brittle bones and myelophthisic anemia.

- Patients with sickle cell disease are prone to osteomyelitis caused by *Salmonella* species.

- End-stage renal failure results in vitamin D deficiency and osteomalacia, also known as renal osteodystrophy.

- Osteogenesis imperfecta is a highly variable disease caused by a defect in type I collagen.

TABLE 19-4. RHEUMATOLOGIC DISORDERS

Disorder	Pathophysiology
Achondroplasia	Mutation in fibroblast growth factor receptor prevents endochondral ossification and limits long bone growth
Gout	Increased uric acid production or decreased uric acid excertion
Osteoarthritis	Degeneration of joint cartilage
Osteogenesis imperfecta	Genetic defects in type I collagen weaken bone
Osteomalacia	Impaired bone mineralization in adults
Osteopetrosis (marble bone disease)	Decreased osteoclast activity, bony invasion of bone marrow leading to myelophthisic anemia
Paget disease	Increased rate of osteoclast activity (perhaps secondary to viral infection of osteoclasts), resulting in increased rates of bone resorption, formation, and mineralization, with consequent deposition of woven rather than lamellar bone
Pseudogout (chondrocalcinosis)	Calcium pyrophosphate deposition
Rheumatoid arthritis	Inflammation of synovial membrane
Rickets	Impaired bone and cartilage mineralization in children

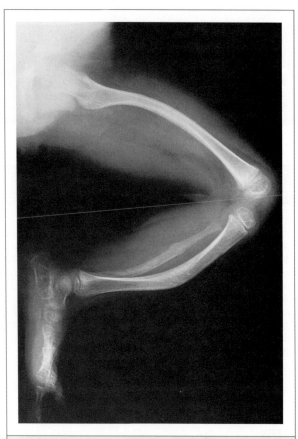

Figure 19-25. Lateral view of the lower extremities shows marked bowing of the bones due to softening and multiple fractures that occur as a result of this congenital bone dysplasia. (From Mettler FA: Essentials of Radiology, 2nd ed. Philadelphia, WB Saunders, 2005.)

CHAPTER 20

VASCULITIDES

Thomas A. Brown, MD, and Sonali J. Shah

INSIDER'S GUIDE TO VASCULITIDES FOR THE USMLE STEP 1

Vasculitides on Step 1 are very straightforward if you know the most common signs and symptoms of each diagnosis. The best way to study for this section is to simply read through the information listed in First Aid (which contains everything that you need to know for boards) and then test yourself with the tables and cases in this chapter. It is advisable that you make a list for yourself of the unique features of each disease (e.g., palpable lower extremity skin rash with Schönlein-Henoch purpura, weak upper extremity pulses in Takayasu's arteritis, unilateral headache in temporal arteritis). These features will most likely be your biggest clues in the clinical vignettes presented to you on boards. You should also be sure to know the unique laboratory features associated with specific vasculitides, such as elevation in perinuclear antineutrophil cytoplasmic antibody (p-ANCA) or cytoplasmic antineutrophil cytoplasmic antibodies (c-ANCA), elevated erythrocyte sedimentation rate (ESR), and hepatitis B seropositivity, as the USMLE loves to test students on these facts.

BASIC CONCEPTS

1. **What are the vasculitides and how do they typically present clinically?**
   The best way to think of the vasculitides is as a group of poorly understood autoimmune disorders involving the blood vessels. They are defined by the presence of leukocytes in the vessel walls, and as inflammatory diseases, they typically present with vague constitutional signs such as fever, malaise, and arthralgias or myalgias. A biopsy of affected blood vessels can be very helpful in making a definitive diagnosis, although obtaining a segment of affected vasculature can be difficult. Although it appears that a majority of the vasculitis syndromes are caused by an immune-mediated mechanism, other possible etiologic factors include drug hypersensitivity reactions and viral infections resulting in immune complex deposition within the vasculature.

2. **Along with constitutional complaints, what clinical signs and patterns of organ involvement suggest a vasculitic syndrome?**
   Palpable nonblanching purpura may indicate vasculitides such as hypersensitivity (leukocytoclastic) vasculitis, Schönlein-Henoch purpura, and microscopic polyangiitis (polyarteritis).

   Mononeuritis multiplex, a clinical picture that arises from simultaneous disease to multiple individual nerves, typically affects sensory and motor function. In the United States, diabetes is the most common cause of this neuropathy, but in the nondiabetic person, it is very suggestive of vasculitis, particularly polyarteritis nodosa (PAN).

   Pulmonary-renal involvement, such as hemoptysis and hematuria, are suggestive of a pulmonary-renal syndrome such as Wegener's granulomatosis or Goodpasture's syndrome.

3. **How are the vasculitides classified?**
   The vasculitides are generally classified by the size and types of blood vessels that are typically affected in patients with each disorder.
   Large vessel vasculitis:
   - Takayasu's arteritis affects the aorta and its major branches.
   - Temporal arteritis, also known as giant cell arteritis, most commonly affects the branches of the external carotid artery, characteristically including the temporal artery.
   Medium-sized vessel vasculitis:
   - PAN affects medium-sized muscular arteries.
   - Kawasaki disease actually affects large, medium-sized, and small arteries, but the most important association is that, if untreated, it can affect the coronary arteries.
   Small vessel vasculitis:
   - Churg-Strauss arteritis affects the arteries of the lungs and of the skin.
   - Wegener's granulomatosis affects medium-sized and small arteries, arterioles, and venules, particularly in the respiratory tract.
   - Cryoglobulinemic vasculitis affects capillaries, arterioles, and venules.
   - Schönlein-Henoch purpura primarily affects venules.
   - Vasculitis that is due to hypersensitivity reaction, secondary to viral infection, or secondary to connective tissue disorder typically affects small vessels.

4. **Cover the right column in Table 20-1 and attempt to describe the "classic presentation" for each of the listed vasculitides.**
   Table 20-1 lists the classic presentations of the vasculitides.

TABLE 20-1. CLASSIC PRESENTATION OF THE VASCULITIDES	
Vasculitis	**Classic Presentation**
Temporal (giant cell) arteritis	Fever, unilateral headache, markedly elevated ESR
Wegener's granulomatosis	Hemoptysis, hematuria, presence of c-ANCA
Kawasaki syndrome	Unexplained fever, maculopapular rash that starts on hands and feet, bilateral conjunctival injection, cervical lymphadenopathy, edema of extremities, and mucosal changes such as strawberry tongue; seen in children
Polyarteritis nodosa	Hepatitis B antigenemia is common, presence of p-ANCA; arterial biopsy reveals inflammation of the tunica media
	Generally affects vessels of the kidney, heart, liver, and GI system
	Does not affect the pulmonary vasculature
Churg-Strauss syndrome	History of asthma, sinusitis, peripheral neuropathy
	Lab tests show eosinophilia
Takayasu's arteritis ("pulseless disease")	Fever, night sweats, arthritis, myalgia, vision problems, different blood pressures in the arms
	Commonly seen in Asian women younger than 40 years of age

Continued

TABLE 20-1. CLASSIC PRESENTATION OF THE VASCULITIDES—continued	
Vasculitis	**Classic Presentation**
Henoch-Schönlein purpura	Abdominal pain, hematuria with red blood cell casts, maculopapular rash on lower extremities (palpable purpura) Most commonly occurs in young children; associated with IgA nephropathy after upper respiratory infection
Thromboangiitis obliterans (Buerger's disease)	Young male smoker with distal extremity cold intolerance

c-ANCA, cytoplasmic antineutrophil cytoplasmic antibodies; ESR, erythrocyte sedimentation rate; GI, gastrointestinal; IgA, immunoglobulin A; p-ANCA, perinuclear antineutrophil cytoplasmic antibodies.

CASE 20-1

A 75-year-old Caucasian woman is evaluated for a 1-week history of anorexia, fatigue, and severe headache. She denies any recent visual problems or photophobia.

1. **What are the main considerations in your differential diagnosis?**
Constitutional complaints such as anorexia and fatigue are suggestive of malignancy, depression, infection, and vasculitis. The headache could be caused by a migraine, meningitis, primary or metastatic cancer, subdural hematoma, or vasculitis. However, for boards, headache in an adult over 50 in the absence of fever or head trauma is temporal arteritis until proved otherwise.

CASE 20-1 continued:

Physical examination is significant for right-sided scalp tenderness. Laboratory tests reveal a markedly elevated erythrocyte sedimentation rate (ESR).

2. **What is the likely diagnosis?**
Temporal arteritis or giant cell arteritis (GCA). Temporal arteritis occurs almost exclusively in patients older than 50. Women are more likely than men to be affected, and rates are highest in whites. Unilateral headache and scalp tenderness are classic for temporal arteritis, as is the elevated ESR. Temporal arteritis also commonly presents with jaw pain. Vision impairment or blindness may result in the most serious cases.

   The name temporal arteritis is derived from the fact that the disease preferentially targets the extracranial branches of the carotid arteries, frequently affecting the superficial temporal artery. The ophthalmic, vertebral, and the carotid arteries may also be affected.

3. **What does the elevated erythrocyte sedimentation rate imply?**
The ESR and C-reactive protein (CRP) are the most widely used indicators of the acute-phase protein response. Although these measurements lack specificity (being elevated in vasculitides, infections such as endocarditis, and malignancies), they are useful because the acute-phase protein response may reflect the presence and intensity of an inflammatory process.

   Specifically, the ESR represents the rate at which the erythrocytes fall through the plasma, which depends largely upon the plasma concentration of fibrinogen, a protein that is seen in higher concentration during an inflammatory process.

4. **In temporal arteritis, what events lead to inflammation of the artery?**

It is likely that T cells and macrophages enter the artery wall via the vasa vasorum. How they become activated and targeted is as yet unknown. CD4$^+$ T cells release interferon (IFN)-γ, and macrophages release interleukins (IL-1, IL-6) and platelet-derived growth factor (PDGF). IFN-γ mediates the inflammatory response in the vessel wall, IL-6 is largely responsible for systemic signs of inflammation, and PDGF promotes proliferation of smooth muscle cells and intimal hyperplasia. This intimal hyperplasia leads to occlusion of the arterial lumen, ultimately leading to the symptoms of ischemia experienced by the patient.

CASE 20-1 continued:

The patient is started on high-dose steroids, and the following day a biopsy of a 3-cm section of the right side of the temporal artery returns as negative for signs of inflammation.

5. **Why might it still make sense to treat this patient?**

Temporal arteritis affects the temporal artery in a segmental fashion, and this could explain a negative biopsy result even in the presence of the disease. Furthermore, in some cases, GCA may affect other extracranial branches of the carotid artery and spare the superficial temporal artery. Therefore, if the clinician has a high index of suspicion for temporal arteritis, the patient should be treated regardless of biopsy results (making biopsy of questionable clinical value).

6. **What severe complication of this disorder may be avoided by initiating immunosuppressive therapy as soon as possible?**

Partial or total blindness can occur suddenly and without warning. This is caused by occlusion of the ophthalmic artery, leading to ischemia of the optic nerve. Blindness may be preceded by amaurosis fugax, which is transient visual loss, often with heat or exercise. Blindness is usually permanent but can be prevented by adequate treatment with corticosteroids, making timely diagnosis and treatment of GCA crucial.

As demonstrated in this case, patients with GCA are treated with high-dose steroids to prevent blindness.

7. **What other symptomatic manifestations may be expected as a result of arterial inflammation in patients with giant cell arteritis?**

Decreased blood flow in the extracranial branches of the carotid arteries caused by inflammation of those vessels can lead to symptoms such as jaw claudication, especially with prolonged talking or chewing causing an increase in oxygen demand. Occasionally, respiratory symptoms such as coughing can be seen with GCA and are believed to be a result of inflammatory involvement of branches of the pulmonary artery.

In a subset of patients, the predominant symptoms of GCA may be the constitutional signs of systemic inflammation, such as fever, fatigue, and anorexia. Fatigue is often also noted in patients with more typical presentations, such as headache or scalp tenderness. This is evidence that immune activation is not necessarily limited to vascular lesions. Patients with GCA have elevated levels of circulating monocytes, which produce IL-1 and IL-6, and the latter is a potent inducer of the acute-phase response. Release of IL-6 therefore not only leads to the elevation of the ESR that is seen in these patients but also helps explain the nonspecific systemic symptoms.

8. **How can response to corticosteroids be monitored?**

Remember the ESR? The drop in ESR or CRP, along with the clinical response, can be used to gauge effectiveness of corticosteroid therapy.

9. **What other disease is giant cell arteritis associated with?**
   Polymyalgia rheumatica (PMR) consists of pain for at least 4 weeks in the muscles of the neck, shoulder, and pelvic girdle. PMR is often considered to be a form of GCA that lacks the fully developed vasculitis. Like GCA, PMR responds to steroid therapy.

STEP 1 SECRET

Temporal arteritis is a favorite on the USMLE. Be on the lookout for symptoms of unilateral headache, jaw claudication, vision problems, and joint pain (polymyalgia rheumatica association).

SUMMARY BOX: TEMPORAL ARTERITIS

- Symptoms include headache, scalp tenderness, or jaw claudication, as well as constitutional signs such as fever, fatigue, and weight loss.

- Potential complications include ischemic optic neuropathy leading to sudden partial or complete permanent blindness.

- This disease is an inflammatory process that typically involves the walls of the extracranial branches of the carotid arteries.

- Definitive diagnosis is made by biopsy of the superficial temporal artery, which demonstrates granulomatous infiltration of the arterial wall in patients with the disease. Biopsy has a high false negative rate because of the possibility of skip lesions.

- Erythrocyte sedimentation rate (ESR) and C-reactive protein (CRP) will typically be elevated in patients with giant cell arteritis.

- In most cases, corticosteroids should be started immediately.

- This disease is generally seen in adults older than 50, often Caucasian women.

CASE 20-2

A 4-year-old girl is evaluated for a 5-day history of high fever and a desquamating rash of her palms and soles with swelling of her hands and feet (Fig. 20-1). Examination is significant for cervical lymphadenopathy, injected conjunctiva, and "cherry-red" lips with fissuring and crusting. Laboratory evaluation reveals an elevated ESR and increased number of platelets.

1. **What are the considerations in your differential diagnosis?**
   The desquamating rash is concerning for staphylococcal scalded skin syndrome, in which epidermolytic toxins are produced by an infection by *Staphylococcus aureus*. Children are at increased risk for this because of their lack of immunity.
   The presentation is also concerning for toxic shock syndrome, in which superantigen toxins from streptococcal or staphylococcal infections (often following use of tampons or contraceptive devices) are produced. These toxins overstimulate the immune system, resulting in fever, a rash that may be desquamating, and myriad other signs and symptoms.

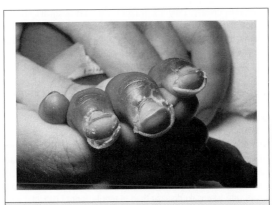

Figure 20-1. Kawasaki disease. (From Shah BR, Laude TA: Atlas of Pediatric Clinical Diagnosis. Philadelphia, WB Saunders, 2000.)

Scarlet fever is another concern in this child. Scarlet fever is an exotoxin-mediated disease associated with streptococcal pharyngitis, impetigo, or other streptococcal infections. It is characterized by fever, rash, and a "strawberry tongue."

Finally, because this is the vasculitis chapter, we need to consider Kawasaki syndrome (also called mucocutaneous lymph node syndrome), an acute febrile systemic illness of childhood affecting medium-sized vessels. It is more common in Asian children and can also present with many of the previously mentioned symptoms.

CASE 20-2 continued:

The attending physician is not interested in an impressive differential diagnosis but rather wants a specific diagnosis for the child.

2. **What is your diagnosis?**
   Kawasaki disease could explain all of this girl's symptoms. The diagnosis of Kawasaki disease requires unexplained fever for at least 5 days, accompanied by at least four of the five following criteria:
   1. Bilateral conjunctivitis
   2. Oral mucous membrane changes, such as cracked lips or "strawberry tongue"
   3. Peripheral extremity changes such as palmar erythema or edema of the hands and feet
   4. Polymorphous rash
   5. Cervical lymphadenopathy

   If these conditions are not strictly met, the patient may have an "atypical Kawasaki disease," which can potentially lead to the same long-term complications as may occur in patients who meet the criteria.

   It may be helpful to remember the other term for Kawasaki disease: mucocutaneous lymph node syndrome. This name is derived from the typical signs and symptoms, which include *muco*sal inflammation, *cutaneous* maculopapular rash, and *lymph node* enlargement, all with an unexplained high fever.

3. **What is the major concern in patients with this disease who do not receive adequate therapy?**
   Lesions of the coronary arteries are responsible for the majority of morbidity and fatality cases associated with this disease. Coronary artery aneurysms occur in 20% to 25% of untreated

children with Kawasaki disease. Only 4% of those who were adequately treated (see later discussion for treatment) developed aneurysms. Coronary artery inflammation can lead to myocardial inflammation, arrhythmias, or death. In fact, roughly 1% of all children who develop Kawasaki disease will die because of rupture of a coronary artery aneurysm or as a result of coronary thrombosis and infarction. Pericardial effusions are seen in approximately 20% of cases, and myocarditis can lead to tachycardia. Otherwise, the course of this disease is self-limited, with fever and acute manifestations lasting an average of 12 days without therapy.

4. What is the pathogenesis of Kawasaki disease?

Overactivation of immune competent cells and an overproduction of cytokines cause endothelial cell injury and blood vessel wall damage. Neutrophils, plasma cells producing IgA, and monocytes are all seen in increased numbers in patients with Kawasaki disease. It is possible that a virus or a bacterial superantigen could be involved in eliciting this overactivation of the immune system, but this has not yet been confirmed. It is known that nitric oxide (NO) levels are higher in patients with Kawasaki disease than in febrile control patients, and that NO levels are highest in patients who develop coronary artery lesions, suggesting that NO plays some role in the inflammatory response that is responsible for the pathogenesis of Kawasaki disease.

5. How is this disease treated?

Intravenous immunoglobulins and high-dose aspirin therapy are given to prevent coronary aneurysms.

6. Describe the epidemiology of this disease.

This is a disease of unknown cause that is seen in children and is most common in Asian populations. Eighty percent of cases occur in children younger than 5 years of age, with the peak incidence at 2 years of age. The disease is more common in boys than in girls. Interestingly, there is a twofold increased risk in a child who has at least one parent who was affected as a child, suggesting a possible genetic component to the disease. Seasonal variation in incidence, with increased incidence in late winter and early spring, and the "epidemic" nature of the disease suggest some environmental component.

SUMMARY BOX: KAWASAKI DISEASE

- The diagnosis requires unexplained fever for at least 5 days, accompanied by at least four of the five following criteria:

  1. Bilateral conjunctivitis

  2. Oral mucous membrane changes, such as cracked lips or strawberry tongue

  3. Peripheral extremity changes such as palmar erythema or edema of the hands and feet

  4. Polymorphous rash

  5. Cervical lymphadenopathy

- Potential complications include coronary artery aneurysms, which can lead to myocardial infarction (MI) or fatal arrhythmias.

- Patients are treated with intravenous immunoglobulin (IVIG) infusion.

- This is a disease of the pediatric population, with 80% of cases occurring in patients under the age of 5. The disease is more common in boys than in girls and has its highest prevalence in Asian populations.

CASE 20-3

A 40-year-old man is evaluated for a 1-year history of recurrent ear and sinus infections and headache. He has a history of pollen allergy and assumed that the sinus congestion resulted from increased allergies this season. Recently, however, he began to notice blood-tinged sputum and a slight cough.

1. **What is your differential diagnosis?**
   Upper airway involvement and constitutional complaints (anorexia, fatigue, weakness) are suggestive of a variety of conditions. Recurrent sinusitis with hemoptysis due to acute bronchitis is one possibility, but this seems unlikely. Other diagnoses to consider include Churg-Strauss syndrome, Wegener's granulomatosis, Goodpasture's syndrome, and bronchogenic carcinoma.

   He may simply be experiencing a difficult-to-eradicate sinus infection, and the recent hemoptysis is due to acute bronchitis, the most common cause of hemoptysis. However, other diagnoses to consider include the Churg-Strauss syndrome, which is a systemic vasculitis that occurs in the setting of allergic rhinitis, asthma, and eosinophilia. Pulmonary infiltrates may occur. Asthma generally precedes this disease by many years, and the allergic nasal and sinus disease are generally not destructive.

   Another vasculitic syndrome that should be considered is Wegener's granulomatosis. Patients with Wegener's granulomatosis will often present with sinus, tracheal, or ear complaints. Goodpasture's syndrome (also known as anti–glomerular basement membrane disease) is a pulmonary renal syndrome that can also present with cough and hemoptysis.

   Finally, pulmonary vascular disorders, such as pulmonary embolism (PE) or elevated pressure in the pulmonary vasculature, can lead to hemoptysis, although nothing else in this patient's history so far would indicate PE or pulmonary hypertension.

CASE 20-3 continued:

A chest x-ray study reveals bilateral nodular and cavitary infiltrates, as shown separately. Laboratory workup is significant for an elevated ESR and the presence of antineutrophil cytoplasmic antibodies (c-ANCA) directed against proteinase 3 (PR3).

2. **What is the likely diagnosis?**
   The presentation of upper and lower respiratory airway symptoms with a workup significant for cavitary infiltrates and elevated inflammatory biomarkers with positive c-ANCA is classic for Wegener's granulomatosis.

3. **What causes disease manifestations?**
   Antibodies to neutrophil cytoplasmic antigens lead to aseptic inflammation and granuloma formation. Inflammation causing vascular injury leads to damage in the respiratory tract and kidneys, specifically causing glomerulonephritis. Granuloma formation occurs both within arterial walls, causing further vasculitic damage, and outside vascular structures, causing granulomatous lesions that may cavitate and damage pulmonary tissue.

4. **What is the usual progression of symptoms in this disease? What other organ systems will likely become involved?**
   Approximately 85% of patients with Wegener's granulomatosis will eventually develop pulmonary disease. Symptoms include cough, hemoptysis, and dyspnea. Upper airway involvement may lead to epistaxis or nasal septum perforation. About 75% will develop glomerulonephritis, which will almost always be asymptomatic until the development of advanced uremia.

   A diagnosis of Wegener's granulomatosis prior to the 1970s meant that the patient had a 50% 5-month survival rate, and 82% of patients died within a year of diagnosis. Besides pulmonary involvement and glomerulonephritis, musculoskeletal symptoms can occur, usually consisting of severe pain that is disproportionate to the signs of inflammation. Peripheral nerves can also be affected in some cases.

5. **How is Wegener's granulomatosis treated?**
The current therapy recommended for Wegener's granulomatosis has become the standard for severe vasculitides with significant organ involvement. This consists of a combination of cyclophosphamide and prednisone. Doses are increased until symptoms are reduced and until the leukocyte count returns to normal values. The prednisone is then tapered gradually. Cyclophosphamide is continued, often for a year after symptomatic improvement, although long-term daily cyclophosphamide therapy is associated with bladder cancer and with myelodysplasia. Long-term immunosuppressive therapy also makes patients susceptible to opportunistic disease.

SUMMARY BOX: WEGENER'S GRANULOMATOSIS

- Initial symptoms may include sinus congestion, headache, epistaxis, and hemoptysis. Consider this diagnosis in the differential for a patient with suspected allergy or upper airway infection that appears intractable.

- Often results in necrotizing granuloma formation in the lungs (resulting in hemoptysis) and in the kidneys (resulting in crescentic glomerulonephritis).

- Chest x-ray may show cavitary nodules. Erythrocyte sedimentation rate (ESR) is typically elevated. Diagnosis can often be made by a positive cytoplasmic antineutrophil cytoplasmic antibodies (c-ANCA) test.

- Patients are treated with a combination of cyclophosphamide and prednisone. Therapy is extremely effective, and prednisone is typically tapered after symptomatic improvement. Cyclophosphamide may be continued for a longer period, although the risk of bladder cancer or opportunistic disease makes this a dangerous medication over a lengthy period of time.

- This disease is generally seen in whites, and it can affect people of any age.

CASE 20-4

A 27-year-old man is evaluated for a 5- to 6-week history of fever, myalgias, fatigue, anorexia, and postprandial abdominal pain. He also complains of painful paresthesias of the hands. His girlfriend adds that she has noticed him dragging his right foot lately. He denies a history of tick bites or unprotected sexual intercourse. Workup reveals that he is positive for hepatitis B surface antigen (HBsAg), although to his knowledge he has never been diagnosed with hepatitis. An arterial biopsy shows inflammation of the tunica media.

1. **What is the diagnosis?**
Polyarteritis nodosa (PAN) is a necrotizing vasculitis affecting small- to medium-sized arteries with a predilection for the arteries supplying peripheral nerves, skin, the gastrointestinal (GI) tract, and the kidneys. Greater than 80% of people with PAN develop neuropathy, often in the pattern of mononeuritis multiplex (see later discussion). This neuropathy explains the tingling in this patient's hand and the footdrop. The postprandial abdominal pain or "intestinal angina" is also classic for PAN.

2. **What is the significance of the positive hepatitis B surface antigen in this patient?**
   About 20% of cases of PAN are associated with hepatitis B viral infection. Other microbial pathogens may be a factor in many of the remaining cases, although no definitive links have been established with any infectious agent other than hepatitis B.

   It is believed that immune complex depositions with antigens may be a cause of the disease. Inflammatory cells, predominantly neutrophils, form an infiltrate in arterial walls, which eventually leads to fibrinoid necrosis and varying degrees of intimal proliferation. Occlusion and thrombosis of arteries may result, leading to tissue ischemia and the symptoms and complications that have been described here.

   The lesions of PAN are segmental and favor the branch points of the smaller arteries. A key pathologic feature is the absence of granulomas or granulomatous infiltration.

STEP 1 SECRET

Hepatitis B association with polyarteritis nodosa is a commonly tested fact on Step 1.

CASE 20-3 continued:

The patient returns to the clinic several weeks later for evaluation of severe hand pain. Examination of his hands reveals severe digital cyanosis and edema, as shown in Figure 20-2.

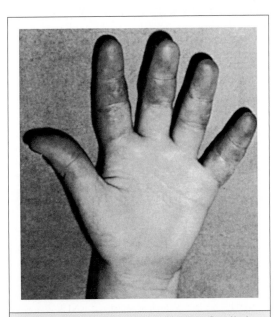

Figure 20-2. Marked digital cyanosis and swelling. (From Harris ED, Budd RC, Genovese MC, et al: Kelley's Textbook of Rheumatology, 7th ed. Philadelphia, WB Saunders, 2005.)

3. **What are the dermatologic manifestations of polyarteritis nodosa?**
The rash on this patient's foot is livedo reticularis, a mottled blue-red discoloration that may affect large areas of the legs, arms, or abdomen. Splinter hemorrhages may also be seen. Later in the course of this disease, skin involvement is typically in the form of gangrene of the digits following occlusion of the arteries in the hands or feet. GI tract involvement is typically evidenced by postprandial periumbilical pain. Potential life-threatening consequences include rupture of mesenteric aneurysms and perforation of ischemic bowel. Finally, renal involvement, which is almost always seen on autopsy, presents as renin-mediated hypertension caused by occlusion of interlobar renal vessels.

4. **How can the diagnosis of polyarteritis nodosa be confirmed?**
ANCA will be elevated in patients with PAN, as they are in patients with Wegener's granulomatosis, discussed previously. Immunofluorescent staining will be in a perinuclear (p-ANCA) pattern rather than a cytoplasmic (c-ANCA) pattern, and this usually corresponds to antibodies against myeloperoxidase (MPO). Finally, an arterial biopsy would reveal inflammation of the tunica media and an inflammatory infiltrate without granulomas (Table 20-2).

TABLE 20-2.	TESTS CONFIRMING WEGENER'S GRANULOMATOSIS AND POLYARTERITIS NODOSA
Wegener's Granulomatosis	**Polyarteritis Nodosa**
Cytoplasmic staining—c-ANCA	Perinuclear staining—p-ANCA
Antibodies to proteinase-3	Antibodies to myeloperoxidase (MPO)

c-ANCA, cytoplasmic antineutrophil cytoplasmic antibodies; p-ANCA, perinuclear antineutrophil cytoplasmic antibodies.

CASE 20-4 continued:

The patient is placed on high doses of corticosteroids for his PAN.

5. **Given the high-dose steroids, what prophylaxis needs to be considered?**
Prophylaxis against *Pneumocystis jirovecii* with trimethoprim-sulfamethoxazole should be considered.

SUMMARY BOX: POLYARTERITIS NODOSA

- Initial symptoms are usually nonspecific and may include unintentional weight loss, myalgias, fatigue, and fever. This will be followed weeks or months later with signs of organ involvement and diffuse ischemic damage. More specific signs and symptoms may then manifest, such as peripheral nerve damage leading to mononeuritis multiplex, mottling of the skin called livedo reticularis, gastrointestinal (GI) involvement leading to postprandial periumbilical pain, and stenosis of the renal arteries leading to renin-induced hypertension.

- The most dangerous complications include rupture of mesenteric aneurysms and ischemic bowel perforation.

- Diagnosis is based on clinical suspicion, positive p-ANCA staining pattern, and arterial biopsy demonstrating neutrophilic infiltration of the arterial walls.

- Patients are treated with corticosteroids.

CASE 20-5

A 41-year-old Caucasian woman is evaluated for a two-week history of fatigue, diffuse myalgias, anorexia, and unintentional weight loss. She was found to be very mildly anemic, and iron supplementation therapy was begun. She is presenting to the emergency department today with a new, very distinct complaint. She states that since she began to feel fatigued weeks ago, she became more interested in her personal health, attempting to exercise every day and taking her own blood pressure (BP) before and after her morning walks. Yesterday she was unable to get a BP reading in her left arm prior to exercising. Her BP in her right arm was 110/60 mm Hg, per her report. She had assumed that there had been some problem with the BP cuff, but the same thing happened again this morning. She could not obtain a BP from her left arm, and her right arm read 100/60 mm Hg. She also states, somewhat fearfully, that her left arm feels cool today, and that in retrospect, her left arm has frequently been "tingly" over the past week.

1. **What is the likely diagnosis in this patient?**
   Given the problem obtaining a BP in this patient's left arm and the coolness in the left extremity, consider involvement of the arch of the aorta or occlusion of the arteries of the upper extremity. This vascular compromise would also explain the tingling in the arm. Other, nonvascular explanations of paresthesias, such as brachial plexus damage, would not explain the difficulty in obtaining the BP. The patient has no severe back pain, which would raise concern for a ruptured aortic aneurysm. The onset late in life makes a congenital coarctation of the aorta unlikely. Given the very specific presentation, Takayasu's arteritis should be considered.

2. **What is Takayasu's arteritis?**
   This is a vasculitis of the large elastic arteries, including the aorta and its main branches. It can also affect the coronary and pulmonary arteries. Inflammatory injury to the arterial wall leads to aneurysm formation or occlusion of the arteries, leading to the symptoms of decreased blood flow to the upper extremity(ies) in this patient. Takayasu's arteritis is also known as pulseless disease, due to the possibility of losing the pulse in one or both upper extremities.
   The cause of this disease is unknown. Granulomas and giant cells are characteristically found in the media of the large elastic arteries, and the adventitia is usually profoundly thickened. Destruction of the media by granulomatous inflammation leads to replacement with fibrotic tissue and subsequent aneurysm formation. Thickening of the adventitia, on the other hand, leads to occlusion of the vascular lumen.

3. **What makes this patient different from the typical presentation of Takayasu's arteritis?**
   Although a different BP in the two upper extremities is a classic presentation for Takayasu's arteritis, this patient does not demonstrate the typical epidemiologic features of this disease. This disease is most common among Asian women (specifically those of Japanese, Chinese, or Korean descent; incidence is also relatively high among Indian women). Furthermore, it is a disease of adolescent girls and young women. Some diagnostic criteria for the disease require that the patient be younger than 40 years of age at onset. Our patient, as a 41-year-old Caucasian woman, is therefore atypical.

4. **Ischemic complication due to vascular involvement of the arch of the aorta and its major branches led to this patient's symptoms. What other symptoms can be expected from further ischemia in a patient with Takayasu's arteritis?**
   The carotid and vertebral arteries can also be involved, leading to symptoms including headache, syncope, or visual disturbance. Stroke can sometimes occur. The following may also be seen:
   - Involvement of the coronary arteries can produce classic symptoms of myocardial ischemia.
   - Involvement of the renal arteries can cause renin-induced hypertension, which is classically the presenting symptom in some specific ethnic groups, such as Indians.
   - Involvement of the mesenteric arteries is less common, but when present it leads to symptoms such as nausea and vomiting.
   - Progressively enlarging aneurysms can occur, typically along the aorta. These are frequently asymptomatic, however.

5. **How is the diagnosis made?**
   In this patient, physical examination would include listening for a bruit over the subclavian arteries and documenting a lower BP in the left arm as compared with the right. Noninvasive magnetic resonance angiography would then be indicated to confirm the diagnosis and to document the extent of arterial wall inflammation. The effects of therapy are usually monitored by documenting change in arterial wall inflammation on angiography as well as monitoring the diameter of the aortic root.

6. **How is this disease treated?**
   Corticosteroids are used for the management of patients with Takayasu's arteritis. The initial dose is usually 60 mg of prednisone per day, and this is tapered as appropriate while monitoring arterial involvement as described previously. Methotrexate may be used to enable a lower dose of steroids to be given.

SUMMARY BOX: TAKAYASU'S ARTERITIS

- Diagnosis is made by clinical suspicion and finding of the perinuclear antineutrophil cytoplasmic antibody (p-ANCA) staining pattern. Initial symptoms are usually nonspecific systemic complaints such as fatigue, myalgias, and weight loss. This will be followed by ischemic symptoms secondary to vascular occlusion. The arch of the aorta and its major branches are usually involved, leading to the classic presenting symptom of the absence of a pulse in one or both upper extremities. This is primarily a disease of young Asian women. Think of this disease immediately if the patient is an Asian woman under the age of 40 presenting with symptoms of arm claudication.

- Diagnosis is confirmed by angiography, which also allows monitoring of disease progression.

- Patients are treated with corticosteroids.

CHAPTER 21

BACTERIAL DISEASES

Thomas A. Brown, MD, and Sonali J. Shah

INSIDER'S GUIDE TO BACTERIAL DISEASES FOR THE USMLE STEP 1

There is no better way to say it: the USMLE *loves* bacterial diseases! This is one of the highest-yield subjects on the examination, so you must know it well! Our book has divided microbiology into two chapters, but you should note that the breakdown of the examination is not likely to be evenly distributed among bacteria, viruses, fungi, and parasites. Bacterial diseases are tested far more commonly than the other three types, but recently, fungal diseases have been heavily represented on many students' forms. Fungal diseases are discussed more in Chapter 22.

As you may know, microbiology is not inherently difficult, but it does take time to learn. The most effective way to study for microbiology on the USMLE is to introduce yourself to this material early on, preferably during your microbiology class in medical school. This is one subject for which multiple resources may be quite helpful to you. For those of you seeking to combine your medical school education with boards studying, we recommend using *Clinical Microbiology Made Ridiculously Simple* and *Microcards* when you first begin learning the material. Pull the highest-yield facts from these already high-yield materials and write them into First Aid. You can then study from your annotated copy of First Aid and the cases in this book once your focus shifts entirely to boards.

How should you be expected to know which facts are the most important to learn for boards? That is why you purchased this book! As always, we will be pointing this information out along the way. However, you should keep in mind that the USMLE will expect you to know the major diseases and toxins associated with each and every medically important bacterial species. The Step 1 places heavy emphasis on the mechanisms of various bacterial toxins as well as the associated characteristics of individual bacterial species that can be helpful in identifying and differentiating among them in the laboratory.

BASIC CONCEPTS

1. **What makes an organism gram-positive or gram-negative?**
   Both gram-positive and gram-negative organisms have an internal cell membrane and cell walls made of peptidoglycan. However, gram-negative bacteria have much thinner cell walls and, in addition, have an outer membrane outside the cell wall. Gram-positive organisms have techoic acid in their cell walls, and gram-negative organisms have lipopolysaccharide (endotoxin) (Fig. 21-1).

2. **Why are gram-negative infections more likely to produce bacterial sepsis?**
   The outer membrane of gram-negative organisms (see previous question) contains lipid A, an endotoxin that is part of the lipopolysaccharide in the cell wall of gram-negative bacteria. Lipid A gets released upon bacterial death and has potent proinflammatory effects.

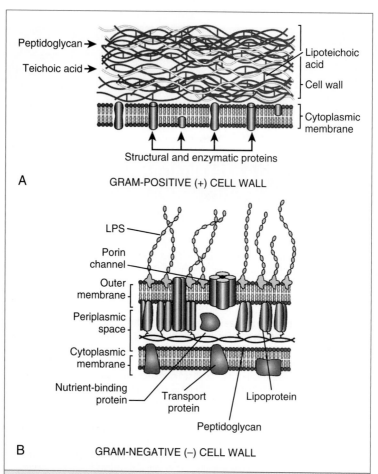

Peptidoglycan →
Teichoic acid →

Lipoteichoic acid
Cell wall

Cytoplasmic membrane

Structural and enzymatic proteins

A   GRAM-POSITIVE (+) CELL WALL

LPS
Porin channel
Outer membrane
Periplasmic space
Cytoplasmic membrane
Nutrient-binding protein
Transport protein
Lipoprotein
Peptidoglycan

B   GRAM-NEGATIVE (–) CELL WALL

Figure 21-1. Structure of the cell wall in gram-positive and gram-negative bacteria. **A,** Gram-positive bacteria have a thick peptidoglycan layer that contains teichoic and lipoteichoic acids. **B,** Gram-negative bacteria have a thin peptidoglycan layer that is connected by lipoproteins to an outer membrane. LPS, lipopolysaccharide. (From Rosenthal K, Tan J: Rapid Review Microbiology and Immunology, 2nd ed. Philadelphia, Mosby, 2007.)

3. **Describe the mechanism by which lipid A causes toxicity?**
Lipid A activates macrophages to secrete interleukin 1 (IL-1) and tumor necrosis factor (TNF), both of which are referred to as acute-phase cytokines. Lipid A also stimulates the release of nitric oxide (NO) from endothelial cells. Large amounts of lipid A may lead to shock and intravascular coagulation via this stimulatory effect (Fig. 21-2).

4. **What are exotoxins?**
Exotoxins are proteins released by both gram-positive and gram-negative bacteria during their normal life cycle. Exotoxins released into food can cause poisoning, as in *Bacillus cereus* and *Staphylococcus aureus* food poisoning. Pyrogenic exotoxins released by *S. aureus* and *Streptococcus pyogenes* can cause rash, fever, and toxic shock syndrome. Enterotoxins act

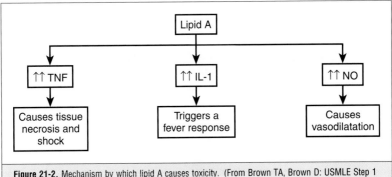

Figure 21-2. Mechanism by which lipid A causes toxicity. (From Brown TA, Brown D: USMLE Step 1 Secrets. Philadelphia, Hanley & Belfus, 2004.)

on the gastrointestinal system, whereas neurotoxins act on nerves or motor end plates. For example, infectious diarrhea is caused by enterotoxins released by *Vibrio cholerae*, *Escherichia coli*, *Campylobacter jejuni*, and *Shigella dysenteriae*.

5. **What is a capsule and what purpose does it serve?**
   Certain species of bacteria produce a slippery outermost covering called a capsule. This covering consists of high-molecular-weight polysaccharides, which help the bacteria to evade phagocytosis by neutrophils and macrophages. Note that *Bacillus anthracis* has a proteinaceous capsule which consists of D-glutamic acid. The capsule is not essential for growth and serves only in a protective capacity. The most common medically relevant encapsulated organisms are **S**treptococcus pneumoniae, **K**lebsiella pneumoniae, **H**aemophilus influenzae type b, **P**seudomonas aeruginosa, **N**eisseria meningitidis, and **C**ryptococcus neoformans (a fungus).

   Remember that **S**ome **K**illers **H**ave **P**erfectly **N**asty **C**apsules. This mnemonic will help you recall the encapsulated organisms that are important to know for boards.

   Note: In the Quellung reaction, which tests for the presence of encapsulated bacteria, encapsulated bacteria will swell when exposed to specific antibodies. The latex agglutination assay and India ink stain are two other methods for detecting capsular presence.

STEP 1 SECRET

Although the Quellung reaction and several other techniques in this book may be clinically outdated, you should remember that many of the physicians who author boards questions will have relied upon this technology during the course of their careers and will thus expect you to know the names and basic principles behind these tests. As a general rule, you should focus on learning the techniques listed in this book and in First Aid. You are *not* expected to know complex or cutting-edge technologies that are not mentioned in your USMLE study resources.

6. **What sort of individuals are susceptible to infection by encapsulated bacteria?**
   Because the spleen normally sequesters encapsulated bacteria, patients who have undergone splenectomy are at a greater risk for incurring infection by encapsulated bacteria.

7. Identify the Gram stain and the morphology of the organisms in Table 21-1.

TABLE 21-1. BACTERIAL IMAGES

Image	Gram Stain and Morphology
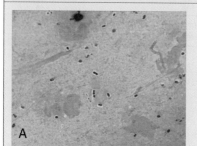 Gram stain of a sputum sample infected with *Streptococcus pneumoniae*.	Gram-positive cocci in pairs: *S. pneumoniae*
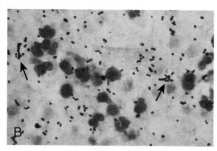 Expectorated sputum with gram-negative rods in a patient with *Klebsiella pneumoniae* pneumonia.	Gram-positive cocci (staining purple in a color image) in chains: *Staphylococcus aureus*
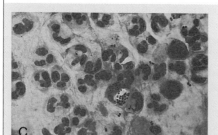 Sputum smear, stained with Gram stain, shows many neutrophils and intracellular gram-negative diplococci, suggestive of *Neisseria meningitidis* infection (oil immersion).	Gram-negative cocci (staining pink in a color image) in pairs: *Neisseria* spp.

TABLE 21-1. BACTERIAL IMAGES—continued	
Image	**Gram Stain and Morphology**
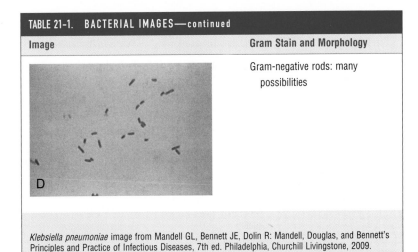	Gram-negative rods: many possibilities

Klebsiella pneumoniae image from Mandell GL, Bennett JE, Dolin R: Mandell, Douglas, and Bennett's Principles and Practice of Infectious Diseases, 7th ed. Philadelphia, Churchill Livingstone, 2009. Images of *Streptococcus pneumoniae, Neisseria meningitidis*, and gram-negative rods from McPherson RA, Pincus MR: Henry's Clinical Diagnosis and Management by Laboratory Methods, 22nd ed. Philadelphia, WB Saunders, 2011.

8. Cover the two columns on the right in Tables 21-2 through 21-9 to test your knowledge of the properties of the clinically relevant bacteria listed in the left column.

TABLE 21-2. GRAM-POSITIVE COCCI		
Organism	**Associated Disease(s)**	**Pearls to Remember**

Staphylococcus aureus	Cellulitis
	Acute endocarditis
	  (in previously normal valve)
	Osteomyelitis
	Pneumonia
	Carbuncles/furuncles
	Stye (hordeolum)
		Toxin-mediated diseases:
		Staphylococcal toxic shock
		Scalded skin syndrome
		Staphylococcal
		  gastroenteritis
		Note: Like all staphylococcal species, *S. aureus* is catalase-positive—but it also is coagulase-positive.

Staphylococcus epidermidis	Prosthetic valve endocarditis	Normal skin flora Novobiocin-sensitive
Staphylococcus saprophyticus	Cystitis in young women Second most common cause of UTI (behind *E. coli*)	Novobiocin-resistant

Continued

TABLE 21-2.   GRAM–POSITIVE COCCI—continued

Organism	Associated Disease(s)	Pearls to Remember
Streptococcus agalactiae (group B streptococci)	Neonatal pneumonia, meningitis, sepsis Chorioamnionitis	Normal vaginal flora β-Hemolysis Bacitracin-resistant
Streptococcus pneumoniae	Pneumonia Meningitis Sinusitis Otitis media	Bile-soluble Optochin-sensitive α-Hemolysis See Case 21-1 for more details
Streptococcus pyogenes (group A streptococci)	Pharyngitis Impetigo Erysipelas Cellulitis Necrotizing fasciitis Rheumatic fever Poststreptococcal glomerulonephritis	Remains largely sensitive to penicillin β-Hemolysis Bacitracin-sensitive
Enterococcus spp.	UTI Bacteremia/sepsis Endocarditis Abdominal abscess	Part of normal bowel flora that causes disease when host is immunocompromised or gastrointestinal tract has been breached α- or γ-Hemolysis
Viridans streptococci	Dental caries (*S. mutans*) Subacute bacterial endocarditis (*S. sanguis*)	Normal oral flora α-Hemolysis Optochin-resistant

UTI, urinary tract infection.

TABLE 21-3.   GRAM–POSITIVE BACILLI

Organism	Associated Disease(s)	Pearls to Remember
Bacillus anthracis	Cutaneous anthrax (most common form) Pulmonary anthrax	Painless black eschars with cutaneous anthrax Wool-sorters at risk for pulmonary anthrax ("wool-sorter's disease) Spore-forming

TABLE 21-3.   GRAM-POSITIVE BACILLI—continued

Organism	Associated Disease(s)	Pearls to Remember
Corynebacterium spp.	Diphtheria Granulomatous lymphadenitis Pneumonitis Pharyngitis Skin infections Endocarditis	Normal skin flora Pseudomembrane or esophageal web Toxin causes disease and is encoded by β-prophage Metachromatic granules ADP ribosylation of EF-2
Listeria monocytogenes	Listeriosis	Perinatal/neonatal infections Immunocompromised persons at risk Raw milk and dairy products

ADP, adenosine diphosphate; EF-2, elongation factor.

TABLE 21-4.   GRAM-NEGATIVE COCCI

Organism	Associated Disease(s)	Pearls to Remember
Neisseria meningitidis (meningococcus)	Meningitis Septicemia Waterhouse-Friderichsen syndrome	Has a capsule Purpuric nonblanching rash Vaccine available See Case 21-8
Neisseria gonorrhoeae (gonococcus)	Infects superficial mucosal surfaces lined with columnar epithelium: *Urethra*: urethritis (gonorrhea) *Vagina*: vulvovaginitis in young girls *Rectum*: proctitis *Conjunctiva*: ophthalmia neonatorum	No vaccine Main cause of infectious arthritis in sexually active persons Prepubescent vaginal epithelium is columnar because not yet acted on by estrogen to become squamous

BASIC CONCEPTS IN ANTIBACTERIAL PHARMACOLOGY

1. **What are the β-lactam antibiotics and what is their mechanism of action?**
    The β-lactam antibiotics include the penicillins, cephalosporins, and carbapenems (imipenem, meropenem). By virtue of their β-lactam chemical moiety, they all inhibit bacterial cell wall synthesis. Resistance to these antibiotics is mediated by bacterially synthesized β-lactamase enzymes that destroy the β-lactam ring (Fig. 21-3).

TABLE 21-5. ENTERIC GRAM–NEGATIVE RODS

Organism	Associated Disease(s)	Pearls to Remember
Campylobacter jejuni	Enteritis	Present in animal feces
Escherichia coli	Enteritis	Normal gut flora
	UTI	*E. coli* O157:H7—a particularly
	Meningitis	virulent pathologic strain
	Peritonitis	associated with HUS
	Mastitis	See Case 21-2
	Septicemia	
	Gram-negative	
	pneumonia	
	HUS	
Salmonella spp.	Food-borne illness	Osteomyelitis in patients with
	Typhoid fever	sickle cell anemia
	(*Salmonella typhi*)	
Shigella spp.	Shigellosis (bacterial	Bloody diarrhea
	dysentery)	Fecal oral route of transmission
		Low inoculum
		required
		Toxin-mediated
Helicobacter pylori	Peptic ulcer disease	Positive urea breath test due to
	Gastritis	presence of enzyme urease
	Duodenitis	Lives in stomach but common in
	Gastric cancer	duodenal ulcers
	Mucosa-associated	Triple treatment:
	lymphoid tissue (MALT)	amoxicillin, clarithromycin,
	lymphoma	and proton pump
		inhibitor

HUS, hemolytic uremic syndrome; UTI, urinary tract infection.

TABLE 21-6. OTHER GRAM–NEGATIVE RODS

Organism	Associated Disease(s)	Pearls to Remember
Bordetella pertussis	Pertussis (whooping cough)	Highly contagious; spread by coughing and nasal drops
Brucella spp.	Brucellosis (also called "undulant fever")	Transmitted via contaminated or unpasteurized milk

TABLE 21-6. OTHER GRAM-NEGATIVE RODS—continued

Organism	Associated Disease(s)	Pearls to Remember
Francisella tularensis	Tularemia ("rabbit fever")	Reservoir in rabbits; transmitted by tick Symptoms/signs similar to those of plague Culture, drainage contraindicated owing to high virulence
Haemophilus influenzae	Meningitis (type b) Bacteremia Cellulitis Pneumonia Sinusitis	Type b encapsulated and more virulent Vaccine available for type b strain
Pseudomonas aeruginosa	Pneumonia in cardiac failure patients External otitis Osteomyeltis in diabetics Endocarditis UTI Hot tub folliculitis	Think *Pseudomonas* infection in burn patients and intravenous drug users Can cause black skin lesions Cultures make blue-green pigment Has endotoxin A Resistant to many antibiotics
Legionella pneumophila	Legionnaire's disease Pontiac fever	*Legionnaire's disease*: acute pneumonia with multisystem involvement; from water source, so no person-to-person spread *Pontiac fever*: similar to flu
Yersinia pestis	Bubonic plague	Transmitted by fleas from rodents to humans Black buboes
Yersinia enterocolitica	Enterocolitis	Pseudoappendicitis Seen in nursery schools

2. **Why are clavulanic acid and sulbactam added to some penicillins?**
These agents inhibit β-lactamase, thereby reducing resistance of bacterial species to the penicillins.

3. **What is the antibacterial spectrum of the various subclasses of penicillins and cephalosporins (Table 21-10)?**
About 10% of people receiving penicillin will have a hypersensitivity reaction. Approximately 10% to 20% of people with a penicillin allergy will also have a hypersensitivity reaction to cephalosporins. There is no cross-reactivity between penicillins and aztreonam.

TABLE 21-7. ANAEROBES

Organism	Associated Disease(s)	Pearls to Remember
Clostridium perfringens	Anaerobic cellulitis Gas gangrene (myonecrosis) Food poisoning	Crepitus is associated with gas gangrene Alpha toxin (lecithinase)
Clostridium tetani	Tetanus	Exotoxin that causes spastic paralysis by blocking glycine release from Renshaw cells in spinal cord Vaccine is available
Clostridium botulinum	Botulinism	Food poisoning that causes flaccid paralysis Preformed toxin prevents release of ACh Classic scenario from consumption of dented canned goods or honey
Clostridium difficile	Pseudomembranous colitis	Caused by antibiotic use, especially clindamycin or ampicillin Treat with metronidazole or oral vancomycin

ACh, acetylcholine.

TABLE 21-8. SPIROCHETES

Organism	Associated Disease(s)	Pearls to Remember
Borrelia burgdorferi	Lyme disease	See Case 21-5
Borrelia recurrentis	Relapsing fever	Organism switches surface proteins to evade immune response, leading to intermittent fevers
Treponema pallidum	Syphilis	See Case 21-4
Leptospira interrogans	Leptospirosis	Transmitted by water that is contaminated by animal urine through cracks in the skin, eyes, or mucous membranes

TABLE 21-9. INTRACELLULAR ORGANISMS

Organism	Associated Disease(s)	Pearls to Remember
Mycoplasma pneumoniae	Atypical ("walking") pneumonia	No cell wall Treat with macrolides Blood shows IgM "cold agglutinins" Chest radiograph demonstrates diffuse interstitial infiltrates; radiographic changes often more extensive than expected from patient's symptoms
Chlamydia trachomatis	Urethritis Pelvic inflammatory disease Blindness Lymphogranuloma venereum Neonatal conjunctivitis	See Case 21-7 Treat neonates with erythromycin eye drops for conjunctivitis
Chlamydia psittaci	Psittacosis (flu-like syndrome)	Transmitted from bird droppings via aerosol
Chlamydia pneumoniae	Atypical pneumonia	Transmitted via aerosols
Mycobacterium tuberculosis	Tuberculosis	See Case 21-6
Mycobacterium leprae	Leprosy (Hansen's disease)	*Tuberculoid form*: milder with few organisms in lesions *Lepromatous form*: severe with many organisms in lesions Grows in cool temperatures, so affects distal sites Treat with dapsone
Rickettsia rickettsii	Rocky Mountain spotted fever	Rash that starts on palms and soles and migrates centrally (centripetal migration) Weil-Felix test results positive for rickettsial diseases

Notice that the first-generation cephalosporins are similar in spectrum to the natural penicillins, and that the third-generation cephalosporins are similar in spectrum to the extended-spectrum penicillins. Knowing this general pattern helps in understanding selection of antimicrobial therapy.

4. **What is the antibacterial spectrum of the fluoroquinolones and what is their mechanism of action?**
   This class has a broad spectrum of activity, including both gram-positive and gram-negative organisms. They also cover *Pseudomonas*, making them fairly similar in spectrum to the antipseudomonal penicillins. These antibiotics work by inhibiting bacterial DNA synthesis by inhibiting the bacterial topoisomerase (DNA gyrase) protein.

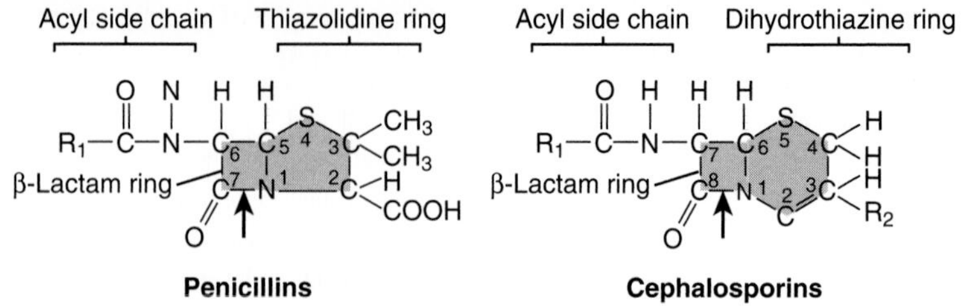

Figure 21-3. General structure of penicillins and cephalosporins. (From Rosenthal K, Tan J: Rapid Review Microbiology and Immunology, 2nd ed. Philadelphia, Mosby, 2007.)

TABLE 21-10. β-LACTAMS

Drug Class	Examples	Coverage
Natural penicillins	Penicillin V (oral) Penicillin G (intravenous) Benzathine penicillin	Mostly gram-positive
Extended-spectrum penicillins	Ampicillin Amoxicillin (oral)	Gram-positive and increased gram-negative
Antistaphylococcal penicillins	Dicloxacillin Cloxacillin	*Staphylococcus aureus*
Antipseudomonal penicillins	Ticaracillin Piperacillin	Increasing gram-negative coverage, including *Pseudomonas*
Penicillin plus beta-lactamase inhibitor	Ampicillin-sulbactam (Unasyn) Amoxicillin–clavulanic acid (Augmentin) Piperacillin-tazobactam (Zosyn)	β-Lactam–resistant bacteria
First-generation cephalosporins	Cephalexin Cefotetan Cefazolin	Mostly gram-positive
Second-generation cephalosporins	Cefuroxime Cefaclor Cefoxitin	Mostly gram-positive
Third-generation cephalosporins	Ceftazidime Ceftriaxone	Penetrates the blood-brain barrier Ceftazidime covers *Pseudomonas*
Aztreonam	Aztreonam	Gram-negative rods

5. **What is the spectrum and mechanism of action of the macrolides?**
   These antibiotics have good gram-positive coverage, and several members of this class are effective against intracellular organisms. They work by inhibiting bacterial protein synthesis.

6. **What is special about the tetracyclines?**
   These drugs are the most important agents for the treatment of intracellular organisms. They also work by inhibiting bacterial protein synthesis.

7. **What are the mechanism of action and spectrum of the aminoglycosides?**
   These are irreversible inhibitors of protein synthesis that are generally only effective against gram-negative rods. However, they may be used in combination with penicillins for enterococcal endocarditis (a gram-positive organism).

8. **How does chloramphenicol work and why is it not used more often?**
   This antibiotic also inhibits protein synthesis, but because of the risk of aplastic anemia it is not commonly used in industrialized nations.

9. **Why is trimethoprim commonly given in combination with sulfamethoxazole, as TMP-SMX?**
   Because these agents inhibit folic acid synthesis at different steps, their combination is synergistic.

10. **Cover the two columns on the right of Table 21-11 and describe the mechanism of action and mechanism of bacterial resistance for the antimicrobial agents listed in the left column.**

TABLE 21-11. MECHANISMS OF DRUG ACTION/RESISTANCE		
Drug Class	**Mechanism of Action**	**Mechanism of Resistance**
Penicillin, cephalosporin, aztreonam	Inhibit transpeptidase and stimulation of autolysins	Formation of β-lactamases that break the β-lactam ring
Vancomycin	Inhibits cell wall synthesis by binding D-alanine	D-Alanine replaced with D-lactate
Tetracyclines	Bind to the 30S subunit of the bacterial ribosome, inhibiting protein synthesis	Decreased transport into the cell and increased transport out of the cell
Aminoglycosides	Impairs proper assembly of the ribosome, causing the 30S subunit to misread the genetic code	Acetylation, adenylation, or phosphorylation
Clindamycin	Binds 50S subunit to prevent peptide bond formation	
Chloramphenicol	Reversibly inhibits protein synthesis by binding to the 50S subunit	Acetylation
Linezolid	Binds to 50S subunit to prevent protein synthesis	

Continued

TABLE 21-11.	MECHANISMS OF DRUG ACTION/RESISTANCE—continued	
Drug Class	Mechanism of Action	Mechanism of Resistance
Macrolides	Bind to 50S subunit of ribosome, inhibiting translocation	Methylation
Fluoroquinolones	Inhibit DNA gyrase, preventing DNA replication	
Trimethoprim	Inhibits folic acid synthesis by inhibiting dihydrofolate reductase	
Sulfonamides	Inhibit folic acid synthesis by being a structural analog (competitive inhibitor) of PABA, a precursor of folic acid in bacteria	Modifications of PABA enzyme and increased synthesis of PABA
Metronidazole	Converts to a toxic metabolite that prevents cell wall synthesis	
Polymyxins	Interact with phospholipids to disrupt the bacterial cell wall	

PABA, para-aminobenzoic acid.

11. Cover the right column in Table 21-12 and describe the adverse effects for each of the antimicrobial agents listed in the left column.

TABLE 21-12.	ADVERSE DRUG EFFECTS
Drug	Adverse Effects
β-Lactams	Hypersensitivity Diarrhea Cephalosporins have 10-20% cross-reactivity in penicillin-allergic patients
Tetracyclines	Gastrointestinal upset Discolors teeth in children Toxicity in patients with renal impairment Photosensitivity Affects bone growth in children
Aminoglycosides	Nephrotoxicity and ototoxicity
Macrolides	Gastrointestinal distress Acute cholestatic hepatitis Prolonged QT interval
Fluoroquinolones	Damages cartilage in young children Tendon rupture in adults

TABLE 21-12.	ADVERSE DRUG EFFECTS—continued
Drug	**Adverse Effects**
Chloramphenicol	Aplastic anemia Gray baby syndrome
Trimethoprim	Mimics folic acid deficiency (megaloblastic anemia, leukopenia, granulocytopenia)
Sulfonamides	Allergic reactions Hemolysis in glucose 6-phosphate deficiency Photosensitivity
Vancomycin	Nephrotoxicity and ototoxicity Thrombophlebitis Red man syndrome (prevented by antihistamines)
Metronidazole	Disulfiram-like reaction with concurrent alcohol intake Metallic taste

STEP 1 SECRET

The list of antibiotics to know for Step 1 is quite extensive, and students often wonder how in depth their knowledge must be to learn this subject for boards. Our best guess is that you should expect anywhere from one to three questions on antibiotics. First Aid has a great review of this topic, but there is still quite a bit of information in these pages. If you can learn it all, great! If you find yourself short on time, go for the highest-yield points. For each antibiotic you should therefore learn this information *in the following order*:

- Mechanism of action and mode of resistance

- Unique side effects and toxicity symptoms: Note that we said you should learn the *unique* side effects of each drug. Boards will not test you on the fact that certain antibiotics can cause occasional gastrointestinal (GI) upset or headache. These symptoms are characteristic of too many drugs to make for good test questions. Focus on the toxicities listed in Table 21-12.

- Clinical uses: Note that you should know the general uses for each drug (e.g., vancomycin is used for gram-positive organisms only, aminoglycosides for serious gram-negative infections, aztreonam for gram-negative rods, metronidazole and clindamycin for anaerobes) but you do not necessarily need to learn the individual organisms affected by every antibiotic. We do not mean to imply that this material is not important for your clinical years or fair game for boards, but it is less likely to be tested than the previous two points. However, you should be sure to know which drugs can be used for select bacterial species—namely, *Pseudomonas*, methicillin-resistant *Staphylococcus aureus* (MRSA), and *Enterococcus*.

CASE 21-1

A 64-year-old man is evaluated for a 3-day history of productive cough, fever, and chills. He describes his phlegm as "rust colored" and notes that his ribs hurt when he takes a deep breath. On examination, the patient is febrile with a temperature of 101.5° F and an O_2 saturation of 89%. Crackles are heard in the right lower posterior lung field. Laboratory workup reveals a significant leukocytosis. Chest x-ray study and sputum culture are pending.

1. **What is the most likely diagnosis?**
   The combination of fever, chills, pleuritic chest pain, hypoxemia, and productive cough is very suggestive of pneumonia. Furthermore, the rust-colored sputum suggests streptococcal pneumonia.

STEP 1 SECRET

Gram-positive diplococci and rust-colored sputum are common buzzwords for *Streptococcus pneumoniae*. Salmon-colored sputum, on the other hand, is associated with *Staphylococcus aureus*. You should know the buzzwords associated with various microorganisms. We will draw attention to these buzzwords throughout the microbiology chapters.

2. **What defense mechanisms prevent pneumonia in the healthy individual?**
   The respiratory tract has many defenses in place to prevent access to the lungs by potential pathogens. The nasal hairs, mucosa, and dynamics of airflow all act early to prevent inhalation of microorganisms. The epiglottis and cough reflex both act to prevent particulate matter from traveling into the deeper airways. The respiratory tract is lined with mucus until the terminal bronchioles are reached. This mucus is propelled upward by the ciliated epithelium, eliminating foreign material as expectorant. The last line of defense is in and around the alveolar complex and is composed of macrophages, neutrophils, immunoglobulin, and complement. These components will become hyperactive during an infectious process because many of their triggers are foreign antigens.
   Note: Any state that alters the level of consciousness (anesthesia, seizure, intoxication, sedation, and neurologic disorders such as coma) predisposes to aspiration pneumonia due to suppression of the cough reflex. The organisms causing this type of infection are usually anaerobes from the mouth or refluxed gastric contents.

3. **Why might a patient in the intensive care unit who is intubated be at increased risk for developing pneumonia?**
   Mechanical ventilation bypasses the normal host defenses (e.g., mucociliary clearance) for preventing contamination of the sterile lower respiratory segments. For each day on mechanical ventilation, it is estimated that the patient has a 1% chance of acquiring nosocomial pneumonia. The expected duration of intubation must therefore be a consideration in deciding whether or not to place a patient on mechanical ventilation.

4. **Why is it important to distinguish between community-acquired and nosocomial pneumonia?**
   There is generally a different spectrum of organisms that cause these two types of pneumonia, so empirical selection of antibiotics is different. The most common pathogens causing community-acquired pneumonia include *S. pneumoniae*, *H. influenzae*, *Legionella pneumophila*, and *Mycoplasma pneumoniae*. The most common pathogen causing nosocomial pneumonia is *S. aureus*.

5. **What is atypical ("walking") pneumonia, and is the patient in this case more likely have a typical or an atypical pneumonia?**
   Atypical or "walking" pneumonia has a more insidious onset than what has been described in this case. It is characterized by headache, nonproductive cough, low-grade fever, and a nonspecific diffuse interstitial infiltrate on x-ray study that looks worse than might be expected from the patient's appearance. Atypical pneumonia is generally caused by viruses or intracellular bacteria such as *L. pneumophila*, *M. pneumoniae*, and species of *Chlamydia* such as *Chlamydia psittaci*. *M. pneumoniae* is the classic causative organism and can be differentiated from other causes based upon a high titer of cold agglutinins (IgM). Most of the bacterial causes can be treated with a macrolide or tetracycline, our favorite drugs for intracellular bugs.

This patient most likely has a typical pneumonia based on the rapidity of onset and productive cough.

Note: The term "cold agglutinins" refers to the fact that IgM antibodies will bind to red blood cells (RBCs) at low temperatures and cause them to agglutinate, or stick together. This can be demonstrated at the bedside when a blood sample becomes clumpy when placed in ice and fluid again when rewarmed. Boards commonly test students on the association between cold agglutinins and *M. pneumoniae*.

CASE 21-1 continued:

Chest x-ray film is shown in Figure 21-4A. Sputum Gram stain reveals large numbers of slightly elongated, gram-positive cocci in pairs and chains (Fig. 21-4B).

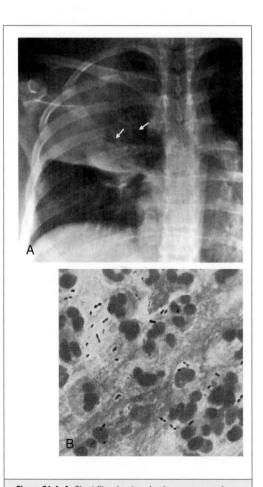

Figure 21-4. A, Chest film showing classic pneumococcal pneumonia *(arrows).* **B,** Gram-stained sputum from a patient with pneumoccal pneumonia at 1000 × magnification. (**A** from Brown TA, Brown D: USMLE Step 1 Secrets. Philadelphia, Hanley & Belfus, 2004. **B** from Mandell GL, Bennett JE, Dolin R: Principles and Practice of Infectious Diseases, 6th ed. Philadelphia, Churchill Livingstone, 2005.)

6. **What is the diagnosis?**
   The sputum Gram stain showing gram-positive diplococci is suggestive of streptococcal pneumonia infection. For the sake of completeness, the chest x-ray film shows opacification (consolidation) of the right upper lobe, consistent with a lobar pneumonia.

STEP 1 SECRET

Although interpretation of complex chest x-ray films is beyond the purview of the second-year medical school curriculum, you should be able to recognize some common chest x-ray findings such as lobar and interstitial pneumonia, pneumothorax, pleural effusion, and congestive heart failure (CHF)-associated pulmonary congestion. We recommend that you peruse an anatomy atlas or credible online sites to study these images. Boards are becoming increasingly clinical, and writers will insert pathologic images and perhaps even some radiographs throughout your test. It may not always be necessary to use the provided images to arrive at the correct answer, but you should not take this gamble. You should also be aware that the USMLE Step 1 occasionally inserts pathological and radiographical images as answer choices to its questions, so you would be wise to prepare for this possibility.

7. **How should this patient be treated pharmacologically?**
   Although penicillin G has been first-line therapy for community-acquired pneumonia, a rising incidence of penicillin resistance among strains of *S. pneumoniae* often necessitates the use of an alternative agent such as ceftriaxone. Notice that as a third-generation cephalosporin, ceftriaxone can cover the more common gram-positive *and* gram-negative organisms that lead to community-acquired pneumonia (e.g., pneumococci and *H. influenzae*, respectively).

8. **Use Table 21-13 to quiz yourself on the most common causes of pneumonia in different age groups.**

TABLE 21-13.   CAUSES OF PNEUMONIA BY AGE

Neonates (0-6 Weeks)	Children (6 Week–18 Years)	Adults (18-40 Years)	Adults (40-65 Years)	Elderly (>65 Years)
Group B streptococci	Viruses Mycoplasma	*Mycoplasma* *C. pneumoniae*	*S. pneumoniae* Haemophilus influenzae	*S. pneumoniae* Viruses Anaerobes
Escherichia coli	Chlamydia pneumoniae *Streptococcus pneumoniae*	*S. pneumoniae*	Anaerobes Viruses Mycoplasma	*H. influenzae* Gram-positive rods

9. **Use Table 21-14 to quiz yourself on the important characteristics of the organisms that are known to cause pneumonias.**

TABLE 21-14.   CHARACTERISTICS OF ORGANISMS THAT CAUSE PNEUMONIA

Streptococcus pneumoniae

Seen in:	Community-acquired pneumonia
Stain	Gram-positive
Morphology	Diplococci
Catalase	Negative
Hemolysis	Alpha
Optochin	Sensitive
Quellung reaction	Positive
Bile solubility	Soluble
Sputum	Rust-colored

Staphylococcus aureus

Seen in:	Nosocomial pneumonias
Stain	Gram-positive
Morphology	Cocci in clusters
Catalase	Positive
Coagulase	Positive
Hemolysis	Beta

Klebsiella spp.

Seen in:	Alcoholics
	Diabetics
	Aspirations
Stain	Gram-negative
Morphology	Rods
Lactose fermentation	Positive
Sputum	Red currant jelly

Pseudomonas aeruginosa

Seen in:	Cystic fibrosis
Stain	Gram-negative
Morphology	Rod
Lactose fermentation	Negative
Oxidase	Positive

Group B Streptococci

Seen in:	Neonates
Stain	Gram-positive
Morphology	Chains
Catalase	Negative
Hemolysis	Beta
Bacitracin	Resistant

Continued

TABLE 21-14. CHARACTERISTICS OF ORGANISMS THAT CAUSE PNEUMONIA—continued

Mycoplasma spp.	
Seen in:	Atypical pneumonias
Stain	None
Growth medium	Eaton's agar
Blood test	Cold agglutinins
Escherichia coli	
Seen in:	Neonates
Stain	Gram-negative
Morphology	Rod
Lactose fermentation	Positive
Chlamydia pneumoniae	
Seen in:	Atypical pneumonia
Stain	Giemsa

SUMMARY BOX: PNEUMONIA

- Nosocomial infection is most commonly caused by *Staphylococcus aureus*.

- Atypical pneumonia has a more insidious onset, with a classic clinical presentation of headache, nonproductive cough, and a nonspecific diffuse interstitial infiltrate on x-ray film that looks worse than would be expected from the patient's condition. Common causes include *Legionella pneumophila*, *Mycoplasma pneumoniae*, and *Chlamydia psittaci*.

- "Red currant jelly sputum" is suggestive of *Klebsiella pneumoniae*.

- For a patient on a respirator, there is a 1% risk per day of acquiring nosocomial pneumonia.

CASE 21-2

A 26-year-old woman presents to your office complaining of severe diarrhea for the past day. She informs you that her bowel movements are watery with small stool particles, and she denies the presence of blood. She just returned from a week-long trip to Mexico, where she drank only bottled water supplemented with ice from her hotel room. She has no other complaints or problems. Examination is remarkable for tachycardia and dry mucous membranes.

1. **What is the most likely diagnosis?**
   This patient is most likely suffering from traveler's diarrhea. Despite her best efforts to drink only bottled water, she has made a very common mistake among travelers: she used ice made with local water. Use Table 21-15 to review the types of *E. coli* and the syndromes they cause.

2. **What other types of diarrhea can be caused by *Escherichia coli*?**
   Enterohemorrhagic *E. coli* (EHEC) and enteroinvasive *E. coli* (EIEC) both cause a dysentery-like syndrome with fever and bloody stools. Enteropathogenic *E. coli* (EPEC) is a common cause of diarrhea in infants, and enteroadherent *E. coli* is another cause of traveler's diarrhea.

TABLE 21-15. *ESCHERICHIA COLI* STRAINS

Strain	Syndrome
Enterotoxigenic	Traveler's diarrhea
Enteroadherent	Traveler's diarrhea
Enteropathogenic	Infantile diarrhea
Enterohemorrhagic	Bloody diarrhea; hemorrhagic colitis and hemolytic uremic syndrome
Enteroinvasive	Bloody diarrhea (dysentery)
Enteroaggressive	Persistent diarrhea in children and HIV-infected patients

HIV, human immunodeficiency virus.

3. **What is the difference between osmotic and secretory diarrhea? Name a cause for each type.**

Secretory diarrhea is caused by *active secretion* of fluids by the intestines. Examples of this type of diarrhea are *V. cholerae* (Fig. 21-5) and enterotoxigenic *E. coli* (ETEC), the cause of traveler's diarrhea.

Osmotic diarrhea is caused by osmotically active agents within the gut lumen that result in passive movement of water into the intestinal lumen along osmotic gradients. An example in which this may occur is nutritional malabsorption (e.g., in celiac sprue or pancreatic insufficiency), in which the osmotically active nutrients pull water into the intestines.

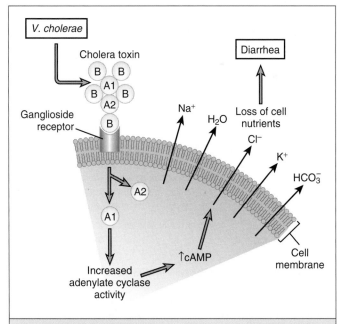

Figure 21-5. Mechanism of cholera toxin, an A-B type toxin. cAMP, cyclic adenosine monophosphate. (From Rosenthal K, Tan J: Rapid Review Microbiology and Immunology, 2nd ed. Philadelphia, Mosby, 2007.)

4. **What predisposes to *Clostridium difficile* colitis and what sort of diarrhea does this cause?**
   The use of antibiotics such as ampicillin and clindamycin must be carefully monitored to avoid inducing *C. difficile* colitis, also known as pseudomembranous colitis. Pseudomembranous colitis occurs when a member of the normal intestinal flora (*C. difficile*) proliferates in excess after elimination of competitor species following antibiotic use, resulting in superinfection. This bacteria is associated with two exotoxins, referred to as toxins A and B, that result in secretory diarrhea and damage the gut mucosa. Detection of Toxin B in the stool can be used to confirm *C. difficile* infection.

5. **How is diarrhea treated?**
   Generally, supportive therapy to replace lost fluids and electrolytes is all that is needed. For the more serious bugs such as those causing bloody diarrhea, broad-spectrum antibiotics may be helpful although this runs the risk of inducing *C. difficile* infection (Tables 21-16 and 21-17).

TABLE 21-16. CAUSES OF WATERY DIARRHEA

Infectious Agent	Comments	Treatment
ETEC	Causes traveler's diarrhea and is an important cause of diarrhea in children younger than 2 years of age in the developing world; heat-labile toxin acts on adenylate cyclase, heat-stable toxin acts on guanylate cyclase	Fluid and electrolyte replacement
Vibrio cholerae	Acts on G protein to stimulate adenylate cyclase, leading to increased Cl^- release into lumen of gut; possible "rice water" diarrhea	Fluid and electrolyte replacement
Giardia (protozoan)	Transmitted by cysts in water and diagnosed by trophozoites in stool	Metronidazole
Norwalk virus	A calcivirus	Fluid and electrolyte replacement
Rotavirus	Fatal diarrhea in children	Fluid and electrolyte replacement
Cryptosporidium (protozoan)	Can be severe in AIDS	None

AIDS, acquired immunodeficiency syndrome; ETEC, enterotoxigenic *Escherichia coli*.

TABLE 21-17. CAUSES OF BLOODY DIARRHEA

Infectious Agent	Comments	Treatment
Shigella	Low inoculum (10^1); nonmotile; transmitted by 4 Fs (fingers, food, feces, flies); does not invade beyond gut mucosa	TMP-SMX
Salmonella	Higher inoculum (10^5); motile; transmitted from animal products, especially poultry and eggs; can become disseminated	TMP-SMX
EHEC	Shiga-like toxin that can cause hemolytic uremic syndrome (HUS), especially O157:H7	Fluid and electrolyte replacement (with glucose)
EIEC	Signs/symptoms similar to those of shigellosis; begins as watery and can proceed to bloody diarrhea	
Campylobacter	"Thermophilic" (optimal growth temperature is 42° C); characteristic comma or S shape; oxidase- and catalase-positive	Usually self-limiting; give fluid and electrolyte replacement
Clostridium difficile	Causes pseudomembranous colitis; can be seen after the administration of clindamycin or ampicillin	Metronidazole or oral vancomycin
Yersinia enterocolitica	Transmitted via pet feces, milk, or pork; causes day care outbreaks with symptoms/signs similar to those of appendicitis, called "pseudoappendicitis"	Fluid and electrolyte replacement (although antibiotics are indicated if infection is invasive)
Entamoeba histolytica (protozoan)	Transmitted by cysts in water	Metronidazole

EHEC, enterohemorrhagic *Escherichia coli*; EIEC, enteroinvasive *Escherichia coli*; TMP-SMX, trimethoprim-sulfamethoxazole.

SUMMARY BOX: DIARRHEA

- Diarrhea can usually be treated by replacing lost fluids and electrolytes (supportive therapy).

- Antibiotics such as clindamycin therapy increase the risk of *Clostridium difficile* colitis.

- Strains of *Escherichia coli* that cause watery diarrhea include enterotoxigenic, enteroaggregative, and enteropathogenic types.

- Strains of *E. coli* that cause bloody diarrhea include enterohemorrhagic and enteroinvasive types.

CASE 21-3

A 65-year-old woman with a history of hypertension and rheumatic fever as a child is evaluated for a 2- to 3-week history of night sweats, fever, malaise, and myalgias. Cardiac auscultation reveals a previously undetected faint diastolic murmur. Findings on inspection of the fingers and funduscopic examination are as shown in Figures 21-6 and 21-7. Echocardiogram and blood culture results are pending.

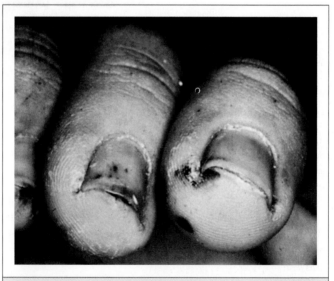

Figure 21-6. Finger inspection of patient in Case 21-3. (From Korzeniowski OM, Kaye D: Infective endocarditis. In Braunwald E [ed]: Heart Disease, 4th ed. Philadelphia, WB Saunders, 1992.)

1. **What is the most likely diagnosis?**
   This case describes the presentation of acute bacterial endocarditis, an infection of the endothelial lining of the heart (Fig. 21-8).

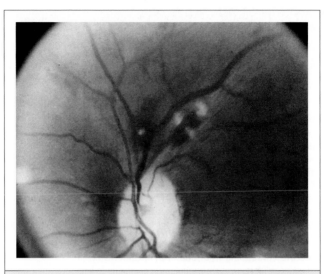

Figure 21-7. Fundoscopic examination of patient in Case 21-3. (From Korzeniowski OM, Kaye D: Infective endocarditis. In Braunwald E [ed]: Heart Disease, 4th ed. Philadelphia, WB Saunders, 1992.)

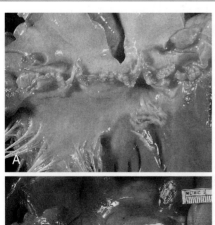

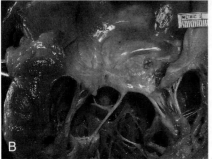

Figure 21-8. A, Acute rheumatic endocarditis. Gross photograph of an aortic valve with small vegetations (verrucae) along the lines of valve closure. **B,** Chronic rheumatic endocarditis. Gross photograph of a mitral valve with massive fibrosis and distortion of the leaflets and fusion of the chordae tendineae. (From King T: Elsevier's Integrated Pathology. Philadelphia, Mosby, 2007.)

2. **What are the major risk factors for developing endocarditis?**
   The major risk factor for the development of endocarditis is a structurally abnormal heart valve causing aberrant flow streams. Common structural abnormalities are *prosthetic valves* or *native valve lesions, calcifications, rheumatic heart disease*, and *congenital abnormalities*. A majority of infections occur in the left side of the heart (the mitral valve is the most frequently affected valve in bacterial endocarditis, but the aortic valve may also be involved), but with intravenous (IV) drug use, right-sided tricuspid valve lesions may occur as a result of introduction of the pathogens into the venous system. Bacterial species associated with IV drug abuse include *S. aureus* and *P. aeruginosa*. *Candida albicans* is a fungal cause of right-sided endocarditis.

3. **What are the clinical signs of bacterial endocarditis?**
   Bacterial endocarditis commonly presents with low-grade to high fever, new-onset heart murmur, chills, night sweats, weight loss, fatigue, and mild anemia of chronic disease. The timeline of this presentation depends on whether the endocarditis is acute or subacute. Bacterial endocarditis also presents with Roth's spots (white dots on the retina surrounded by areas of hemorrhage; see Fig. 21-7), Osler's nodes (painful, elevated lesions on the pads of the fingers and toes), Janeway lesions (painless, flat discolorations on the palms and soles), and splinter hemorrhages (see Fig. 21-6). Roth's spots, Osler's nodes, Janeway lesions, and splinter hemorrhages are all manifestations of small bacterial emboli (Table 21-18).

TABLE 21-18. SYMPTOMS AND SIGNS OF BACTERIAL ENDOCARDITIS

Symptom/Sign	Description
Fever	Can be spiking
Roth spots	Retinal hemorrhages with pale, white centers composed of fibrin
Osler's nodes	Tender, raised lesions of finger or toe pads
Murmur	New or changing due to valvular damage
Janeway lesions	Nontender erythematous macules on palms or soles
Anemia	Anemia of chronic disease
Nail bed hemorrhages	Often called splinter hemorrhages and can be seen under the nail bed; due to microemboli blocking smaller vessels
Emboli	Can lead to stroke or gangrene of distal extremities

4. **What are the clinical signs of rheumatic fever?**
   Rheumatic fever is a sequela of *S. pyogenes* (group A, β-hemolytic) pharyngitis. Acute rheumatic fever most commonly occurs in children but has been seen in adults. The symptoms of acute rheumatic fever usually occur 2 to 3 weeks following pharyngitis, making prompt treatment of *S. pyogenes* pharyngitis an important part of rheumatic fever prevention. Table 21-19 lists the clinical manifestations of acute rheumatic fever, although not all need to be present to make this diagnosis.

Note: Aschoff bodies are the pathognomonic histologic finding in rheumatic heart disease. They are found in the myocardium and consist of regions of fibrinoid necrosis with mononuclear and multinucleated giant cell infiltrates (Fig. 21-9). Also, the antistreptolysin O (ASO) titer is used to detect a recent *S. pyogenes* infection and should be elevated in cases of acute rheumatic fever.

TABLE 21-19. ACUTE RHEUMATIC FEVER

Symptom/Sign	Description
Migratory arthritis	Multiple joint involvement, but each only for a short period of time; arthritis usually the initial manifestation
Carditis	New or changing murmurs may appear; pericardium, epicardium, myocardium, and endocardium all affected; may see cardiomegaly on radiologic studies
Chorea	"St. Vitus dance"—sudden, nonrhythmic, purposeless movement; also can see muscle weakness and emotional outbursts
Subcutaneous nodules	Most commonly seen over bony prominences; nonpainful and noninflammatory
Erythema marginatum	A rash similar to that of Lyme disease, in which the erythematous region extends outward as the center becomes pale, forming a ring; most often seen on trunk and not the face; occurs early in the disease and persists throughout its course

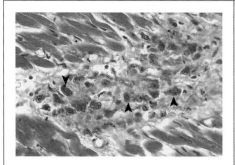

Figure 21-9. Microscopic appearance of an Aschoff body in a patient with acute rheumatic carditis; there is central necrosis with a circumscribed collection of mononuclear inflammatory cells, some of which are activated macrophages (Anitschkow cells) with prominent nucleoli (*arrowheads*). (From Kumar V, Cotran R, Robbins S: Robbins Basic Pathology, 8th ed. Philadelphia, WB Saunders, 2008.)

STEP 1 SECRET

Rheumatic fever is a high-yield diagnosis for Step 1. You should be able to identify Figure 21-9 as an Aschoff body, a pathognomonic finding in this disease.

5. **Which bacteria are most commonly associated with bacterial endocarditis?**
    Endocarditis can be classified into acute or subacute types depending on the time course. Acute infections occur within days to weeks and patients are extremely sick during this time; they are most often due to *Streptococcus* or *Staphylococcus*. Subacute infections present with milder symptoms and are characterized by a consistently low-grade illness for 3 to 4 weeks; they are frequently caused by *Streptococcus viridans* and group D streptococci such as *Streptococcus bovis* (Table 21-20).
    Note: Bacterial endocarditis that occurs soon after prosthetic valvular surgery is commonly due to *Staphylococcus epidermidis* and is believed to result from intraoperative contamination.

TABLE 21-20. ACUTE VERSUS SUBACUTE ENDOCARDITIS

Characteristic	Acute	Subacute
Organisms	*Staphylococcus aureus*	*Streptococcus viridans* (*S. sanguis*) after dental procedures
Onset	Rapid (days → weeks)	Insidious (3-4 weeks)
Clinical manifestations	Severe sickness	Mild sickness
Vegetation size	Large	Smaller
Types of valves affected	Previously normal valves	Damaged or congenitally abnormal valves

6. **What drugs could be used to treat this patient?**
    Because acute endocarditis can be caused by *Streptococcus* species as well as *S. aureus*, the drug chosen will need to cover both of these organisms. If there is no suspicion of methicillin-resistant *S. aureus* (MRSA), then either oral dicloxacillin (PO) or IV nafcillin would work on both, but if there is suspicion of MRSA, then IV vancomycin would be the drug of choice.

7. **How does bacterial endocarditis differ from Libman-Sacks endocarditis?**
    Libman-Sacks (LS) endocarditis, which is seen in systemic lupus erythematosus (SLE), is an aseptic inflammation of the heart valves. The vegetations typically involve both sides of the valve, whereas the vegetations occur primarily on the "downstream" side of the valve in bacterial endocarditis. Finally, the vegetations in LS endocarditis will not embolize.

SUMMARY BOX: ENDOCARDITIS

- Any structural abnormality can predispose to endocarditis.

- The valves of the left side of the heart are most commonly affected, except in intravenous (IV) drug users, in whom the right side of the heart is commonly involved.

- *Staphylococcus aureus* is the most common cause of acute bacterial endocarditis, and *Streptococcus viridans* is an important cause of subacute endocarditis.

- Libman-Sacks endocarditis is seen in systemic lupus erythematosus (SLE), does not contain bacteria, and will not embolize.

CASE 21-4

A 20-year-old man is evaluated for a new genital lesion. The patient returned from spring break last week and noticed a painless ulcer on his scrotum. He is quite concerned and admits to several instances of unprotected intercourse. On examination, there is a well-demarcated, 2-cm painless lesion with a raised border on the shaft of the penis (Fig. 21-10). The remainder of the examination is unremarkable.

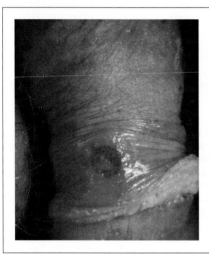

Figure 21-10. Physical examination of patient in Case 21-4. (From Habif TP: Clinical Dermatology, 4th ed. Edinburgh, Mosby, 2004.)

1. **What is the likely diagnosis?**
   Syphilis is caused by the organism *Treponema pallidum*. The organism enters the body through broken epithelium or direct mucosal contact. The classic syphilitic chancre has a clean, nonpurulent base with a sharply defined border, as shown in Figure 21-10.

2. **Based on this man's presentation, in which "stage" of syphilitic infection is he most likely to be?**
   Syphilis progresses through three stages: primary, secondary, and tertiary. This patient displays the classic painless genital chancre of primary syphilis, which appears 3 to 6 weeks after contact. This lesion is highly infectious and continuously sheds motile spirochetes. The primary stage will last 4 to 6 weeks and then resolve, often fooling patients that they are cured.

3. **What stage of syphilis would you suspect in a patient with a diffuse maculopapular rash?**
   This presentation is classic for secondary syphilis. The secondary stage of syphilis will begin approximately 6 weeks after the primary chancre has healed. This phase is characterized by a generalized maculopapular rash with or without the fleshy, painless genital warts termed *condylomata lata*. The secondary stage of syphilis resolves in 6 weeks and enters the latent phase. If the infection is not treated, it will progress to tertiary syphilis in approximately one third of these patients.

STEP 1 SECRET

You should know which bacteria and viruses cause genital lesions and whether these lesions are painful or painless. Remember that the two bugs associated with painful genital lesions are HSV-2 (genital herpes) and *Haemophilus ducreyi*. An easy way to keep this in mind is to remember that "those with *genital herpes do cry* (ducreyi) in pain." By contrast, infections associated with syphilis, gonorrhea, chlamydia, lymphogranuloma venereum, human papillomavirus (HPV), trichomoniasis, and bacterial vaginosis are painless.

CASE 21-4 continued:

This patient does not seek treatment and presents to your office 10 years later with a regurgitant murmur heard best over the right second intercostal space and an ataxic gait.

4. **What is the likely diagnosis?**
   This patient is presenting with symptoms of tertiary syphilis. This stage can develop anywhere from 5 to 35 years after the initial infection. Tertiary syphilis is a systemic disease with three major components: granulomatous change (gummas), cardiovascular syphilis, and neurosyphilis. Inflammatory destruction is the pathophysiologic mechanism that is inherent to all three components. Know that cardiovascular syphilis may result in aortic valve insufficiency and aortic aneurysm, and neurosyphilis can cause *tabes dorsalis*, a condition that causes dorsal column disease of the spinal cord and subsequent ataxia.

5. **Use Table 21-21 to quiz yourself on the three stages of syphilitic infection.**

6. **What diagnostic tests could be done to definitively diagnose syphilis in this man?**
   Direct visualization by darkfield microscopy can be done during the active phases of stage 1 and stage 2 syphilis. This is conducted by obtaining a sample from the lesion and observing the motile spirochetes. Serologic tests were also developed to satisfy the need for a syphilis screen. The Venereal Disease Research Laboratory (VDRL) and the rapid plasma reagin (RPR) tests were developed to detect antibodies present against certain components released after cell death. These tests are nonspecific treponemal tests and, if positive, require a more specific measure, the fluorescent treponemal antibody absorption (FTA-ABS) test. The key point is that the VDRL and the RPR tests are effective for screening high-risk patients. The VDRL test is easier and less expensive, so it is usually done first. However, it can have false positive results because it cross-reacts in the presence of various drugs, viruses, and rheumatologic diseases (e.g., SLE). The VDRL test will become positive in late primary syphilis and becomes negative again in late secondary syphilis. In addition to being more specific, the FTA-ABS test also becomes positive earlier and stays positive longer. Therefore, the FTA-ABS test can be used to diagnose tertiary syphilis and to confirm a positive screening VDRL test (Table 21-22).

7. **How would you treat this patient?**
   Fortunately, syphilis is one of the easiest diseases to treat. Administer penicillin G, and if the patient is penicillin-allergic, offer tetracycline or doxycycline. It is important to remember that only primary and secondary syphilis can be cured with medication. Antibiotics do nothing for tertiary syphilis.

TABLE 21-21. STAGES OF SYPHILIS

Parameter	Primary	Secondary	Tertiary	Congenital
Timing	3 weeks of incubation followed by emergence of papule	Weeks to months after emergence of papule	1-30 years after primary infection (because of latent period between secondary and tertiary)	Transmitted to fetus
Characteristic symptoms/signs	Painless papule on genitals	Disseminated disease with constitutional symptoms; possible rash that can involve palms and soles; condylomata lata are white lesions on genitals; most infectious stage	Gummas (granulomas), aortitis, tabes dorsalis (neurosyphilis of dorsal columns), Argyll Robertson pupil (constriction to accommodation but not to light)	Stillbirth; "saber shins," saddle-nose deformity, deafness
Treatment	Penicillin G	Penicillin G	None	Symptom-dependent

TABLE 21–22. SYPHILIS TESTS

Test	Use
Darkfield microscopy	Test of choice when a chancre is present and a biopsy of the lesion can be taken for direct observation
VDRL	First test used when secondary syphilis is suspected; may need to be confirmed by FTA-ABS testing due to high number of false positives
FTA-ABS	Test of choice for tertiary syphilis; used to confirm a positive result on VDRL test

FTA-ABS, fluorescent treponemal antibody absorption; VDRL, Venereal Disease Research Laboratory.

8. **Later that night, the patient calls you at home with serious concerns about a reaction to penicillin. He states that several hours after being treated he developed a new rash, along with fever, headache, and muscle aches. What are you concerned about in this patient?**
   This patient has likely suffered from a common reaction to the penicillin treatment of syphilis known as the Jarisch-Herxheimer reaction. This side effect of treatment is due to the immune system's reaction to the lysis of treponemes. When exposed to the tremendous load of foreign antigens, the body releases IL-1 and TNF-α, causing fever and possibly shock. This entity should not be confused with an allergy to penicillin and requires only treatment of symptoms and close monitoring.

SUMMARY BOX: SYPHILIS

- The chancre seen in primary syphilis will appear 3 to 6 weeks following exposure.

- The second stage of syphilis is characterized by a rash on the palms of the hands and the soles of the feet and the emergence of condylomata lata.

- The third stage of syphilis can occur years after the primary infection and can cause aortitis, tabes dorsalis, and Argyll Robertson pupil.

- Syphilis is treated with penicillin.

- Venereal Disease Research Laboratory (VDRL) assay is used as a screening test and, if positive, diagnosis is confirmed with fluorescent treponemal antibody absorption (FTA-ABS) test

CASE 21-5

A frantic mother has brought her 8-year-old son in for an emergent visit. She is concerned about an enlarging rash located on the child's back. She adds that he has been complaining of a flu-like illness since the family's return from a hiking trip in New England, during which he was bitten by a tick. On examination you appreciate a large, well-demarcated 20-cm erythematous rash with central clearing (Fig. 21-11) and some regional adenopathy.

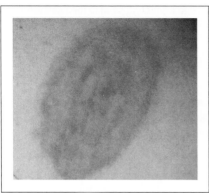

Figure 21-11. Lesion from patient in Case 21-5. Note the variation in color and target–like appearance of the lesion. The bite site is visible in the center. (Courtesy of Dr. Steven Luger, Old Lyme, Connecticut.)

1. **What is the most likely diagnosis?**
   Lyme disease, caused by the spirochete *Borrelia burgdorferi*, is most likely. This bug is transmitted from the bite of an *Ixodes* tick, endemic to the woodlands of New England. The image in Figure 21-11 shows an expanding erythematous lesion known as erythema chronicum migrans.
   Note: The *Ixodes* tick is the vector for *B. burgdorferi* (Lyme disease), *Babesia* (babesiosis), and *Anaplasma phagocytophilum* (granulocytic ehrlichiosis). Treponemal diseases include Lyme disease, syphilis, and yaws.

STEP 1 SECRET

The USMLE commonly asks students about vectors for various bacterial and parasitic infections. Coinfection with Lyme disease and babesiosis is a particular favorite because both bugs share the same vector.

2. **What stage of Lyme disease would you suspect in this child?**
   Our patient has manifestations consistent with stage 1 or "early localized" Lyme disease. Lyme disease is similar to syphilis in that both illnesses are caused by the dissemination of an infectious spirochete and progress through three stages: early localized stage, an early-disseminated stage, and a late stage (stages 1, 2 and 3, respectively). This patient is in stage 1, which consists of the expanding erythematous lesion known as erythema chronicum migrans. A flu-like syndrome and regional adenopathy often accompany the rash of stage 1 Lyme disease.

3. **How would your diagnosis change if this patient presented with a similar history but had complaints of various painful swollen joints and a diffuse macular rash all over his body?**
   He would then mostly likely be suffering from stage 2 or early disseminated Lyme disease. This stage is characterized by the spread of *B. burgdorferi* to four components of the body: joints, heart, nervous tissue, and skin. Migratory musculoskeletal pains occur and usually affect the large joints such as the knee. These joints become swollen and tender. Cardiac complications can vary, ranging from conduction block to myocarditis, and neural issues range from viral meningitis to nerve palsies, most classically a bilateral Bell's palsy. The skin lesions of stage 2 Lyme disease are similar to stage 1 rashes but are smaller and more widely distributed over the body surface.

4. **If this patient does not receive appropriate treatment, what is the likelihood that the infection will progress to stage 3 Lyme disease?**
The late stage of Lyme disease (stage 3) occurs in only 10% of untreated patients and is characterized by the development of a chronic arthritis, which involves multiple large joints and a progressive central nervous system (CNS) disease (Table 21-23).

TABLE 21-23. STAGES OF LYME DISEASE

Stage	Characteristic Symptoms
Early local (stage 1)	Erythema chronicum migrans; flu-like symptoms; occurs within 1 month of tick bite
Early systemic (stage 2)	Monoarticular or oligoarticular arthritis, Bell's palsy or other cranial nerve palsy, and atrioventricular conduction blocks; can occur days to months after tick bite
Late (stage 3)	Migratory polyarthritis and neurologic symptoms; occurs months to years after initial infection

5. **What is the treatment for Lyme disease? Name a preventive measure that can be taken.**
Lyme disease is effectively treated with doxycycline. Later stages of Lyme disease should be treated with ceftriaxone. Recently, an effective vaccine has been developed.
   Note: Lyme disease is most commonly transmitted during the summer, so the vaccine should be given in the spring.

6. **Describe the *Ixodes* life cycle.**
Remember, the *Ixodes* tick is only the vector for the infectious spirochete *B. burgdorferi*. The *Ixodes* life cycle extends over 2 years. Eggs are laid in the spring and will develop into larvae that feed in the summer, preferably on mice. The mice act as the reservoir for *B. burgdorferi*, and it is here that *Ixodes* acquires the spirochete that it can later transmit. *Ixodes* is dormant in the fall and winter and will become a nymph in the following spring. It will feed on a mouse or a human (but note that the human is not necessary for the life cycle of the tick) and *Borrelia* can be transmitted at this time. After feeding, the tick becomes an adult and will mate, often on a deer (Fig. 21-12).

SUMMARY BOX: LYME DISEASE

- Lyme disease is caused by a spirochete, *Borrelia burgdorferi*, and is carried by the tick *Ixodes*.
- Treatment of Lyme disease is with doxycycline.
- Early local Lyme disease is characterized by a bull's-eye target–like rash and flu-like symptoms that occur within 1 month of the tick bite.
- Early systemic disease can manifest as articular disease, Bell's palsy, and heart block.
- Later stages of Lyme disease may manifest as migratory arthritis and neurologic symptoms.

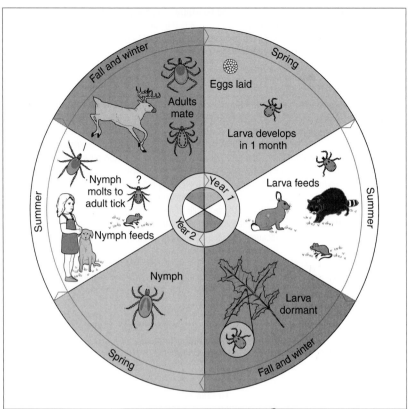

Figure 21-12. Life cycle of *Ixodes scapularis* (also known as *Ixodes dammini*). (Adapted from an illustration by Nancy Lou Makris in Rahn DW, Malawista SE: Lyme disease. West J Med 154(6):708, 1991.)

CASE 21-6

While you are in Pakistan on a medical mission, a patient presents with an 8-week history of fever, night sweats, and a productive cough, at times tinged with blood (hemoptysis). He has lost 20 lb during this time and has been generally fatigued and weak. A chest x-ray film reveals a pulmonary infiltrate, and a purified protein derivative (PPD) skin test is positive. The patient reports that the same test was negative a year ago. A sputum stain for acid-fast bacilli is positive.

1. **What is the presumptive diagnosis?**
   He has tuberculosis (TB), caused by *Mycobacterium tuberculosis*. Note that this is a presumptive rather than a definitive diagnosis because several other occasionally pathogenic mycobacteria such as *Mycobacterium avium-intracellulare* (MAC) can produce a similar clinical presentation and positive acid-fast stain result.

2. **How is this disease primarily transmitted?**
   Aerosolization of contaminated respiratory secretions (e.g., coughing) spreads the disease.

3. **Why is the acid-fast stain required to visualize this bacterium?**

Mycobacterium does not stain well with the Gram stain because it contains mycolic acids in its cell wall rather than peptidoglycan. However, it does stain well with the acid-fast stain, which is why it is referred to as an acid-fast bacterium.

Note: Acid-fast bacteria are visualized with Ziehl-Neelsen stain, and *M. tuberculosis* is grown on Lowenstein-Jensen agar.

4. **Does this patient most likely have primary tuberculosis, latent tuberculosis, or recrudescent (secondary) tuberculosis?**

Because his previous PPD test was negative, he most likely has primary TB, which results from initial infection with the organism. More specifically, he probably has a "progressive" primary infection, in which symptoms manifest. This latter distinction is made because most patients who become infected with the mycobacterium do not develop symptoms. Latent TB develops after symptoms have resolved from primary TB (if there were any symptoms) and is due to tubercle bacilli residing in macrophages. Recrudescent TB develops after some form of immunologic compromise that allows the latent tubercle bacilli to begin proliferating again (Fig. 21-13).

Note: About 10% of patients infected with TB in the United States will eventually have a recrudescence. Miliary TB occurs when the bacilli are transmitted and cause foci of infection throughout the body.

A Ghon complex refers to a region of the lung and associated perihilar lymph nodes that have been exposed to TB and have become granulomatous. A Ghon complex indicates that there has either been an exposure to TB that the body was able to resolve immunologically or that there is a current primary infection.

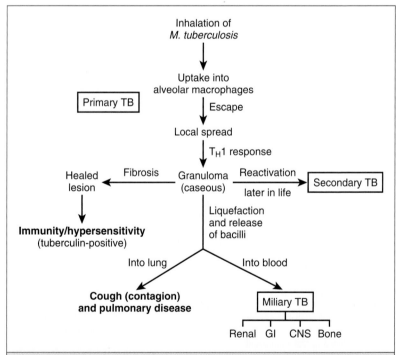

Figure 21-13. Pathogenesis and clinical course of tuberculosis (TB) caused by *Mycobacterium tuberculosis*. CNS, central nervous system; GI, gastrointestinal. (From Rosenthal K, Tan J: Rapid Review Microbiology and Immunology, 2nd ed. Philadelphia, Mosby, 2007.)

5. **What are the first-line drugs for treating tuberculosis and why are they always used in combination?**
These drugs include isoniazid (also used for prophylaxis), rifampin, ethambutol, streptomycin, and pyrazinamide. They are used in combination because there is a high incidence of resistance to these drugs. In the United States, in fact, about 10% to 15% of isolates have resistance to one these drugs even before treatment is started.

6. **If this patient is treated with isoniazid as part of his regimen, why should he also receive supplemental pyridoxine (vitamin B$_6$)?**
One of the main side effects of isoniazid is a peripheral neuropathy, which is caused by the drug stimulating pyridoxine excretion and creating a relative pyridoxine deficiency. Remember that one of the features of pyridoxine deficiency is peripheral neuropathy.
   Note: Isoniazid is well known for its hepatotoxicity. It can even cause a full-blown hepatitis with nausea, vomiting, jaundice, and right upper quadrant pain. Isoniazid is also known to cause a lupus-like syndrome and can lead to hemolysis in glucose-6-phosphate dehydrogenase deficiency. It is an inhibitor of the P-450 system.

7. **If this patient is treated with rifampin as part of his regimen, why may he need larger doses of opioid analgesics for pain control in other illnesses/injuries?**
Rifampin induces hepatic P-450 enzymes, including those that metabolize opioids.

8. **Three weeks after starting a therapeutic regimen with rifampin and isoniazid the patient complains of orange urine. What is probably causing this?**
This is a well-known and common side effect of rifampin. Rifampin also often turns sweat, tears, and contact lenses an orange color.

9. **If this patient begins complaining of vision problems, what would you suspect is the cause?**
Ethambutol has a side effect of optic neuropathy (decreased visual acuity and color blindness).

10. **Why is the standard treatment regimen that this patient will be put on so prolonged?**
Several characteristics of the tubercle bacillus makes it difficult to control quickly. One problem is its intracellular location, where drugs do not penetrate well. In addition, the bacillus is often found in large cavities with avascular centers, into which drugs do not penetrate well either. Finally, the tubercle bacillus has a very slow generation time.

RELATED QUESTIONS

11. **Is cell-mediated immunity or humoral immunity more important for fighting tuberculosis? Why?**
Because the tubercle bacillus resides intracellularly in macrophages, cell-mediated immunity is more important because it targets intracellular pathogens.

12. **How does the purified protein derivative skin (Mantoux) test work?**
PPD is made from the bacterial cell wall of *M. tuberculosis*. When injected into an individual whose immune system has been exposed to the tubercle bacilli, the PPD elicits a type IV hypersensitivity response, which manifests as an indurated area at the site of injection within about 48 hours.

13. **Why is reactivation tuberculosis more likely to occur in the apical lungs rather than in the lower lobes?**
Because mycobacteria are obligate aerobes, the higher oxygen tension in the apex of the lung facilitates their growth there. However, primary infections are more likely to occur in the lower segments where the bacteria are initially deposited.

14. **What type of necrosis is associated with granulomatous cell death in tuberculosis?**
Caseous necrosis, which has a cheesy white appearance. For boards, other types of necrosis include liquefactive (e.g., stroke), coagulative (e.g., MI), fat (e.g., pancreatitis), and gangrenous necrosis (e.g., bacterial infection).
   Note: TB is the only granulomatous disease associated with caseous necrosis. Other granulomatous diseases (e.g., syphilis, cat scratch fever, leprosy, Crohn's disease, CGD, Wegener's granulomatosis, berylliosis, sarcoidosis, systemic fungal infections, *Listeria* infection, and foreign bodies) are noncaseating.

15. **What type of secondary infection can be seen in pulmonary cavitation such as that associated with tuberculosis?**
Aspergillus can colonize in previously formed lung cavities. These colonies are often called "aspergillus balls" or "fungus balls."

16. **How can tuberculosis cause a urinalysis to show microscopic pyuria and hematuria (with red blood cell casts) in the face of a "sterile" culture?**
Hematogenous spread of TB to the kidneys can cause pyelonephritis. TB is notoriously difficult to culture, and the urine is not cultured routinely unless specifically requested.

17. **Why might Pott's disease be suspected in a patient with tuberculosis who has new-onset back pain but denies any trauma that might explain the pain?**
Hematogenous spread of TB to the spine can lead to vertebral osteomyelitis, referred to as Pott's disease.

SUMMARY BOX: TUBERCULOSIS

- Most cases of tuberculosis (TB) in the United States are due to recurrence of latent infections.

- TB is always treated with drug combinations because resistance will develop if only a single drug is given at a time.

- Cell-mediated immunity is the most important defense against TB.

CASE 21-7

A 21-year-old woman presents to your clinic because of abdominal discomfort, which she describes as becoming increasingly severe over the past week. She has also noticed a yellow, malodorous vaginal discharge as well as occasional vaginal bleeding following sex. It is becoming more uncomfortable for her to urinate, but there has been no change in urgency or frequency. She has had three sexual partners over the last 3 months and uses an intrauterine device (IUD) as contraception, which was most recently changed 2 weeks ago.

1. **What is the most likely diagnosis?**
These symptoms most likely point to pelvic inflammatory disease (PID).

2. **What is unique about the chlamydial cell wall?**
The peptidoglycan lacks muramic acid. This renders β-lactam antibiotics useless against *Chlamydia*.

3. **When a sample of infected tissue is stained with Giemsa, where will the chlamydial bacteria be seen?**
Chlamydiae are obligate intracellular organisms because they cannot make their own adenosine triphosphate (ATP), and therefore, they will be seen in the cytoplasm of the infected cell. *Rickettsia* is another example of an obligate intracellular organism.

4. **How is pelvic inflammatory disease transmitted and why can it lead to pelvic discomfort, vaginal discharge, and vaginal bleeding?**
PID is the result of a cervical or vaginal infection that ascends the female reproductive tract to cause endometritis or salpingitis. The inflammation of the uterine lining or the fallopian tubes leads to the pelvic discomfort. The original infection of the lower reproductive tract and the resulting inflammatory response can result in discharge. The infected epithelium is more likely to bleed with even mild contact.

5. **What are the two organisms that could most likely cause her symptoms?**
PID is most likely caused by *Chlamydia trachomatis* or *Neisseria gonorrhoeae*.

6. **What test would you do to differentiate between these two organisms and why?**
A Gram stain would be the best test to differentiate between these two because *C. trachomatis* is an obligate intracellular organism whereas *N. gonorrhoeae* is a gram-negative diplococcus.

7. **How are *Chlamydia trachomatis* and *Neisseria gonorrhoeae* transmitted?**
Both are transmitted by contact with infected genitals, most commonly via sexual contact or at birth.

CASE 21-7 continued:

The laboratory results report the presence of cytoplasmic inclusions but no gram-negative diplococci, leading to the diagnosis of *C. trachomatis* infection.

8. **What should be prescribed as a treatment for your patient?**
Chlamydial infections respond best to tetracyclines. Azithromycin is most often used for *C. trachomatis*. Because patients with *Chlamydia* are at risk for simultaneous gonorrheal infection, you should also treat them with ceftriaxone.

9. **If the patient's current and past partners do not have any symptoms, should they also be considered for treatment?**
Yes. Anyone who has had sexual contact with the patient in the 60 days leading up to her symptoms should also be treated. *C. trachomatis* genital infections are often asymptomatic and are an important reservoir for continuing the infectious cycle. Despite the fact that they can be asymptomatic, chlamydial infections can still lead to sterility in women, most often due to the inflammatory effects on the fallopian tubes (salpingitis).

10. **Why is the fact that the patient was using an intrauterine device significant in this case?**
An IUD may help the infection to ascend from the lower reproductive tract into the endometrium of the uterus when the IUD is inserted.

11. **What are other risk factors for the development of pelvic inflammatory disease?**
Any act that may help the passage of an infection from the lower genital tract into the upper genital tract, including douching, aborting a pregnancy, and parturition, is a risk factor.

12. **If this patient was not using any birth control and had been trying to become pregnant, what other concerns would you need to take into account?**
PID increases the risk of ectopic pregnancy and can also lead to infertility due to scarring of the fallopian tubes as a sequela of the inflammatory response.

13. **What is Reiter's syndrome?**
This autoimmune disease is caused when the antibodyies formed against *C. trachomatis* react against antigens on the urethra, joints, and uveal tract. This results in the classic triad of urethritis, arthritis, and uveitis. Remember that Reiter's syndrome is associated with chlamydial infection.

14. **Describe the unique life cycle of a chlamydial infection.**
Infection begins when an elementary body attaches to and enters an epithelial cell. The elementary body will then transform into a reticulate body, which will divide many times by binary fission. The many reticulate bodies will then be organized into elementary bodies, and it is at this point that the cytoplasmic inclusion bodies may be seen microscopically. The elementary bodies will be released from the cell, and each is then capable of infecting another epithelial cell (Fig. 21-14).

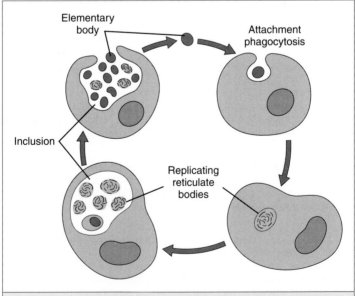

Figure 21-14. Life cycle of *Chlamydia* spp. (From Cohen, Powderly WG, Berkley SF, et al: Infectious Diseases, 2nd ed. Edinburgh, Mosby, 2004.)

15. **What are the serotypes of *Chlamydia trachomatis* that can cause pelvic inflammatory disease?**
PID is caused by serotypes D through K. See Table 21-24 for diseases caused by other *C. trachomatis* serotypes.

TABLE 21-24.	SEROTYPES OF *CHLAMYDIA TRACHOMATIS*
Serotypes	Disease
A, B, C	Blindness in Africa due to chronic infections
D-K	Pelvic inflammatory disease, neonatal pneumonia, neonatal conjunctivitis
L1, L2, L3	Lymphogranuloma venereum

16. **What are the other species of *Chlamydia* and what diseases do they cause?**
Table 21-25 presents the diseases, modes of transmission, and recommended treatment for *Chlamydia* species.

TABLE 21-25. CHLAMYDIAL SPECIES AND ASSOCIATED DISEASES			
Species	Disease	Transmission	Treatment
Chlamydia trachomatis	Reactive arthritis, nongonococcalurethritis (NGU), conjunctivitis, blindness, lymphogranuloma venereum	Sexual or passage through birth canal	Tetracycline or erythromycin (eye drops for neonatal conjunctivitis)
Chlamydia pneumoniae	Atypical pneumonia	Aerosol	Tetracycline or erythromycin
Chlamydia psittaci	Atypical pneumonia with avian reservoir	Aerosol	Tetracycline or erythromycin

SUMMARY BOX: CHLAMYDIA

- *Chlamydia* is an obligate intracellular disease.

- There are two phases of the chlamydial life cycle. The elemental body will infect new cells and the reticulate body will divide within the cell.

- Serotypes L1-3 cause lymphogranuloma venerum (LGV), serotypes A-C cause blindness, and serotypes D-K cause pelvic inflammatory disease (PID).

CASE 21-8

A 20-year-old university music major is brought to your clinic by one of his roommates, who reports that the patient was complaining of a headache last night and was confused when

he was awakened this morning. Upon questioning, the patient knew his name but thought that he was in a different city and that the year was 2008. He reports having a severe headache and asks for the lights to be turned down in the office. His roommate says that he has no history of migraines and that they have known each other for the last 3 years. His temperature is taken and shown to be elevated at 38.7°C. On examination, he has positive Brudzinski and Kernig signs.

1. **What is the most likely diagnosis?**
   This patient most likely has meningitis.

2. **What is the "classic triad" of symptoms associated with meningitis?**
   The classic triad of meningitis is fever, nuchal rigidity, and altered mental status (confusion). However, only about one third of patients with meningitis will present with all three of these symptoms. Photophobia and headache can commonly be seen in meningitis but are not considered part of the triad.

3. **What are the Brudzinski and Kernig signs?**
   The Brudzinski sign is performed by passively flexing the neck while the patient is supine; the test is considered to be positive if the patient spontaneously flexes the hips. The Kernig sign is performed by flexing the hip with the knee flexed and then having the patient extend at the knee while keeping the hip flexed. If the patient is reluctant to fully extend because of nuchal discomfort, the test is positive. Both tests assess for nuchal rigidity secondary to meningeal inflammation.

4. **What are the possible causes for meningitis? What tests can be done to make the diagnosis of meningitis and identify the causative agent?**
   Meningitis can be caused by bacteria, viruses, or fungi. A lumbar puncture should be performed to find the cause. A Gram stain, as well as other laboratory tests, is ordered to assess the cerebrospinal fluid (CSF). Use Table 21-26 to quiz yourself on the different CSF findings for each cause of meningitis.

TABLE 21-26. CEREBROSPINAL FLUID FINDINGS IN MENINGITIS

Infective Agent	WBC Differential	Cell Type	Protein	Glucose	Opening Pressure
Bacterial	↑	PMNs	↑	↓	↑
Viral	Normal	Lymphocytes	Normal	Normal	Normal/↑
Fungal	Normal/↑	Lymphocytes	↑	↓	↑

PMNs, polymorphonuclear neutrophils (leukocytes); WBC, white blood cell.

5. **What are the most common causes of meningitis by age group? Use Table 21-27 to quiz yourself.**

6. **_Haemophilus influenzae_ used to be the most common cause of meningitis in newborns but is now only rarely seen in this age group. Why has this changed?**
   Newborns are now given a vaccine to protect them against _H. influenzae_ type b, but the vaccine is effective only for about the first 2 years of life.

TABLE 21-27. CAUSES OF MENINGITIS BY AGE

0-2 Years	2-18 Years	18-60 Years	60+Years
Escherichia coli	Neisseria meningitidis	N. meningitidis	S. pneumoniae
Group B streptococci	Streptococcus	S. pneumoniae	L. monocytogenes
Listeria	pneumoniae	H. influenzae	N. meningitidis
monocytogenes	Haemophilus	L. monocytogenes	Group B streptococci
	influenzae		H. influenzae

7. **When would be an appropriate time to initiate antibiotic therapy in this patient and what antimicrobial agent could be used?**
    Antibiotic therapy must be initiated immediately when bacterial meningitis is suspected. Based on the age of the patient and the morphology on the Gram stain an appropriate antimicrobial can be chosen. Often a combination of IV vancomycin and ceftriaxone is used because of their central nervous system (CNS) penetration and broad coverage.

8. **A Gram stain of the cerebrospinal fluid shows gram-negative cocci in pairs. What is the most likely cause of the meningitis? Should the roommate and contacts of the patient be notified?**
    N. meningitidis is the most likely causative agent based upon this Gram stain and the patient's age. Contacts of a patient with bacterial meningitis should be treated prophylactically with rifampin.

9. **In a patient with human immunodeficiency virus (HIV), what infective agents may be more likely to cause meningitis than in a patient who has a fully competent immune system?**
    In a patient with HIV, opportunistic infections such as toxoplasmosis, *Cryptococcus,* and JC virus must be considered in the differential diagnosis.

SUMMARY BOX: MENINGITIS

- The classic triad in meningitis is fever, nuchal rigidity, and altered mental status.

- The characteristics of spinal fluid can be used to identify the cause of meningitis.

- Vancomycin and ceftriaxone are often used to treat bacterial meningitis because of their good central nervous system (CNS) penetration.

- Group B streptococci and *Escherichia coli* are important causes of neonatal meningitis.

CHAPTER 22

VIRAL, PARASITIC, AND FUNGAL DISEASES

Thomas A. Brown, MD, and Sonali J. Shah

INSIDER'S GUIDE TO VIRAL, PARASITIC, AND FUNGAL DISEASES FOR THE USMLE STEP 1

Preparing for microbiology does not end after you master the bacterial diseases that were discussed in the previous chapter. These remaining critters are important, too. Fungi are becoming particularly high-yield on Step 1. In fact, some students report having more questions on fungi than on bacteria, so you should learn this section particularly well. Viruses and protists also show up rather frequently on boards, though not nearly as often as do bacteria and fungi. In comparison, helminths and helminth-related drugs are a relatively low-yield topic. We recommend that you study for this section in the same way that you learned the bacteria in Chapter 21.

BASIC CONCEPTS IN VIROLOGY

1. **What structural components are used to categorize viruses?**
    Viruses can be classified according to the following:
    - Nucleic acid
      □ Ribonucleic acid (RNA) vs. deoxyribonucleic acid (DNA)
      □ Single-stranded vs. double-stranded
      □ Segmented vs. nonsegmented
    - Capsid symmetry (icosahedral vs. helical)
    - Size
    - Presence or absence of an envelope
        There are many RNA viruses; all contain single-stranded RNA (ssRNA) except rotavirus, which contains a double-stranded DNA (dsDNA) genome. They are most easily categorized by their capsid symmetry and nucleic acid polarity. The nucleic acid polarity is either + or − sense; viruses with + sense polarity have RNA strands that function directly as messenger RNA (mRNA). Viruses that contain − sense genomes (like influenza and parainfluenza) rely on RNA-dependent RNA polymerases to make a + sense template for transcription.
        All DNA viruses except the Parvoviridae family contain dsDNA. All are enveloped except Parvoviridae, Adenoviridae, and Papovaviridae. If you can memorize the viruses that are all medically relevant DNA viruses, then you know by default any other virus must contain RNA (Figs. 22-1 and 22-2).

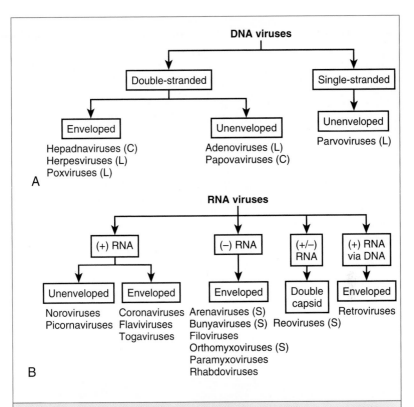

Figure 22-1. Classification of major viral families based on genome structure and virion morphology. **A,** DNA viruses. C, circular genome; L, linear genome. **B,** RNA viruses. S, segmented genome. + or − refers to nucleic acid polarity (see text). (From Rosenthal K, Tan J: Rapid Review Microbiology and Immunology. Philadelphia, Mosby, 2007.)

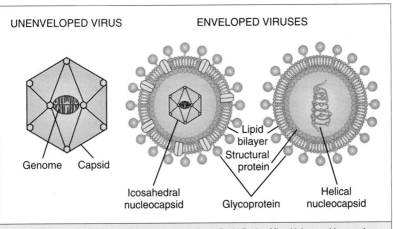

Figure 22-2. Virion structures. (From Rosenthal K, Tan J: Rapid Review Microbiology and Immunology. Philadelphia, Mosby, 2007.)

STEP 1 SECRET

Although it is of little clinical relevance, you are expected to know how to classify viruses according to their genomes (DNA vs. RNA, single- vs. double-stranded, linear vs. circular), capsids (helical or icosadehedral), and presence or absence of a membrane. For instance, you may be given a clinical vignette with a question that asks, "The causative agent of this patient's disease is _____." Instead of naming viruses, you might see answer choices that reflect the composition of the virus (e.g., "a dsDNA virus with a circular genome"). Remember, the USMLE testmakers love to ask second- and third-order questions!

Unfortunately, the only way to learn this information is simply to memorize it. Tricks and mnemonics are of great use here.

Of the DNA viruses, any virus core name ending with an "a" (papilloma, polyoma, hepadna) has a circular genome, and the rest are linear (adeno, parvo, pox, herpes). All of these viruses have double-stranded genomes except parvovirus, because it is the smallest DNA virus ("parvo" is derived from the Latin word for small). All of the DNA viruses replicate in the nucleus except poxvirus, which is large enough to carry its own DNA-dependent RNA polymerase. Enveloped viruses include hepadnavirus, herpesviruses and poxvirus; the rest are naked. You can remember this because poxvirus is large, so it has an envelope, and the other two enveloped DNA viruses both begin with "H."

2. Name the disease associated with each DNA virus listed in Table 22-1.

TABLE 22-1. DNA VIRUSES

Family	Member Virus(es)	Disease(s)
Parvoviridae	Parvovirus B19	Fifth disease, aplastic anemia, arthritis, hydrops fetalis in utero
Herpesviridae	Herpes simplex virus types 1 and 2 (HSV1 and HSV2)	Oral and genital lesions Temporal lobe encephalitis
	Varicella-zoster virus (VZV)	Chickenpox (varicella), herpes zoster
	Epstein-Barr virus (EBV)	Infectious mononucleosis
	Cytomegalovirus (CMV)	CMV retinitis, congenital deafness
	Human herpesvirus types 6 and 7 (HHV6 and HHV7)	Roseola infantum (exanthema subitum)
	HHV8	Kaposi sarcoma in HIV infection
Poxviridae	Variola	Smallpox
	Molluscum contagiosum virus	Umbilicated papules (spread among wrestlers and sexual partners)
Hepadnaviridae	Hepatitis B	Hepatitis
Adenoviridae	Adenovirus	Conjunctivitis, pneumonia, gastroenteritis and pharyngitis

TABLE 22–1.	DNA VIRUSES—continued	
Family	Member Virus(es)	Disease(s)
Papovaviridae	Human papillomavirus (HPV)	Serotypes 16, 18 cause cervical dysplasia
	JC virus	Progressive multifocal leukoencephalopathy

HIV, human immunodeficiency virus.

3. **Cover the right-hand column in Table 22-2, and using the clinical description given, name the most likely virus.**

TABLE 22–2.	CLASSIC CLINICAL MANIFESTATIONS OF INFECTION WITH DIFFERENT VIRUSES
Description	Virus(es)
Rash with "slapped cheek" appearance	Parvovirus B19
Descending maculopapular rash, Koplik's spots	Measles (rubeola) virus
Typically causes gastroenteritis but may cause paralysis by destruction of anterior horn cells	Poliovirus
Cervical cancer in sexually active smoker	HPV (serotypes 16,18)
Parotitis, orchitis, and possible sterility in males	Mumps virus
Cataracts leading to blindness in newborns	Rubella virus
Painful vesicular lesions in dermatomal pattern; virus remains dormant in dorsal root ganglion	Varicella-zoster virus
Acute retinitis in patient with AIDS	CMV
Genital warts	HPV (serotypes 6, 11)
Painful genital vesicular lesions	HSV2 (occasionally HSV1)
Hepatitis in pregnant women, with high mortality rate	Hepatitis E virus
Fatigue, splenomegaly, and atypical lymphocytosis in a teenager; positive heterophile antibody test result	Epstein-Barr virus (EBV)
Gastroenteritis on cruise ship	Norwalk virus
Common cause of gastroenteritis in children	Rotavirus
Common cold viruses	Coronaviruses, rhinoviruses
Most common cause of bronchiolitis in children	RSV
Segmented genome can undergo reassortment, causing epidemic shift pneumonia	Influenza A virus

Continued

TABLE 22-2. CLASSIC CLINICAL MANIFESTATIONS OF INFECTION WITH DIFFERENT VIRUSES—continued	
Description	Virus(es)
Severe encephalitis after an animal bite; intracytoplasmic Negri bodies in neurons	Rabies virus
Neonatal encephalitis	HSV or CMV

AIDS, acquired immunodeficiency syndrome; CMV, cytomegalovirus; HPV, human papillomavirus; HSV, herpes simplex virus; RSV, respiratory syncytial virus.

BASIC CONCEPTS IN PARASITOLOGY

1. **What are protozoa?**
   Parasites can be classified as protozoa or metazoa. Protozoa are single-celled eukaryotic organisms. The medically important protozoa and their associated diseases are listed in Table 22-3.

TABLE 22-3. PROTOZOA COMMONLY CAUSING DISEASE IN HUMANS	
Protozoan	Associated Disease
Entamoeba histolytica	Amebic dysentery (may cause sterile, "flask-shaped" liver abscess)
Giardia lamblia	Giardiasis (foul-smelling diarrhea after drinking contaminated water)
Cryptosporidium spp.	Diarrhea in immunocompromised person
Trichomonas vaginalis	Trichomoniasis (vaginitis with green discharge)
Plasmodium falciparum, Plasmodium vivax, Plasmodium ovale, Plasmodium malariae	Malaria; spread by *Anopheles* mosquito (only *P. vivax* and *P. ovale* cause recurrent infection due to liver hypnozoite stage) Treat with primaquine to eradicate; adverse reaction in patients with G6PD deficiency is hemolytic anemia
Toxoplasma gondii	Toxoplasmosis (from cat feces) Can cause intracerebral infection in HIV infection
Leishmania spp.	Leismaniasis (cutaneous and visceral)
Trypanosoma brucei	African sleeping sickness (African trypanosomiasis) Transmitted by tsetse fly
Trypanosoma cruzi	Chagas disease (American trypanosomiasis), reduviid kissing bug Dilated cardiomyopathy, dementia, and megacolon

G6PD, glucose-6-phosphate dehydrogenase; HIV, human immunodeficiency virus.

2. **What is the difference between cestodes, nematodes, and trematodes?**
They are all helminths (worms). Cestodes are flatworms (tapeworms), nematodes are roundworms, and trematodes are flukes.

3. **Cover the left column in Table 22-4, and from the description of the infection at the right, name the helminth that causes it.**

TABLE 22-4. HELMINTHS COMMONLY CAUSING DISEASE IN HUMANS	
Helminth	Manifestation(s)/Mechanism(s) of Infection
Cestodes (Flatworms)	
Taenia solium (pork tapeworm)	Infection from eating pork leads to intestinal worm; infection from egg ingestion causes cysts to encrust in brain
Taenia saginatum (beef tapeworm)	Transmitted by undercooked beef (mostly asymptomatic)
Diphyllobothrium latum (fish tapeworm)	Extremely long intestinal tapeworm that causes vitamin B_{12} deficiency and anemia; can be acquired by eating raw fish
Echinococcus granulosus	Ingestion of eggs in dog feces, causing cysts in liver, lungs, and brain Rupture of cysts causes allergic reaction
Nematodes (Roundworms)	
Enterobius vermicularis (pinworm)	Anal itching with white worms visible in perianal region; positive result on Scotch tape test
Ascaris lumbricoides (giant roundworm)	Intestinal infection, but worms pass from intestine to lungs Marked eosinophilia Eggs have rough, bumpy surface
Ancylostoma duodenale or *Necator americanus* (hookworms)	Larvae directly penetrate the skin and attach to intestinal mucosa, causing chronic blood loss and anemia
Trematodes (Flukes)	
Schistosoma hematobium	Hematuria after swimming in the Nile Egg has small terminal spine Increased risk of bladder squamous cell cancer
Schistosoma mansoni or *Schistosoma japonicum*	Free-swimming cercariae released from snails infect the human host Eggs are antigenic and induce granuloma formation Pipestem fibrosis of liver
Clonorchis sinensis	Biliary obstruction in patient from southeast Asia
Paragonimus westermani	Transmitted by eating raw crab meat, resulting in gastrointestinal and pulmonary disease

BASIC CONCEPTS IN MYCOLOGY

1. **What are the two morphologic types of pathogenic fungi?**
   Filamentous mold and unicellular yeast are the two morphologic types. An example of a filamentous mold is *Aspergillus*. Inhalation of spores, often found in hay and dead organic matter, is responsible for allergic bronchopulmonary aspergillosis, angioinvasive aspergillosis, and pneumonia with "fungus balls." The pathognomonic microscopic appearance of *Aspergillus* is septate hyphae with a 45-degree branching pattern (Fig. 22-3). Other pathogenic filamentous molds include *Mucor* and *Rhizopus*, which branch at wide angles.

   Cryptococcus neoformans is a unicellular (yeast), encapsulated fungus that can cause cryptococcal meningitis in immunocompromised patients. The capsule is antiphagocytic, is responsible for conferring virulence, and characteristically excludes India ink.

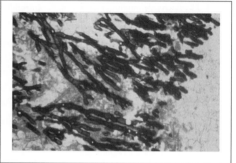

Figure 22-3. *Aspergillus* in tissue showing acute–angle branching, septate hyphae (Grocott's methenamine silver stain, × 1000). (From Murray P, Rosenthal K, Pfaller M: Medical Microbiology, 6th ed. Philadelphia, Mosby, 2009.)

STEP 1 SECRET

You should know the appearances of all the medically relevant fungi. It is common for the USMLE testmakers to ask students to identify fungi based on images.

2. **What is meant by the term *dimorphic fungi*?**
   Dimorphic fungi can exist in either the filamentous mold form or the unicellular yeast form, depending on conditions. In the environment, they live as mold, and in the host as yeast. As a general rule of thumb, all dimorphic fungi are responsible for systemic infections that mimic tuberculosis (i.e., they often lead to granuloma formation). The exception to this rule is *Candida albicans*, which does not result in granulomas.

   Histoplasma capsulatum and *C. albicans* are both dimorphic fungi that can cause pathogenic infections. *H. capsulatum* causes an atypical pneumonia (occasionally with cavitations) endemic to the Ohio and Mississippi river valleys. *C. albicans* causes a variety of mucocutaneous and systemic infections (thrush, intertrigo, diaper rash, paronychia, vaginitis, urinary tract infections [UTIs], endocarditis in intravenous [IV] drug users, and pneumonia). Treat superficial *Candida* infections with nystatin, and systemic infections with fluconazole or amphotericin B.

   Note: Certain systemic fungal infections typically occur only in patients with severely compromised immune systems, especially with defects in cell-mediated immunity. These fungi include *C. albicans, C. neoformans,* and *Aspergillus fumigatus*.

3. **How do the antifungal "-azole" agents work?**
   These agents all inhibit the synthesis of ergosterol, a key component of fungal cell membranes. Examples of this class of drug are ketoconazole, itraconazole, and miconazole.
   Note: Ketoconazole inhibits hepatic enzymes, as well as adrenal and gonadal steroid synthesis. This latter effect may explain the frequent reversible gynecomastia that develops in men who take this drug.

4. **What is the mechanism of action for amphotericin B and nystatin?**
   Both of these agents bind to ergosterol in the fungal membrane, creating pores that affect membrane permeability and stability. Note that amphotericin B is very nephrotoxic and can cause distal (type 1) renal tubular acidosis.

5. **Cover the right-hand column in Table 22-5 and determine the most likely fungal organism based on the clinical description in column 1.**

TABLE 22-5. CLINICAL MANIFESTATIONS OF FUNGAL INFECTIONS	
Description	**Fungal Pathogen(s)**
Diffuse interstitial markings on chest radiograph in HIV-seropositive patient who presents with shortness of breath Positive silver staining Responds to trimethoprim-sulfamethoxazole	*Pneumocystis jirovecii*
Thrush in cancer patient receiving high-dose chemotherapy	*Candida albicans*
Signs and symptoms of meningitis in an HIV-infected patient Positive India ink staining of CSF obtained by lumbar puncture	*Cryptococcus neoformans*
Lung granulomas in former or present resident of Ohio River Valley Intracellular yeast	*Histoplasma capsulatum*
Tinea cruris, corporis, and pedis Hyphae on KOH preparation	*Trychophyton, Epidermophyton,* or *Microsporum*
Lung granulomas in San Joaquin Valley (coccidioidomycosis) Spherule with endospores	*Coccidioides* spp.
Fungus ball in cavitary lung lesion Can be angioinvasive	*Aspergillus*
Systemic mycoses involving lungs, bone, and skin Broad-based, budding yeast	*Blastomyces*
Ascending lymphangitis after puncture with a thorn	*Sporothrix schenkii*

Continued

TABLE 22-5. CLINICAL MANIFESTATIONS OF FUNGAL INFECTIONS—continued	
Description	**Fungal Pathogen(s)**
Severe rhinocerebral infection in diabetic ketoacidosis	Agents of mucormycosis (any of several different fungi)
Nonseptate hyphae with wide 90-degree branching pattern	Angioinvasive fungi

CSF, cerebrospinal fluid; HIV, human immunodeficiency virus; KOH, potassium hydroxide.

CASE 22-1

A 45-year-old woman presents to the clinic with complaints of a flu-like illness. The patient is currently employed as a nurse and has recently had to take several days off for sick leave. She states that approximately 1 month ago she started feeling fatigued and feverish. Soon she developed an "achy" abdominal pain in the right upper quadrant (RUQ). Last week she noticed that her urine was darker than usual.

1. **With this initial history, what is your differential diagnosis?**
   There are several causes of acute RUQ pain—biliary disease (colic, cholecystitis, ascending cholangitis), acute pancreatitis, peptic ulcer disease, dyspepsia, lower lobe pneumonia, or an atypical presentation of myocardial infarction. In a 45-year-old woman, a gallstone should be high on your differential list. Her complaint of darkened urine suggests conjugated bilirubinuria and is further support for an obstruction. It is also possible that this clinical picture could be caused by an intrahepatic process.

CASE 22-1 continued:

On further questioning, you learn that she is quite concerned about being infected with human immunodeficiency virus (HIV) due to a needlestick exposure a few months earlier. On examination you appreciate a jaundiced, ill-appearing woman with RUQ tenderness to palpation. You remind yourself about Charcot's triad (fever, jaundice, and RUQ pain) and realize that she has all three features.

2. **How does the preceding information alter the differential diagnosis?**
   Given the needlestick exposure, the concern now should be an infection such as HIV or, even more likely, hepatitis B. One would want to check liver enzymes and serologic findings for viral hepatitis as well as HIV at this point. These tests may also help clarify whether her pain is related to gallbladder disease and if an abdominal ultrasound is necessary.

CASE 22-1 continued:

Alanine aminotransferase (ALT) and aspartate aminotransferase (AST) are markedly elevated, but the alkaline phosphatase and γ-glutamyltransferase (GGT) are within normal limits. The hepatitis serologic assays return positive for hepatitis B core IgM antibody (HBcAb IgM) and hepatitis B surface antigen (HBsAg).

3. **What is the diagnosis?**
   She has acute hepatitis B infection. Hepatitis B can be acute or chronic (>6 months). Acute hepatitis B often manifests weeks to months after infection with constitutional symptoms, RUQ abdominal pain, and jaundice. Because hepatitis B can be transmitted parenterally, she was likely infected by the needlestick.

4. **Why are the aspartate aminotransferase and alanine aminotransferase values elevated in this patient?**
   Hepatitis is an inflammatory disease of the liver. The viral particles infect hepatocytes, and in an effort to clear the infection, the host immune system destroys infected cells. Hepatocyte necrosis causes a massive leakage of hepatic enzymes. The AST and ALT are markers of hepatocyte death, *not liver function*. Thus, the phrase "transaminitis" indicates an increased AST and ALT. In comparison, a "cholestatic" pattern suggests an obstructive process (intra- or extrahepatic) with elevated alkaline phosphatase and GGT.

5. **What are the three different antigens in a hepatitis B panel?**
   Surface antigen (HBsAg), the core antigen (HBcAg), and the e antigen (HBeAg) are the three types (Fig. 22-4 and Table 22-6).

6. **Which antibody shows up first in acute hepatitis B virus infection?**
   HBcAb IgM is the first to be made. The presence of this antibody and the HBsAg indicates acute infection. The presence of this antibody and absence of HBsAg indicates a recent, resolved acute infection. Note that nearly 95% of all acute hepatitis B infections are resolved; in contrast, only 15% to 45% of hepatitis C infections are resolved. Thus, hepatitis C is more likely to cause chronic disease.

7. **What is the "core window" in hepatitis B infections?**
   The core window is the time frame in which HBsAg has disappeared but HBsAb has not yet appeared. HBcAb IgM will be positive and is essential for diagnosis of acute infection.

8. **Can hepatitis B surface antibody IgG indicate active infection?**
   No. The presence of HBsAb indicates resolution of infection and immunity.

9. **Which of the serologic tests would be positive 6 months after hepatitis B vaccination?**
   Only the surface antigen is used to vaccinate, so 6 months later the only antibody present would be HBsAb.

10. **Based on serologic values how can we differentiate those who have been vaccinated and those who have cleared an infection?**
    Only those patients who have cleared an infection will have antibody to the core antigen (HBcAb) in addition to surface antigen (HBsAb). Those who have been vaccinated make antibody to the surface antigen only and will not have been exposed to the core antigen, because it is not part of the vaccine. They will only have HBsAb.

11. **What other viruses cause hepatitis and what is their usual course of infection?**
    Hepatitis A, C, D, and E viruses are all RNA viruses. Hepatitis B virus is the only DNA virus that commonly causes hepatitis. Hepatitis A and E cause acute infections and are transmitted by the fecal-oral route, typically through contaminated water or food. Hepatitis B, C, and D can cause acute or chronic infections and are transmitted sexually, parenterally (IV drug use,

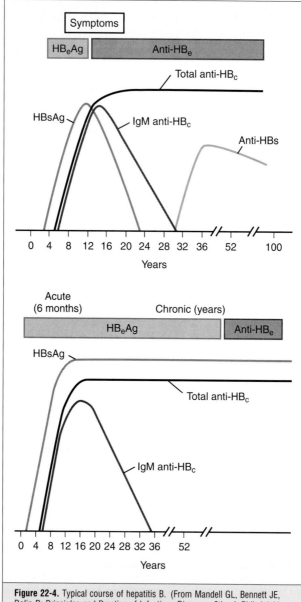

Figure 22-4. Typical course of hepatitis B. (From Mandell GL, Bennett JE, Dolin R: Principles and Practice of Infectious Diseases, 6th ed. Philadelphia, Churchill Livingstone, 2005.)

transfusion, or needle-stick), and vertically (mother to baby). Remember that the "chronic" viruses are so labeled because they persist beyond 6 months; it is important to realize that any of the hepatitis viruses can cause an acute infection with the classic presenting signs. Hepatitis D is a uniquely defective virus: It requires coinfection with hepatitis B before it can cause disease. Thus, a serum test for anti-hepatitis D Ab is indicated only if the HBsAg is positive.

TABLE 22-6. SEROLOGIC MARKERS IN HEPATITIS B INFECTION

Marker	Abbreviation	Significance
Hepatitis B surface antigen	HBsAg	Indicates active infection (acute or chronic)
Hepatis B surface antibody	HBsAb	Indicates successful eradication of infection or immunized status
Hepatitis B core antibody IgM	HBcAb IgM	First antibody produced in acute hepatitis B infection
Hepatitis B e antigen	HBeAg	Indicates high level of viral infectivity

IgM, immunoglobulin M.

12. **How is viral hepatitis treated?**
    Hepatitis A is treated with passive immunization through the administration of pooled IgG and supportive care. A vaccine is available. Active hepatitis B is treated with interferon-α and the reverse transcriptase inhibitor lamivudine. The hepatitis B vaccine is now routinely administered to children and high-risk individuals such as yourself (health care workers). Hepatitis C is treated with combination therapy consisting of interferon-α and ribavirin. There is currently no vaccine available for hepatitis C. The best treatment for hepatitis D consists of the prevention of hepatitis B infection. At this time hepatitis E is treated with supportive care (Table 22-7).

TABLE 22-7. HEPATITIS VIRUSES

Virus	Mode of Transmission	Time Course	Treatment
Hepatitis A virus	Fecal-oral	Acute	Pooled intravenous immunoglobulin (IVIG); vaccine for travelers to endemic areas
Hepatitis B virus	Usually sexual contact, but also parenteral and vertical transmission	Chronic (>6 months)	Vaccine for persons at high risk. Interferon alfa and lamivudine
Hepatitis C virus	Usually parenteral transmission, but also sexual contact and vertical	Chronic	Interferon alfa and ribavirin
Hepatitis D virus	Sexual contact, parenteral and vertical	Chronic	Prevention of hepatitis B infection through vaccination
Hepatitis E virus	Fecal-oral	Acute	Symptomatic relief

SUMMARY BOX: HEPATITIS

- Charcot's triad is the constellation of fever, jaundice, and right upper quadrant pain.

- Hepatitis is considered to be acute if symptoms persist for less than 6 months, and chronic if symptoms persist for more than 6 months.

- Patients vaccinated against hepatitis B will have only hepatitis B surface antibody (HBsAb). Patients who have cleared an active infection will have both HBsAb and hepatitis B core antibody (HBcAb).

- Elevated aspartate aminotransferase (AST) and alanine aminotransferase (ALT) suggest hepatocellular damage. Elevated alkaline phosphatase or γ-glutamyltransferase (GGT) suggests a "cholestatic" or intra- or extrahepatic obstructive process.

- See Chapter 7 for a more detailed analysis of hepatitis B.

CASE 22-2

A 51-year-old Mexican-American man presents to the emergency department in a moderately stuporous condition with new-onset seizure and headache. He is confused and is unable to answer questions. His wife describes an approximate 1-month history of worsening headache that has not been relieved with ibuprofen. Three days prior to admission, he awoke feeling nauseated in the middle of the night and collapsed on the way to the bathroom. He was found unconscious on the bedroom floor and regained consciousness minutes later. On the day of admission, the patient complained of an acrid, burning smell at breakfast, and his right arm began to twitch uncontrollably. He then slumped in his chair and seized violently.

1. **What is the differential diagnosis for new-onset seizure in adults?**
   New-onset seizure in an adult is an ominous sign. It can be associated with a space-occupying lesion, head trauma, medications, alcohol withdrawal, illicit drug use, or intracranial infection.

CASE 22-2 continued:

On admission, the patient is obtunded and oriented to person only. His speech is disorganized and incoherent. He is afebrile with no lymphadenopathy or nuchal rigidity. Further history is elicited from his wife. It turns out that his daughter has recently been treated for a *Taenia solium* infection.

2. **What is the significance of a close contact with previous taeniasis?**
   Humans can serve as the intermediate or definitive host, depending on which stage of the parasite is ingested. Taeniasis is caused by consumption of cysticerci (larvae) in undercooked pork, with subsequent growth of the adult tapeworm in the intestine. Thus, the patient's daughter most likely ate infected meat and represents the index case. When ova shed in the feces of a human carrier are ingested, a distinct disease, cysticercosis, develops. Here, the organism disseminates hematogenously and encysts in the skin, striated muscle, and brain.

3. **How is the diagnosis of neurocysticercosis made?**
   Diagnosis is typically made clinically on the basis of radiographic findings, symptomatology, and exposure history. Images can show a single lesion that is often calcified, serving as a substrate for seizures, or hundreds of lesions distributed diffusely through the cortex. There are serologic tests for antiparasite antibodies, but they are somewhat unreliable and rarely available in endemic areas. Examination of the stool for parasite eggs may detect concurrent taeniasis, but a positive finding is not diagnostic of cysticercosis.

CASE 22-2 continued:

The patient is given IV lorazepam for seizure prophylaxis. Blood work and chest x-ray film are unrevealing. A computed tomography (CT) scan of the head shows viable cysts as diffuse radiolucent defects (small arrow in figure) and as calcified (nonviable) cysts (large arrow in figure) (Fig. 22-5).

Based on unequivocal radiographic evidence, his possible exposure history in an endemic area, and clinical symptoms of new-onset seizures, the diagnosis of neurocysticercosis is made. Stool sample for *Taenia solium* ova is positive, indicating active gastrointestinal (GI) infection.

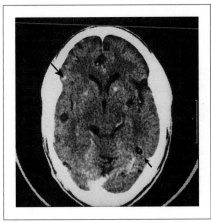

Figure 22-5. Computed tomography head scan demonstrating cysts in patient from Case 22-2. (From Cohen J, Powderly WG, Berkley SF, et al: Infectious Diseases, 2nd ed. Edinburgh, Mosby, 2004.)

4. **How is neurocysticercosis managed?**
Treatment depends on clinical presentation and the number of cysts. Asymptomatic disease is not treated. Symptomatic neurocysticercosis with few parenchymal lesions is managed only with anticonvulsant therapy. Cysticidal agents like albendazole and praziquantel, paired with prophylactic IV corticosteroids, are reserved for symptomatic disease with a high burden of cysts.

CASE 22-2 continued:

An infectious disease (ID) consult suggests that the patient should be started on IV dexamethasone to limit the anticipated inflammatory response to antihelminth therapy. Within 12 hours, the patient's mental status improves. His 15-day course of albendazole, a cysticidal agent, is initiated.

5. **What does neurocysticercosis look like pathologically?**
The brain parenchyma is infiltrated with fluid-filled cysts surrounded by a dense fibrotic capsule. Inflammation is scant and mainly lymphocytic (Fig. 22-6).

6. **What is the epidemiology of neurocysticercosis?**
Neurocysticercosis is the most common parasitic disease of the central nervous system (CNS). It is caused by the cestode *Taenia solium*, a parasite endemic to Central and South America, sub-Saharan Africa, and parts of Asia. It is the leading cause of late-onset seizure in these regions. Infections in the United States have also been reported, primarily in large urban centers among immigrants and travelers.

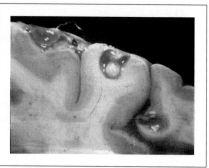

Figure 22-6. Neurocysticercosis. (Photograph from *A Pictorial Presentation of Parasites: A Cooperative Collection* prepared and edited by H. Zaiman.)

SUMMARY BOX: NEUROCYSTICERCOSIS

- Parasites can be divided into two broad categories—protozoa and metazoa. Protozoa are single-celled eukaryotic organisms, such as *Plasmodium*, *Giardia*, and *Entamoeba*. Metazoa are the worms (cestodes, nematodes, and flukes).

- The -bendazole drugs (mebendazole, thiabendazole) are used to treat roundworm infections. Flukes, such as *Schistosoma* and *Clonorchis*, are treated with praziquantel. Flatworms (*Taenia* species and *Diphyllobothrium*) can be treated with praziquantel or niclosamide.

CASE 22-3

A 35-year-old man with acquired immunodeficiency syndrome (AIDS) presents to the emergency department complaining of fever, stiff neck, and a mild but persistent headache. One month ago he experienced an upper respiratory tract infection that resolved on its own without specific therapy. A chest x-ray film at that time was normal. Over the last 48 hours he has vomited twice, and he complains that it hurts his eyes to go outside because "it is too bright." He denies night sweats or recent weight loss. Examination is significant for nuchal rigidity and positive Kernig's and Brudzinski's signs. Laboratory tests from his last visit show a CD4 count of 105 (normal is 500-1500).

1. **What diagnosis do you suspect?**
   Fever, nuchal rigidity, and photophobia are classic for meningitis. The causes of meningitis vary considerably based on age and immune status, and it is important to know likely pathogens in the different age groups (Table 22-8).
   In immunocompromised patients, CNS symptoms can be caused by cytomegalovirus (CMV) encephalitis, toxoplasmosis, cryptococcosis, CNS lymphoma, and progressive multifocal leukoencephalopathy (PML). CMV typically occurs in HIV patients with a CD4 count below 50. PML is a rare, typically fatal development in AIDS patients following recrudescence of JC virus (a polyomavirus). It presents with signs of increased intracranial pressure and focal neurologic deficits, rather than true meningismus, as described here. Primary CNS lymphoma is almost always accompanied by night sweats and weight loss. In this patient the clinical picture is best accounted for by toxoplasma encephalitis or cryptococcal meningitis.

TABLE 22-8. CAUSES OF MENINGITIS IN DIFFERENT AGE GROUPS

Newborns (0-6 months)	Children	Adults	Elderly
Group B streptococci	Pneumococci	Pneumococci	Pneumococci
E. coli	N. meningitidis	N. meningitidis	E. coli
Listeria	Haemophilus influenzae type b	Enterovirus (echovirus, coxsackievirus B)	Listeria
	Enterovirus (echovirus, coxsackievirus B)		

Note: For purposes of review, Kernig's sign is positive when a straight leg raise in the supine position elicits severe neck pain. Brudzinski's sign is positive when passive flexion of the neck causes involuntary knee and hip flexion (to reduce stress on the spine).

CASE 22-3 continued:

A head CT scan is performed and no contraindications to lumbar puncture are identified. An elevated opening pressure is noted.

2. **How do the cerebrospinal fluid findings differ among viral, fungal, and bacterial meningitis?**
See Table 22-9 for a comparison of these findings.

TABLE 22-9. CEREBROSPINAL FLUID FINDINGS IN MENINGITIS

Infection	Color	WBC Differential	Glucose	Protein
Viral (aseptic)	Clear	Increased lymphocytes	Normal	Normal
Fungal	Clear	Increased lymphocytes	Low	Normal to elevated
Bacterial	Cloudy	Predominantly neutrophils	Low	High ($>$40 mg/dL)

WBC, white blood cell.

CASE 22-3 continued:

Cerebrospinal fluid (CSF) analysis reveals a lymphocytosis, with normal to mildly decreased glucose and slightly elevated CSF protein. Gram stain is negative. Serum is negative for toxoplasma antibodies, ruling out previous exposure. An India ink preparation of the CSF is as shown in Figure 22-7.

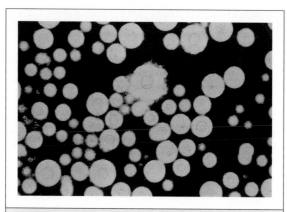

Figure 22-7. India ink preparation of cerebrospinal fluid revealing encapsulated cryptococci. (From Andreoli TE: Cecil Essentials of Medicine, 4th ed. Philadelphia, WB Saunders, 1997.)

3. **What is the diagnosis?**
   The most likely diagnosis based on clinical presentation and CSF analysis is cryptococcal meningitis. The India ink stain (see Fig. 22-7) shows encapsulated cryptococci; note the large capsules surrounding the smaller organisms More commonly, a latex agglutination assay for the cryptococcal capsular antigen is done. *Cryptococcus* can also be cultured on Sabouraud's agar.

4. **What is aseptic meningitis?**
   Aseptic meningitis is an inflammation of the meninges caused by nonbacterial pathogens. Over 80% of aseptic meningitis diagnoses are due to viral infections (commonly by enteroviruses such as echovirus and coxsackievirus B), but other causes include mycobacteria, fungi, rickettsiae, spirochetes, malignancy, and medications (e.g., IV immunoglobulin and Bactrim).

5. **Why is the distinction between aseptic meningitis and bacterial meningitis important?**
   The prognosis and treatment vary tremendously depending on whether the cause of the meningitis is viral, fungal, or bacterial. Acute bacterial meningitis can be a life-threatening disease and often responds well to antibiotics. Fungal meningitis likewise requires emergent therapy. In contrast, aseptic viral meningitis is usually self-limited. After 48 hours of negative CSF cultures, patients will be taken off empiric antibiotics and monitored for any change in course. Viral encephalitis, in which both the meninges and the brain parenchyma itself become inflamed, frequently has devastating outcomes.

6. **What is the treatment of cryptococcal meningitis?**
   The preferred treatment regimen for cryptococcal meningitis is amphotericin B plus the antimetabolite 5-flucytosine for induction therapy. Maintenance therapy requires a minimum of 10 weeks of fluconazole; depending on the severity of infection, fluconazole may also be continued for life if well tolerated

SUMMARY BOX: MENINGITIS

- Causes of meningitis vary by age group.

- *Pneumococcus*, *Neisseria meningitidis*, and enteroviruses are responsible for a majority of infections in both children and adults.

- In newborns and the elderly, *Listeria* and gram-negative bacteria such as *Escherichia coli* are more likely the cause of meningitis.

- Before the routine immunization of infants with the Hib vaccine (a capsular polysaccharide conjugated to diphtheria toxoid), *Haemophilus influenzae* type b (Hib) was also a leading cause of neonatal meningitis.

- Immunocompromised patients are susceptible to the standard bacterial and viral causes of meningitis, in addition to *Cryptococcus neoformans*, an encapsulated yeast.

- Azoles inhibit ergosterol synthesis; polyenes (amphotericin B and nystatin) bind ergosterol in the fungal cell membrane, creating pores.

CASE 22-4

A 6-year-old boy is evaluated for a 2-day history of headache, runny nose, and nausea. He also complains of diffuse muscle aches but denies neck stiffness or photophobia. He does not know of any sick contacts but was recently transferred to a new elementary school. Examination is significant for low-grade fever and pink and edematous ("boggy") nasal turbinates but is otherwise unrevealing. A rapid flu test is negative.

1. **Are you concerned, given the history, examination, and laboratory test findings?**
   This is a common story for young children. The cause of new-onset fever accompanied by headache and nausea varies significantly. This clinical picture could be caused by something as commonplace as a viral infection (respiratory vs. gastroenteritis) or an ear infection as well as something more serious like meningitis. Influenza should be eliminated from the differential if there is a high index of suspicion with a rapid flu test, as well as ear infections and meningitis by clinical examination. With these findings negative, reassurance and clinical follow-up may be all that is necessary.

CASE 22-4 continued:

Several days later an erythematous macular rash develops in the malar distribution. His abdomen and extremities are also covered diffusely by a reticular pattern. No desquamation is noted. Antistreptolysin O (ASO) titer is negative.

2. **What is the most likely diagnosis now?**
   Erythema infectiosum is most likely. Given the description of the diffuse rash, it is important to rule out exotoxin-mediated scarlet fever with an arteriosclerosis obliterans ASO titer, in addition to rarer vasculitic entities like Kawasaki disease, with clinical examination and history (absence of desquamation, conjunctivitis, and cervical lymphadenopathy).

3. **What is erythema infectiosum?**
   Erythema infectiosum is a self-limited illness most often affecting school-aged children. It is a viral exanthem also known as fifth disease or slapped cheek disease, caused by parvovirus B19. The virus infects erythroid progenitor cells in the bone marrow and peripheral blood leads to, causing defective erythropoiesis.

Often it presents as a biphasic illness, with a viremic period marked by fever, headache, and myalgia. Up to a week later, the characteristic slapped cheek rash can appear and evolve to include the whole body. The illness may persist for several weeks to months and is exacerbated by stress, increased physical activity, and exposure to sun.

4. **What are the other viral exanthems?**
   - First disease: rubeola (measles)
   - Second disease: varicella (chickenpox)
   - Third disease: rubella (German measles)
   - Fourth disease: scarlet fever
   - Fifth disease: erythema infectiosum (parvovirus)
   - Sixth disease: roseola (exanthem subitum)

5. **What are other clinical manifestations of parvovirus B19 infection?**
   Remember the other presentations of B19 as the three As (anemia, arthritis, and abortion):
   - Aplastic *anemia* (transient anemic crisis): usually causes pure red blood cell aplasia but can also affect other hematopoietic cell lines. Severe anemia most often occurs in patients with extant hematologic abnormalities such as sickle cell disease, thalassemia, and hereditary spherocytosis. Severity varies, and transfusions are occasionally necessary.
   - *Arthritis:* chronic monoarticular or pauciarticular in nature. Symptoms are usually symmetric and involve the small joints of the hands, knees, and feet. The arthritis is nondestructive.
   - *Abortion:* in pregnant women, parvovirus can cause miscarriage, intrauterine fetal death, and nonimmune hydrops fetalis. When infection occurs before 20 weeks' gestation, outcomes are worse.

6. **Describe the structure of the B19 virion. How is it transmitted?**
   Parvovirus B19 is a nonenveloped ssDNA virus. It is transmitted primarily by respiratory aerosols but can also pass hematogenously and transplacentally. Approximately 50% to 70% of Americans older than 18 years of age are seropositive.

7. **How is infection diagnosed?**
   Serologic testing for B19-specific IgM is used to detect acute infection. Detectable levels can be found within 7 to 10 days of exposure and remain elevated for several months. Another method to diagnose acute infection is detection of B19 DNA by polymerase chain reaction (PCR). This test, however, has the drawback of remaining positive for several years and does not reliably indicate acute infection.

8. **What is the treatment for parvovirus infection?**
   There is no specific treatment for B19 infection. Passive immunity via immunoglobulin transfer may be beneficial to compromised hosts with chronic infection but plays no role in acute disease. Currently, there is no vaccine available. Prevention of disease by good infection control practices is the best method to decrease transmission.

SUMMARY BOX: PARVOVIRUS B19

- Parvovirus B19 is a single-stranded DNA virus that infects early-stage red blood cells (RBCs).

- It first presents as fever, nausea, and myalgia, with subsequent development of the slapped cheek rash characteristic of erythema infectiosum.

- Other clinical manifestations include aplastic anemia, arthritis, and abortion.

- Diagnose with serum immunoglobulin (Ig) M levels or polymerase chain reaction (PCR).

CHAPTER 23

PHARMACOLOGY AND TOXICOLOGY

Khoshal Latifzai, Thomas A. Brown, MD, and Sonali J. Shah

INSIDER'S GUIDE TO PHARMACOLOGY AND TOXICOLOGY FOR THE USMLE STEP 1

We recognize that pharmacology and toxicology are not trivial boards subjects. Each section has its own extensive list of drugs to know, and after a while, it can become very overwhelming. We hope that the following list of tips will help you prepare for this subject with the minimum amount of stress:

- Although there are no shortcuts for learning all the drugs that you are expected to know for boards, you do not necessarily need to know an extensive amount of information about each and every drug. If a drug pops up over and over again in First Aid and in your question bank software, you should learn more about it because it has a greater chance of showing up on your exam. For example, the USMLE is not likely to ask you about the adverse effects of an infrequently used drug such as bosentan, but you will be expected to know its use and basic mechanism of action. On the other hand, you should know the mechanism of action, uses, adverse effects, and toxicity treatment for a drug such as digitalis, which is commonly used in practice and shows up repeatedly within the context of boards questions.

- Focus on unique aspects and properties of the drugs you learn. Boards are not as likely to ask you about whether a drug causes headache or gastrointestinal (GI) upset because these reactions are quite common. You will be tested on drugs that cause seizures, sexual dysfunction, reflex tachycardia, or pulmonary fibrosis however.

- You should expect to have a few questions on the fundamental principles of pharmacology included in the Basic Concepts section of this chapter. The equations for pharmacology are particularly high-yield. It is a great idea to practice using these equations as much as possible. You may consider writing these on your marker board immediately before you begin your exam.

- Do not try to cram pharmacology. The more you practice, the better you will get at classifying drugs by groups and acquiring a feel for the drug categories that are most important to know for Step 1. Five-star topics include drugs of the autonomic nervous system (ANS). In fact, you should expect to get three to five questions on your exam specifically about ANS drugs. Four-star topics include antibiotics, analgesics, and cardiovascular and neurologic/psychiatric drugs.

BASIC CONCEPTS

1. **How does the route by which a drug is administered affect its metabolism?**
Most drugs that are taken orally enter the bloodstream at the level of the portal circulation, and encounter the liver almost immediately. Here, they undergo first-pass metabolism, which renders them less efficacious than if they had reached their target organs first. First-pass metabolism can be circumvented by administering the medication parenterally

(e.g., intravenously, intramuscularly, or subcutaneously). Because the drug is able to reach its target faster and relatively unaltered, its onset of action is more rapid. In comparison with the oral route, the advantage of parenteral administration is that the clinician is able to observe the effects of the drug almost instantaneously and manage dosing appropriately. Disadvantages include elicitation of undesired effects that accompany rapid delivery, and the need for frequent dosing in cases in which a sustained effect is desired.

Other routes of delivery include inhalation (rapid effect, targeted delivery); intrathecal (into the cerebrospinal fluid [CSF]); sublingual (rapid onset, avoids first-pass metabolism); rectal (half of the delivered drug will undergo first-pass metabolism); topical (for local effect); and transdermal (sustained delivery).

The concentration of a drug in the body is dependent on the route of administration because this influences the bioavailability (F) of the drug. A drug administered intravenously has 100% bioavailability (F=1), but drugs administered orally have F < 1. You should know how to calculate the concentration of a drug based on dose administered, bioavailability, and volume of distribution (V_D), which is the volume of the compartment into which a drug is distributed. V_D is dependent on the molecular weight and hydrophilicity of the drug.

$$\text{Concentration} = \text{Dose} \times F/V_D$$

2. **What does the Henderson-Hasselbalch equation mean?**
   A simple rule of pharmacology is that for a drug to move as freely as possible across various membranes in the body, it must be uncharged. Most drugs are either weak acids (i.e., uncharged while they still have their proton), or weak bases (i.e., uncharged in their conjugate acid form). How much of a medication ends up being uncharged in solution depends on the drug (specifically, the pK_a of the drug) and the pH of the solution. If given a list of drugs that are weak acids and asked which will readily cross the blood-brain barrier, simply subtract the pK_a of the drug from the pH of the solution. For whichever choice this number is most negative, that is the drug that will primarily end up being uncharged at that pH. If given a list of weak bases and asked the same question, again subtract the pK_a from the pH. This time, however, the more positive this number, the more of that drug is in the uncharged form. This simplification is derived from the Henderson-Hasselbalch equation:
   For acids (the acid itself is uncharged):

   $$pH = pK_a + \log\,[\text{conjugate base}]/[\text{acid}]$$

   For bases (the conjugate acid is uncharged):

   $$pH = pK_a + \log\,[\text{conjugate acid}]/[\text{base}]$$

   Look at these equations and convince yourself of the reason that the preceding simplification holds true.

3. **What is the difference between zero-order kinetics and first-order kinetics?**
   After a certain period of time in the body, most drugs are inactivated in the liver. Enzymes carry out this biotransformation in one of two ways: first-order kinetics or zero-order kinetics. If a drug is metabolized according to zero-order kinetics, this means that a constant amount of drug is metabolized in a given period of time regardless of the initial dose or half-life of the drug. In other words, enzymes metabolize the same amount of drug per unit time and do not respond to increased workload by increasing their rate of work. The only drugs that you should know are metabolized by zero-order kinetics are ethanol, phenytoin, and aspirin in high doses.

In first-order kinetics, a constant *fraction* of a drug dose is metabolized per unit time. If the concentration of the drug is steadily increased, metabolic enzymes increase the rate at which they work in order to abide by the rule of metabolizing a certain fraction per unit time. First-order kinetics takes half-life into account (see question 4).

4. **What is half-life?**
The half-life ($t_{1/2}$) of a drug refers to the amount of time required for half of a drug dose to be metabolized. Half-life can be calculated according to the following formula:

$$t_{1/2} = 0.7 \times V_D/Cl$$

where Cl = the clearance of a drug. Clearance refers to the volume of blood from which a drug is removed per unit time.
After one half-life, 50% of a drug will disappear. After two half-lives, another 50% of the remaining drug dose will disappear (75% of the original dose). After four half-lives, 94% of the original drug dose will have been metabolized. For boards, you should know that steady state is reached after four to five half-lives.

5. **What is the difference between loading dose and maintenance dose and how is this affected by liver and renal disease?**
Loading dose is the higher dose of drug that is given at the start of a treatment course prior to starting the patient on a lower maintenance dose. Loading dose is calculated using the formula:

Loading dose = Target plasma concentration $\times$ V_D/F

where V_D is the volume of distribution and F is the bioavailability of the drug.
Maintenance dose is calculated using the formula:

Maintenance dose = Target plasma concentration $\times$ Cl/F

where Cl is the clearance of the drug.
You will notice that loading dose takes volume of distribution into account while maintenance dose takes clearance into account. Because clearance is altered in renal and liver disease, maintenance dose must be decreased in these patients, but loading dose is unaffected.

6. **What is therapeutic index?**
Therapeutic index is used as a tool to measure the safety and efficacy of a drug. Therapeutic index is calculated using the formula:

Therapeutic index = Median lethal dose/Median effective dose

The higher the therapeutic index, the safer the drug. Drugs with low therapeutic indices include phenobarbital, theophyline, digoxin, and warfarin (Coumadin). These drugs must therefore be monitored closely in patients who receive them.
Therapeutic window refers to the difference between the median lethal dose and the median effective dose of a drug.

7. **What are the differences between competitive and noncompetitive inhibitors?**
Competitive inhibitors bind to the same active site of an enzyme as the substrate of interest. In competitive inhibition, the enzyme is bound to either the substrate or the inhibitor at any given point. This is because the inhibitor closely resembles the substrate. Competitive inhibition can be overcome by overwhelming the system with increasing concentrations of substrate, which compete with the inhibitor for the active site of the catalytic enzyme. On the other hand, *noncompetitive inhibitors* bind

to alternate sites of the enzyme than the substrate itself. They do not resemble the substrate, but binding of the noncompetitive inhibitor to the enzyme of interest distorts the enzyme such that it can no longer bind to the substrate. Noncompetitive inhibition is often irreversible and cannot be overcome by saturating the system with increasing concentrations of substrate.

SUMMARY BOX: BASIC CONCEPTS

- Drugs administered orally are susceptible to first-pass metabolism, whereas the parenteral route largely bypasses this mechanism.

- The Henderson-Hasselbalch equation can be used to determine the proportion of a drug that ends up being uncharged after being dissolved in solution. This is important because it is the uncharged form of a medication that is able to cross lipid barriers in the body.

- When you hear first-order kinetics, think fractions; when you hear zero-order kinetics, think constant amounts.

- Half-life refers to the time required to metabolize half the amount of drug. A drug reaches steady state after four to five half-lives.

- Volume of distribution refers to the volume of the compartment into which a drug is distributed. Clearance refers to the volume of blood from which a drug is completely removed per unit time.

- You should know the formulas listed in the preceding questions.

CASE 23-1

A 2-year-old girl is evaluated for a 2-day history of fever, vomiting, and diarrhea. Since being given over-the-counter medications this morning she has become increasingly sleepy. Examination is significant for fever, tachycardia, tachypnea, hypotension, somnolence, and decorticate posturing. Urgent workup reveals normal electrolytes, normal head computed tomography (CT) scan, stool positive for rotavirus antigen, and markedly elevated liver enzymes.

1. **Given the preceding clinical picture, what is the most likely explanation for this patient's presentation?**
   This patient appears to have started out with a viral gastroenteritis that was then compounded with an over-the-counter medication, which is now causing confusion, somnolence, and fulminant hepatitis. Given this presentation, the most likely culprit is acetylsalicylic acid (Aspirin) exposure, which led to Reye syndrome (fulminant hepatitis and cerebral edema). Aspirin is a nonsteroidal anti-inflammatory drug (NSAID) that is contraindicated in children for this exact reason. To treat this patient, one needs to alkalinize the urine (bicarbonate is commonly used) to facilitate aspirin excretion from the body. Consider the pharmacologic principles by which this process occurs: Ionized species can be trapped in urine and eventually excreted, but neutral substances are reabsorbed into the bloodstream. Aspirin is a weak acid and is thus ionized in an alkaline environment from $RCOOH \leftrightarrow RCOO^- + H^+$. This ionized form is then excreted in the urine. In the instance that a patient consumes large quantities of a weak base (e.g., amphetamines), the base can be ionized using an acid.

2. **What are the pharmacotherapeutic actions of aspirin and other nonsteroidal anti-inflammatory drugs?**
   Aspirin and other NSAIDs have anti-inflammatory, antipyretic, and analgesic actions. Because of its potency as an anti-inflammatory, aspirin is the NSAID to which all other NSAIDs are

typically compared. These other NSAIDs include ibuprofen, indomethacin (drug of choice for a gouty flare or for closing a patent ductus arteriosus), ketorolac, and naproxen.

3. **What is the mechanism of action of NSAIDs?**
   Injurious stimuli induce involved cells to release arachidonic acid. The two general pathways by which arachidonic acid is broken down in the body are referred to as the cyclooxygenase (COX) and the lipoxygenase (LOX) pathways. NSAIDs play a role in inhibiting the COX pathway, thus reducing prostaglandin production. Prostaglandins are local hormones that are proinflammatory, heighten sensitivity to painful stimuli, and alter the hypothalamic temperature setting so as to promote fever.

4. **What are some side effects of NSAIDs, and what alternative medications exist that circumvent these side effects?**
   The COX pathway is run by one of two isozymes, depending on where in the body the reaction is taking place. COX-1 is the isozyme involved almost anywhere in the body, whereas COX-2 is typically active at the site of inflammation. Ideally, selective inhibition of the latter would achieve the goal of decreasing inflammation. NSAIDs in general are not selective for COX-2 and thus cause effects in other tissues as well. These other sites include platelets (where inhibition of thromboxane A_2 leads to inability of these cells to aggregate into a clot), and gastric mucosa (where reduction of prostaglandins PGE_2, PGF_2, and PGI_2 compromises the protective lining of the stomach and increases acid secretion, thus predisposing to ulcers).

   Selective COX-2 inhibitors (e.g., celecoxib) do exist that purportedly have less renal and intestinal toxicity. Alternatively, acetaminophen may be given to patients with a coagulopathy or a history of gastric ulcers.

5. **If given the choice of aspirin or acetaminophen, which would you administer to a child with a fever.**
   Aspirin given to a child during a viral infection can lead Reye syndrome, which can be fatal. To avoid this possibility, always pick acetaminophen over aspirin for children. The exception to this rule is Kawasaki disease. Children suffering from this condition should be treated with high-dose aspirin to prevent coronary aneurysm.

SUMMARY BOX: NONSTEROIDAL ANTI-INFLAMMATORY DRUGS AND REYE SYNDROME

- Nonsteroidal anti-inflammatory drugs (NSAIDs) are used therapeutically for their anti-inflammatory, antipyretic, and analgesic actions.

- They produce their effects by inhibiting the cyclooxygenase (COX) pathway, thus reducing prostaglandin production. Prostaglandins are involved in pain, inflammation, and fever.

- There are two versions of the COX pathway, and because NSAIDs are not selective in which of these they inhibit, side effects involving the gastrointestinal (GI) system and coagulability are not uncommon.

- Aspirin is an NSAID that is contraindicated in children because it causes Reye syndrome, which is marked by fulminant hepatitis and cerebral edema. Acetaminophen is a better alternative in this patient population.

CASE 23-2

A 14-year-old obtunded boy is brought to the emergency department by his friends, who subsequently leave without providing a history. Vital signs reveal a heart rate of 45 beats/ min, respiratory rate (RR) of 8 breaths/min, and oxygen saturation of 90% on room air. Examination is significant for pinpoint pupils. There is no sign of trauma. He does not smell of alcohol, no needle track marks are evident, and there is no indication of an irritated or perforated nasal septum. The patient has several chewed-up pieces of plastic in his possession that resemble pharmacologic dermal patches.

1. On the basis of the preceding information, what can be the cause of this patient's presentation?
   The patient is likely intoxicated on a substance that is depressing his mental status and his cardiorespiratory status, and inducing pinpoint pupils. The substance was likely introduced into his bloodstream sublingually given the chewed-up dermal patches that were recovered. Given this presentation, the culprit is likely to be an opioid that is available in a transdermal form (e.g., fentanyl).

2. What is the mechanism of action of opioids?
   There are four types of opioid receptors: μ, κ, σ, and δ. The μ-receptors in particular are concentrated in central and peripheral pain pathways and account for the analgesic effects of opioids. When opioids bind these receptors, the cell becomes hyperpolarized, and it becomes difficult to reach the firing threshold. As a result, release of neurotransmitters that are associated with the perception of pain (e.g., substance P) is hindered, and the painful stimulus is not conducted through the nervous system.
   In addition to their analgesic effects, opioids also have anxiolytic effects. It is this ability to relieve anxiety and induce a state of euphoria that has led to the illicit use of opioids. Among the family of opioids, heroin ranks toward the top in terms of being able to cross the blood-brain barrier, possibly explaining its use as an illicit agent.

TABLE 23-1.	OPIOIDS
Agent	**Description**
Morphine	A natural substance
Codeine	A natural substance
	A fraction of the potency of morphine (less potential for abuse)
	Can be taken orally (a common ingredient in cough syrup for its antitussive properties)
Heroin	A derivative of morphine, but altered to increase potency threefold
	Eventually gets converted back to morphine while in the body
	Because heroin is lipid-soluble, it crosses the blood-brain barrier faster than morphine
Methadone	Synthetic
Meperidine	Synthetic
Fentanyl	Synthetic
	80 times more potent than morphine

3. **List a few members of the opioid family.**
See Table 23-1.

TABLE 23-2. OPIOID INTOXICATION

Structure/System Affected	Manifestations
Eyes	Miosis ("pinpoint pupils") due to stimulation of the parasympathetic outflow to the eye
Central nervous system	Confusion, obtundation, euphoria
Lungs	Central respiratory depression resulting in hypercapnic respiratory failure, which can be life-threatening
Intestines	Constipation

4. **What are some signs/symptoms of opioid intoxication? Is it life-threatening?**
See Table 23-2.

5. **How can an opioid overdose be reversed?**
Because opioid intoxication is life-threatening, cases of overdose need to be rapidly treated. To this end, naloxone is a competitive antagonist that quickly (in seconds to minutes) displaces opioids already bound to receptors. Note that the administration of naloxone may cause intense pain in opiate-dependent patients.

6. **What is the difference between naloxone and naltrexone?**
Naltrexone has a longer duration of action and is therefore better suited for long-term management of opioid dependence (rather than acute cases of intoxication, for which naloxone would be a better option). Because the euphoria associated with alcohol dependence is also related to stimulation of opioid receptors, naltrexone can be used to manage alcohol depen dence as well.

7. **What role can methadone play in treating opioid dependence?**
Methadone is a long-acting opioid that reduces the patient's pain to a tolerable level so that he or she can function relatively normally. However, methadone does not cause the euphoric symptoms that drew the patient to opioids in the first place. The patient is then weaned off methadone slowly. Because the withdrawal symptoms of methadone are not as severe and take longer to develop compared with other opioids, the process is more tolerable.

8. **What are signs/symptoms of opioid withdrawal?**
Gooseflesh skin, abdominal pain, and diarrhea can all occur. Withdrawal is *not* life-threatening.

SUMMARY BOX: OPIOIDS

- Opioids bind μ-receptors that are located on the neuronal cell surface. This hyperpolarizes the cell and blunts its ability to conduct painful stimuli. In addition to their analgesic effects, opioids are also anxiolytics.

- Some common opioids are morphine, codeine, heroin, methadone, meperidine, and fentanyl.

- Signs and symptoms of opioid intoxication include miosis, obtundation, euphoria, respiratory depression, and constipation.

- Opioid intoxication can be reversed with naloxone in an acute setting, whereas opioid dependence can be addressed with naltrexone and methadone.

- Opioid intoxication is life-threatening, whereas withdrawal is not.

CASE 23-3

A 22-year-old man with no prior medical history is brought to the emergency department after he had a seizure on the floor of his office nearly an hour ago. His coworkers describe him as a very energetic individual who regularly forgoes sleep in order to excel at his job. He is not taking any medications, and there is no recent history of head trauma. Examination reveals a diaphoretic and confused young man with a heart rate of 140 beats/min, dilated but reactive pupils, and an eroded nasal septum. No focal neurologic deficits or needle-track marks can be appreciated.

1. **Given this clinical picture, what is the most likely explanation for this patient's presentation?**
    This is a young man brought in because he had a seizure recently. His tachycardia, hyperthermia, dilated pupils (mydriasis), and perforated nasal septum suggest cocaine intoxication, likely by inhalation.

2. **What is the mechanism of action of cocaine?**
    Cocaine acts both centrally and peripherally to block the reuptake of norepinephrine, serotonin, and dopamine. When this occurs centrally, the result is an increase in mental awareness, hallucinations, delusions, and paranoia. At high-enough doses, tremors, convulsions, and even death can result from these effects. When reuptake of these neurotransmitters is blocked peripherally, sympathomimetic effects (tachycardia, hypertension [HTN], and pupillary dilation) can occur as a result.

3. **The net effects of cocaine on the body can mimic those of which other illicit drug?**
    It should be apparent that cocaine is a stimulant, similar to amphetamines.

4. **What is the explanation for development of tolerance to cocaine use?**
    The euphoric effects of cocaine are due to prolongation of dopaminergic effects. Over the long term, however, dopamine levels become depleted, and the person craves more cocaine to achieve the same degree of euphoria (this phenomenon is called tolerance). Put another way, dopamine levels become depleted but the threshold at which dopamine causes euphoria remains the same. To reach that same threshold, more cocaine is needed to elicit dopamine release.

5. **Aside from tolerance and dependence, what are some other adverse effects of cocaine?**
    Cocaine can cause cardiac arrhythmias (manage with propranolol) and seizures (manage with diazepam). As with use of other stimulants, cocaine use is followed by post-use "crash" in which the person is physically and emotionally depressed.

AMPHETAMINES

6. **How does the mechanism of action of amphetamines differ from that of cocaine?**
    As mentioned, amphetamines are stimulants, similar to cocaine. Unlike cocaine, however, instead of inhibiting reuptake of neurotransmitters, amphetamines induce release of catecholamines. Think of the two drugs as being analogous to filling a kitchen sink: the amount of water in the sink (i.e., the amount of the neurotransmitter in the synaptic cleft) can be increased in one of two ways: the drain can be plugged (similar to what cocaine does), or the faucet can be turned on high (what amphetamines do).

    When amphetamines act centrally, the result is a release of dopamine. Dopamine increases mental awareness, while decreasing fatigue, appetite, and the need for sleep. Because of these effects, amphetamines can be used therapeutically to treat depression, an abnormally high appetite, and narcolepsy. Paradoxically, they can also be used to treat hyperactivity (attention-deficit/hyperactivity disorder [ADHD]) in children. When amphetamines act peripherally, the result is a release of norepinephrine that causes tachycardia, HTN, and pupillary dilation.

7. **What are some adverse effects of amphetamines?**
    Through their effects on the central nervous system (CNS), amphetamines can cause insomnia, irritability, tremor, and panic. Long-term use can lead to development of psychosis (i.e., hallucinations, delusions, loose thought process) that resembles schizophrenia.

    Through their peripheral effects, amphetamines can cause cardiac arrhythmias, HTN, headache, diaphoresis, anorexia, and diarrhea.

LYSERGIC ACID DIETHYLAMIDE (LSD)

8. **What is the mechanism of action of LSD and its effects on the body?**
    Lysergic acid diethylamide (LSD) is a serotonin agonist. It stimulates the sympathetic nervous system and causes tachycardia, HTN, pupillary dilation, and other similar effects. It also causes *visual* hallucinations of bright colors (in contrast with opioids, for which *tactile* hallucinations predominate). These hallucinations can be treated with antipsychotics (e.g., haloperidol).

PHENCYCLIDINE (PCP)

9. **What is the mechanism of action of phencyclidine and its resultant effects on the body?**
    Phencyclidine (PCP) inhibits the reuptake of dopamine, serotonin, and norepinephrine. The result is a feeling of numbness, staggering gait, slurred speech, rigidity, and *hostile* behavior.

    PCP derivatives have some clinical value. An example is ketamine, which is used to produce anesthesia without loss of consciousness. A major side effect of ketamine is hallucinations and bad dreams (after all, it is still a PCP derivative). Its use is not recommended in children.

TETRAHYDROCANNABINOL (THC)

10. **What is the mechanism of action of tetrahydrocannabinol and its resultant effects on the body?**
    Tetrahydrocannabinol (THC) is an ingredient in marijuana. Although its mechanism of action is unknown, it does cause a feeling of euphoria, drowsiness, xerostomia, visual hallucinations, conjunctival injection (red eyes), impaired judgment, and increase in appetite.

SUMMARY BOX: COCAINE, AMPHETAMINES, AND OTHER ILLICIT DRUGS

- Cocaine blocks the reuptake of norepinephrine, serotonin, and dopamine. This results in an increase in mental awareness, hallucinations, delusions, paranoia, tremors, convulsions, and even risk of death (typically from myocardial infarction or fatal cardiac dysrhythmia).

- The effect of cocaine on the body is very similar to that of amphetamines. Instead of blocking reuptake, however, amphetamines induce the release of catecholamines.

- Lysergic acid diethylamide (LSD) is a serotonin agonist that stimulates the sympathetic nervous system to cause tachycardia, hypertension, mydriasis, and visual hallucinations.

- Phencyclidine (PCP) inhibits reuptake of serotonin and catecholamines, thus causing numbness, ataxia, slurred speech, and hostile behavior.

- Tetrahydrocannabinol (THC) is a component of marijuana and is responsible for inducing euphoria, drowsiness, xerostomia, visual hallucinations, conjunctival injection, and increase in appetite.

CASE 23-4

A 26-year-old woman with an unremarkable medical history is evaluated for a several-hour history of confusion, dizziness, blurred vision, dyspnea, and nausea/vomiting. These symptoms started this morning after she drank herbal tea that was prepared using leaves from a foxglove plant. Examination is significant for an irregular heart rate of 52 beats/min, confusion, and normally reactive pupils. An electrocardiogram (ECG) shows what is termed paroxysmal atrial tachycardia with a 2:1 atrioventricular (AV) heart block. Blood work shows a moderately elevated potassium level of 5.7 mEq/L.

1. **Based on this presentation, what is the likely culprit?**
   This patient became acutely symptomatic after ingesting extracts from a foxglove plant. A reader who is familiar with the pharmaceutical uses of this plant can quickly infer that this is a case of digitalis toxicity. Even if the reader is unfamiliar with this use, physical examination of this patient nonetheless points to cardiac manifestations (bradyarrhythmia, heart block) and (hyperkalemia, both of which suggest digitalis toxicity).
   Digitalis belongs to a class of drugs called cardiac glycosides. Because most members of this class are derived from the *Digitalis lanata* plant (foxglove), the class as a whole is sometimes referred to as digitalis glycosides. Included in this group are digitoxin and digoxin. In terms of their action, glycosides are considered ionotropes, which are drugs that increase cardiac contractility by increasing intracellular calcium.
   Note: Because there is no sign of hemodynamic instability, and because the associated arrhythmia will likely resolve with supportive measures, there is no need to administer antiarrhythmics (e.g., lidocaine, atropine) at this point.

2. **What is the mechanism of action of digitalis?**
   Cardiomyocytes have pumps embedded in their membranes that transport sodium out of the cell in exchange for potassium. Digitalis inhibits this pump (the Na/K-ATPase [adenosine triphosphatase] pump). As a result, the amount of intracellular sodium accumulates, and the cell comes to rely on a "backup system" of exporting the extra sodium. This "backup system" is a

sodium-calcium exchanger that is also embedded in the cell membrane, and transports sodium out of the cell in exchange for calcium. The increase in intracellular calcium means that calcium influx during depolarization of the cell no longer has to be very significant to trigger calcium release from the sarcoplasmic reticulum (i.e., calcium-induced calcium release is "easier" to achieve). Owing to the phenomenon of excitation-contraction coupling in cardiomyocytes, the hyperexcitable cell is now able to contract more readily and, together with other similar cells, return the ejection fraction of the heart toward normal. With increased output, sympathetic stimulation to the heart and peripheral vasculature begins to taper: heart rate slows, and peripheral resistance decreases.

3. What are clinical indications for using glycosides?
Glycosides increase the force of contraction (+ inotropic effect) and are therefore well suited for treatment of heart failure. They also slow conduction velocity through the AV node (- chronotropic effect) by increasing vagal tone and are therefore used to treat supraventricular tachycardias such as atrial fibrillation, atrial flutter, and atrial tachycardia.

4. What are some adverse effects of glycosides?
Because glycosides have an affinity for extravascular proteins, they tend to get widely distributed in the body, and are thus difficult to dose (especially when being coadministered with other medications). For this reason, cases of glycoside toxicity are not uncommon.

Recall that digitalis prevents the cell from exporting Na and importing K (i.e., it blocks the Na/K-ATPase pump). The repercussion of having increased intracellular Na has been described earlier, as it directly results in the therapeutic use of this medication.

The consequence of having abnormal serum K is that it can lead to arrhythmias and even complete heart block. Notice the words in the previous sentence ("abnormal" serum K rather than "increased" or "decreased" serum K). The reason for this is that intuitively, one would expect serum K to rise once the Na/K pump is blocked, and indeed this is what happens in *acute* cases of overdose. However, in practice, patients are rarely taking digitalis alone because it is not a drug of first resort. Patients will typically also be taking thiazide or loop diuretics, both of which expel K from the body through the renal system. Therefore, in chronic cases of digitalis toxicity, it is hypokalemia (rather than hyperkalemia) that causes cardiac dysrhythmias. This is why one should consider either potassium-sparing diuretics or potassium supplements in patients on long-term glycoside regimens.

SUMMARY BOX: GLYCOSIDES AND DIGITALIS TOXICITY

- Cardiac glycosides are a group of ionotropes that increase cardiac contractility by increasing intracellular calcium levels.

- Digitalis is a prominent member of this group and increases intracellular calcium indirectly by inhibiting the Na/K-ATPase (adenosine triphosphatase) pump.

- Glycosides are well suited for treating heart failure and tachyarrhythmias because of their positive inotropic and negative chronotropic effects.

- Because glycosides are not easy to dose appropriately, toxicity is not uncommon.

- Cases of toxicity should be managed with an aim toward normalizing electrolyte imbalances.

CASE 23-5

A 3-year-old child is brought to the emergency department by his parents. He is crying and drooling and is unable to complete his words due to shortness of breath. Seated on his mother's lap, he is doubled over and holding his abdomen. You note that he has significant stridor and a hoarse voice. His parents report that they found their son beside some cleaning products being used in the renovation of their house. They are uncertain as to what chemical he ingested, how much, or the duration of exposure. After finding the child, they immediately removed his chemical-soaked clothes and drove him to the hospital. En route, he had two episodes of blood-tinged emesis.

1. In general terms, how does a caustic agent damage tissue?

   Most caustic agents are either acidic or alkaline and damage tissue directly by chemical means (i.e., they either donate or accept a proton, and thus disrupt bonds native to the tissue). The pH of a substance is directly related to how corrosive it will be should it come into contact with tissue, and substances with pH <2 or >12 are especially notorious.

   Exposure to caustic agents is a fairly common occurrence, more so than poisonings by any other single class of drugs. The typical patient tends to be a child, and the usual route of exposure is via accidental ingestion. If the subject is an adult, then the likelihood of its being an intentional occurrence and an attempt at suicide is much higher.

2. How do alkaline agents damage cells, tissues, and organs?

   Alkaline substances (e.g., drain cleaners, bleach, products containing ammonia) emulsify fat and cause protein to become soluble. A predictable outcome of this is that cell membranes are destroyed, and liquefactive necrosis occurs. This is a very rapid process that generates a considerable amount of heat. Because the means of exposure typically involves ingestion, the pharynx and esophagus are heavily damaged. These organs become edematous and remain so for 1 to 2 days, thus posing a risk for airway obstruction during this period. As the damaged areas become scarred over the next month or so, anatomy of the involved organs can be altered due to stricture formation. Organ perforation can be another outcome.

3. How do acidic agents damage cells, tissues, and organs?

   Acidic substances (e.g., toilet bowl cleaners, metal cleaners) typically cause proteins to denature, which results in coagulative necrosis (contrast this with the liquefactive necrosis caused by alkaline substances). As with alkaline substances, the usual means of exposure here is also ingestion. However, unlike ingestion of alkaline substances, the organ most heavily damaged in this case is usually the stomach (as opposed to the pharynx or esophagus). The damaged coagulated area will slough off in 3 to 4 days, with scar tissue forming soon thereafter. In the interim, however, there is a possibility of organ perforation.

4. If you encountered the preceding patient in the emergency department, what are the next few steps that would need to be addressed immediately in order to arrive at a favorable outcome?

   Although the caustic agent was introduced into the gastrointestinal (GI) tract, stridor is a respiratory symptom, and it is an indication of airway narrowing. Therefore, a primary objective is to secure the airway, and for that, intubation may be required.

   Contrary to one's impulsive urge, emesis should not be induced, as this will simply re-expose the already damaged areas to the irritant. Instead, it is best to extract the corrosive substance using suction through a nasogastric tube. Dilution, using water or milk, is another viable option. Neutralization with a weak acid or a weak base should be avoided, because this can produce a high amount of heat and induce vomiting. Activated charcoal will not necessarily be helpful due to poor adsorption and interference with future attempts at direct visualization (using an endoscopic camera) of the damaged areas.

SUMMARY BOX: CAUSTIC AGENTS

- Alkaline substances include drain cleaners, bleach, and ammonia-containing products. These agents cause liquefactive necrosis by emulsifying fat and causing protein to become soluble. If swallowed, risk of damage to and perforation of the airway and esophagus is high.

- Acidic substances include toilet bowl cleaners and metal polishes. These agents cause coagulative necrosis by denaturing proteins. If ingested, risk of damage to and perforation of the stomach is high.

- Cases of ingestion should be managed by gastric suction and dilution (not emesis).

CASE 23-6

A 58-year-old man is brought to the emergency department with complaints of headache, dizziness, drowsiness, excessive fatigue, and two episodes of fainting. These symptoms started 2 days ago. He denies recent trauma or dehydration. He has no history of neurologic deficits or metabolic anomalies. His past medical history is notable for congestive heart failure (CHF), which has been well controlled and without issues for the last 3 years. He also has a history of hypertension (HTN), which persists despite being on beta blockers. He was seen 3 or 4 days ago by his primary care physician, who prescribed verapamil in addition to his beta blocker. He is not on any other medication. The patient has no allergies. The review of systems is otherwise negative. Physical examination is notable for a heart rate of 44 beats/min and a blood pressure (BP) of 110/70 mm Hg.

1. **What is likely causing this patient's symptoms?**
   This patient, who has a history of chronic HTN, is being forced to function at a much lower perfusion pressure and evidently is unable to do so. Because beta blockers alone were not sufficient in controlling his HTN, his regimen was supplemented with verapamil (a calcium channel blocker [CCB]), which is the likely cause of his bradycardia, relative hypotension, and other symptoms. A different CCB would have been a better choice in this case (see following questions).

2. **What is the mechanism of action of calcium channel blockers?**
   The concentration of intracellular calcium is important when considering any excitable cell in the body. In muscle cells specifically, there is a concept of calcium-induced calcium release. CCBs block the L-type calcium channel (the one in the cell membrane, *not* the one associated with the sarcoplasmic reticulum). By decreasing the initial influx of calcium into the cell, the likelihood of a massive release of calcium from the sarcoplasmic reticulum is also decreased. The net effect of this phenomenon is interference with the excitation-contraction couplet that is typical of myocytes, and resultant relaxation of these cells. In the heart, this effect translates into lower cardiac output. Peripherally, calcium channel blockade results in decreased vascular resistance.

3. **What are the different types of calcium channel blockers?**
   CCBs are divided into three different classes based on chemical properties. Names of these classes are less important than the members themselves. The three members that are important to know are verapamil, diltiazem, and nifedipine. Aside from their different classes, a feature that directly influences their eventual clinical application is their site of action.
   Verapamil predominantly exerts its effects at the level of the heart, but in practice it also influences the peripheral vasculature. Verapamil's effects on the heart include dilation of the coronary arteries and decrease in contractility. It also slows the heart by suppressing conduction through the sinoatrial (SA) and AV nodes. Peripherally, it causes dilation of the arteries, with a resultant drop in BP. Clinically, verapamil is used to treat/prevent angina, arrhythmias, and HTN. Its

use should be avoided in those with a history of CHF because it not only slows the rate of contraction but also decreases contractility, thus precipitating failure. Moreover, its combined use with beta blockers should be avoided, because this can lead to profound bradycardia and hypotension.

Diltiazem has more influence at the level of peripheral vasculature than of the heart. Diltiazem does not decrease contractility to the same extent as is typical with verapamil. Peripherally, it decreases BP by inducing vasodilation of the arteries. Its clinical indications are more or less the same as those for verapamil, although its side effect profile is relatively more benign.

Nifedipine is much more influential at the level of peripheral vasculature than of the heart. It is able to decrease BP but causes reflex tachycardia by stimulating the baroreceptor reflex as well. For this reason, it would have been the most ideal CCB for this patient because it would have supplemented the beta blocker in decreasing BP without suppressing the heart's compensatory response (Table 23-3).

TABLE 23-3. CALCIUM CHANNEL BLOCKERS

Agent	Site of Action	Effect	Clinical Indication(s)
Verapamil	Heart/vasculature	Dilates coronary arteries, decreases cardiac contractility, suppresses SA/AV nodes Causes peripheral vasodilation without reflex tachycardia (due to its negative chronotropic/inotropic effects on the heart)	Vasospastic (Prinzmetal's) angina Obstructive (exertional) angina Arrhythmias (especially supraventricular tachyarrhythmias) Hypertension
Diltiazem	Vasculature > heart	Dilates coronary arteries, suppresses SA/AV nodes Causes peripheral vasodilation without reflex tachycardia (due to its suppression of SA/AV nodes)	Vasospastic (Prinzmetal's) angina Obstructive (exertional) angina Arrhythmias (especially supraventricular tachyarrhythmias) Hypertension
Nifedipine	Vasculature	Dilates coronary arteries Causes peripheral vasodilation with reflex tachycardia (no chronotropic/inotropic effects on the heart)	Vasospastic (Prinzmetal's) angina Not useful in obstructive (exertional) angina because reflex tachycardia increases oxygen demand Ideal for hypertension with bradycardia because it causes a reflex tachycardia

AV, atrioventricular; SA, sinoatrial.

4. **What are some general side effects of calcium channel blockers?**
Although CCBs are fairly selective for cardiomyocytes and vascular smooth muscle, they do have limited activity at GI smooth muscle, which usually manifests as constipation. Their vascular effects in the brain can cause headaches. Excessive hypotension may manifest as generalized fatigue.

SUMMARY BOX: CALCIUM CHANNEL BLOCKERS

- Calcium channel blockers (CCBs) block the L-type calcium channel, thus decreasing the initial influx of calcium into the cell and hampering the excitation-contraction couplet. With less contractility, the output of the heart decreases, as does peripheral resistance with relaxation of vascular smooth muscle.

- Commonly used CCBs include verapamil, diltiazem, and nifedipine.

- Verapamil is more selective for the heart than for the peripheral vasculature and is used to treat/prevent angina, arrhythmias, and hypertension.

- Diltiazem is used for the same indications as for verapamil and has the advantage of a more benign side effect profile.

- Unlike verapamil, nifedipine is more selective for the peripheral vasculature than for the heart and is used to treat hypertension. A common side effect of nifedipine is reflex tachycardia, which is mediated by the baroreceptor reflex.

CASE 23-7

An otherwise healthy 35-year-old man is brought to the emergency department by his coworker who found him to be excessively drowsy and slurring his speech when he showed up to work this morning. The friend mentions that the patient's past medical history is notable for anxiety and insomnia, for which he was prescribed an unknown medication recently. There is no history of trauma, neurologic or metabolic anomalies, or alcohol/drug abuse. On physical examination, the patient has a heart rate of 55 beats/min, BP of 120/70 mm Hg, RR of 9, and a temperature of 37° C. The remainder of the examination is unremarkable.

1. **Given the preceding presentation, which types of items are at the top of the differential diagnosis and would be worth exploring?**
This patient presents in a generally depressed cognitive state, and his vital signs are similarly somewhat diminished. The process appears to be acute in onset, but there is no history of trauma, and the patient is afebrile. This history immediately moves injuries, infections, and chronic processes down the differential list, and shifts other items such as alcohol intoxication, hypoglycemia, and medication involvement up the list. History also reveals that he was recently started on pharmacologic therapy for his anxiety and insomnia. Medications typically used for this purpose tend to be general depressants (e.g., Xanax) that if misused could precipitate a presentation similar to this one. This patient should have his blood glucose checked as well as his levels of alcohol and other depressants (e.g., barbiturates and benzodiazepines).

2. **What is the mechanism of action of benzodiazepines?**
Benzodiazepines bind sites on the cell membrane that are adjacent to but separate from γ-aminobutyric acid (GABA) receptors. Their presence enhances the affinity that GABA receptors have for their ligand, GABA. This translates into a higher frequency of GABA-(GABA receptor) interaction, and therefore more frequent opening of chloride channels in the cell membrane. The chloride influx hyperpolarizes the cell, making it "more difficult" to reach the firing threshold. The end effect is that benzodiazepines enhance the actions of a major inhibitory neurotransmitter in the CNS—namely, GABA—and bring about depressive effects overall.

Incidentally, if this patient were a woman, and if the history were more fitting, then intoxication with a different GABAergic substance would be very high on the differential list. The name of this agent is γ-hydroxybutyrate, commonly referred to by its acronym GHB, and it is a metabolite of GABA. GHB acts as a fast-acting sedative-hypnotic that is a popular choice as a drug of abuse and has also been implicated as a date rape drug.

3. **What are a few clinical indications for using benzodiazepines?**
See Table 23-4.
One means of categorizing benzodiazepines is based on their duration of action (Table 23-5).

TABLE 23-4. BENZODIAZEPINES	
Indication/Use	**Comments**
Anxiolytic	Alprazolam (Xanax) helps calm patients with intense fear of flying before boarding plane
Sedative-hypnotic	Induces sleep
Anticonvulsant	Diazepam and lorazepam can terminate seizures and are used for treatment of status epilepticus Clonazepam may be used for long-term treatment of epilepsy
Alcohol withdrawal	Chlordiazepoxide, diazepam, and oxazepam can be used in acute withdrawal

TABLE 23-5. CATEGORIES OF BENZODIAZEPINES BASED ON DURATION OF ACTION	
Short-acting	Triazolam, oxazepam (Serax), midazolam (Versed)
Intermediate-acting	Clonazepam (Klonopin), alprazolam (Xanax), temazepam (Restoril), lorazepam (Ativan), estazolam
Long-acting	Chlordiazepoxide (Librium), diazepam (Valium)

4. **What are some common adverse effects of benzodiazepines?**
Given that benzodiazepines are generally depressants, it is no surprise that they can produce oversedation, predisposing the patient to falls, fractures, or work injuries; cause cognitive impairment (e.g., memory loss); exacerbate respiratory problems (e.g., emphysema); and lead to dependence. Given the risk of dependence, benzodiazepines should not be prescribed for prolonged durations.

Benzodiazepine intoxication can be reversed with flumazenil (a GABA receptor blocker); withdrawal should be treated symptomatically using long-acting benzodiazepines.

5. What are symptoms of benzodiazepine intoxication and withdrawal?
See Table 23-6.

TABLE 23-6.	BENZODIAZEPINE INTOXICATION AND WITHDRAWAL
Intoxication	Slurred speech, drowsiness, decreased respiratory rate and tidal volume, bradycardia
Withdrawal	Shaking, diaphoresis, anxiety, irritability, insomnia, cardiac palpitations, painful abdominal cramps

SUMMARY BOX: BENZODIAZEPINES

- Benzodiazepines and barbiturates are general depressants.

- Benzodiazepines bind sites adjacent to γ-aminobutyric acid (GABA) receptors and enhance the affinity that GABA receptors have for their ligand, GABA. This results in a chloride influx that hyperpolarizes the cell and accounts for depressive effects of the drug on the body.

- This depressive effect can be therapeutic to persons with anxiety, insomnia, or seizures, or those experiencing alcohol withdrawal.

- Benzodiazepines are usually grouped based on duration of action, and the longer-acting agents can be used to treat those dependent on the shorter-acting benzodiazepines.

- Side effects include oversedation, memory loss, respiratory depression, and dependence.

- The antidote for benzodiazepine intoxication is flumazenil.

CASE 23-8

You are on call overnight, and are paged about a 54-year-old patient who is reportedly having a grandmal seizure. The patient underwent an uncomplicated emergent appendectomy ~72 hours earlier. Over the last 48 hours, the nursing staff reports the patient to have deteriorated from being fairly pleasant soon after his operation to being quite anxious, diaphoretic, tremulous, and unable to sleep. More recently, the patient is said to have been experiencing visual and auditory hallucinations. His past medical history is notable for a simple hand fracture sustained during a bar fight; he is not currently on any medications, nor does he have any allergies. He has no history of prior seizures. He lives alone and is unemployed and twice divorced. A comparison of his day-to-day vital signs shows that his heart rate, BP, and temperature have been progressively increasing over the last 48 hours.

1. Given his recent uncomplicated hospital course and his benign past medical history, what condition is this patient likely experiencing?
This patient has no history of epilepsy and is not taking any medications that would predispose him to seizures. On the other hand, he has several risk factors for depression and substance abuse (e.g., living alone, inability to hold a job or establish close relationships). The most likely cause of his seizure is alcohol withdrawal syndrome, which usually presents 2 to 3 days after a chronic alcohol abuser stops his intake of alcohol. Symptoms of

withdrawal can range from insomnia and tremulousness to severe complications such as seizures and even delirium tremens.

2. **What are the symptoms of acute alcohol toxicity and how can these effects be explained at the molecular level?**
Alcohol has a depressive effect on the brain. It impairs motor function, cognition, judgment, speech, respiration, and it disinhibits behavior.

   At the molecular level, think of the brain as being a teeter-totter that is balanced by an inhibitory neurotransmitter (GABA) at one end and an excitatory neurotransmitter (glutamate) at the other end. Alcohol enhances the effects of GABA on the $GABA_A$ receptor and blunts the effects of glutamate on the N-methyl-D-aspartate (NMDA) receptor (thus weighing the teeter-totter in favor of a net inhibitory effect).

   If exposure to alcohol is chronic, then the brain will enact certain compensatory measures in an attempt to reestablish balance. On the GABA end, the brain will downregulate the number of $GABA_A$ receptors, and on the glutamate end, the brain will upregulate the number of NMDA receptors. Not only is more alcohol needed to attain the same degree of inhibitory effect (i.e., tolerance), but if alcohol exposure is halted suddenly, then there will be pronounced hyperexcitability due to the increased number of NMDA receptors (i.e., withdrawal).

3. **What are symptoms of chronic alcohol abuse?**
Hepatic manifestations are fairly common with chronic exposure and include fatty liver, hepatitis, cirrhosis, and liver failure. Other findings include pancreatitis, nutritional deficiencies, peripheral neuropathy, and cerebellar degeneration.

4. **What is the relationship between alcohol and benzodiazepines in terms of their effect on the brain?**
They both enhance the effects of GABA on the $GABA_A$ receptor (i.e., they are cross-reactive). As described earlier, if the duration of exposure to alcohol is prolonged, then the number of $GABA_A$ receptors will be downregulated to reestablish homeostasis. As a result, just as a chronic abuser of alcohol builds a tolerance to alcohol so that a higher and higher dose is required to achieve the same effect, the same patient will require a higher than normal dose of benzodiazepines to achieve sedation in a medical setting (i.e., cross-tolerance).

   The notion of cross-reactivity between alcohol and benzodiazepines can be used therapeutically to manage alcohol withdrawal. For example, an intermediate-acting benzodiazepine (e.g., lorazepam) can be used as a substitute for alcohol to ameliorate the hyperexcitable state that is characteristic of alcohol withdrawal. Once the teeter-totter is balanced, the intermediate-acting benzodiazepine can be tapered slowly or replaced with a long-acting benzodiazepine (e.g., chlordiazepoxide) that has less abuse potential. Eventually, the number of $GABA_A$ and NMDA receptors will be recalibrated to levels present prior to alcohol exposure, and the benzodiazepines can be stopped altogether.

5. **How is alcohol metabolized in the body?**
Most of the metabolism occurs in the liver, where alcohol is oxidized by alcohol dehydrogenase (ADH) to acetaldehyde, which in turn is oxidized by aldehyde dehydrogenase (aldehyde-DH) to acetate. So remember:

$$Alcohol \rightarrow Acetaldehyde \rightarrow Acetate$$

metabolized by ADH and aldehyde-DH, respectively.

Disulfiram is a drug used to manage alcoholism. It inhibits aldehyde-DH, thus causing accumulation of acetaldehyde. Acetaldehyde in turn causes nausea, vomiting, severe headaches, and flushing. Polymorphisms in acetaldehyde dehydrogenase result in accumulation of acetaldehyde and are common especially among people of Asian descent.

SUMMARY BOX: ALCOHOL

- Alcohol has a depressive effect on the brain by enhancing the effects of γ-aminobutyric acid (GABA) on the GABA$_A$ receptor and blunting the effects of glutamate on the *N*-methyl-D-aspartate (NMDA) receptor.

- Long-term exposure leads to compensation (downregulation of GABA$_A$ receptors and upregulation of NMDA receptors). As a result, more alcohol is required to achieve the same level of depression, and if the supply of alcohol is suddenly halted, then the system tilts toward hyperexcitability because excitatory receptors (NMDA receptors) outnumber inhibitory receptors (GABA receptors).

- Alcohol withdrawal syndrome usually presents 2 to 3 days after a chronic abuser stops intake. Symptoms include insomnia, tremulousness, seizures, and even delirium tremens.

- Chronic exposure can damage the liver, pancreas, and the nervous system, potentially leading to nutritional deficits.

- Those with a tolerance to alcohol will have cross-tolerance to benzodiazepines given their similar site of action. This cross-reactivity can be used therapeutically to treat those withdrawing from alcohol.

- In the liver, alcohol → acetaldehyde → acetate, through alcohol dehydrogenase (ADH) and aldehyde-DH, respectively.

- Disulfiram can be used to manage alcoholism. It inhibits aldehyde-DH, thus causing accumulation of acetaldehyde, which causes nausea, vomiting, severe headaches, and flushing.

CASE 23-9

A 52-year-old woman is brought to the emergency department by ambulance 3 hours after an apparent suicide attempt by ingestion of medication. Her symptoms include nausea, vomiting, and right upper quadrant pain. Her past medical history is positive for depression and chronic alcohol abuse. Her physical examination reveals normal vital signs and some mild tenderness in her right upper quadrant. A serum panel is positive for acetaminophen, but levels are below the toxic threshold.

1. **Given this presentation, which other laboratory values would prove informative? Should this patient be treated based on the information provided?**
   Acetaminophen is metabolized in liver, and one of its byproducts (NAPQI) is toxic to hepatocytes. Therefore, any time a toxic level of this drug is ingested, liver necrosis is a real danger. Fortunately, NAPQI can be inactivated by glutathione, which is an antioxidant regenerated in the body by the enzyme glutathione reductase. However, patients whose reserves of glutathione are decreased (e.g., alcoholics, diabetics) or those who ingest massive quantities of acetaminophen that overwhelm the glutathione system are at risk for hepatocyte damage by NAPQI. To assess the degree of damage to the liver, determining levels of liver function enzymes and a coagulation panel would be informative. Moreover, although this patient's serum level of acetaminophen is below the toxic threshold, given her past history of alcohol abuse, treating her with *N*-acetylcysteine can prevent liver failure. Recall that *N*-acetylcysteine replenishes glutathione supply.

2. **Is acetaminophen considered a nonsteroidal anti-inflammatory drug?**
   Acetaminophen is not considered an NSAID. Acetaminophen acts centrally (in the CNS) to inhibit prostaglandin synthesis, whereas NSAIDs inhibit the same pathway in peripheral tissues. This difference in location accounts for the analgesic/antipyretic effects of acetaminophen and the anti-inflammatory effects of NSAIDs.

3. **What is the mechanism of action of acetaminophen?**
Cell membranes are composed of fatty acids, and one of these fatty acids is arachidonic acid. When the membrane is damaged, arachidonic acid begins to be broken down along one of two pathways—the COX pathway or the LOX pathway. The COX pathway results in prostaglandin production; the LOX pathway produces leukotrienes.

Prostaglandins are among a handful of molecules that mediate inflammation, pain, and fever. If the objective is to decrease inflammation, pain, and fever, then inhibiting the COX pathway is a good start. Acetaminophen reversibly inhibits this pathway. Ibuprofen and aspirin (both NSAIDs) act on the same enzyme, albeit peripherally. Steroids (e.g., hydrocortisone, prednisone) inhibit a different enzyme, phospholipase A_2, that plays a role earlier along this same pathway.

SUMMARY BOX: ACETAMINOPHEN

- Acetaminophen is not considered a nonsteroidal anti-inflammatory drug (NSAID). Acetaminophen acts in the central nervous system (CNS), whereas NSAIDs act in peripheral tissues.

- When the cell membrane is damaged, arachidonic acid begins to be broken down along one of two pathways: the cyclooxygenase (COX) or the lipoxygenase (LOX) pathway. The COX pathway results in prostaglandin production, which mediates inflammation, pain, and fever. Acetaminophen reversibly inhibits the COX pathway.

- Acetaminophen is metabolized in liver, and toxic levels of the drug can cause liver necrosis.

- The antidote to toxic levels of acetaminophen is *N*-acetylcysteine

CASE 23-10

A 74-year-old man with Alzheimer's disease is brought to the emergency department by ambulance. His grandson had found him on the bathroom floor, along with a half-empty bottle of his "Alzheimer's medication." The patient apparently ingested the medication within the last 3 hours, as this was the last time his grandson saw the patient before finding him unconscious. He reports his grandfather to have vomited a few times prior to being found, and several pills could be seen in the vomitus. The patient's other symptoms include diaphoresis, hypersalivation, and urinary incontinence. Physical examination is notable for a low heart rate and RR, mydriasis, and fasciculations.

1. **Given this patient's presentation, which group of medications is the likely culprit?**
Alzheimer's disease is thought to be due in part to a deficiency of acetylcholine (ACh) in the CNS. One way of managing an ACh deficiency is to employ a group of medications generally referred to as cholinergics. In the case of Alzheimer's disease specifically, this means using drugs that are able to cross the blood-brain barrier and block acetylcholinesterase (AChE), thus decreasing the rate of breakdown of ACh. A few AChE inhibitors used in this way include donepezil, rivastigmine, and tacrine.

If AChE inhibitors are used in excessive amounts, however, ACh levels can reach toxic proportions. This in turn can cause more global effects due to the interaction of ACh with nicotinic receptors (fasciculations, muscle weakness), as well as muscarinic receptors (e.g., nausea, vomiting, diarrhea, urinary incontinence, mydriasis, diaphoresis, hypersalivation, bradycardia, hypotension).

Using an anticholinergic agent such as atropine to reverse these effects is a reasonable therapeutic approach.

2. **In general terms, how is the nervous system organized?**
The nervous system can be divided according to function (sensory/motor) or anatomy (central/peripheral). For discussion of anticholinergics, it is best to adopt the former approach and consider only the motor half of the nervous system.

The motor branch can be further categorized into autonomic and somatic nervous systems (ANS and SNS, respectively). SNS and ANS can also be viewed in terms of either anatomy or function. In terms of function, the SNS is the voluntary portion of the nervous system, whereas the ANS is the involuntary portion. In terms of anatomy, the SNS is relatively simple in that a single neuron leaves the CNS and travels directly to the target organ where it delivers ACh to a nicotinic receptor that is located on striated muscle.

In terms of anatomy, the ANS is a bit more specialized than the SNS in that instead of relying on a single neuron, it involves two neurons connecting the CNS to target organs. These two neurons are connected to each other via a synapse. The specifics of this synapse are easy to remember because its anatomy is very similar to that of the SNS; that is, it always involves delivery of ACh to a nicotinic receptor.

The anatomic feature that really sets the ANS apart from the SNS is how the postsynaptic neuron delivers the message from the synapse to the target organ. In fact, the ANS is divided into three groups based on the anatomy of this second neuron:
1. Parasympathetic division delivers ACh to muscarinic receptors.
2. Sympathetic division delivers norepinephrine to adrenergic receptors.
3. Third division is actually partially endocrine and delivers epinephrine (from the adrenal medulla) to an adrenergic receptor (Table 23-7). Because this division also involves a catecholamine as its primary neurotransmitter, it is usually considered part of the sympathetic nervous system. The sympathetic nervous system is discussed more extensively in a separate chapter.

TABLE 23-7. ORGANIZATION OF THE NERVOUS SYSTEM

Nervous System		
Sensory	**Motor**	
Autonomic nervous system (ANS)	Sympathetic nervous system (SNS)	
Involuntary	Voluntary	
2 neurons/1 synapse	1 neuron/no synapse	
Synapse $=$ ACh $\rightarrow$ Nct	ACh $\rightarrow$ Nct (at NMJ)	
Parasympathetic	**Sympathetic**	**Endocrine**
ACh $\rightarrow$ M	NE $\rightarrow$ Adr	Epi (from adrenals) $\rightarrow$ Adr

ACh, acetylcholine; Adr, adrenergic; Epi, epinephrine; M, muscarinic; Nct, nicotinic receptor; NE, norepinephrine; NMJ, neuromuscular junction.

3. **Which neurotransmitter can be said to be pivotal to the function of the entire motor nervous system?**
ACh is the lone neurotransmitter in the SNS and thus the only means of connecting the two neurons in a typical ANS pathway. If its release is hindered (as occurs in botulinum toxicity), the entire motor nervous system can be blocked, thus producing flaccid paralysis.

4. **Is there a way to selectively affect the parasympathetic nervous system?**
   Yes, by stimulating/inhibiting muscarinic receptors, which are exclusive to this branch of the ANS. The two most common stimulants include bethanechol (used to induce urination in nonobstructive urinary retention) and pilocarpine (used to reduce intraocular pressure in glaucoma).

   The two most common antimuscarinics are atropine and ipratropium. Atropine drips can be used in the eye to induce mydriasis (cholinergic input into the eye causes myosis or pinpointing; if this function is blocked by antimuscarinics, then sympathetic input goes unchecked to induce mydriasis or dilation). Atropine is typically used during evaluations for corrective lenses. At high doses, atropine causes tachycardia by blocking muscarinic receptors at the SA node. Ipratropium is a derivative of atropine and comes in an inhaled form that is used to treat asthma and chronic obstructive pulmonary disease (COPD).

5. **What is one way to reduce the side effects of a drug that stimulates both nicotinic and muscarinic receptors?**
   By limiting its physical distribution in the body, one can localize the effects of a drug that would otherwise act on a global level. An example of this approach is using carbachol eye drops to reduce intraocular pressure.

6. **Are there nicotinic receptor blockers that are selective for the autonomic nervous system or somatic nervous system rather than blocking the entire motor nervous system?**
   Yes. Nicotinic receptor antagonists that are selective for the ANS (those receptors located in synapses) are called ganglionic blockers. Unfortunately, their effect is still too expansive to serve an effective therapeutic role. An example of such a blocker is nicotine, which initially depolarizes the postsynaptic neuron (resulting in hypertension (HTN), tachycardia, and increased peristalsis) before blocking the nicotinic receptors (which causes a drop in BP, heart rate, and GI motility).

   Nicotinic receptor blockers that are selective for receptors located on skeletal muscle (i.e., are SNS-selective) are called neuromuscular blocking agents. There are two classes of neuromuscular blockers—depolarizing and nondepolarizing. Depolarizing neuromuscular blockers bind the sodium ion channel at the neuromuscular junction (NMJ), thereby prolonging depolarization and preventing the myocyte from repolarizing. The net effect of this inability to repolarize is flaccid paralysis. An example of a depolarizing blocker is succinylcholine, which is employed in brief procedures (e.g., endotracheal intubations just prior to surgical procedures).

   Nondepolarizing neuromuscular blockers compete with ACh (i.e., they are competitive antagonists). The parent compound for nondepolarizing blockers is curare, and as a result, drugs in this class have some variation of this word incorporated into their names (e.g., tubocurarine). These agents typically serve as part of general anesthesia to achieve skeletal muscle relaxation during surgical procedures. Their effects can be overcome by increasing the concentration of their competitor (ACh). This can be done with AChE inhibitors (e.g., neostigmine or edrophonium) (Table 23-8).

TABLE 23–8. ACETYLCHOLINE AGONISTS AND ANTAGONISTS		
Category	**Muscarinic Receptors**	**Nicotinic Receptors**
Agonist	Bethanechol, pilocarpine Carbachol	Nicotine
Antagonist	Atropine, ipratropium	Nicotine (a ganglionic blocker), succinylcholine (a depolarizing neuromuscular junction blocker), tubocurarine (a nondepolarizing neuromuscular junction blocker)

7. **How can a cholinergic drug help diagnose myasthenia gravis?**
   Myasthenia gravis is a neuromuscular disease marked by autoantibodies that occupy ACh
   receptors at the NMJ (type II hypersensitivity reaction). The typical patient tends to fatigue
   unusually quickly with increasing activity. The reason for this is that the autoantibodies that
   occupy ACh receptors prevent the neurotransmitter from contacting its target, and ACh is
   degraded by AChE before it has a chance to displace the autoantibody. Ptosis and diplopia are
   common initial findings. Weakness in proximal muscles and the diaphragm often follows.
   Patients may also present with dysphagia to solids and liquids.

   With use of fast-acting AChE inhibitor such as edrophonium, the exposure time of the receptor
   to ACh is increased, and the autoantibodies are therefore displaced. A completely fatigued patient
   may then momentarily regain his or her strength and energy. This is in contrast with a genuinely
   fatigued patient, who will not respond because the muscle itself is fatigued. This test, called the
   Tensilon test, is used to diagnose myasthenia gravis. Pyridostigmine is used for long-term
   treatment of myasthenia gravis.

STEP 1 SECRET

Myasthenia gravis is a popular Step 1 topic. Be on the lookout for patients who experience muscle
fatigue with increasing use (in contrast with Lambert-Eaton syndrome). Note that myasthenia
gravis is also associated with thymoma, which may be presented to you on a chest x-ray.

SUMMARY BOX: CHOLINERGICS/ANTICHOLINERGICS

- The motor branch of the nervous system is divided into the somatic nervous system (SNS) and
  the autonomic nervous system (ANS).

- SNS is voluntary and is designed so that a single neuron leaves the central nervous system (CNS)
  and travels directly to striated muscle, delivering acetylcholine (ACh) to a nicotinic receptor.

- ANS is involuntary, and it uses two neurons and a synapse to connect the CNS to target organs.
  In the synapse, ACh is delivered to a nicotinic receptor. There are three variations on how
  the message is then delivered from the synapse to the target organ:

  □ The parasympathetic division can deliver ACh to muscarinic receptors.

  □ The sympathetic division can deliver norepinephrine to adrenergic receptors.

  □ The neuroendocrine division can deliver epinephrine (from the adrenal medulla) to an
    adrenergic receptor (this division is usually considered part of the sympathetic nervous
    system).

- Botulinum toxin inhibits release of ACh, which is pivotal to both SNS and ANS, thus causing
  flaccid paralysis.

- Muscarinic receptors are exclusive to the parasympathetic branch of the ANS. The two most
  common stimulants of these receptors are bethanechol (used to induce urination in nonobstructive
  urinary retention) and pilocarpine (used to reduce intraocular pressure in glaucoma).

- The two most common antimuscarinics are atropine and ipratropium. Atropine drips can be used
  in the eye to induce mydriasis. At high doses, atropine causes tachycardia by blocking
  muscarinic receptors at the sinoatrial (SA) node. Ipratropium can be inhaled to treat asthma and
  chronic obstructive pulmonary disease (COPD).

- Nicotinic receptor blockers that are ANS-selective are called ganglionic blockers.

- Nicotinic receptor blockers that are SNS-selective are called neuromuscular blockers.

- Depolarizing neuromuscular blockers bind the sodium ion channel at the neuromuscular junction, and prolong depolarization at the expense of repolarization, thus causing flaccid paralysis. An example is succinylcholine (employed in brief procedures such as intubation).

- Nondepolarizing neuromuscular blockers are competitive ACh antagonists. These are derivatives of curare and are employed in general anesthesia to achieve skeletal muscle relaxation during surgical procedures. Their effects can be overcome by increasing the concentration of their competitor (ACh). This can be done with acetylcholinesterase (AChE) inhibitors (e.g., neostigmine or edrophonium).

CASE 23-11

A 48-year-old woman is brought to the emergency department (ED) by her son, who found her to be unarousable this morning from last night's sleep. There is no history of trauma or drug abuse. Her past medical history is notable for insomnia, for which she was started on secobarbital recently. Her son brought the pill bottle to the ED with him, and all the pills are accounted for. She takes no other medication and has no known allergies. When questioned, the patient's son notes that his mother did have a few beers last night, although was not overtly intoxicated. Physical examination reveals a somnolent woman with slurred/unintelligible speech, constricted pupils, diminished deep tendon reflexes, a heart rate of 48 beats/min, BP of 100/60 mm Hg, and a RR of 8.

1. **Given this clinical picture, what scenario best explains this patient's presentation?**
   This patient has a history of insomnia and was therefore recently started on a barbiturate (secobarbital). To this, she added another depressant (alcohol) and is now presenting with CNS, respiratory, and cardiac depression.
   Although alkalinizing her urine using intravenous bicarbonate may help rid the body of secobarbital, there is no specific antidote to barbiturates. In this case, the best approach is to monitor her respiration (and intubate if warranted) and prevent cardiovascular collapse (give intravenous fluids and possibly administer ionotropics/vasopressors such as dopamine or norepinephrine).

2. **What is the mechanism of action of barbiturates?**
   Although their binding site is different, barbiturates act very similarly to benzodiazepines in that they potentiate the effect of GABA on the chloride channel. The result is a hyperpolarized cell that is less excitable. However, instead of increasing the frequency of chloride channel opening as benzodiazepines do, barbiturates increase the duration for which the channel is open.
   In addition, barbiturates also diminish activity of the excitatory neurotransmitter glutamate. Barbiturates do this by blocking a type of glutamate receptor that is found almost exclusively in the CNS. Although its actual name is much longer (and relatively unimportant), this receptor is commonly referred to by the acronym AMPA.

3. **What are some common indications for using barbiturates?**
   Although barbiturates have largely been replaced by benzodiazepines due to the better side effect profile and less abuse potential of the latter, barbiturates continue to have uses in some clinical settings. For example, they are still used in induction of anesthesia, as anticonvulsants to treat seizures, and as anxiolytics, and they have also been useful in treating alcohol withdrawal and insomnia.

One means of categorizing barbiturates is based on the duration of action—long-acting, short-acting, or ultrashort-acting. Phenobarbital is a long-acting agent that can be used to treat seizures on a long-term basis; pentobarbital is short-acting and used as a sedative-hypnotic; thiopental is ultrashort-acting and used to induce anesthesia.

4. **What are some common adverse effects of barbiturates?**
Similar to benzodiazepines, barbiturates are generally depressants. At the level of the CNS, this manifests as drowsiness. In cases of overdose, respiratory depression due to blockade of the body's response to hypoxia/hypercapnia is also a very real risk. At toxic doses, barbiturates can also cause severe bradycardia to the point of causing a shock-like condition. In contrast with benzodiazepines, there is no pharmacologic treatment for barbiturate overdose. Treatment consists of symptom management.

As noted earlier, barbiturates do have hypnotic/anxiolytic effects that can precipitate dependence and abuse. On withdrawal, symptoms such as tremors, anxiety, seizures, delirium, and cardiac arrest can result. This ability to cause death with both intoxication and withdrawal is a feature that really sets barbiturates and benzodiazepines apart from other drugs of abuse and is all the more reason not to combine the two with other general depressants such as alcohol.

STEP 1 SECRET

Barbiturates and benzodiazepines are commonly encountered drugs on Step 1. You should know their mechanisms of action, clinical uses, and adverse effects and treatment for overdose.

SUMMARY BOX: BARBITURATES I

■ Barbiturates act very similarly to benzodiazepines: they potentiate the effect of γ-aminobutyric acid (GABA) on the chloride channel. The result is a hyperpolarized cell that is less excitable. Barbiturates also diminish activity of the excitatory neurotransmitter glutamate by blocking AMPA, a type of glutamate receptor.

■ Barbiturates are used in induction of anesthesia, as anticonvulsants to treat seizures, as anxiolytics, and for treatment of alcohol withdrawal and insomnia.

■ Barbiturates are grouped on the basis of their duration of action. Phenobarbital is a long-acting agent (used to treat seizures on a long-term basis), pentobarbital is short-acting (used as a sedative-hypnotic); thiopental is ultrashort-acting (used to induce anesthesia).

■ Adverse effects include drowsiness, respiratory depression, and severe bradycardia.

■ Barbiturates do have hypnotic/anxiolytic effects that can precipitate dependence and abuse. On withdrawal, symptoms such as tremors, anxiety, seizures, delirium, and cardiac arrest can result.

CASE 23-12

A 22-year-old man is brought to the emergency department by his parents, who report that he recently ingested his father's antihypertensive medication in an apparent suicide attempt. His past medical history is notable for depression and asthma. On physical examination, the patient is bradycardic, hypotensive, tachypneic, and in respiratory distress. The patient's mental status is also depressed.

1. **Given this presentation, to which group of antihypertensives does the likely culprit belong?**

   Very few antihypertensive medications precipitate respiratory crisis in a patient with a history of asthma. From that standpoint, the drug in question is likely a beta blocker (more on beta blockers later). Management of this patient requires intravenous fluid, adrenergic agents, and inotropic/chronotropic drugs that bypass the β-receptors altogether and work to restore heart rate and BP. If this patient's respiratory crisis is unresponsive to β-agonists, endotracheal intubation may be warranted as well.

2. **In the sympathetic nervous system, what are the two types of neurotransmitters and the two main adrenergic receptors?**

   The two main neurotransmitters are norepinephrine (NE) and epinephrine (Epi). Both are derived from the amino acid tyrosine through the following steps (Fig. 23-1):

   Phenylalanine → Tyrosine (tyrosine hydroxylase) → Dopa (dopa decarboxylase) → Dopamine (dopamine β - hydroxylase) → Norepinephrine (methylation) → Epinephrine

   The two main types of receptors in the sympathetic nervous system are α-adrenergic receptors and β-adrenergic receptors. Dopaminergic receptors also exist but are not the predominant subtype.

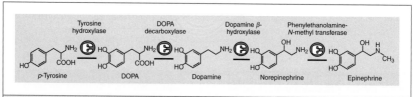

Figure 23-1. Synthesis of neurotransmitters. Pathways of synthesis of neurotransmitters are simple. (From Baynes J, Dominiczak M: Medical Biochemistry, 2nd ed. Philadelphia, Mosby, 2005.)

STEP 1 SECRET

You should memorize the steps in this pathway for synthesis of neurotransmitters, as it is very important for boards.

3. **Describe α-receptors in terms of their distribution in the body and a few of their agonists/antagonists.**

   There are actually two types of α-adrenergic receptors: α_1 and α_2.

   α_1-Receptors are located in the radial muscle of the eye (causes mydriasis), smooth muscle of the vasculature (causes vasoconstriction), and in the penis (causes ejaculation). An example of an α_1-agonist is phenylephrine, which is used to treat nasal congestion by inducing vasoconstriction. An example of an α_1-blocker is prazosin, which is used to treat HTN and benign prostatic hyperplasia (BPH) by causing smooth muscle relaxation.

   α_2-Receptors are located centrally, and stimulating them actually inhibits norepinephrine release from synaptic vesicles. As a result, these receptors can be regarded as part of the inhibitory arm of the sympathetic nervous system. α_2-Agonists include clonidine and α-methyldopa. Clonidine is used to treat severe HTN, nicotine withdrawal, heroin withdrawal, alcohol dependence, and migraines. α-Methyldopa is used to treat HTN. An example of an α_2-blocker is mirtazapine, which is used in the treatment of depression. By inhibiting the inhibitory arm of the sympathetic nervous system, it increases catecholamine activity (Table 23-9).

TABLE 23-9. α–ADRENERGIC RECEPTORS

Category	α_1-Receptors	α_2-Receptors
Agonists	Phenylephrine	Clonidine, α-methyldopa
Antagonists	Prazosin, terazosin	Mirtazapine
	Phentolamine, phenoxybenzamine	

4. **Describe β-receptors in terms of their distribution in the body and a few of their agonists/antagonists.**
    There are also two types of β-adrenergic receptors: β_1 and β_2.
    β_1-Receptors are located in the heart, and stimulating them increases cardiac output by increasing conduction velocity and contractility. An agonist selective for this receptor is dobutamine, which is used to increase cardiac output in CHF. Blocking these receptors decreases cardiac output and hence BP. A few antagonists selective for this receptor are metoprolol, esmolol, and atenolol.
    β_2-Receptors are located in the lungs, and stimulating them causes dilation of the bronchi. An example of a selective agonist is albuterol, which is used in the management of asthma. Blocking these receptors can constrict the airways and precipitate an asthma attack in those predisposed to such an event. Because there is little therapeutic advantage to selectively blocking these receptors, there are few such agents available. The drugs that do happen to block these receptors do so as a side effect of their nonselective β-blocking activity. These agents include temalol, nadolol, and propranolol, and all are contraindicated in asthmatic patients (Table 23-10).

TABLE 23-10. β–ADRENERGIC RECEPTORS

Category	β_1-Receptors	β_2-Receptors
Agonists	Dobutamine	Albuterol
	Isoproterenol	
Antagonists	Metoprolol, esmolol, atenolol	
	Temalol, nadolol, propranolol	

SUMMARY BOX: BARBITURATES II

- The two main neurotransmitters in the sympathetic nervous system are norepinephrine (NE) and epinephrine (Epi).

- The two predominant types of receptors in the sympathetic nervous system are α- and β-adrenergics.

- There are two types of α-adrenergic receptors: α_1 and α_2.

  □ α_1-Receptors are located in the radial muscle of the eye (causes mydriasis), in the smooth muscle of the vasculature (causes vasoconstriction), and in the penis (causes ejaculation). Phenylephrine is an α_1-agonist (used to treat nasal congestion). Prazosin is an α_1-blocker (used to treat hypertension and benign prostatic hyperplasia [BPH]).

  □ α_2-Receptors are located centrally, and stimulating them inhibits norepinephrine release from synaptic vesicles. Clonidine (used to treat severe hypertension, nicotine withdrawal, heroin withdrawal, alcohol dependence, and migraines) and α-methyldopa (used to treat hypertension) are α_2-agonists. Mirtazapine is an α_2-blocker (used in the treatment of depression).

- There are also two types of β-adrenergic receptors: β_1 and β_2.

  □ β_1-Receptors are located in the heart, and stimulating them increases cardiac output. Dobutamine is a β_1-agonist (used to manage CHF). Metoprolol, esmolol, and atenolol are β_1-blockers (used to treat hypertension).

  □ β_2-Receptors are located in the lungs, and stimulating them causes dilation of the bronchi. Albuterol is a β_2-agonist (used to manage asthma). Temalol, nadolol, and propranolol are nonselective beta blockers, which are contraindicated in asthmatic patients because they can precipitate an asthma attack.

CASE 23-13

A 40-year-old farmer arrives at the emergency department complaining that he cannot breathe. Physical examination reveals pulse of 48 beats/min and BP of 94/58 mm Hg. He also demonstrates excessive lacrimation, salivation, and pinpoint pupils.

1. **What is the likely cause of this man's symptoms?**
   Organophosphate poisoning is most likely. Organophosphates are components of insecticides, and toxicity is often suspected in farmers who present with symptoms of excessive cholinergic release.

STEP 1 SECRET

Organophosphate poisoning in a farmer is one of the most commonly encountered clinical vignettes on Step 1.

2. **How does organophosphate poisoning result in this patient's symptoms?**
   Organophosphates are AChE inhibitors. AChE is an enzyme that is responsible for degradation of ACh. Inhibition of AChE results in accumulation of ACh. Excessive ACh results in the **DUMBBELSS** symptoms:
   - **D**iarrhea
   - **U**rination
   - **M**iosis
   - **B**radycardia

- **B**ronchospasm
- **E**xcitation of skeletal muscles (muscle fasciculations, twitches, and trembling)
- **L**acrimation
- **S**alivation
- **S**weating

3. **What is the treatment for organophosphate poisoning?**
   Atropine and pralidoxime are used. Atropine is a cholinergic antagonist, which directly inhibits ACh receptors. Pralidoxime is used to regenerate AChE.
   Note: Atropine toxicity is treated with physostigmine, an indirect agonist of ACh (inhibits AChE).

4. **Atropine administration alone relieves which of the DUMBBELSS symptoms?**
   Excitation of skeletal muscle is not relieved by atropine. The synapses at the NMJ are nicotinic receptors, and atropine is a muscarinic antagonist. Therefore, atropine will not block the nicotinic receptors at the NMJ.

STEP 1 SECRET

Question 4 is a perfect example of the type of tricky question you can expect to see on boards. At first, you may panic when arriving at this question because you may have not seen the answer directly in a textbook. However, if you take a deep breath and just think about what the question is asking, you will realize that you can integrate and apply your knowledge to arrive at the correct answer. The purpose of boards, after all, is to see if you can apply the basic science knowledge you have gained in the first and second years of medical school toward clinical problem solving.

SUMMARY BOX: BARBITURATES III

- Organophosphate poisoning results in acetylcholinesterase inhibition.
- Excessive acetylcholine (ACh) release results in the DUMBBELSS symptoms listed in question 2.
- Organophosphate overdose is treated with atropine and pralidoxime.

CHAPTER 24

BEHAVIORAL SCIENCES

Thomas A. Brown, MD, and Sonali J. Shah

INSIDER'S GUIDE TO BEHAVIORAL SCIENCES FOR THE USMLE STEP 1

Behavioral sciences often are overlooked by medical students taking the USMLE Step 1, but in our opinion, this is a huge mistake. Most students say that they wish they had studied more for this section, because it is often a huge score booster for those comfortable with the material. Expect to see multiple questions that will present ethical dilemmas and then ask you what you would do in those situations. The ideal way to prepare for such questions is to practice reading through as many ethical scenarios as possible! In other words, your best resources will be the cases in this chapter and those presented to you in question bank software programs. Other high-yield behavioral sciences topics include developmental milestones and the physiology and pathophysiology of sleep. You should also know about informed consent, advanced directives, and care for minors. Be sure to pay special attention to exceptions for any rules that apply to ethical situations.

CASE 24-1

A 37-year-old man presents to a psychiatrist for evaluation of symptoms he believes might be depression. He reports trouble sleeping for the last 6 months, stating he never feels rested after 7 to 8 hours of sleep. He also notices decreased concentration at work.

1. **What are the considerations in the differential diagnosis?**
   Depression, sleep apnea, sleep disorders (dyssomnias), adjustment disorder, hypothyroidism, chronic renal failure, anemia, dementia, substance abuse or withdrawal, and anxiety should be considered.

   He has had relationship troubles with his wife and is recently divorced. He reports that her primary reason for leaving him was that he no longer seemed to care about her, as he never wanted to go out or do the things they used to do. She even went so far as to accuse him of having an affair. They stopped sleeping in the same room 2 years ago because his excessive snoring, with intermittent bursts of awakening short of breath, kept her up at night. He says he just doesn't have energy to do things anymore. He also relates having been recently reprimanded at work for falling asleep. On examination, he is a moderately obese, otherwise healthy-appearing middle-aged man. His mental status examination is unremarkable. He denies any thoughts of suicide, appetite disturbances, or feelings of guilt or hopelessness. He does feel like he has had depressed mood since his wife has left.

2. **In addition to a diagnosis of adjustment disorder with depressed mood, what sleep-related disorder likely explains most of this patient's problem?**
This patient is suffering from *sleep apnea* and would appropriately be diagnosed with a breathing-related sleep disorder. These patients are often obese, and a collar size greater than 17 inches should be a red flag; presumably, the weight of the fat around the neck collapses the airway. Sleep is often interrupted at night because of the occluded airway, leading to excessive daytime sleepiness and fatigue. Chronic poor sleep can lead to irritability, poor concentration, and the need to "nap" during the day.

STEP 1 SECRET

Associate "excessive daytime sleepiness" with narcolepsy and obstructive sleep apnea. Both diseases are favorites on the USMLE.

3. **What treatment can be employed to allow this man to sleep at night?**
The therapy used to allow these patients to sleep involves pressurizing the airway to keep it patent. The patient wears a mask that provides positive airway pressure to keep the airway from being obstructed. Positive airway pressure is only one treatment option for those patients who suffer from obstructive sleep apnea, as does this man. As always, lifestyle modifications are important as well. This patient should be encouraged to lose weight, which should reduce the compressive forces on the airway and thereby decrease the airway obstruction. Uvuloplasty or nasal surgery may also be indicated.
Note: Sleep studies will show apneic episodes with increasing breathing effort against an obstructed airway, frequent arousals, and decreased rapid eye movement (REM) sleep.

SUMMARY BOX: SLEEP APNEA

- Obstructive sleep apnea may be associated with loud snoring, difficulty concentrating, poor memory, and waking up feeling unrested after sleep.

- Sleep studies will show apneic episodes, frequent arousals, and decreased rapid eye movement (REM) sleep.

- Depending on the case, treatment may consist of lifestyle modifications and nasal continuous positive airway pressure (CPAP).

CASE 24-2

A 29-year-old woman presents following an automobile accident in which she fell asleep at the wheel. She notes that she frequently falls asleep during the day and feels rested after these episodes.

1. **What are the considerations in the differential diagnosis?**
Sleep deprivation, primary hypersomnia, narcolepsy, sleep apnea, substance abuse or withdrawal, hypothyroidism, and anemia are considerations.
In addition, she states that sometimes she awakens but is utterly "unable to move a muscle." She states she has always been able to fall asleep quickly. She denies any use of drugs or

medications. You excuse yourself to answer a page and find her asleep when you return to your office. On awakening she is startled at first but then seems to regain her orientation and asks, "What is wrong with me?"

2. **What is the likely diagnosis and what would be the expected electroencephalographic findings?**
   This patient has *narcolepsy.* The electroencephalogram (EEG) in a sleep study would likely show a decreased REM latency, meaning she rapidly progresses into REM sleep. This accounts for the restfulness these patients feel upon falling asleep.
   Note: Patients with primary hypersomnia have a completely normal sleep architecture.

3. **Which treatment is available for patients with narcolepsy?**
   A regimen of a regular schedule of forced naps during the day can be a successful treatment for some patients. In severe cases of narcolepsy, amphetamines such as methylphenidate (Ritalin) are also used in the treatment of narcolepsy. These agents cause the release of norepinephrine, dopamine, and serotonin, but all have some abuse potential. A newer agent, modafinil, has been added that has lower abuse liability. Modafinil appears to selectively decrease somnolence in narcoleptic patients; however, the mechanism of action is unknown.

4. **What are the stages of sleep and what happens physiologically in these stages?**
   Sleep is divided into non-REM (NREM) and REM sleep. NREM sleep is divided into four stages, each being a deeper sleep. The stages are further described as fast wave or slow wave sleep. The earliest two stages are fast wave sleep and stages 3 and 4 are termed slow wave sleep based on the EEG appearance of brain waves. REM refers to rapid conjugate eye movement. As a person falls asleep, he passes through stages 1 to 4 and then enters REM sleep the first time, normally after approximately 90 minutes. The first REM episode lasts typically less than 10 minutes, and then the person cycles through the stages again, with further REM episodes of about 15 to 40 minutes each.
   Physiologically, during NREM sleep, a person's pulse, respiration rate, and blood pressure are decreased and show less minute-to-minute variation. Resting muscle tone is relaxed somewhat, and there are episodic body movements during NREM sleep. Males do not experience erection, and blood flow, including cerebral circulation, is somewhat lower. By contrast, REM sleep is characterized by higher pulse rate, respiratory rate, and blood pressure; EEG patterns are similar to those of one who is awake. REM sleep is also termed paradoxical sleep because of its similarities on EEG to a person who is awake. Men will experience partial or full erection. Additionally, a person in REM sleep experiences near total skeletal muscle paralysis, and movement is quite rare. Abstract and surreal dreams occur during this phase of sleep. Most REM sleep occurs in the last one third of the night.

5. **In Table 24-1, cover the columns to the right, and for each stage of sleep listed in the left column, name the EEG appearance and describe the frequency and voltage of the waves seen:**

TABLE 24-1. ELECTROENCEPHALOGRAPHIC (EEG) CHARACTERISTICS OF SLEEP STAGES

State	EEG Appearance	Frequency	Voltage
Awake	β waves	Random fast waves	Low
Eyes closed	α waves	8-12 cycles/sec	Low
Stage 1	θ waves	3-7 cycles/sec	Low

Continued

TABLE 24-1. ELECTROENCEPHALOGRAPHIC (EEG) CHARACTERISTICS OF SLEEP STAGES—continued

State	EEG Appearance	Frequency	Voltage
Stage 2	Sleep spindles	12-14 cycles/sec	Low
	K complexes	Slow, triphasic waves	High
Stage 3	δ waves	0.5-2.5 cycles/sec	High
Stage 4			
REM sleep	β waves	Random fast waves	Low

REM, rapid eye movement.

6. **How do nightmares differ from night terrors?**
   Nightmares occur almost exclusively in REM sleep. Patients who experience nightmares are able to recall the events of these frightening events, which usually involve threat to life, security, or self-esteem. Upon awakening, the person rapidly becomes oriented. *Night terrors* occur in deep NREM sleep (stages 3 and 4). Often, the person wakes with a panicky scream. These patients are often unresponsive upon awakening, have amnesia for the episode, and show signs of autonomic arousal, such as tachycardia, tachypnea, and diaphoresis. Night terrors can be treated with benzodiazepines.

7. **An 82-year-old woman complains that her sleep patterns have changed as she has aged. What changes in sleep are typical as people age?**
   Though this is somewhat controversial, for the purpose of boards you should assume that as people age, they experience a decrease in the amount of time in slow wave sleep (stages 3 and 4) and REM sleep. This typically results in a reduced need for time spent sleeping. Insomnia is common in the elderly population.

8. **This woman had been given a benzodiazepine to assist her sleep, which improved for a while, but now she complains of poor sleep once more. Why have her sleep problems returned?**
   She is experiencing tolerance to the effects of her medication. Benzodiazepines may be used for short-term management of insomnia, especially when there is an identifiable precipitant, but not for long-term management, because tolerance and dependence may result. Reevaluation should follow a 7- to 10-day trial of a benzodiazepine, and other agents should be considered.

9. **How do benzodiazepines manifest their pharmacologic effect?**
   Benzodiazepines are agonists of γ-aminobutyric acid (GABA) receptors, which are bound to chloride channels. GABA is the primary inhibitory neurotransmitter in the central nervous system (CNS). This CNS inhibition leads to decreased alertness, drowsiness, and less agitation.

10. **Why would this be another reason benzodiazepines should be avoided in the elderly population?**
    The aged population has a markedly increased (about 25%) incidence of falls when given these types of medications, due to drowsiness and impaired balance. This effect would be especially concerning in this elderly postmenopausal woman, who may have underlying osteopenia or frank osteoporosis. Additionally, the geriatric population is more sensitive to this effect and should be started on a lower dose initially.

11. There are now a number of drugs other than benzodiazopines that also act on the γ-aminobutyric acid benzodiazepine receptor and that reach hypnotic effects with less tolerance and less daytime sedation. What are some examples of these?

    Zaleplon, zolpidem, and eszopiclone are examples of these drugs.

    Note: Sedating antidepressants such as trazodone and nefazodone (remember the zzzzzzzz group) may also be used.

12. When evaluating a person for sleep problems, perhaps the first and most important step is to make sure that the patient has good sleep hygiene. What does good sleep hygiene entail?

    - No alcohol
    - No caffeine or nicotine
    - Regular exercise (but not too late in the day)
    - Relaxing activity before bed (e.g., bath, reading)
    - Only sleep and sex in the bedroom (no TV)
    - No clockwatching
    - No daytime naps
    - No late meals

SUMMARY BOX: SLEEP DISTURBANCE

- Narcolepsy: daytime sleepiness, sleep attacks, decreased rapid eye movement (REM) latency, rested after sleep

- Primary hypersomnia: excessive somnolence (>1 month), normal sleep architecture

- Treatment for narcolepsy and primary hypersomnia: methylphenidate or modafinil

- Insomnia: difficulty initiating or maintaining sleep

- Nonbenzodiazepines acting at the benzodiazepine γ-aminobutyric acid (GABA) receptor may be the best treatment for insomnia because they allow for hypnotic effects with less tolerance and less daytime sedation.

CASE 24-3

An 80-year-old man with severe pulmonary disease requires a lung transplant. Soon after the surgery, the patient develops respiratory failure, which requires him to receive mechanical ventilation. When the patient's family asks the doctor how long the patient will require ventilation, the physician responds that he is unsure, but that it is likely to be maintained for an extended period of time. The patient's wife expresses to you that her husband has told her many times that he would not wish to be kept alive on mechanical ventilation. At this moment the patient's oldest son, who currently supports his parents, demands that his father be kept on mechanical ventilation until an alternative solution can be found.

1. What should the physician do?

   The physician should terminate mechanical ventilation, according to the patient's own wishes.

2. What are advance directives?

   Advance directives are instructions provided by a patient in anticipation of the need for a decision to be made regarding his own medical care. They can be oral, written (e.g., living will), or in the form of a durable power of attorney. A durable power of attorney is responsibility assigned to a person by the patient to make medical decisions on his or her behalf in the event that he/she loses the capacity to do so. Statements made to others by the patient can qualify as oral advance directives. They gain more validity if they were repeated, heard by multiple persons, and recent. Although oral advance directives provide more flexibility than written directives, problems may arise from inaccurate communication of the patient's wishes or deviations in interpretation.

3. **How is competence (decision-making capacity) defined?**
The patient must be informed (provided with adequate insight regarding all options), able to make and communicate a stable choice, and free from the influence of others. The decision cannot result from delusions or hallucinations.

4. **What is substituted judgment?**
If a medical decision must be made on behalf of an incompetent patient who does not have any advance directives in place, the rule of substituted judgment can be used. The physician and the patient's family members can make a decision for the patient based on *what they would expect that the patient would have wanted*. The personal wishes of the physician or family members should not affect this decision.

SUMMARY BOX: ADVANCED DIRECTIVES

- A patient is considered to be competent if he/she is informed, able to make and communicate a stable decision, and is free from the influence of delusions, hallucinations, or other individuals.

- Advanced directives can be written, oral, or in the form of a durable power of attorney.

- Substituted judgment can be applied whenever an incompetent patient does not have any advanced directives in place. In this circumstance, the physician and the patient's family can make a decision on behalf of the patient according to what they expect the patient would have wanted.

CASE 24-4

A 15-year-old girl comes into your office asking for birth control. She admits that her parents do not know that she is sexually active, and she implores you not tell them.

1. **What should you do?**
Write the prescription and agree not to tell her parents but discuss the risks and benefits of using oral contraceptives with the patient. You should also encourage the patient to communicate with her parents.

2. **What are the rules regarding parental consent for minors?**
Parental consent is required for minors under the age of 18, unless the minor is emancipated (married, self-supporting, or in the military). There are, however, several situations in which parental consent is not required. These situations include emergencies, prescription of oral contraceptives, pregnancy-related medical care, and treatment of sexually transmitted diseases (STDs) or drug problems.

SUMMARY BOX: CONSENT FOR MINORS

- Parental consent must be obtained unless the minor is emancipated.

- Exceptions to this rule include emergency situations, drug abuse, pregnancy-related medical care, prescription of oral contraceptives, or treatment of sexually transmitted diseases (STDs).

CASE 24-5

A patient comes into your office with depressive symptoms. You work with her over the next few months to treat her for her depression. During a follow-up visit, she expresses her gratitude for your devotion and assistance and says she would like to make it up to you by taking you out to dinner. She winks, and you understand that she intends it to be a date. Although you do not admit it to her, you find that you are indeed attracted to her as well.

1. **What do you do?**
   It is *never* acceptable for you to have a romantic relationship with your patients. You should politely decline her invitation and continue to see her as your patient. It is not necessary to refer her to another physician if you can continue to be professional, but it would be a good idea to invite a chaperone into the office.

2. **Is it a good idea for you to be honest and tell her that you cannot have a relationship with her while she is your patient?**
   No. This would send the message that if your professional relationship were terminated, you would be willing to pursue a personal relationship with her.

STEP 1 SECRET

Whenever the USMLE asks you what to do in a situation similar to the one in Case 24-5, they will often try to entice you with an answer choice that suggests you refer the patient to another physician. For the purpose of boards, this will almost *never* be correct. The correct choice will require you to be an active participant in the solution.

SUMMARY BOX: THE PHYSICIAN-PATIENT RELATIONSHIP

- The physician-patient relationship should never extend beyond professional boundaries. Under no circumstances is it acceptable to pursue a romantic relationship with a patient.

- In the instance that a patient breaches this boundary, your best course of action is to continue to see the patient but to clarify the professional nature of your relationship. It is not necessary to refer the patient to another physician, but you may want to bring a chaperone into the office during future appointments with this patient.

CASE 24-6

A patient confides to you that he has been cheating on his wife and now suspects that he may be infected with human immunodeficiency virus (HIV). You perform the appropriate tests, which all turn out to be positive. You tell the patient that you will treat him for HIV, but that it is his responsibility to tell his partner. He immediately breaks down and tells you that he cannot tell his wife and all other sexual partners because his wife will leave him once she finds out that he acquired HIV while cheating on her.

1. **What do you do?**
   Patients who are HIV-positive have a duty to protect their sexual partners from acquiring the infection. If the patient fails to do so, the physician is legally allowed to inform the patient's partner.

2. **Under what other conditions is it acceptable to violate patient confidentiality?**
   Patient confidentiality should be maintained unless the patient is at significant risk for suicide or poses a risk to another individual. The physician can also intervene in the instance of child or elder abuse.
   Note: The *Tarasoff* decision provides physicians with the legal ability to warn a targeted victim and notify the appropriate officials if a patient poses significant risk to another individual.

SUMMARY BOX: PATIENT CONFIDENTIALITY

- Patient confidentiality should be maintained unless a patient is at risk for suicide or harming another individual.

- It is the responsibility of the patient to warn any sexual partners if he/she acquires a life-threatening sexually transmitted infection such as human immunodeficiency virus (HIV). If the patient fails to protect his/her sexual partners from acquiring the infection, the physician is entitled to inform them directly.

CASE 24-7

A 70-year-old obese man with a history of congestive heart failure and newly diagnosed depression comes into your office because he can no longer sustain an erection. He seems upset, because this is greatly affecting his sex life. He admits that he is too embarrassed to discuss this problem with his wife.

1. **What is the differential diagnosis for this patient's sexual dysfunction?**
   Drug effects (beta blockers, selective serotonin reuptake inhibitors [SSRIs], ethanol), diseases (atherosclerosis, depression, diabetes, decreases in testosterone levels), and psychological effects (e.g., performance anxiety) can lead to sexual dysfunction.
   Given this man's history of congestive heart failure, it is likely that he has been taking beta blockers for some time. He was also newly diagnosed with depression and may have been given an SSRI. Side effects of both of these drugs include sexual dysfunction. This man's age and obesity put him at risk for atherosclerosis and diabetes, which can also contribute to sexual dysfunction. Performance anxiety must be included in the differential diagnosis, particularly if he can sustain erections at certain times of the day (e.g., in the absence of his partner). As the physician, you should include this question in your medical history taking.

2. **What changes occur in the elderly with regard to sexual health?**
Men are slower to achieve erections and ejaculation and have longer refractory periods. After menopause, women experience vaginal dryness and irritation. Unless patients are on particular medications, libido does *not* decrease. Never assume that your elderly patients are not interested in sex. If you do not include sexual health in your history and physical examination, they may be too timid to bring up their concerns on their own!

SUMMARY BOX: SEXUAL HEALTH IN THE ELDERLY

- Elderly men may be slower to achieve erections/ejaculation and may experience increased refractory time.

- Postmenopausal women may experience vaginal dryness and irritation.

- For the purpose of boards, sexual interest does not decrease in the elderly.

- Sexual dysfunction may be attributed to drug effects, disease, or psychological effects.

CASE 24-8

A 24-year-old patient comes into your office with flu-like symptoms. You suspect a viral infection and tell the patient to rest and take plenty of fluids. He becomes irritated with this advice and demands that you prescribe him antibiotics so that he can get over his sickness before his vacation the following week. You hesitate because you know that antibiotics would be of no benefit to the course of this patient's illness.

1. **What should you do?**
Ask the patient why he feels he needs the antibiotics, and politely explain why you feel that it is unnecessary to prescribe them. The patient may become argumentative, and you should do your best to avoid conflict but always keep in mind that it is your decision whether or not to prescribe medication to a patient. Avoid writing unnecessary prescriptions.

SUMMARY BOX: PATIENT-REQUESTED PRESCRIPTIONS

- Avoid writing a prescription for a patient if you as the physician do not consider the medication to be an appropriate treatment.

CASE 24-9

You are working alongside a second-year resident during your inpatient medicine rotation. Over the past 2 weeks, you have noticed abrupt changes in the resident's dress and behavior. He often arrives to work late and ungroomed. You have also noticed that his breath frequently smells like alcohol. You suspect that he has been drinking heavily before and after work to take the edge off his day.

1. **What do you do?**
   It is your responsibility to protect patients from receiving inadequate or negligent care from an impaired or incompetent medical professional. You should inform the attending physician in charge of the resident of your suspicions. Do not attempt to confront the resident yourself. In this situation it is better to leave the attending in charge of getting the resident the help that he may need.

2. **What is the CAGE questionnaire?**
   The CAGE questionnaire is a widely used method for screening for alcohol abuse. You are expected to know this acronym for boards. If a patient responds with "yes" to more than one of the following questions, the patient should be examined further for alcoholism.
   - Have you ever felt like you should **C**ut down on your drinking?
   - Are you ever **A**nnoyed by people criticizing you for drinking?
   - Have you ever felt **G**uilty because of your drinking?
   - Have you ever needed a drink first thing in the morning (**E**ye-opener) to get out of bed or start your day?

SUMMARY BOX: ALCOHOL ABUSE

- It is your responsibility to protect patients from receiving care from any medical professional who is under the influence of alcohol or drugs.

- If you suspect that a colleague has been abusing drugs or alcohol, inform that person's immediate supervisor (resident in the case of a medical student, attending physician in the case of a resident).

- The CAGE questionnaire is often used as a screening tool for alcoholism. You should know the components of this acronym (see text).

CASE 24-10

A mother brings her 2-year-old child to the pediatrician's office for a well-child visit. She is concerned that her child still does not speak in full sentences. She also says that despite numerous attempts, she has been unable to toilet-train her child even though her neighbor's 2-year-old child has had success.

1. **Is this child developing normally?**
   Yes. You should know the developmental milestones listed in Table 24-2.

2. **What should you tell this concerned parent?**
   The mother should be told that every child develops differently, but that her child is on track for normal development. Do not automatically dismiss the mother's concerns; be sure that she feels comfortable coming to you if she notices "anything else that she considers unusual."

SUMMARY BOX: DEVELOPMENTAL MILESTONES

- You should know the information listed in Table 24-2. This is a high-yield topic for boards.

TABLE 24-2.   DEVELOPMENTAL MILESTONES

Age	Gross Motor	Fine Motor	Language	Other
Birth-3 months	Rolls over (3 months)	Rooting reflex	—	Orients to voice
3-6 months	Sits up (6 months)	Puts hands together (3 months)	Strings syllables together	Social smile
		Passes items (6 months)		Moro reflex disappears
6-9 months	Crawls	—	—	Feeds self
				Stranger anxiety
12 months	Walks	Stacks 3 blocks	Speaks 1-3 words	Drinks from a cup
15 months	Runs	—	Speaks 6 words	Babinski reflex disappears
	Walks backward			Separation anxiety
18 months	Climbs stairs	Stacks 4 blocks	Combines words	Brushes teeth with help
	Kicks ball			
2 years	Jumps (upward)	Stacks 6 blocks	Uses 2-word sentences	Washes hands
3 years	Jumps (forward)	Stacks 9 blocks	Completely understandable	Brushes teeth
	Rides tricycle	Draws circles and dashes		Plays board games
				Toilet training
				Develops gender identity
4 years	Hops on one foot	Copies stick figure	—	Dresses self
				Plays cooperatively and with imaginary friends
5 years	—	Draws squares and triangles	—	Identifies colors
		Ties shoes		Counts to 5

CASE 24-11

A 24-year-old patient with type 1 diabetes is admitted to the hospital after an insulin overdose that resulted in hypoglycemic seizures. You go in to see the patient once she is stabilized. You ask her whether she uses her insulin regularly, and she tells you that she gives herself injections twice a day according to the doctor's instructions. When you ask her how much insulin she injects, she shrugs and tells you that it varies, depending on the food she eats. You ask her to clarify, and she tells you, *"I give myself less if I skip meals and more whenever I eat junk food."*

1. **How should you handle this situation?**

   This is a clear example of a noncompliant patient who is not properly following the instructions of her treatment plan. Not only is this patient administering her insulin incorrectly, but she is not adhering to a proper diabetic diet. The most important thing to remember when dealing with a noncompliant patient is that scolding will be ineffective in preventing future mishaps (and will never be the correct answer on boards!). Instead, you must have a discussion with the patient to figure out the reason for the noncompliance and work together to fix the problem.

   Note: In severe cases, patients may be dismissed by a physician for noncompliance. For the purpose of boards, this is not likely to be the correct answer.

2. **How can compliance be increased in the future?**

   As mentioned previously, it is crucial to determine the reason for the patient's noncompliance. Therefore, it is important to figure out whether this patient is neglecting the physician's instructions because (a) she does not understand them, (b) it is difficult for her to adhere to them, or (c) she does not know the importance of following them. If you get the feeling that a patient does not understand the directions, do your best not to embarrass the patient. Instead, tell the patient that this could happen to anyone and simplify your instructions. Have the patient repeat the instructions back to you when you are done so that you know she has understood correctly. Write the instructions down whenever possible. This is especially important to consider whenever the patient is not a native English speaker.

   Sometimes, it is difficult for a patient to adhere to the treatment plan. Insulin, for example, must be refrigerated. Consider a scenario in which a diabetic travels a lot for work and does not always have access to a refrigerator. He or she might skip insulin dosages frequently. Once again, simplify the treatment regimen whenever possible.

   It is also a good idea to make sure that the patient understands why it is important to follow a specified treatment plan. Perhaps this patient does not understand why junk food is especially harmful to a diabetic, or why skipping meals can lead to hypoglycemia. Perhaps she does not understand the reason behind regulated insulin doses. Educating the patient will most likely motivate her to follow the treatment plan correctly.

   Do not attempt to scare the patient into complying with a treatment plan. (For example, it is unethical to show the patient graphic pictures of gangrene and say, "This will happen to you if you don't shape up!")

SUMMARY BOX: THE NONCOMPLIANT PATIENT

- Nonadherence is a common hurdle faced by all physicians.

- Patients should not be scolded for their noncompliance. It is more important to determine the reason for the noncompliance and attempt to fix the problem.

- Never use scare tactics in an attempt to improve a patient's compliance.

CASE 24-12

A 68-year-old man is brought to your office by his wife because of abdominal pain, jaundice, and unintentional weight loss. A computed tomography (CT) scan of the abdomen reveals adenocarcinoma of the head of the pancreas. When you walk into the office to break the news to the patient, his wife asks to speak to you alone outside. The two of you step out of the office and she confesses that she has a feeling you are returning with bad news. "Please tell me first," she begs. "If it's really bad I know my husband won't be able to handle it. If I know what it is, I can help break the news to him in time."

1. **How should you handle this situation with the patient's wife?**
    It is unlawful to disclose a patient's medical information to family or friends without the permission of the patient. Therefore, you should avoid revealing any information to the patient's wife at this time. You should, however, find out why the patient's wife is so concerned about her husband's ability to handle the news. Her concerns will perhaps guide your approach to handling this patient.

2. **What should you say to the patient when you walk into the room?**
    You should tell the patient that you have some news to discuss with him and politely dismiss his wife for the time being. At this point, you can ask the patient whether he would like his wife to be present. If he agrees, you can invite her back into the room. Asking the patient's permission for his wife to remain in the room in her presence might pressure his decision.

SUMMARY BOX: DISCLOSURE OF PATIENT INFORMATION

-   It is unlawful to disclose any patient information to family or friends without explicit permission from the patient.

-   Always ask to speak to a patient privately before discussing confidential medical information in front of others.

CASE 24-13

A 45-year-old patient comes into your office with his wife and complains that he has been experiencing a frequent sensation of his "legs falling asleep." His discomfort causes an urge to constantly move his limbs because he feels much better when he is active. His wife testifies that her husband continually jerks his legs in his sleep. This activity disrupts both his and her sleep patterns, and both profess feeling tired throughout the day.

1. **What is the most likely diagnosis?**
    Restless legs syndrome (RLS) is a disorder of unknown etiology that causes a constant urge to move in attempt to relieve unpleasant sensations in the lower limbs. It has been linked to several conditions, including Parkinson's disease, rheumatoid arthritis, diabetes, kidney failure, and iron deficiency anemia. Use of certain medications may also trigger RLS. However, RLS can be idiopathic in nature.

2. **What are the most common symptoms of restless legs syndrome?**
Symptoms include an unpleasant sensation in the legs, urge to constantly move, relief upon movement, and worsening of symptoms when inactive. Typical leg movements associated with RLS are jiggling, pacing, tossing, rubbing, and stretching. Limb movements often occur during sleep.

3. **How is restless legs syndrome treated?**
Although there is no direct cure for RLS, the treatment plan involves correcting the underlying cause of the condition whenever possible. Treatment also focuses on symptom relief, and includes sleep improvement, alcohol avoidance (alcohol may trigger RLS symptoms), walking, and heat/cold packs on the affected limbs.

SUMMARY BOX: RESTLESS LEGS SYNDROME

- Restless legs syndrome (RLS) is associated with a constant urge to move in response to an unpleasant sensation in the legs.

- There is no direct treatment for RLS. Focus on treating the underlying cause of the disease and providing patients with symptom relief.

CHAPTER 25

BIOSTATISTICS

Thomas A. Brown, MD, and Sonali J. Shah

INSIDER'S GUIDE TO BIOSTATISTICS FOR THE USMLE STEP 1

Like behavioral sciences, biostatistics is a subject that most medical students do not spend nearly enough time studying because it appears to be "common sense." Unfortunately, students often miss a lot of straightforward biostatistics questions because of lack of practice. Biostatistics is one of the highest-yield boards subjects and an easy way to earn points on your exam if you take the time to understand the concepts. This chapter introduces you to the types of questions you are likely to see on your exam and prepares you to solve them in the most efficient manner possible.

Note that you will be given a whiteboard to use during your exam prior to the start of your test. You may take up to 5 minutes before you begin your exam to write anything you would like on your whiteboard. Throughout the chapter, the formulas that students find most helpful to add to their whiteboard are highlighted. It would be a good idea to review these formulas and the information you plan to include on your whiteboard the day before your exam.

BASIC CONCEPTS

TEST CHARACTERISTICS

1. **What does the sensitivity of a diagnostic test measure?**

   Sensitivity is a measure of how effectively a diagnostic test can detect the disease in a patient who truly has the disease (true positive). In other words, sensitivity measures the proportion of individuals with a disease who test positive for it.

   Sensitivity can be calculated by dividing the number of true positives by the total number of people tested with the disease: true positives/(true positives + false negatives), or $a/(a+c)$ in the 2×2 table (Table 25-1). You can also calculate sensitivity by subtracting the false negative rate from 1 (i.e., sensitivity $= 1 -$ false negative rate); however, you will seldom be given the false negative rate on boards.

TABLE 25-1. SAMPLE 2×2 TABLE			
		Presence of Disease	
		+	**−**
Test Result	**+**	True positives (a)	False positives (b)
	−	False negatives (c)	True negatives (d)

STEP 1 SECRET

Practice setting up these tables whenever you encounter a biostatistics problem that involves sensitivity or specificity. They will help you immensely on the USMLE. It might also be helpful to copy this table onto your whiteboard before the start of your exam.

2. **What does the specificity of a diagnostic test measure?**
   The *specificity* of a diagnostic test is a measure of how effectively the test can detect the absence of disease in a patient without the disease (true negative). It is an indication of how "specific" a positive test result is to the disease it is designed to detect. The greater the number of different conditions that cause a positive test result other than the disease the test is designed to detect, the less specific the test.
   Specificity can be calculated by dividing the number of true negatives by the total number of people tested who do not have the disease: true negatives/(true negatives + false positives), or $d/(b+d)$ in the 2×2 table). Specificity is also equal to $1 -$ false positive rate.

3. **Quick terminology review: Cover the right column in Table 25-2 and define each of the terms in the left column.**

TABLE 25-2.	BASIC TERMINOLOGY
Term	**Definition**
True positive	A positive test result in someone who truly has the disease
False positive	A positive test result in someone who truly does not have the disease
True negative	A negative test result in someone who truly does not have the disease
False negative	A negative test result in someone who truly does have the disease

4. **How does the sensitivity of a test relate to its specificity?**
   Sensitivity and specificity move in opposite directions as test parameters change. In other words, as sensitivity increases, specificity decreases, and vice versa. This occurs because, in order to improve the sensitivity of a test (i.e., detect more people with a disease of interest), the limits on what results are considered to be positive must be made less stringent. In detecting more people with the disease, the test will therefore also yield positive results in more people without the disease.
   For example, the rheumatoid factor (RF) is often used to aid in the diagnosis of rheumatoid arthritis (RA). RF is positive in 70% of patients with RA. If you want to catch more cases of patients with RA, you can use the erythrocyte sedimentation rate (ESR). The ESR is positive in 90% of patients with RA. However, with this increased sensitivity comes decreased specificity. ESR is very nonspecific and can be positive in any inflammatory process, from pneumonia to temporal arteritis. Given its high sensitivity, a negative ESR is helpful in ruling out inflammatory disease (see later discussion).
   SPIN and SNOUT are useful mnemonics. SPIN tells us that specific tests rule in disease. That is, the more specific a test, the more likely it is that a positive result indicates real disease. SNOUT tells us that sensitive tests rule out disease. That is, the more sensitive a test, the more likely that a negative result rules out disease. In serious diseases that can be treated effectively if detected, a greater sensitivity is desired (often at the expense of specificity).
   SPIN: **SP**ecific tests rule **IN**
   SNOUT: **S**e**N**sitive tests rule **OUT**

5. **What information is given by the relative risk?**

   The *relative risk* (RR) is a ratio that compares event rates in one group versus another. It can be calculated by dividing the probability of occurrence of disease (incidence) in the exposed group by the probability of occurrence of disease in the unexposed group.

   For example, in the 2×2 table (Table 25-3), the probability of lung cancer in smokers is 90/100 or .90. The probability of lung cancer in nonsmokers is 10/100, or .10. Therefore, the RR for smoking is .90/.10, or 9. An RR of 9 implies that smokers are 9 times more likely to get lung cancer than nonsmokers.

   An RR of >1 means that the event is more likely to occur in the exposed group. An RR of <1 means the event is less likely to occur in the unexposed group. An RR of 1 means that there is no difference between the groups.

TABLE 25-3. SMOKING EXPOSURE AND LUNG CANCER

		Lung Cancer	
		+	−
Smoking Exposure	+	90	10
	−	10	90

6. **What information is given by the odds ratio?**

   The *odds ratio* (OR) also compares event rates between two groups but is calculated by comparing odds rather than probabilities.

   For the preceding example, the OR can be calculated by dividing the odds of smokers' developing lung cancer (90:10) by the odds of nonsmokers' developing lung cancer (10:90), as follows:

   $$OR = \frac{90/10}{10/90} = \frac{90 \times 90}{10 \times 10} = \frac{9}{1}$$

   As with RR, an OR of 1 means the event was equally likely in both groups, an OR of >1 means the event was more likely to occur in the exposed group, and an OR of <1 means the event was more likely to occur in the unexposed group.

   You must know that RR and ORs are used for different types of tests. RR is used for cohort studies and randomized controlled trials (study types that measure risk of outcome based on exposure status) because those studies allow for calculation of the percentages of participants that are affected. ORs are usually used in case-control studies, which approximate odds of exposure based on rates of outcome occurrence in which percentages cannot be calculated. You will read more about types of tests later in this chapter.

   The RR and ORs for one study may be drastically different (as in the preceding example) for common events but approximate each other for rare events.

7. **What is the difference between probability and odds and how are they measured?**

   Probability is measured along a continuum from 0 to 1, where 0 means the event is certain not to happen and 1 means the event is certain to happen.

   Odds are measured along a continuum from 0 to infinity.

   Probabilities can be easily converted to odds, and vice versa.

$$\text{Odds} = \text{Probability}/1 - \text{Probability}$$

and

$$\text{Probability} = \text{Odds}/1 + \text{Odds}$$

If the pretest probability of a certain diagnosis is 90%, then the odds are $.9/1 - .9 = 9$ (sometimes stated as "9 to 1").

8. **What is the positive predictive value? negative predictive value?**

   The *positive predictive value* (PPV) is the probability that, given a positive test result, the disease in question is actually present. The *negative predictive value* (NPV) is the probability that disease is absent if there is a negative test result. If a 2×2 table is provided, the PPV can be calculated by dividing the number of true positives by the total number of positive test results ($a/a + b$) and the NPV can be calculated by dividing the number of true negatives by the total number of negative test results ($d/c + d$) (Table 25-4).

   Because a 2×2 table is not normally provided, the PPV can also be calculated if the sensitivity and specificity of the test and the prevalence of the disease being tested are known, as discussed later.

   What happens to the positive and negative predictive values as disease incidence changes? This is the type of question you might see on boards— is the reason why setting up the 2×2 table can be so helpful. If disease incidence increases, the numbers in the left column (true positives [TP] and false negatives [FN]) will both increase. Because $PPV = TP/(TP + FP)$, PPV will increase if the number of TP increase. NPV, on the other hand, will decrease as incidence increases because FN increase in value. Recall that $NPV = TN/(TN + FN)$, where $TN =$ true negatives.

TABLE 25-4. CALCULATING PREDICTIVE VALUES USING THE 2×2 TABLE			
		Presence of Disease	
		+	**−**
Test Result	**+**	True positives (a)	False positives (b)
	−	False negatives (c)	True negatives (d)

9. **What is the positive likelihood ratio?**

   The positive likelihood ratio (PLR) reflects how much a positive test result increases the probability of disease being present. The higher the ratio, the more likely it is that disease is present. This ratio is calculated as the sensitivity divided by $1 -$ specificity. For example, if the sensitivity is 85% and the specificity is 90%, the PLR is $0.85/(1 - 0.9) = 8.5$. Consequently, the more sensitive and specific the test is, the higher the PLR. The PLR is now widely used in evidence-based medicine because of the ease with which it can be used to calculate the PPV of a test.

10. **How is the positive likelihood ratio used to calculate the positive predictive value?**

    This is done by converting the prevalence of a disease to an odds ratio (e.g., 20% to 1:4) and then multiplying the first part of the ratio by the PLR ($8.5 \times 1:4 = 8.5:4$). Then the ratio is converted back to a percentage: $8.5/(8.5 + 4) = 0.68$ or 68%.

    $$\text{Posttest probability} = \text{Pretest probability} \times \text{PLR}$$

Let's assume the pretest probability of coronary artery disease in a 40-year-old man with diabetes who smokes is 20% and that the presence of a "positive" exercise stress test has a PLR of 10.

Expressed in odds, 20% is 1:4, so the PPV of the exercise stress test is calculated as follows:

$$10 \times 1:4 = 10:4, \text{ or } 5:2$$

$$5/(5+2) = 5/7 = .71, \text{ or } 71\%$$

So the probability that this man has coronary artery disease if he has a positive stress test is 71%, which is substantially up from his pretest probability of 20%.

11. **What is meant by the reliability of a test?**
Reliability (precision) is the consistency or repeatability of a test. A test is reliable if it produces the same results each time when the conditions are the same. For example, the SAT exam would be considered reliable if a student could take it more than once and get close to the same score each time. It would not be considered a reliable test if the same student received dramatically different scores on two different days. Precision is improved by reduction in random error. Random error is unpredictable and affects all measurements. It is used to describe any deviations from the true value of a measurement that result from fluctuations in the readings provided by the measurement tool.

12. **What is meant by the validity of a test?**
Validity (accuracy) is a measure of how well a test result corresponds to what it claims to measure. In other words, a test result is considered valid if it closely matches the actual value of whatever is being measured. Note that this actual value is usually estimated using the gold standard test method. Validity is generally reduced through systematic error. For example, an IQ test that depends in part on reading comprehension is invalid because IQ should not depend on literacy. This is a systematic error in designing or conducting the test. Systematic error refers to deviations from the true value of a measurement that result from poor instrument calibration or flawed observation methods.

13. **In statistical analyses of differences between groups, a *P* value is often included to reflect how significant the difference is. What is the meaning of this *P* value?**
At its most basic level, the *P* value reflects the probability that the difference observed between groups could occur by chance alone. For example, if the *P* value is 0.05, there is a 5% chance that the difference observed could have been entirely due to random chance, and not due to whatever intervention was used in the experiment. Nevertheless, most of modern science considers a difference "significant" if there is a <5% ($P < .05$) chance that the difference could have occurred by random chance. Obviously, the smaller the *P* value, the smaller the probability that any difference was due to chance, and with that, the more convincing it is that the intervention evaluated was responsible for the difference.

STEP 1 SECRET

P values are not as high-yield for Step 1 as some other biostatistics-related topics but will be very important for you to understand when interpreting scientific literature. On the other hand, type I and type II errors (see question 14) are commonly-tested boards topics.

14. **What are the differences between type I and type II error? How is power related to type II error?**
Type I (α) error refers to "false positive error." In other words, $\alpha =$ the probability of claiming that a true difference exists between two means when in reality none exists. The "null hypothesis"

(H_0) claims that there is no difference between two means. If a researcher claims a statistical difference between two groups when none exists and falsely rejects the null hypothesis, the researcher has committed a type I error.

By contrast, type II (β) error is "false negative error." It refers to the probability of stating that no difference exists between the means of two values when in fact there truly is a difference. Type II error is an acceptance of the null hypothesis when it should indeed be rejected.

Let's, for instance, say that we wish to determine the factors that influence the difference in the mean USMLE scores observed between two groups of medical students. We hypothesize that time spent studying for the USMLE could be significantly different between the two groups and may thus exhibit a causal relationship with the scores obtained by the students. We devise a method to measure this variable and do not find that this significantly differs between the two groups. If a difference truly exists, we have made a type II error in this case.

The term "statistical power" is a reflection of a study's ability to correctly detect a difference between means when one truly exists. *Power* is equal to $1 - \beta$. This makes good sense, right? Since β is the probability of committing a type II error (not detecting a difference that truly exists), power should inversely correlate with this value.

15. **What are some determinants that can be used to evaluate the existence of a causal relationship between two variables?**
    - Consistency (e.g., the more studies that support the hypothesis, the better)
    - Strength of correlation (e.g., the higher the RR, the better)
    - Biologic plausibility (e.g., colon cancer is unlikely to be caused by ultraviolet light exposure)
    - Temporality (cause must *precede* disease outcome)
    - Supportive experimental studies (e.g., animal studies)
    - Dose-response relationship (e.g., higher exposure leads to more severe phenotype)

16. **What is the difference between prevalence and incidence?**
    Prevalence is the percentage of the population that currently has the disease. For example, 25% of Americans are obese, so the prevalence of obesity is 25%. *Incidence* refers to how many people develop a disease *within a given time frame* (usually annually). Thus, if 300,000 people are newly diagnosed with diabetes each year, the annual incidence of diabetes is 300,000.

17. **How do the incidence and duration of a disease affect its prevalence?**
    The higher the incidence and the longer the duration of the disease, the greater the prevalence. Chronic diseases (e.g., arthritis) are unlikely to rapidly result in death, so their prevalence is high. Diseases that have a short duration (e.g., meningitis), either because they rapidly result in rapid death or because they resolve quickly, will have a low prevalence in the population. Incidence and prevalence are roughly equal in diseases that have a short duration.

MEASURES OF SPREAD

18. **The following sample distribution pattern lists the ages of 11 patients seen by a physician on a given day:**

    1, 2, 3, 3, 3, 4, 5, 5, 7, 8, 80

    A. What are the mean, median, and mode for the ages of the patients seen by the physician on this day?
    The *mean* is simply the average of the sample, which is calculated by adding together all of the results and then dividing by the number of results. In this example, the mean would be 11 (121/11 = 11). The *median* is the number in the middle of the data set when ordered sequentially.

Half of your data should lie above the median and half will lie below. In this example, the number 4 has equal numbers of subjects on either side. In cases in which there is an even number of results, the median is calculated by taking the average of the middle two numbers. The *mode* is the number present with the highest frequency. In this case, the mode is 3.

B. Is the mean or the median more representative of central tendency?

The median is less affected by outliers (e.g., 80) than the mean and is therefore a better representation of central tendency than the mean, particularly for small sample sizes containing multiple outliers. However, keep in mind that because the mean encompasses all individuals in a study, it has much more statistical power than either the median or the mode.

C. Is this sample "skewed" at all and if so, in which direction?

Yes, this sample population is positively skewed to the right because of the outlier value 80. In Figure 25-1, graph A represents a positive skew and graph B a negative skew. Positive skews occur when there are outliers that have a higher value than the numbers closer to the mean. Negative skews occur when the outliers have a lower value then the numbers close to the mean.

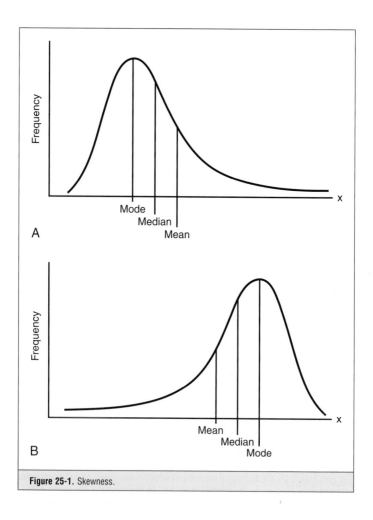

Figure 25-1. Skewness.

STEP 1 SECRET

You may be asked to interpret diagrams like those depicted in Figure 25-1 on boards. The easiest way to remember the difference between positively and negatively skewed data is to make up your own data set to match the figures shown in Figure 25-1A. We will refer to midline as the number along the *x*-axis of the curve that falls in the direct center of the data range. The curve is asymmetrical, with most of the data falling to the left of midline and the tail on the right. If the numbers that this data set represents range from 0 to 100 (midline is 50), this data set could plausibly consist of 20, 20, and 80. The mean of this data set is 40 and the median is 20. Thus, a positive skew has mean > median. The opposite will be true for negatively skewed data (Fig. 25-1B). Here, most of the data falls to the right of midline. This data set could consist of 20, 80, and 80. Here, mean is 60 and median is 80. Negatively skewed data will thus show median > mean. Recall that a normal (gaussian) statistical distribution will have mean = median = mode.

19. **What does the standard deviation of a population represent?**
    The *standard deviation* is a measure of how spread out a test population is. If most of the values are close to the mean, the standard deviation is small. However, if many of the values are far from the mean, the standard deviation is larger. You will not need to calculate the standard deviation, but understand that it is calculated by adding together the differences or "deviations" of each value from the mean and then taking the average of these deviations.

    By definition, if one takes all the members of a population within one standard deviation of the mean (both above and below), these members will constitute 68% of the total population. If two standard deviations from the mean are taken, these members will constitute 95% of the total population. Three standard deviations will contain 99.7% of the data set. However, this is true only if the population falls into a "*normal*" or "bell" curve. Figure 25-2 shows the distribution of a bell curve.

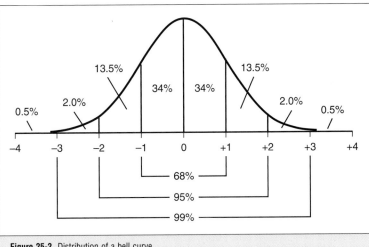

Figure 25-2. Distribution of a bell curve.

STEP 1 SECRET

You are expected to know the bell curve distribution for Step 1. Recall that the data are distributed evenly to both sides! Lots of students get confused by this concept on boards. If, for example, you are asked to calculate how much of the data fall out of the range of two standard deviations in a gaussian distribution, the answer is 5% because 95% of the data will fall within the range of two standard deviations. If you are asked to calculate how much of the data fall *above* two standard deviations, the answer is 2.5% (half of the 5% will fall above two standard deviations and half will fall below). As obvious as this may sound to you, pay close attention to the question being asked! It is easy to fall into these types of traps when you are under pressure on test day.

STUDY DESIGNS

20. **What is meant by the term "bias" and which study design best eliminates bias?**
Bias is *systematic error* that affects one study group more than the other. This differs from *random error*, which typically affects both groups equally and should not adversely affect the study if there are enough participants. Randomized clinical trials control most effectively for bias, whereas a case-control study controls least effectively for bias. Other types of study designs (e.g., cohort, cross-sectional) fall somewhere between these two extremes in their ability to eliminate bias (Table 25-5).

CASE 25-1

In the mid-1800s, London was plagued by recurrent outbreaks of cholera, which extracted a high death toll. Although the cause of these outbreaks was unknown, the prevailing hypothesis was that cholera was spread by "miasmus," a poisonous odor emitted from decaying organic material found in open graves, sewers, and swamps. The now-famous epidemiologist John Snow disagreed with the miasmus theory and postulated instead that cholera was spread by contaminated water. He believed this in part because the initial symptoms of cholera were intestinal in nature and he reasoned that an inhaled poisonous odor would not manifest symptoms in this way.

To study this hypothesis, he reviewed death certificates and plotted addresses for each person in whom the death certificate implied death from cholera infection. On a map of London, he then mapped out where these people had lived prior to their death and compared their location to those who died of causes unrelated to cholera infection. What he found was that the incidence of cholera was much higher in London residences that obtained their water supply from the water company.

1. **What sort of study design was this?**
This was a case-control study because participants were selected on the basis of either having or not having the disease of interest (cholera).

2. **How does a retrospective case-control study differ in design from a retrospective cohort study?**
These studies differ largely with respect to how subjects are classified and selected. In a case-control study, subjects are classified according to the presence or absence of disease. By contrast, in a retrospective cohort study, subjects are classified based on the presence or absence of exposure. Only then is disease status determined.

TABLE 25-5. STUDY DESIGNS

Study Design	Setup	Strengths	Limitations
Cohort study	A "cohort" of subjects is classified according to exposure and then followed to determine the effect of exposure on disease outcome.	■ Relatively easy to set up compared with randomized studies ■ Allows for the study of exposures that are known or suspected to be harmful ■ Establishes a causal relationship between exposure and outcome variables	■ *Confounding variables:* The exposure being studied may *correlate* with the disease outcome but may not be the *cause*. There may be other "confounding" variables that are more causative.
Case-control study	Subjects are classified according to the presence or absence of disease, and correlations are made between past exposures and the presence of disease.	■ Easiest to set up ■ Allows for the study of exposures that are known or suspected to be harmful	■ *Recall bias:* Participants may remember their exposures differently depending on the presence or absence of disease ■ *Interviewer bias:* Interviewers may assume that someone with a disease has been exposed ■ Does not allow for calculation of the relative risk or the percentages of those in the exposed versus unexposed groups who go on to develop disease ■ Confounding variables
Randomized study	Participants are randomly assigned to exposure groups and followed for the development of disease.	■ Provides evidence for cause, and not just correlation, because only one "exposure" is manipulated at a time	■ Costly and time-consuming ■ Cannot be used to study exposures that are known or suspected to be harmful

3. **What are the strengths of a case-control study?**

Case-control studies are relatively easy to set up because the researcher simply has to locate people who have been affected by a disease. Another strength is that case-control studies can be used to look at the effect of exposures that are known or suspected to be harmful. For example, a randomized study could not look at the effect of child abuse on the chances that someone will abuse his or her own children, because it would be unethical and illegal to randomize participants to be abused. However, with a case-control study, a researcher could look at child abusers as well as nonabusers and compare the incidence of abuse in their childhoods.

4. **What are the limitations of a case-control study?**

Although case-control studies are easy to design, they have a number of flaws. As mentioned, case-control studies simply uncover an association between two variables but do not establish a causal relationship. For example, if you did a case-control study and found that those with lung cancer have higher rates of alcoholism, you might conclude that alcoholism leads to lung cancer. However, alcoholics might be more likely than nonalcoholics to smoke cigarettes, and smoking could be the actual cause of their lung cancer.

Another flaw in case-control studies is "recall bias," which is the tendency of those with a disease to exaggerate their exposures and those without a disease to minimize their exposures. For example, a woman with a child who has been born with a birth defect might recall many more chest x-ray studies during her pregnancy than might a woman with healthy children. "Interviewer bias" is also an issue. This occurs when an interviewer assumes a person with the disease has been exposed to risk factors whereas the healthy person has not. For example, the interviewer might ask a person with lung cancer the question "How many packs per day did you smoke?" whereas a healthy person might be asked the question "You never smoked, did you?" Even though both questions ask for similar information, the sense of judgment imposed by the latter may deter the interviewee from providing accurate responses (Table 25-6).

TABLE 25-6.   STATISTICAL BIAS

Bias Type	Definition	Example
Selection bias	General term for nonrandom assignment of participants to various groups within a study	See Berkson's bias.
Berkson's bias	Selection bias performed on hospitalized patients	In studying duration of a disease in hospitalized patients, the subjects may have more severe symptoms or better access to care, which can alter disease course.
Recall bias	Data can be altered by a participant's memory of the tested variable	Administering a survey immediately after a specific incident or 10 years later may alter the accuracy of responses acquired from participants based on recollection of the event.

Continued

TABLE 25-6. STATISTICAL BIAS—continued

Bias Type	Definition	Example
Confounding bias	The effect of an independent variable on a dependent variable is distorted by a third, unmeasured variable	Studying genetic linkage of cancer incidence based on family history without controlling for age, race, gender, or other variables that may independently alter cancer risk may affect findings.
Hawthorne effect	Patients change their normal behavior once they know they are being studied	In using dietary recalls to examine normal fruit and vegetable intake in a population, study participants may change their normal intake of these foods if they know this is being measured.
Lead-time bias	Early detection of a disease is mistaken for increased survival	Diagnosis of breast cancer with a novel technology increases patient survival by 6 months; it is possible that the cancer is simply diagnosed at an earlier stage with the new technology and that disease course is completely unaltered.
Pygmalion effect	Study conclusions are influenced by the researcher's own belief in a specific hypothesis	In studying the effectiveness of using new surgical technology based on surgeon-reported data, if the surgeon believes in the efficacy of the technology, his report may be biased by his own belief.
Observer bias	Observer knows exposure status (not double-blinded)	Researcher reports a reduced incidence of depression in a group that he knows is currently placed on a new SSRI.
Procedure bias	Subjects in different study groups are not treated equally	In a weight loss study in which one group is placed on a diet pill and the second is placed on a placebo, the former group is trained more intensely than the latter; differences in exercise routines may account for some of the observed weight loss.

Continued

TABLE 25-6.   STATISTICAL BIAS—continued

Bias Type	Definition	Example
Sampling bias	Selecting participants who do not represent the makeup of the overall population, so that findings will not be generalizable	In studying factors that contribute to heart attack risk in an upper-middle-class suburban town, subjects may have financial and stress-related factors that do not match those present in the general population but nevertheless influence their risk for heart attack.
Late-look bias	Acquisition of data at an incorrect or inappropriate time	In a survey of patients to study the impact of lupus in a community, patients who have already died from lupus are unable to respond to the survey.

STEP 1 SECRET

Bias occurs when one outcome is favored over another due to systematic error. The various types of statistical bias are commonly tested on Step 1. You should know the types of bias defined in Table 25-6.

5. **What ratio can be used to compare event rates in a case-control study?**
   OR (know this!). Case-control studies cannot be used to calculate the RR of an exposure on the disease outcome or to define the percentage of people with a certain exposure that will go on to develop a disease. This is because the calculation of RR requires the incidence rate, which cannot be calculated from a case-control study because there is no follow-up time. ORs are used for case-control studies, and RR is used for cohort studies

6. **How is the odds ratio calculated?**
   The OR is calculated by dividing the odds of developing the disease for those in the exposed group versus the odds of developing the disease for those in the unexposed group. For example, if John Snow charted the water supply of 100 people who died of cholera and 100 people who died of other causes and found that 80 of the 100 people who died of cholera lived in homes supplied by the water company, but only 10 of the 100 people who died of other causes lived in homes supplied by the water company, then the OR would be calculated as follows:

$$OR = \frac{80/20}{10/90} = \frac{80 \times 90}{20 \times 10} = \frac{7200}{200} = 36$$

An OR > 1 implies that the disease is more likely to occur in the exposed group, so cholera occurred more often in those who received their water supply from the water company. This does not prove that the water was the source of the infection, because there may have been confounding variables that were the actual cause. For example, it may have been that those who lived in homes supplied by the water company were poorer than those who had their own wells, and therefore they had jobs where they were exposed to less sanitary conditions. These unsanitary working conditions, rather than the water in their homes, may have then exposed them to cholera.

SUMMARY BOX: CASE-CONTROL STUDIES

- In a case-control study, subjects are classified according to the presence or absence of disease.

- Strengths of case-control studies are that they are easy to set up and can be used to study exposures that are known or suspected to be harmful.

- Limitations of case-control studies are that they leave room for recall bias, interviewer bias, and confounding variables.

- Case-control studies cannot be used to define relative risk (RR) but can be used to calculate an odds ratio (OR).

CASE 25-2

Blood pressure is monitored regularly in a group of 500 adult men. The mean blood pressure for the group is reported as 130 ± 10 mm Hg, and the coefficient of variation (CV) is noted to be small. The blood pressure measurements within the group are described as having a "normal distribution."

1. **What does the expression "130±10 mm Hg" mean with respect to the distribution of blood pressure in this sample?**
   The "130 mm Hg" refers to the mean blood pressure of the sample, whereas the "10 mm Hg" refers to the standard deviation. A standard deviation of 10 mm Hg implies that 68% of the population had blood pressures within 10 mm Hg of the mean of 130 (i.e., between 120 mm Hg and 140 mm Hg). For 95% of the population of this study, the blood pressure is within two standard deviations of the mean, or within 110 mm Hg and 150 mm Hg. The top 2.5% of the population has a blood pressure above two standard deviations of the mean (>150 mm Hg) and the bottom 2.5% of the population has a blood pressure below two standard deviations of the mean (below 110 mm Hg).

2. **What does it mean when the blood pressure in this population is said to be "normally distributed"?**
   To be normally distributed means that if a plot of the magnitude of the variable being analyzed (in this case, blood pressure) against the frequency of each magnitude is made, the curve takes on a "bell-shaped" form that is well described by a specific mathematical equation, which can be used to accurately calculate the standard deviation. A normal curve (see Fig. 25-2) represents a population in which a majority of people have measurements close to the mean, and the farther from the mean, the fewer people have that measurement. Curves are often assumed to be normal for the sake of easy calculations, but some curves differ largely from a normal curve. For example, if you asked a group of people what temperature they like their coffee, most would say either very hot or very cold. Almost no one would say that they like lukewarm coffee. This study would produce a "bimodal" distribution (Fig. 25-3), with two "humps," which would not fit the normal curve.

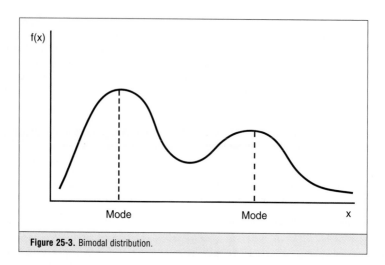

Figure 25-3. Bimodal distribution.

3. **What does a small coefficient of variation for the sample in the blood pressure study imply?**
   The CV is used to express the standard deviation as a percentage of the sample mean. This can be very informative. Standard deviation typically decreases with increasing sample size. For example, this study expresses blood pressure as 130 ± 10 mm Hg. In this study, the $CV = 10/130 \times 100 = 7.6\%$. Smaller sample sizes are associated with larger CVs. For example, if blood pressures were measured in 10 men as opposed to 500, one might get a value such as 130 ± 60 mm Hg. In this case, the CV would equal $60/130 \times 100 = 46\%$. A "good" study will usually have a $CV \le 10\%$.

4. **Quick review: What percentage of the men in this study had a blood pressure in the following ranges?**
   A. 120 and 140 mm Hg
      68%
   B. 110 and 150 mm Hg
      95%
   C. Above 150 mm Hg
      2.5%
   D. Below 110 mm Hg
      2.5%

SUMMARY BOX: NORMAL DISTRIBUTION, STANDARD DEVIATION, AND COEFFICIENT OF VARIATION ✓

- Standard deviation can be used to estimate the percentage of a population that falls into a certain range, as long as the population fits a normal distribution.

- Some populations do not fit the normal distribution.

- Coefficient of variation uses the standard deviation and the sample mean to create an even more informative way to look at the distribution of a population.

CASE 25-3

A 27-year-old man complains of fatigue and general malaise beginning several months earlier. Although his past medical history is unremarkable, his more recent history is significant for the use of intravenous drugs and for unprotected sex with prostitutes. With the patient's consent, you screen him for human immunodeficiency virus (HIV) infection using a test with a reported sensitivity of 95% and specificity of 75%.

1. **Why does it make sense to use a screening test with a high sensitivity, even at the cost of specificity, for this patient?**
   Screening tests in general, and particularly for life-threatening diseases such as HIV infection, should have a high sensitivity so that they will likely detect the disease if it is present. Because screening tests in general must be inexpensive, this high sensitivity may come at the cost of a suboptimal specificity. However, because it is much more important to not miss a life-threatening disease (i.e., few false negatives) than it is to inconvenience (or even traumatize!) someone with a false positive result, this is considered acceptable.

   Not all screening tests have high sensitivity. When used as a single data point, mammograms and Papanicolaou (Pap) smears, for example, have low sensitivity. However, when used on a regular basis (e.g., annually) they become much more effective screening tools because of a high *cumulative* sensitivity.

2. **If this patient tests positive, is it reasonable to tell him that you are 95% confident that he is infected with human immunodeficiency virus?**
   No. Sensitivity and specificity values simply represent how good a test is at ruling in or ruling out a disease, and perhaps whether the test is ideal for screening large populations for a given disease. Although a positive test result will undoubtedly be concerning to the clinician and the patient, with the information provided there is no way of determining if this is a true positive or a false positive result. What is needed to calculate the PPV for this test? That depends on additional information (prevalence of the disease in the specific population within which the patient falls), as discussed in the next case.

3. **What if the test comes back negative? Can you tell this patient that you are 75% confident that he does not have human immunodeficiency virus infection?**
   Again, such a statement cannot be made unless you know the NPV of the test, which was not provided.

4. **Now let's assume that 90-year-old grandma and our young drug-abusing model citizen in this vignette both test positive for human immunodeficiency virus using this test. Are they both equally likely to have the disease?**
   No, and this question addresses the important concept of utilizing screening tests appropriately. The goal of clinicians is to *selectively* screen only those individuals at higher risk for developing a given disease. This is because the PPV of a test depends on the prevalence of the disease in the given population being tested as well as on the specificity and sensitivity of the test. The prevalence of HIV in 90-year-old women is much lower than in young intravenous drug users. Therefore, if the grandmother tests positive for HIV, she is much more likely to have a false positive than our other patient is, because she had a smaller chance of having HIV before we ran the test.

   Consider the havoc that would be created if physicians screened all women starting at the age of 20 for breast cancer by performing annual mammograms. Given that the prevalence of breast cancer in young woman is low, such testing would yield numerous false positives, necessitating unnecessary referrals and expensive workups by specialists, not to mention a lot of unneeded anxiety! Using this same test to screen only women over 40 makes a bit more sense, as the number of true positives will increase and the number of false positives will decrease owing to the increased prevalence of breast cancer with aging.

SUMMARY BOX: LIKELIHOOD RATIOS, PREDICTIVE VALUES, AND PRINCIPLES OF SCREENING

- In general, screening tests should have high sensitivity so as not to miss anyone with the disease.

- The sensitivity or specificity of a test cannot be used to determine the likelihood that a person has a disease if he tests positive or negative for that disease. In order to determine the likelihood of the disease after testing, the positive predictive value or negative predictive value of the test must be calculated.

- The positive and negative predictive values of a test result depend on the prevalence of disease in the population being tested, so a positive test result in a person belonging to a low-risk population may not be as great a predictor of disease as it would be for a person within a more high-risk population.

CASE 25-4

In a town of 1000 individuals, the prevalence of coronary artery disease across all age groups is 20% (as determined by angiography, the "gold standard"). You have created a wonderfully inexpensive screening test that you believe is both highly sensitive and specific for detecting coronary artery disease.

1. **Given the data presented in the 2 × 2 table in Table 25-7, what is the sensitivity of this new test?**
   Sensitivity can be calculated by dividing the number of true positives by the total number of persons tested with the disease, or a/(a+c) in the 2 × 2 table. There were 180 true positives of the 200 patients tested who had disease, yielding a sensitivity of 180/200, or 90%. This means that this test detects (senses) the disease in 90% of people who have the disease.

TABLE 25-7. TESTING FOR CORONARY ARTERY DISEASE

		Coronary Artery Disease	
		+	−
New Test	+	180 (a)	80 (b)
	−	20 (c)	720 (d)

2. **What is the specificity of this new test?**
   Specificity can be calculated by dividing the number of true negatives by the total number of people tested who do not have the disease (true negatives plus false positives), or d/(b+d) in the 2 × 2 table. There were 720 true negatives and 80 false positives, so the specificity of this test is 720/800, or 90%.

3. **What information can be obtained from calculating the positive likelihood ratio?**
   As described in the Basic Concepts section, the PLR reflects how much a positive test result increases the probability of the presence of disease (i.e., indicates posttest probability of disease). The higher the ratio, the more likely it is that disease is present.

This ratio is calculated as the sensitivity divided by 1 − specificity

$$PLR = \text{sensitivity}/1 - \text{specificity}$$

For this example, given that sensitivity and specificity are both 90%, the PLR can be calculated as

$$
\begin{aligned}
PLR &= .90/1 - .90 \\
&= .9/.1 \\
&= 9
\end{aligned}
$$

So a positive test means that this patient's posttest probability is 9 times greater for having the disease than was his pretest probability.

4. **How is the positive likelihood ratio used to calculate the positive predictive value?**
   This calculation can be done if the disease prevalence is known. First, the disease prevalence needs to be converted to a ratio (e.g., 20% to 1:4). Then we multiply the first part of the ratio by the PLR ($9.0 \times 1:4 = 9:4$). Then the ratio is converted back to a percentage $9/(9+4) = .69$, or 69%. So if in this case the prevalence of coronary artery disease was 20% and the PLR was 9, the PPV of the test would be 69%, indicating that someone testing positive would have a 69% chance of actually having coronary artery disease.

5. **If the positive likelihood ratio is not known, what is another way to calculate the positive predictive value?**
   It can be calculated (by using the 2 × 2 table) as the number of true positives divided by the total number of positives (true and false). This calculation requires knowledge of sensitivity and specificity of the test, as well as the prevalence of the disease, to generate the number of true positives and false positives.
   For the preceding example, given the fact that the disease prevalence is 20% and the sensitivity and specificity of the screening test are both 90%, the PPV of a positive test result would equal 69% (see following calculation). So you would tell your patient that he is only 69% likely to have coronary artery disease based on his positive test result.

$$
\begin{aligned}
\text{Positive predictive value} &= TP/(TP + FP) \\
&= 180/180 + 80 \\
&= 69\%
\end{aligned}
$$

6. **How is the negative predictive value calculated?**
   The NPV is the probability that the disease is absent if the test is negative. It is calculated as true negatives divided by both true negatives and false negatives: $TN/(TN + FN)$.

7. **Using the same preceding example for the calculation of the positive predictive value, calculate the negative predictive value.**

$$
\begin{aligned}
\text{Negative predictive value} &= TN/(TN + FN) \\
&= 720/(720 + 20) \\
&= 0.97 \text{ or } 97\%
\end{aligned}
$$

So, 97% of the people in this sample who had a negative test result would not have the disease.

SUMMARY BOX: SENSITIVITY, SPECIFICITY, LIKELIHOOD RATIOS, AND PREDICTIVE VALUES

- Sensitivity and specificity can be calculated from a 2 × 2 table.

- Positive likelihood ratio reflects how much a positive test result increases the risk of disease and can be calculated be dividing sensitivity by 1 − specificity.

- Positive predictive value can be calculated from the positive likelihood ratio or from a 2 × 2 table.

- Negative predictive value can also be calculated from a 2 × 2 table.

CASE 25-5

In the 1940s, a study was performed on employees at a nuclear power plant to determine if an association exists between radiation exposure and cancer rates. In this study 500 employees with high-level radiation exposure and 500 employees with very limited exposure were followed for 10 years, and the incidence rates for cancer were compared in the two groups throughout this time. The results are depicted in the 2 × 2 table shown in Table 25-8.

TABLE 25-8. RADIATION EXPOSURE AND CANCER		Cancer	
		+	−
Exposure	+	50 (a)	450 (b)
	−	5 (c)	495 (d)

1. **What type of study design is this?**
   This is a (prospective) cohort study because individuals are classified on the basis of exposure, not disease (as with a case-control study). Furthermore, this was an ongoing study in which the complications associated with radiation exposure were analyzed as they occurred.

2. **What is the difference between a prospective cohort study and a retrospective cohort study?**
   In a prospective cohort study, individuals with a given exposure are followed over time to see if there is an increased or decreased frequency of disease development. In a retrospective cohort study, a group of individuals who were exposed some time in the past are evaluated to see if they have a higher frequency of the disease. In both cases, the study population is *grouped according to exposure*.

3. **What is the major limitation of cohort studies?**
   Although the groups may be distinct from each other according to the factor being studied, there are many other factors that may be different between the groups and which could be influencing outcome (confounding variables). For example, a cohort study found that people who eat more β-carotene had a lower incidence of lung cancer. However, this did not take into account that people who ate more β-carotene may eat substantially more fruits and vegetables in general, which itself may be protective from cancer. In fact, when a randomized trial was done, β-carotene supplementation actually *increased* the risk of lung cancer.

4. **On the basis of data presented in Table 25-8, what is the relative risk for cancer in the exposed group?**
The RR is determined by comparing incidence rates in exposed individuals (I_E) to incidence rates in nonexposed individuals (I_{NE}), as shown below. Thus, the RR for the employees exposed to radiation is 10 times greater than for the nonexposed employees.

$$RR = \frac{I_E}{I_{NE}} = \frac{a/a + b}{c/c + d} = \frac{50/500}{5/500} = 10$$

5. **What is meant by attributable risk and attributable risk percent? Calculate both for the preceding example.**
Attributable risk (AR), also referred to as the absolute risk, is the incidence of disease in the exposed group caused solely by exposure. It can be calculated by the difference in incidence rates between exposed and nonexposed groups, as shown in the following equation for the preceding example.

$$
\begin{aligned}
AR &= I_E - I_{NE} \\
&= 50/500 - 5/500 \\
&= 45/500 \\
&= 0.09
\end{aligned}
$$

This AR of 0.09 implies that 9% of people exposed to radiation developed cancer as a result of that exposure (i.e., which could be attributed to that exposure).
 The *attributable risk percent* is a measure of the percentage of people who were exposed and developed the disease, and in whom the development of disease was due to the exposure. It can be calculated by dividing the AR by the incidence of disease in the exposed group:

$$
\begin{aligned}
AR\% &= AR/I_E \times 100 \\
&= 0.09/0.10 \times 100 \\
&= 90\%
\end{aligned}
$$

This AR percent of 90% implies that 90% of people who were exposed to radiation and developed cancer developed their cancer as a result of the radiation.
 Absolute risk reduction percent is calculated in the same way as for AR but is used in reference to exposures that *reduce* one's chances of acquiring the disease outcome. For example, if you found a reduction in cholesterol levels in a group taking statins compared with a group not currently on cholesterol-lowering medication, you would use the term "absolute risk reduction" to describe the difference in risk of developing high cholesterol between exposed and unexposed groups.
 Number needed to treat is related to absolute risk reduction. Number needed to treat = 1/absolute risk reduction. In other words, how many participants must gain exposure status to prevent one from developing the disease outcome? *Number needed to harm* is calculated using the same concept, except that it equals 1/AR.

STEP 1 SECRET

You should know how to calculate odds ratio, relative risk, absolute risk reduction, attributable risk, and number needed to treat/harm. These are helpful formulas to add to your whiteboard before the start of your exam!

6. **What experimental design overcomes the shortcomings of the cohort study?**
   The best experimental design, which is the one least susceptible to confounding and bias, is the randomized controlled trial. In this trial design, individuals are randomly allocated to treatment or control groups, thereby reducing considerably the effects of any confounding factors.

   The best kind of randomized study is a double-blind placebo-controlled trial. "Double-blind" refers to the fact that neither the investigator nor the study subjects know who is receiving the treatment. "Placebo-controlled" means that those who do not receive the treatment being tested receive a placebo instead, which should be similar enough to the treatment that the participants cannot tell whether they are receiving the placebo or the treatment.

SUMMARY BOX: COHORT STUDIES

- In a cohort study, participants are classified according to exposure.

- The major limitation of cohort studies is the existence of confounding variables.

- Cohort studies allow for calculation of relative risk.

- Absolute or attributable risk is the risk that can be attributed solely to exposure.

- The best kind of experimental design is a randomized double-blind placebo-controlled trial.

CHAPTER 26

CLINICAL ANATOMY

Stephen B. Marko, Thomas A. Brown, MD, and Sonali J. Shah

INSIDER'S GUIDE TO CLINICAL ANATOMY FOR THE USMLE STEP 1

Students often wonder how to study anatomy for boards. You may have noticed that the anatomy sections of First Aid are rather sparse in comparison with the depth at which you may have studied this subject in your medical school curriculum. Do not interpret this to mean that anatomy will not be present on your examination. Although some students have reported having relatively few anatomy questions, others have found 5 to 6 questions per block. We share this information not to frighten you but, rather, to give you the idea that boards considers anatomy to be important.

Unfortunately, it is much more difficult to prepare for anatomy than it is for some of the other subjects on boards. There is simply too much material for you to be able to learn everything at this point. In consideration of this reality, how should you go about tackling this subject? Simple: Be realistic and do not expect to know it all. Focus on high-yield topics. In other words, this is *not* the time to relearn each branch of every nerve and all of the origins and insertions of every muscle in the body. You are welcome to do this if you would like, but you would be compromising time that you could be spending on more "test-worthy" topics.

The most important thing to keep in mind is that boards anatomy questions are clinically based. You will be given clinical vignettes for which you will be asked to relate patients' symptoms to anatomic lesions and deformities. Expect to see x-ray films, magnetic resonance imaging (MRI) studies, computed tomography (CT) scans, and angiograms. You may be given a question in which you must first determine the site of the lesion based on the patient's symptoms and then locate the deformed structure on a radiograph. Spend some time perusing an anatomy atlas and some credible online sites for these types of images.

No matter how much you prepare for boards, you *will* encounter questions on material that you failed to study. Do not let this frustrate you. Make your best guess and move on. You can still earn a terrific score if you miss these random questions. Center the majority of your study time on the topics with the best odds of appearing on your examination. This chapter will help guide you to high-yield anatomy topics for boards.

Neuroanatomy-specific tips are discussed in Chapter 17.

CASE 26-1

Stanley, a 68-year-old retired soldier, presents to your family medicine clinic with a 2-year history of pain and cramping of the lower extremities (LEs) with walking. This has not been much of a problem, but for the past month, he has noticed pain in his right foot that awakens him from sleep. He has a 50-pack-year smoking history, a 10-year history of type 2 diabetes mellitus, and erectile dysfunction.

1. **What is the differential diagnosis for his foot and lower extremity pain?**
   Peripheral vascular disease (PVD), neurogenic causes (e.g., disk herniation resulting in radiculopathy), arthritis, trauma, diabetic neuropathic pain, and coarctation of the aorta are considerations.

   ## CASE 26-1 continued:

   Upon further questioning, you find that the pain and cramping are absent at rest and begin after about 50 meters of walking. Stopping for about 5 minutes relieves the pain. The right foot pain occurs only at night and is relieved by hanging the foot over the side of the bed. On physical examination, light touch, pinprick, vibration, and temperature sense are intact on the LEs bilaterally. He is noted to have intact femoral pulses, weak popliteal pulses, weak posterior tibial pulses, a weak left dorsalis pedis pulse, and an absent right dorsalis pedis pulse.

2. **What is now the most likely diagnosis?**
   PVD is characterized by claudication symptoms (pain and cramping of the LEs with walking) that appear after a specific walking distance and resolve after a specific duration of rest. The peripheral pulse findings on physical examination also are strongly suggestive of PVD.

3. **Which historical features in this patient increase the likelihood of a peripheral vascular disease diagnosis?**
   Smoking and diabetes mellitus are strong PVD risk factors. Patients with PVD often have evidence of atherosclerosis elsewhere, as demonstrated by this patient's past MI and erectile dysfunction. Other PVD risk factors include hypertension, hypercholesterolemia (most notably increased low-density lipoprotein [LDL]), obesity, sedentary lifestyle, and a family history of atherosclerotic disease.

4. **Why does his nocturnal right foot pain resolve when he hangs the affected foot over the bedside?**
   Rest pain commonly occurs in the feet at night in PVD. When a patient is supine, there is no gravitational assistance in foot blood flow. Reduced blood flow results in ischemia and pain. Hanging the foot over the side of the bed places the foot below the level of the heart; then gravity increases the flow of blood to the ischemic areas, reducing the pain.

5. **Describe the path of arterial blood from the heart to the femoral sheath.**
   Blood leaves the heart through the aortic valve to enter the ascending thoracic aorta, arch of the aorta, and descending thoracic aorta. The thoracic aorta passes through the aortic hiatus of the diaphragm at the level of T12 to become the abdominal aorta. The abdominal aorta bifurcates into the right and left common iliac arteries at the level of L4. Each common iliac artery bifurcates into the internal and external iliac arteries just anterior to the sacroiliac joint. The internal iliac primarily supplies pelvic structures, while the external iliac runs deep to the inguinal ligament to become the common femoral artery.

6. **Outline the borders of the femoral triangle.**
   The femoral triangle is bordered by the inguinal ligament (superiorly), the sartorius (laterally), and the adductor longus (medially). From lateral to medial, it contains the femoral **N**erve, common femoral **A**rtery, femoral **V**ein, femoral canal (**E**mpty space containing lymph nodes that is the site of femoral hernias), and the **L**acunar ligament. The classic mnemonic is **NAVEL** (Fig. 26-1).

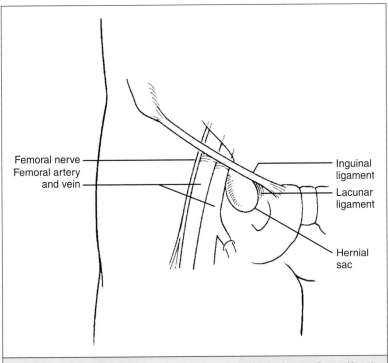

Figure 26-1. Anatomy of the femoral canal. (From Khatri VP, Asensio JA: Operative Surgery Manual. Philadelphia, WB Saunders, 2003.)

7. **Describe the path of arterial blood from the femoral sheath to the feet.**

The common femoral artery quickly bifurcates at the level of the femoral trochanters into the profunda femoris (supplying primarily the thigh) and the superficial femoral artery, which runs through the adductor canal to the popliteal fossa (via the adductor hiatus) to become the popliteal artery. In the posterior compartment of the leg, the popliteal artery bifurcates into the tibiofibular trunk and the anterior tibial artery, which perforates the superior most portion of the interosseous membrane and descends in the anterior compartment until it crosses the ankle joint to become the dorsalis pedis artery, which can be palpated on the dorsum of the foot lateral to the tendon of the extensor hallucus longus. The tibiofibular trunk bifurcates to become the fibular artery, which runs downward in the deep posterior compartment of the leg, and the posterior tibial artery, which can be palpated between the medial malleolus and the calcaneus before bifurcating to form the lateral and medial plantar arteries, which supply the plantar aspect of the foot (Fig. 26-2).

8. **At which sites is arterial plaque formation most likely?**

The most likely sites of plaque formation are arterial branch points, such as the bifurcation of the tibiofibular trunk and anterior tibial artery, and tethered arteries, such as the superficial femoral artery in the adductor canal. Pathophysiologically, the turbulent blood flow occurring at branch points and tethering sites causes shear forces on the endothelium, increasing the likelihood of endothelial damage and potentially leading to atherosclerosis. Such changes are evident in this patient, who appears to show significant bilateral superficial femoral atherosclerotic narrowing (given intact pulses at the femoral triangle and weak pulses at the popliteal fossa) and marked right anterior tibial narrowing (supported by the absence of the dorsalis pedis pulse).

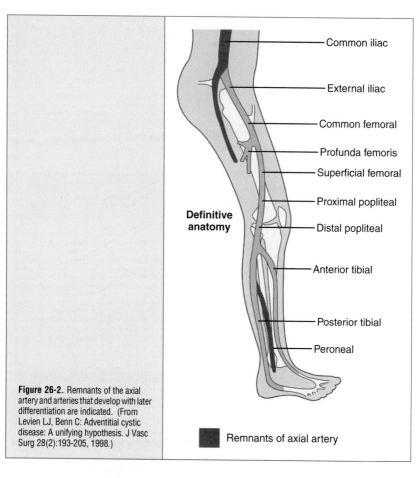

Common iliac

External iliac

Common femoral

Profunda femoris

Superficial femoral

Proximal popliteal

Definitive anatomy

Distal popliteal

Anterior tibial

Posterior tibial

Peroneal

Figure 26-2. Remnants of the axial artery and arteries that develop with later differentiation are indicated. (From Levien LJ, Benn C: Adventitial cystic disease: A unifying hypothesis. J Vasc Surg 28(2):193-205, 1998.)

Remnants of axial artery

9. In Table 26-1, cover the two columns on the right and attempt to list the drug class and mechanism of action for each of the drugs commonly used in treatment of peripheral vascular disease.

TABLE 26–1. SELECTED DRUGS USED TO TREAT PERIPHERAL VASCULAR DISEASE		
Drug	**Class**	**Mechanism of Action**
Aspirin	Nonselective cyclooxygenase inhibitor	Irreversibly inhibits COX-1, decreasing platelet production of thromboxane A_2, a vasoconstrictor and promoter of platelet aggregation
Clopidogrel	$P2Y_{12}$ antagonist	Irreversibly inhibits $P2Y_{12}$, a platelet ADP receptor necessary for activation of the glycoprotein IIb/IIIa pathway of platelet aggregation

TABLE 26-1. SELECTED DRUGS USED TO TREAT PERIPHERAL VASCULAR DISEASE—continued

Drug	Class	Mechanism of Action
Statins (e.g., atorvastatin, rosuvastatin, fluvastatin, lovastatin, pravastatin, simvastatin)	HMG-CoA reductase inhibitors	Inhibit HMG-CoA reductase, the rate-limiting step in endogenous production of cholesterol, to reduce the buildup of cholesterol in atherosclerotic plaques
Cilostazol	Phosphodiesterase III inhibitor	Inhibits cAMP phosphodiesterase III to reduce cAMP degradation, vasodilating peripheral arteries and inhibiting platelet aggregation
Pentoxifylline	Phosphodiesterase inhibitor	Inhibits cAMP phosphodiesterase; increases platelet flexibility and decreases blood viscosity

ADP, adenosine diphosphate; cAMP, cyclic adenosine monophosphate; CoA, coenzyme A; COX-1, cyclooxygenase-1; HMG, hydroxymethylglutarate.

SUMMARY BOX: PERIPHERAL VASCULAR DISEASE

- Peripheral vascular disease (PVD) is caused by atherosclerotic narrowing of peripheral arteries, usually of the lower extremities (LEs).

- Atherosclerotic lesions form preferentially at branch points and sites of tethering, as a result of turbulent blood flow and endothelial shear stress.

- Blood flow to the LE: aorta → common iliac → external iliac → common femoral → profunda femoris (ends in thigh) and superficial femoral → popliteal → anterior tibial (supplies anterior compartment and ends as dorsalis pedis in the dorsum of the foot) and tibiofibular trunk → fibular (supplies lateral compartment) and posterior tibial (supplies posterior compartment) → lateral and medial plantar arteries.

- From lateral to medial, the femoral triangle contains the femoral **N**erve, **A**rtery, **V**ein, canal (**E**mpty space), and the **L**acunar ligament. Remember the acronym **NAVEL**.

CASE 26-2, PART A

Oscar, a 22-year-old college student, presents to the emergency department (ED) after rear-ending a car while driving his new motorcycle. He claims that the major site of impact was his left shoulder, but his head and neck were wrenched to the right as well. He is clearly intoxicated and has managed to sit up, though his left upper extremity (UE) hangs by his side in medial rotation. His forearm is extended and pronated and his wrist is frozen in flexion. The intern on call claims to be able to diagnose Oscar's injury from across the room.

1. **What structure has Oscar injured, and how has it led to his upper extremity position?**
Oscar has torn nerve roots C5 and C6 (or the upper trunk) of the brachial plexus, resulting in a condition known as Erb-Duchenne palsy. His left UE hangs by his side in medial rotation because the C5 component of the axillary nerve is necessary for shoulder flexion and abduction (via the deltoid) and lateral rotation (via the teres minor). His forearm is extended and pronated because C5 and C6 are the main components of the musculocutaneous nerve, which supplies the two major forearm flexors (brachialis and biceps) and the major forearm supinator (biceps). His wrist is flexed because the C6 component of the radial nerve is necessary for wrist extension (via the extensor muscles of the posterior compartment of the forearm).

2. **If Oscar had forced his upper extremity above his head by grabbing the handlebars of the motorcycle to prevent his fall, he may have presented with a loss of sensation and impaired flexion in digits 4 and 5, impaired wrist flexion, hyperextension of the metacarpophalangeal joints, and an inability to abduct and adduct digits 2 to 5. What would be the diagnosis in this situation?**
This pattern of injury is characteristic of a tear of nerve roots C8 and T1 (or a lower trunk tear) of the brachial plexus, a condition known as Klumpke's paralysis. The ulnar nerve is exclusively supplied by C8 and T1 and is responsible for sensory innervation to the fifth digit, the medial half of the fourth digit, and the corresponding palmar surface of the hand. It controls the majority of medial digit flexion (via the medial heads of the flexor digitorum profundus and the flexor digiti minimi muscles) as well as abduction (via the dorsal interossei) and adduction (via the palmar interossei) of digits 2 to 5. It is partially responsible for metacarpophalangeal joint flexion (via the lumbricals of digits 4 and 5) and wrist flexion (via the flexor carpi ulnaris) (Fig. 26-3).

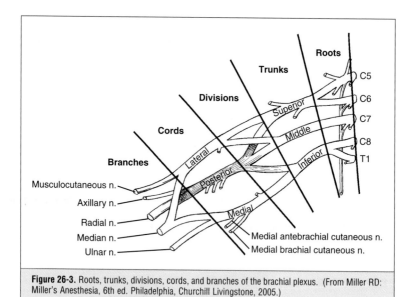

Figure 26-3. Roots, trunks, divisions, cords, and branches of the brachial plexus. (From Miller RD: Miller's Anesthesia, 6th ed. Philadelphia, Churchill Livingstone, 2005.)

CASE 26-2, PART A continued:

One year later, Oscar's wild ways have continued, and he admits to twisting his ankle during an episode of extreme intoxication last weekend. He did not go to the doctor then, as he was a bit embarrassed, and his ankle feels much better. He presents today with an inability to extend his right elbow and right wrist drop since he started using crutches a friend let him borrow.

3. **What structure has Oscar injured this time and how has it led to his upper extremity position?**
A compression injury to the posterior cord of the brachial plexus can occur if underarm crutches are used incorrectly. The inability to extend his wrist is due to a lack of radial nerve (a branch of the posterior cord) input to the posterior compartment of the forearm. The radial nerve also innervates the triceps brachii and anconeus muscles, which are necessary for elbow extension. Pure radial nerve palsies (which often result from injury to the nerve at the spiral groove of the humerus) generally do not affect the triceps, because the branch of radial nerve to the triceps is very close to the origin at the posterior cord, proximal to the spiral groove.

CASE 26-2, PART B

One month later, Oscar's father, George (who happens to be a writer), presents to your clinic with paresthesias and pain involving his lateral palm, digits 1 to 3, and the lateral half of his fourth digit. He tells you that he has been typing long hours over the past few months and now has almost finished his latest masterpiece. On physical examination, you notice mild atrophy of the thenar eminence, a positive Tinel sign (tapping the middle of the wrist crease elicits paresthesias of the lateral hand), and a positive Phalen test (palmar flexion of the wrist for longer than 1 minute results in paresthesias of the lateral hand).

4. **What structure has been injured and how has this happened?**
Repetitive use of the hands—typing, in George's case—can lead to inflammation, swelling, and subsequent compression of the structures within the carpal tunnel. This condition is known as carpal tunnel syndrome, and the pain, paresthesias, and muscle wasting are due to median nerve injury within the tunnel. George's pain and paresthesias have arisen in the distribution of the sensory component of the median nerve, the lateral palm, and the lateral 3½ digits. Because the median nerve also innervates the intrinsic muscles of the thumb, early thenar wasting has occurred.

5. **Outline the contents of the carpal tunnel.**
The carpal tunnel is formed by the eight wrist (carpal) bones and the transverse carpal ligament (flexor retinaculum), which spans from the tubercles of the scaphoid and trapezium to the pisiform and the hook of the hamate. The contents include the four flexor digitorum profundus tendons, the four flexor digitorum superficialis tendons, the flexor pollicis longus tendon, and the median nerve (Fig. 26-4).

6. **Name the muscles of the thenar and hypothenar eminences and describe their function.**
   - *Thenar eminence* (located proximal to the thumb): opponens pollicis, abductor pollicis brevis, and flexor pollicis brevis (all innervated by the median nerve after it passes through the carpal tunnel).
   - *Hypothenar eminence* (located proximal to the fifth digit): opponens digiti minimi, abductor digiti minimi, and flexor digiti minimi (all innervated by the ulnar nerve).
   - *Function*: These two groups have symmetrical function. As their names suggest, each group has a muscle that performs opposition, abduction, and flexion.

7. **Describe the pattern of sensory innervation of the hand.**
   - *Median nerve*: lateral palm, thumb, digits 2 and 3, and lateral half of digit 4.
   - *Ulnar nerve*: medial palm, medial dorsal hand, digit 5, and medial half of digit 4.
   - *Radial nerve*: lateral dorsal hand, extending distally to the proximal interphalangeal (PIP) joint of digits 1 to 3 and the lateral half of digit 4 (Fig. 26-5).

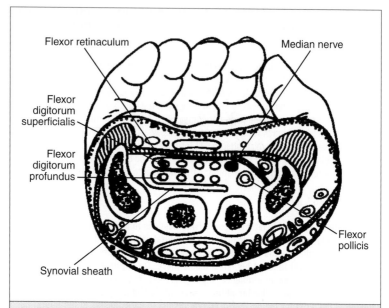

Figure 26-4. Cross-sectional anatomy of wrist. Tendons and median nerve may be compressed by inflammation or infection because they are encompassed by synovial sheath and flexor retinaculum. (From Noble J: Textbook of Primary Care Medicine, 3rd ed. St. Louis, Mosby, 2001.)

CASE 26-2, PART B continued:

As George walks out of the office, he slips on icy steps and falls forward, breaking the fall with his right hand. He immediately feels severe pain in his wrist, and as his distal forearm is very obviously deformed, he carefully walks back into the clinic. You order an x-ray film, and the radiologist remarks that she sees the classic "dinner fork deformity" of a certain fracture commonly seen in patients over the age of 50.

8. **What fracture has George suffered?**
   Colles' fracture is a fracture of the distal radius in which the distal fragment is displaced posteriorly/dorsally. Radiographically, the angle of the radius and the fragment in combination with the angle of the fragment and the hand resembles the curvature of a fork. This fracture is common after the age of 50 and most often occurs when one breaks a fall with an outstretched hand.

CASE 26-2, PART C

Two months later, you are working in the ED again, and you come across another member of the family, 20-year-old Jake. He is a former high school starting pitcher who was getting a lesson from Oscar on how to ride a motorcycle. Unfortunately, he too has taken a nasty fall. The attending at the ED says she is worried about a humerus fracture.

9. **What are the three most common sites of humerus fracture, and which nerve and artery are at risk at each of these sites?**
   See Table 26-2.

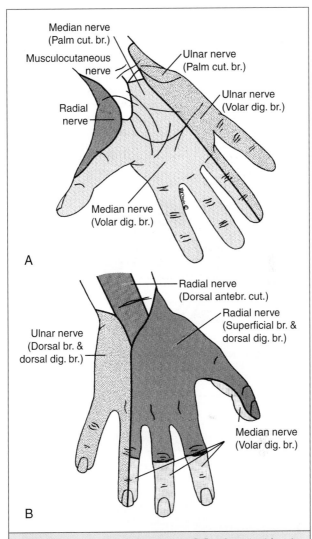

Figure 26-5. Nerves of the hand. **A,** Volar aspect. **B,** Dorsal aspect. antebr. cut., antebrachial cutaneous; cut. br., cutaneous branch; dig. br., digital branch. (From Noble J: Textbook of Primary Care Medicine, 3rd ed. St. Louis, Mosby, 2001.)

Humerus Fracture Site	Nerve	Artery
Surgical neck	Axillary	Anterior and posterior circumflex humeral (branches of the axillary artery)
Midshaft	Radial	Profunda brachii (branch of the brachial artery)
Supracondylar	Median	Brachial

TABLE 26-2. THREE MOST COMMON SITES OF HUMERUS FRACTURE

10. **On reviewing Jake's past medical history, you note that his baseball career was marred by a partially torn rotator cuff. Describe why the rotator cuff makes the glenohumeral joint different from other joints, and name its four components.** Most joints are stabilized primarily by a ligamentous capsule, but the glenohumeral joint is stabilized primarily by the rotator cuff, which consists of the tendons of four muscles—supraspinatus, infraspinatus, teres minor, and subscapularis (Fig. 26-6). This design allows the glenohumeral joint to have the widest range of motion of all joints in the body, at the expense of stability and resistance to injury. The rotator cuff stabilizes the glenohumeral joint by pulling the head of the humerus toward the glenoid fossa of the scapula as other muscles flex, extend, abduct, or adduct the arm. Rapid, forceful, or repetitive movements (such as repeatedly throwing a baseball) can tear the tendons of the rotator cuff, leading to a lack of joint stability, restricted movement, and pain.

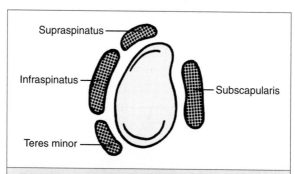

Figure 26-6. Cross-sectional view of the shoulder with humeral head stabilized in shallow scapular glenoid by rotator cuff and capsule. (From Noble J: Textbook of Primary Care Medicine, 3rd ed. St. Louis, Mosby, 2001.)

STEP 1 SECRET

Upper extremity injuries, particularly those that involve the brachial plexus, are popular subjects for Step 1 anatomy questions. You should learn all of the brachial plexus components and the muscles that they innervate. Remember, boards questions usually have a clinical focus! When you study the brachial plexus, spend most of your time reasoning through the various injuries that result from lesions to the different nerves, branches, trunks, divisions, and so on. You are expected to know the most common ways in which these injuries can occur, because it is likely that you will have to deduce this from the stem of the question (e.g., associate frequent computer use with median nerve damage). Lower extremity nerve injuries are also tested on boards but not quite as commonly as upper extremity injuries.

SUMMARY BOX: UPPER EXTREMITY INJURIES

- From proximal to distal, the brachial plexus consists of:
  - Five roots: C5 through T1
  - Three trunks: superior, middle, and inferior

- Six divisions: three anterior and three posterior

- Three cords: lateral, posterior, and medial

- Five major branches: musculocutaneous, axillary, radial, median, and ulnar

- The musculocutaneous nerve innervates the flexors of the elbow.

- The axillary nerve innervates the deltoid and teres minor muscles as well as the long head of the triceps brachii.

- The radial nerve innervates the extensors in the arm and forearm.

- The ulnar nerve innervates the medial heads of the flexor digitorum profundus, the flexor carpi ulnaris, medial lumbricals, interossei, and hypothenar muscles.

- The median nerve innervates the anterior forearm muscles not innervated by the ulnar nerve, the lateral lumbricals, and the thenar muscles.

- The blood supply to the upper extremity (UE) is from the brachial artery, the continuation of the axillary artery after it crosses the teres major.

- The carpal tunnel consists of the eight carpal bones and the transverse carpal ligament. It contains the median nerve and the tendons of the long flexors of the digits.

- The rotator cuff consists of the tendons of four muscles: supraspinatus, infraspinatus, teres minor, and subscapularis.

CASE 26-3. PART A

You are working in an outpatient pediatrics clinic, and your next patient is a 14-day-old infant who was born 2 weeks prematurely. The mother has no complaints, and you proceed to examine the child. The infant is mildly diaphoretic, and you notice a continuous (both systolic and diastolic) "machinery murmur," auscultated best at the second left intercostal space.

1. **What is the most likely diagnosis?**
Patent ductus arteriosus (PDA) is likely.

2. **What is the utility of the ductus arteriosus?**
In utero, this connection between the aorta and the pulmonary artery acts as a right-to-left shunt. It allows the majority of oxygenated blood (which has entered the right side of the heart through the route of placenta → umbilical vein → ductus venosus → inferior vena cava) to bypass the developing (nonfunctioning) lungs and enter the systemic circulation. Just after birth, the ductus arteriosus normally closes and undergoes fibrotic degeneration to become the ligamentum arteriosum (Fig. 26-7).

3. **What causes the ductus arteriosus to close after birth?**
During life as a fetus, circulating prostaglandins and a low blood P_{O_2} keep the ductus arteriosus open. Blood P_{O_2} rises when breathing is initiated, signaling the newborn's ability to obtain oxygenated blood from the lungs rather than from the umbilical vein. Along with rising P_{O_2}, falling levels of prostaglandins act to close the ductus arteriosus. In the event that the ductus arteriosus remains patent after birth, it can often be closed by administering a drug that blocks the production of prostaglandin E_2, such as the COX inhibitor indomethacin. Alternatively, in the event that a baby is born with a congenital defect such as transposition of the great vessels, it is necessary to keep the ductus arteriosus open until the transposition can be surgically fixed. This can be achieved by administering alprostadil, a prostaglandin E_1 analog.

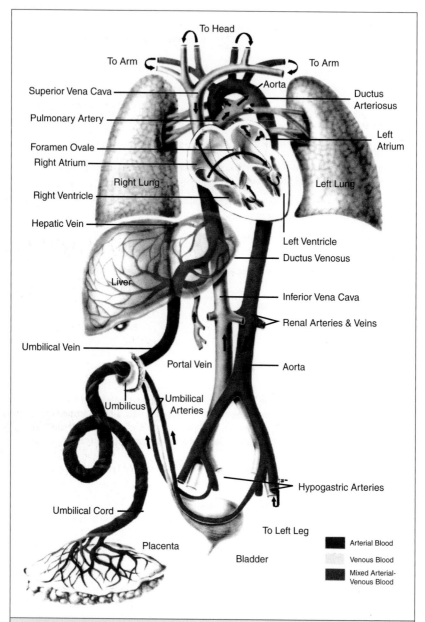

Figure 26-7. Course of fetal circulation in late gestation. Note the selective blood flow patterns across the foramen ovale and the ductus arteriosus. (From Miller RD: Miller's Anesthesia, 6th ed. Philadelphia, Churchill Livingstone, 2005.)

CASE 26-3, PART B

It is a slow morning on your cardiology rotation when Rick, a 32-year-old man with a history of factor V Leiden and deep venous thrombosis (DVT), is brought by ambulance to the ED apparently suffering from a stroke. He has no history of atrial fibrillation, valvular disease, or MI. On cardiac auscultation, you hear a mild systolic ejection murmur and wide, fixed splitting of S_2. Neurology confirms that Rick has had an ischemic stroke, and a transesophageal echocardiogram (TEE) reveals interatrial blood flow.

4. **What is the most likely diagnosis?**
   Atrial septal defect (ASD) is most likely. A thromboembolic stroke is relatively rare in patients without atrial fibrillation, valvular disease, or a past MI. Although factor V Leiden produces a hypercoagulable state, it is much more likely to cause DVT than a left-sided heart or arterial thrombus. The physical examination and TEE study findings strongly support ASD, so Rick's stroke was most likely caused by a paradoxical embolus (in which an embolus of venous origin that traveled through the ASD and then to the cerebral vasculature).

5. **Is atrial septal defect the most common congenital heart defect?**
   No. Ventricular septal defect (VSD) is the most common. ASD is the second most common congenital heart defect, and PDA is the third.

6. **What are the three most common types of atrial septal defect?**
   1. *Ostium secundum defect*
      Ostium secundum defect is the most common type of ASD. The atrial septum is formed by the septum primum and the septum secundum. In ostium secundum defect, there is usually excessive absorption of the septum primum, inadequate growth of the septum secundum, or enlargement of the foramen ovale (the opening at the inferior margin of the septum secundum). A subtype of ostium secundum defect is patent foramen ovale, in which the septum primum and septum secundum fail to fuse. This common defect may allow interatrial blood flow (note that this is physiologic in fetal life).
   2. *Ostium primum defect*
      In ostium primum defect, the septum primum fails to fuse with the endocardial (atrioventricular [AV]) cushion. This is often due to an endocardial cushion defect, commonly associated with Down syndrome. Note that the endocardial cushion is the point of fusion for the atrial septum, ventricular septum, mitral valve, and tricuspid valve, and the magnitude of the defect determines the pathology. For instance, partial ostium primum defect causes an interatrial connection, but complete ostium primum defect causes an AV connection.
   3. *Sinus venosus defect*
      Normally, the atrial septum develops completely to the left of the sinus venosus, the structure that is to become the superior and inferior venae cavae and part of the right atrium. In this rare defect, the septum develops anterior to the sinus venosus, allowing interatrial flow via the sinus venosus (Fig. 26-8).

7. **How might atrial septal defect lead to right-sided heart failure?**
   Left-sided heart pressures are higher than right-sided heart pressures, so an ASD allows for left-to-right shunting of blood. This increases flow volumes through the right side of the heart, leading to right ventricular (and atrial) dilation, increased stroke work, decreased pumping ability, and eventually right-sided heart failure.

8. **What is the dreaded late complication of atrial septal defect?**
   Eisenmenger's complex refers to a situation in which inappropriately increased right-sided heart flow and pressure damage the pulmonary vasculature, causing small vessel fibrosis to develop. The fibrotic vasculature further increases pulmonary hypertension and does not

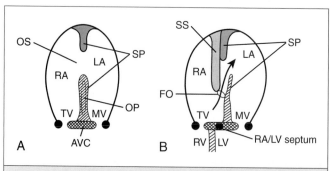

Figure 26-8. Development of atrial septum. **A,** The septum primum (SP) grows down from the roof of the primitive common atrium to meet the atrioventricular cushions (AVCs) and divides the primitive common atrium into right atrium (RA) and left atrium (LA). The defect below the growing free lower edge of SP is called ostium primum (OP)—shown here as a dotted oval. The septum primum has reached the AVCs, which have developed into tricuspid (TV) and mitral (MV) valves. The drawing shows that the upper part of the SP has (normally) degenerated to leave the large *ostium secundum* (OS) or fossa ovale defect. **B,** A second interatrial septum—septum secundum (SS)—grows to the *right* of the SP. The upper portions of the two septa fuse and a portion of the upper part degenerates to form the OS. The lower edge of the SS grows downward to partially cover the OS but does not reach the AVCs. A valve-like opening—*foramen ovale* (FO)—is there by established, permitting a shunt from RA to LA but *not* in the reverse direction. The FO persists during fetal life (during which it transmits an essential right-to-left shunt), but after birth it usually seals off by fusion of the lower part of SP with SS. Note that the interventricular septum separates right ventricle (RV) from left ventricle (LV). The interventricular septum meets AVCs to the *right* of the atrial septum, so that one portion of the AVC separates RA from LV. This portion later forms the upper part of the interventricular septum, and it is through this portion that the Gerbode defect occurs. (From Grainger RG, Allison D, Adams A: Grainger & Allison's Diagnostic Radiology: A Textbook of Medical Imaging, 4th ed. Philadelphia, Churchill Livingstone, 2001.)

contribute to gas exchange, causing the right side of the heart to increase its output. Eventually, right-sided heart pressures become high enough to reverse the shunt of ASD to right-to-left shunt, resulting in cyanosis and heart failure.

CASE 26-3, PART C

You are in the newborn nursery on the first day of your inpatient pediatrics rotation, and the neonatology fellow invites you in to see an infant. The infant is obviously cyanotic but seems to be having no respiratory difficulty other than mild tachypnea.

9. **What are the five cardiogenic causes of cyanosis in a newborn?**
   These five causes are known as the five Ts: **T**etralogy of Fallot, **T**ransposition of the great vessels, **T**runcus arteriosus, **T**ricuspid atresia, and **T**otal anomalous pulmonary venous return.

CASE 26-3, PART D

On cardiac auscultation, you hear a 3/6 systolic crescendo-decrescendo murmur at the second left intercostal space and a loud S_2 at the fourth left intercostal space. The fellow shows you the infant's chest radiograph, which shows a "boot-shaped" heart, signifying right ventricular hypertrophy.

10. **What is the most likely diagnosis?**
    Tetralogy of Fallot is the congenital heart defect most likely to cause cyanosis in infants. The murmurs of tetrology of Fallot vary depending on the degree of pulmonary stenosis and the extent of the

VSD. In this case, the pulmonary stenosis murmur overshadows any VSD murmur that might be appreciable. The loud S_2 is due to the closure of the aortic valve. Recall the four components of this disease: VSD, overriding aorta, pulmonary stenosis, and right ventricular hypertrophy.

11. **How does tetralogy of Fallot cause cyanosis?**
Pulmonary stenosis causes a high resistance to flow through the pulmonary trunk. Coupled with concentric right ventricular hypertrophy, this leads to high right-sided heart pressures, causing right-to-left flow through the VSD (Fig. 26-9). When a critical proportion of deoxygenated blood is shunted through the VSD and mixed with oxygenated blood, cyanosis appears. It is classically seen first in the fingers and lips.

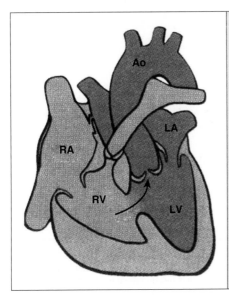

Figure 26-9. Schematic diagram of the most important right-to-left shunts (cyanotic congenital heart disease). Tetralogy of Fallot. Diagrammatic representation of anatomic variants, indicating that the direction of shunting across the ventricular septal defect (VSD) depends on the severity of the subpulmonary stenosis. Arrow indicates the direction of the blood flow. AO, aorta; LA, left atrium; LV, left ventricle; RA, right atrium; RV, right ventricle. (Courtesy of William D. Edwards, M.D., Mayo Clinic, Rochester, MN.)

12. **What is the cause of tetralogy of Fallot?**
Unequal partitioning of the primitive truncus arteriosus by the truncoconal ridges misplaces the infundibular septum, the structure that divides the two ventricular outflow tracts. The anterosuperior displacement of the infundibular septum causes pulmonary stenosis in addition to causing the aorta to override the VSD that results from failure of the truncoconal ridges to fuse with the muscular interventricular septum. Stenosis of the pulmonary trunk increases afterload, leading to concentric right ventricular hypertrophy, seen on a radiograph as a "boot-shaped" heart.

SUMMARY BOX: CONGENITAL HEART DEFECTS

- The ductus arteriosus connects the pulmonary artery to the aorta and allows blood to bypass the developing lungs during fetal life.

- The patency of the ductus arteriosus is maintained by low P_{O_2} and prostaglandin E_2. It can be pharmacologically closed with indomethacin or kept open with alprostadil.

- During fetal life, blood also bypasses the developing lungs via the foramen ovale, which is appropriately patent at this time.

- Atrial septal defect (ASD) can be recognized on cardiac auscultation by a mild systolic ejection murmur and wide, fixed splitting of S_2.

- Ventricular septal defect (VSD) is the most common congenital heart defect.

- Eisenmenger's complex refers to a right-to-left shunt (resulting in cyanosis) that occurred because a left-to-right shunt (VSD, ASD, or patent ductus arteriosus [PDA]) caused right-sided heart overload and pulmonary hypertension, leading to high right-sided heart pressures and shunt reversal.

- Tetralogy of Fallot is characterized by VSD, overriding aorta, pulmonary stenosis, and right ventricular hypertrophy. It is the most common cause of right-to-left cyanotic shunt in infants.

CASE 26-4, PART A

John, a 19-year-old college freshman, presents to the ED with severe neck stiffness and a headache. His temperature is 38.8° C and he has been experiencing chills. According to friends, he has become increasingly confused in the past 24 hours.

1. **What is the differential diagnosis for John's symptoms?**
   Meningitis, encephalitis, mass lesion of brain (abscess or tumor), and subarachnoid hemorrhage are possible.

CASE 26-4, PART A continued:

Upon further questioning of his friends, it is discovered that John was suffering from an upper respiratory tract infection during the 3 days prior to his current illness. On examination, Brudzinski's sign (flexion of the neck with the patient supine elicits pain and involuntary hip and knee flexion) and Kernig's sign (when the hip is flexed, attempted extension of the knee elicits pain and is difficult due to hamstring stiffness) are positive.

2. **What is the most likely diagnosis and what is the next step to confirm this suspicion?**
   He most likely has meningitis, which can be confirmed by lumbar puncture (LP).

3. **At what spinal level should a lumbar puncture be performed? Why?**
   In adults, the needle should be inserted between the spinous processes of L4 and L5. The space between L3 and L4 is also an acceptable choice, because the conus medullaris (the terminal portion of the spinal cord) usually ends near the superior border of L2. Recall that the cauda equina continues below this level, but the free-floating nature of the nerve bundles in the cerebrospinal fluid (CSF) makes them less likely to sustain puncture damage. It should be noted that in children, an LP should be performed only between L4 and L5, because the spinal cord in children can extend to L3.

4. **Through what major structures and spaces, from superficial to deep, should the needle pass in a lumbar puncture?**
   Skin → subcutaneous tissue → spinal ligaments (supraspinous ligament, interspinous ligament, and ligamentum flavum) → epidural space → dura mater → arachnoid mater → subarachnoid space (from which CSF can be drawn).

5. Describe the three layers of the meninges.

1. *Dura mater*

This outermost layer is fused to the inside of the skull via the periosteal dural layer. The dura is double-layered in the skull, allowing cranial compartmentalization and investment of the venous sinuses. In contrast, it is single-layered within the vertebral canal, where it is separated from the sides by the epidural space. The dural sac extends to S2 and is attached to the coccyx via the filum terminale externum.

2. *Arachnoid mater*

This layer is fused to the inner surface of the dura and sends trabeculae to the outer surface of the pia. Between the arachnoid and the pia (the subarachnoid space) lies the CSF.

3. *Pia mater*

This is essentially the outermost layer of the brain, spinal cord, and nerve roots, as it cannot be separated from them. It invests the blood vessels of the brain and spinal cord. The pia continues after the conus medullaris as the filum terminale internum (which is not part of the cauda equina, because it does not contain any axons) until the end of the dural sac at S2, where it is invested with dura to become the filum terminale externum, terminating at the coccyx (Fig. 26-10).

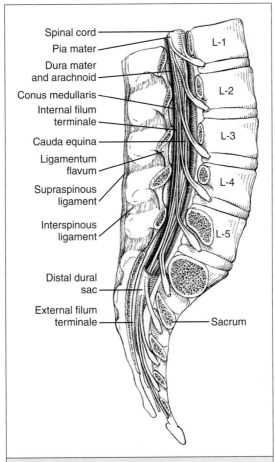

Figure 26-10. Spinal cord anatomy. Notice the termination of the spinal cord (i.e., conus medullaris) at L1-L2. (From Miller RD: Miller's Anesthesia, 6th ed. Philadelphia, Churchill Livingstone, 2005.)

6. **What cerebrospinal fluid findings would you expect to find with different causes of meningitis?**
See Table 26-3.

TABLE 26-3. CEREBROSPINAL FLUID FINDINGS IN MENINGITIS

Pathogenic Category	Cell Type	Pressure	Protein	Sugar
Bacterial	PMN	↑	↑	↓
Tuberculosis	Lymphocyte	↑	↑	↓
Fungal	Lymphocyte	↑	↑	↓
Viral	Lymphocyte	Normal/↑	Normal/↑	Normal

PMN, polymorphonuclear neutrophil (leukocyte).

7. **What are the most common causes of meningitis by age group?**
See Table 26-4.

TABLE 26-4. COMMON CAUSES OF MENINGITIS BY AGE GROUP

0-6 Months	6 Months–6 Years	6 Years–60 Years	60+ Years
Group B streptococci	*Neisseria meningitidis*	*N. meningitidis*	Gram-negative rods
Escherichia coli	Enteroviruses	Enteroviruses	*S. pneumoniae*
Listeria monocytogenes	*Streptococcus pneumoniae*	*S. pneumoniae*	*L. monocytogenes*
	Haemophilus influenzae type b	Herpes simplex virus (HSV)	

STEP 1 SECRET

The information in Tables 26-3 and 26-4 is high-yield for Step 1, and this knowledge will earn easy points for you if you take the time to learn it well. The causes of meningitis in Table 26-4 are not listed in any particular order, although you should note that *Haemophilus influenzae* is becoming an increasingly rare cause of meningitis secondary to vaccination. The mnemonic for recalling the common causes of meningitis by age group is **GEL MESH, MESH GeLS,** where each word represents a separate age group (see Table 26-4).

CASE 26-4, PART B

Ava, a 1-month-old girl, presents for a well-child checkup. She is developmentally normal for her age. On examination, a tuft of hair overlying a 1-cm darkly pigmented patch is found at the level of L5. There is no evidence of any neurologic deficits.

8. **What disorder of neurologic development can be characterized by these findings?**
Spina bifida occulta is a disorder in which the posterior neural tube fails to close, resulting in a failure of midline vertebral arch closure with intact dura. There are no associated neurologic deficits.

9. **What are the other significant disorders related to a failure of posterior neural tube closure?**
A. *Spina bifida cystica—meningocele*
Failure of posterior midline closure of both the vertebral arch and the dura mater. The arachnoid mater herniates through the defect, creating a cyst. Neurologic deficits may or may not occur.
B. *Spina bifida cystica—meningomyelocele*
Failure of posterior midline closure of both the vertebral arch and the dura mater, but the defect is wide enough to allow spinal cord herniation with the arachnoid. Neurologic deficits are level-dependent but usually include paralysis of some degree.
C. *Rachischisis*
Because of an underlying inability of the neural folds to fuse, the spinal cord fails to roll into a round structure, and the posterior neural tube is unable to close. This results in exposure of the flattened spinal cord. This defect may be restricted to a small area or it may be extensive. As with the three types of spina bifida, rachischisis is thought to develop as a result of multiple genetic lesions coupled with environmental factors, with maternal folate deficiency during fetal organogenesis being the most prominent example.

CASE 26-4, PART C

> Jeremy, a 64-year-old carpenter, presents with severe lower back pain. Most of the pain is localized to a single spot in his lower back, but he has ill-defined pain and tingling that begins in the left gluteal region and courses down the lateral side of his left LE to his foot. He also has experienced left LE weakness. He reports that all of these symptoms started 3 days ago, coming on suddenly while he was working in his yard. On physical examination, passive right straight leg raise causes moderate pain in the distribution [on the left] as described here.

10. **What is the most likely diagnosis?**
Jeremy has suffered an intervertebral disk herniation. This is supported by his severe, acute-onset lumbar back pain (upward of 90% of disk herniations involve the L4/L5 or L5/S1 disks), unilateral motor deficit, and pain and tingling that follow a spinal nerve distribution.

11. **Describe intervertebral disk anatomy and how herniation usually occurs.**
The nucleus pulposus is the central elastic cartilaginous portion of the disk. It is surrounded by the anulus fibrosus, which consists of concentric rings of fibrocartilage. With age, the nuclei pulposi become thin and lose their elasticity and the annuli fibrosi degenerate. This makes the disk more likely to herniate, an action characterized by the nucleus pulposus breaking through a localized weakness in the anulus fibrosus. Herniations usually occur in the posterolateral direction, because this is a site of relative anulus fibrosus thinness and there is no support from the anterior or posterior longitudinal ligaments of the vertebral column. Posterolateral disk herniations occur proximal to the intervertebral foramina through which the spinal nerves pass, potentially compressing the spinal nerves and leading to radiculopathy (Fig. 26-11).

12. **Describe the pattern of nerve compression seen in intervertebral disk herniations.**
Recall the scheme for numbering spinal nerves: The cervical spinal nerves C1 to C7 exit the spinal canal superior to the vertebra with the same number. The naming scheme changes at C8, which exits inferior to C7. Thereafter, the spinal nerve roots exit below the vertebra with the same number (the L1 spinal nerve exits below the L1 vertebra). Despite the change within this

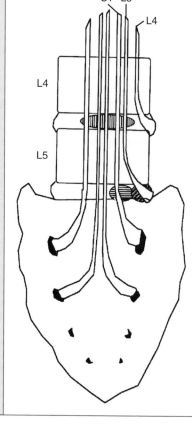

Figure 26-11. Lumbosacral disk herniation. The most common posterolateral herniation compresses the nerve root traveling downward to emerge one level below the level of the exiting root. Hence, L5-S1 herniation most commonly compresses the descending S1 root (*horizontal hatching*). More lateral herniation may compress the root exiting at the level of herniation (*diagonal hatching*). A large central herniation may compress multiple bilateral descending roots of the cauda equina (*vertical hatching*). (From Goetz CG: Textbook of Clinical Neurology, 2nd ed. Philadelphia, WB Saunders, 2003.)

numbering scheme, disk herniations tend to compress the nerve root with the same number as the vertebra below the intervertebral disk. For example, C4/C5 disk herniations result in compression of the C5 nerve root, and L4/L5 disk herniations result in compression of the L5 nerve root. This relationship is maintained because of the increasingly acute angles at which the spinal nerves come off the spinal cord as it descends (Fig. 26-12). However, this change in angle and the presence of the cauda equina allow for multiple nerve compressions to occur with a relatively medial herniation in the lower lumbar region (e.g., an L5/S1 herniation can compress both the L5 and S1 nerves).

SUMMARY BOX: SPINAL CORD AND VERTEBRAL COLUMN

- The best site for a lumbar puncture (LP) is the L4/L5 interspace, well below the end of the spinal cord at L2.

- In performing an LP, the needle should pass through the three spinal ligaments, epidural space, dura, and arachnoid to reach the subarachnoid space, which contains the cerebrospinal fluid (CSF).

- The three layers of the meninges (superficial to deep) are dura mater, arachnoid mater, and pia mater.

- Spina bifida is a disorder in which the posterior neural tube fails to close.

  □ Spina bifida occulta is the least severe subtype, followed by meningocele, and then by meningomyelocele.

- Intervertebral disk herniation:

  □ Occurs when the central nucleus pulposus herniates through the anulus fibrosus.

  □ Usually occurs in the posterolateral direction, where support from the anterior and posterior longitudinal ligaments is lacking.

  □ Usually occurs in the lower lumbar region.

  □ Often results in compression of the nerve root named for the vertebra below the intervertebral disk.

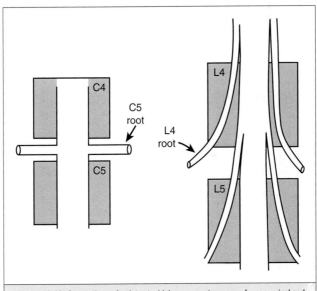

Figure 26-12. Comparison of points at which nerve roots emerge from cervical and lumbar spine. (From Kikuchi S, Macnab I, Moreau P: Localisation of the level of symptomatic cervical disc degeneration. J Bone Joint Surg 63B:272, 1981.)

CASE 26-5

Alexander, an 18-year-old college student, presents with a 1-month history of an intermittent bulge in the right side of his scrotum. He has recently started bodybuilding and states that the bulge is more likely to appear during workouts and less likely to appear while he is lying down. There is no associated pain or scrotal erythema or edema. On physical examination, the scrotum does not transilluminate, and a soft structure can be reduced through the superficial inguinal ring.

1. **Describe the characteristics of the most likely diagnosis.**

   Indirect inguinal hernia is characterized by a protrusion of parietal peritoneum and viscera through a part of the abdominal wall lateral to the inferior epigastric vessels. The viscera exit the abdominal cavity via the deep inguinal ring and enter the scrotum via the superficial inguinal ring, passing through the entirety of the inguinal canal. Recall that parietal peritoneum envelops the testicles during their descent out of the abdomen into the scrotum, eventually forming the tunica vaginalis. During the descent, the cavity of the tunica vaginalis is connected to the peritoneal cavity by the processus vaginalis, which is normally obliterated in the perinatal period. In certain cases, a persistent processus vaginalis remains, forming a potential space within the spermatic cord through which indirect inguinal hernias can protrude. Note that this etiology makes indirect inguinal hernias congenital (Fig. 26-13).

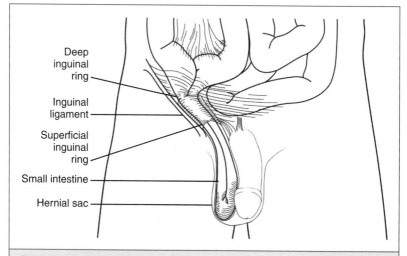

Figure 26-13. Indirect inguinal hernia. (From Roberts JR: Clinical Procedures in Emergency Medicine, 4th ed. Philadelphia, WB Saunders, 2004.)

2. **What differentiates a direct from an indirect inguinal hernia?**

   A direct inguinal hernia is characterized by protrusion of parietal peritoneum and viscera through Hesselbach's triangle, bordered laterally by the inferior epigastric artery, medially by the lateral margin of the rectus abdominis, and inferiorly by the inguinal ligament. The hernia sac is usually composed of transversalis fascia, and although it may pass through a portion of the inguinal canal, it rarely enters the scrotum and is not within the spermatic cord (Fig. 26-14). Most direct inguinal hernias are acquired.

STEP 1 SECRET

Differentiating between the various classes of hernias is commonly tested on Step 1. You should understand the relationship of the different hernia types to their respective anatomic borders.

3. **Describe the structure of the inguinal canal.**

   The inguinal canal is an inferomedially directed passageway that connects two openings, the deep and the superficial inguinal rings. The deep inguinal ring is in the transversalis fascia, just lateral to the inferior epigastric vessels. The superficial inguinal ring is in the external oblique aponeurosis

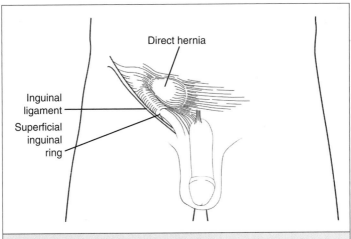

Figure 26-14. Direct inguinal hernia. (From Roberts JR: Clinical Procedures in Emergency Medicine, 4th ed. Philadelphia, WB Saunders, 2004.)

and lies just superolateral to the pubic tubercle. Two walls, a roof, and a floor delineate the canal formed between these two rings. Its major constituents are as follows: The transversalis fascia forms the posterior wall, the external oblique aponeurosis forms the anterior wall, the internal oblique and transversus abdominis muscles form the roof, and the inguinal ligament forms the floor. It should be noted that the layers of the spermatic cord are applied via passage of the testicles through the inguinal canal. Consequently, the internal spermatic fascia is continuous with the transversalis fascia, the cremasteric fascia is continuous with the internal oblique, and the external spermatic fascia is continuous with the external oblique aponeurosis.

4. **Discuss the major contents of the spermatic cord.**
   - *External spermatic fascia*: Continuation of the external oblique aponeurosis.
   - *Cremasteric muscle and fascia*: Continuation of the internal oblique muscle and fascia; draws testes superiorly, often in response to cold temperatures.
   - *Internal spermatic fascia*: Continuation of the transversalis fascia.
   - *Vas deferens*: Transports sperm from the epididymis to the ejaculatory duct.
   - *Testicular artery*: Supplies testes and epididymis (testicular torsion is a medical emergency because twisting of the spermatic cord leads to occlusion of this artery).
   - *Pampiniform plexus*: A venous network that drains into the right and left testicular veins. The venous blood of the pampiniform plexus is cooler than the adjacent blood from the testicular artery. This countercurrent flow cools the blood destined for the testes, maintaining an intratesticular temperature just below core body temperature.
   - *Genital branch of the genitofemoral nerve*: Supplies sensory innervation to the anterior aspect of the scrotum and supplies motor innervation to the cremaster muscle.
   - *Ilioinguinal nerve*: This nerve pierces the internal oblique muscle to enter the inguinal canal, thereafter traveling on the surface of the spermatic cord, rather than within it, to supply some sensory innervation to the superior aspect of the scrotum and root of the penis.
   - *Other*: Autonomic nerve fibers and lymphatic vessels that drain to the para-aortic (lumbar) and preaortic lymph nodes are also present.

5. **Which lymph nodes are the most likely site of first metastasis in testicular cancer? Why is this the case?**
   Testicular lymphatic fluid drains directly to the preaortic and para-aortic (lumbar) lymph nodes. Recall that during embryogenesis, each developing gonad arises from a combination of

mesoderm and mesothelium called the gonadal ridge, which lies just medial to the mesonephros (itself, lying medial to the metanephros, which develops into the kidney). Thus, the testes (and ovaries) develop markedly superior to their position in adult life. Consequently, the blood supply and lymphatic drainage of the testes are located closer to the kidneys than to any structures of the pelvis. For example, the two testicular arteries branch directly from the aorta just inferior to the origin of the renal arteries. It should be noted that, in contrast with testicular cancer, cancer of the scrotum initially metastasizes to the superficial inguinal lymph nodes.

STEP 1 SECRET

You should expect to get a question regarding the sites of local metastasis for various types of cancers. The USMLE is especially fond of the fact that testicular and ovarian cancers metastasize to the para-aortic lymph nodes.

6. **After a vasectomy, by what means does a male produce an ejaculate that does not include sperm? Include a summary of the path of sperm from spermatogenesis to exit from the urethra.**
Normally, sperm pass from their point of origin in the seminiferous tubules to the epididymis and onward into the vas deferens. The two vasa deferentia merge with the outlets of the two seminal vesicles to form the ejaculatory duct. The ejaculatory duct feeds into the prostatic urethra, where the prostate gland deposits its secretions. The prostatic urethra leads to the penile urethra, where the bulbourethral glands deposit their secretions. From the penile urethra, the ejaculate exits the body (Fig. 26-15). In a vasectomy, the vasa deferentia are ligated bilaterally, so

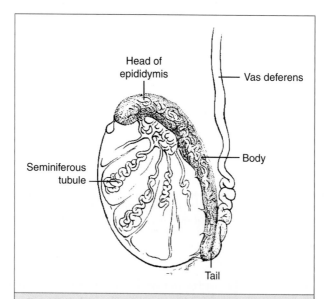

Figure 26-15. Testis and epididymis. One to three seminiferous tubules fill each compartment and drain in the rete testis in the mediastinum. Twelve to 20 efferent ductules become convoluted in the head of the epididymis and drain into a single coiled duct of the epididymis. The vas is convoluted in its first portion. (From Retik A, Vaughan E Jr, Wein A, Walsh P: Campbell's Urology, 8th ed. Philadelphia WB Saunders, 2002.)

sperm cannot pass into the ejaculatory duct, and most of them degenerate in the proximal vas deferens and epididymis. The secretions of the seminal vesicles, prostate, and bulbourethral glands enter the system distal to the ligation points at the vas deferens, and these secretions are ejaculated without sperm, which nominally contributes very little to the volume of normal ejaculate. Thus, the volume of ejaculate is not noticeably changed by vasectomy.

7. **Describe the neurologic basis for erection, emission, and ejaculation.**
   In the unaroused state, arteriovenous anastomoses allow most of the blood from the deep artery of the penis to bypass the helicine arteries within the corpora cavernosa. Upon sexual stimulation, parasympathetic input to the helicine arteries causes vasodilation and vessel straightening, greatly increasing blood flow to the corpora cavernosa, which become engorged. As the corpora cavernosa increase in volume, they compress the obliquely exiting veins against the tunica albuginea, blocking outflow of blood. Blood drainage is also restricted by contraction of the ischiocavernosus and bulbospongiosus muscles, causing a complete *erection* to occur. *Emission* occurs via sympathetic input, which causes contraction of the smooth muscle of the epididymis, vas deferens, seminal vesicles, and prostate (effectively delivering sperm and secretions to the prostatic urethra). *Ejaculation* is a mixed autonomic and somatic response. As the sympathetic system closes the internal urethral sphincter to guard against backflow, the parasympathetic system causes peristalsis of the urethral muscle while the pudendal nerve causes contraction of the bulbospongiosus muscle to propel the semen forward.

8. **Name the most common drugs used for treatment of erectile dysfunction and outline their mechanism of action.**
   Sildenafil (Viagra), vardenafil, and tadalafil are the drugs most commonly used to treat erectile dysfunction.
   Sexual stimulation normally results in parasympathetic-mediated endothelial cell nitric oxide (NO) release within the helicene arteries of the corpora cavernosa. NO diffuses to the adjacent vascular smooth muscle, where it causes vasodilation through a multistep pathway. NO directly activates guanylyl cyclase to produce cyclic guanosine monophosphate (cGMP). This activates protein kinase G (PKG), which then activates myosin light-chain phosphatase (MLCP), which dephosphorylates myosin light chains, leading to arterial smooth muscle relaxation and increased blood flow to the corpora cavernosa.
   Sildenafil, vardenafil, and tadalafil inhibit cGMP-specific phosphodiesterase-5 (PDE-5), which breaks down cGMP. Note that these drugs do not act in the absence of sexual stimulation, which is the initial event that causes helicene NO to be produced. Given their mechanism of action, it should be noted that these drugs should not be administered with nitrates, as hypotension may result. Note that the commercial warnings of priapism represent an exceedingly rare side effect. In fact, the most common cause of drug-induced priapism is trazodone, a selective serotonin reuptake inhibitor used to treat depression.

SUMMARY BOX: HERNIAS AND MALE REPRODUCTIVE FUNCTION

- Indirect inguinal hernia: Protrusion begins lateral to the epigastric vessels, runs through deep inguinal ring into inguinal canal, and often enters scrotum. It is congenital.

- Direct inguinal hernia: Protrusion begins medial to the epigastric vessels, bypasses deep inguinal ring into inguinal canal, and rarely enters scrotum. It is acquired.

- Inguinal canal: begins with the deep inguinal ring and ends with the superficial ring.

  □ Anterior wall: external oblique aponeurosis

- Posterior wall: transversalis fascia

- Roof: internal oblique and transversus abdominis muscles

- Floor: inguinal ligament

■ Spermatic cord: invested in layers continuous with the abdominal muscles as it passes through the inguinal canal; contents include external and internal spermatic fascia, cremaster muscle and fascia, vas deferens, testicular artery, pampiniform plexus, nerves, and lymphatics.

- Testicular lymphatic drainage is to the preaortic and para-aortic (lumbar) lymph nodes.

- Path of sperm: seminiferous tubules → epididymis → vas deferens → ejaculatory duct → urethra → urethral meatus.

- Erection is achieved by the parasympathetic nervous system, emission by the sympathetic nervous system, and ejaculation by mixed autonomic and somatic input.

- Erectile dysfunction drugs work by inhibiting phosphodiesterase-5 (PDE-5).

CASE 26-6

Carlos, a 24-year-old fishing guide, presents with intermittent scrotal enlargement, which he first noticed a few months ago. He relates that the left scrotum is larger than the right and that the swelling decreases significantly when he lies down. Occasionally, he experiences an aching scrotal pain and "heaviness." On review of systems, you discover that Carlos and his wife have been seen in the fertility clinic, as they have failed to conceive after 15 months of trying.

1. **What is the differential diagnosis for Carlos's symptoms?**
   Indirect inguinal hernia, varicocele, hydrocele, hematocele, testicular cancer, and infection (epididymitis or infection of the scrotal skin) are all considerations. Testicular torsion and trauma should be ruled out but are much less likely, given that the onset is not acute.

CASE 26-6 continued:

Carlos is found to be afebrile and in no acute distress. He is not currently having testicular pain. Upon scrotal palpation, the left side feels like there is a bundle of worms superior to the testicle. The scrotum becomes less tensely swollen when Carlos moves from the upright to the supine position. The scrotum does not transilluminate. You are unable to appreciate a hernia sac or any focal testicular masses.

2. **Which of the possibilities is now the most likely diagnosis?**
   Varicocele is most likely. The infertility, aching scrotal pain and heaviness, and "bag of worms" on testicular palpation suggest this diagnosis.

3. **Outline varicocele pathophysiology. Be sure to explain why varicocele is more likely to occur on the left than on the right and how this condition may have led to Carlos's inability to have children.**
   A varicocele refers to a varicosity (dilated and tortuous veins) of the pampiniform plexus. The exact cause is still debated, but there are at least three important factors. Recall that the left testicular vein drains into the left renal vein, which then crosses between the superior mesenteric artery and aorta to drain into the inferior vena cava (IVC). The angle of the testicular-renal vein junction is large enough to disturb flow, which may result in backpressure

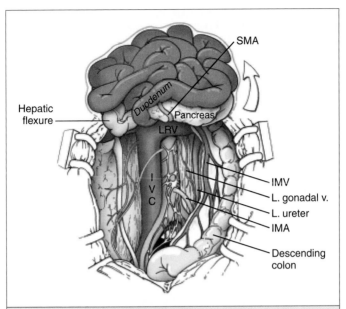

Figure 26-16. The retroperitoneal space has been exposed. The duodenum has been kocherized; its second, third, and fourth portions have been reflected superiorly, along with the pancreas and the superior mesenteric artery (SMA). The entire right colon has been mobilized and exteriorized. IMA, inferior mesenteric artery; IMV, inferior mesenteric vein; IVC, inferior vena cava; LRV, left renal vein. (From Wein AJ, Kavoussi LR, Novick AC, et al: Campbell-Walsh Urology, 9th ed. Philadelphia, WB Saunders, 2007.)

down into the pampiniform plexus. Likewise, because it runs between two arteries, the left renal vein is subject to compression (nutcracker syndrome), which results in backpressure into the distal renal vein, left testicular artery, and left pampiniform plexus (Fig. 26-16). However, though more rare, varicocele can occur on the right side as well (the right testicular vein drains directly into the IVC at an acute angle and has no major compression points), so it is likely that defective valves in the testicular veins play a role in the development of varicocele on both sides. This condition results in some degree of venous stasis in the pampiniform plexus, thus decreasing its ability to cool the arterial blood en route to the testes. The high intratesticular temperatures decrease sperm production and quality.

4. **Describe the difference between hydrocele and hematocele.**
   Hydrocele is a collection of excess nonsanguineous fluid within the tunica vaginalis. It can be caused by a persistent processus vaginalis that communicates between the cavity of the tunica vaginalis and peritoneal cavity, orchitis, epididymitis, corditis, or it can be idiopathic. Scrotal transillumination is often seen on physical examination.
   Hematocele occurs when injury to the spermatic vessels leads to hemorrhage into the cavity of the tunica vaginalis.

CASE 26-6 continued:

Carlos undergoes surgical correction of his varicocele. He goes on to have three children and is so pleased with how you treated him that his entire family has transferred to your care. His father, Miguel, a 65-year-old bartender, first presents to your office with apparent cirrhosis and portal hypertension. He has been feeling extremely fatigued for the past 3 days. In the office, he is jaundiced and tachypneic and has a 2/6 systolic flow murmur. You quickly send him to the ED, where he is admitted for melena and anemia. Upper endoscopy reveals bleeding esophageal varices.

5. **What are esophageal varices?**
Dilated esophageal veins. The esophageal venous system is one of the sites of portacaval (portal-systemic) anastomosis. Esophageal vein dilation occurs because of high portal pressures that force venous flow into the systemic circuit in higher volumes than normal.

6. **How do the esophageal veins connect the portal and systemic venous systems?**
To reach portal circulation, the esophageal veins drain into the left gastric vein. The left gastric vein feeds directly into the portal vein. To reach systemic circulation, the esophageal veins drain into the veins of the azygous system. Other portacaval anastomoses include:
   - Superior rectal veins (portal) with inferior and middle rectal veins (systemic) (dilation can lead to hemorrhoids)
   - Paraumbilical veins (portal) with superficial epigastric veins (systemic) (dilation can lead to caput medusae)
   - Various branches of the colic veins (portal) with the retroperitoneal veins of Retzius (systemic)
   - Branches of the splenic vein (portal) with the left renal vein (systemic)

7. **Outline the flow of blood to the superior vena cava through the veins of the azygous system.**
The azygous system primarily drains the posterior walls of the thorax (via intercostal and vertebral veins) and the abdomen (via ascending lumbar and vertebral veins). It also receives the mediastinal, bronchial, and esophageal veins. The azygous system is infamous for variability, but in general, the primary vein is the azygos vein, which runs vertically along the right anterolateral aspect of the vertebral column within the thorax. Note that the right ascending lumbar vein becomes the azygos vein as it crosses the diaphragm. The azygos vein ends by arching over the hilum of the right lung to drain into the superior vena cava. The left ascending lumbar vein drains posterior abdominal structures before ascending through the diaphragm to become the hemiazygos vein. It drains posterior thoracic structures as it continues up to T9 along the left anterolateral aspect of the vertebral column, which it then crosses to drain into the azygos vein. The accessory hemiazygos vein drains from a variable level between T2 and T4 down to T8, where it crosses the vertebral column and drains into the azygos vein (Fig. 26-17).

SUMMARY BOX: ASYMMETRIES OF THE VENA CAVA

- A varicocele is characterized by varicose veins of the pampiniform plexus.

- Hydrocele and hematocele differ in that these result from fluid and blood, respectively, in the cavity of the tunica vaginalis.

- The right gonadal (testicular or ovarian) vein drains directly into the inferior vena cava (IVC), and the left gonadal vein drains into the left renal vein.

- The left renal vein runs between the superior mesenteric artery and the abdominal aorta.

- The esophageal veins are one of the five major anastomoses that connect the systemic (via the azygous system) and portal (via the left gastric vein) systems.

- The azygous system, headlined by the azygos vein on the right and the hemiazygos and the accessory hemiazygos veins on the left, is the main venous drainage of the posterior walls of the thorax and abdomen.

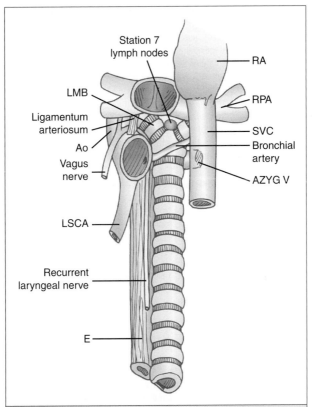

Figure 26-17. Anatomic structures at the carinal level as seen from the surgeon's perspective standing at the patient's head. AO, aorta; AZYG V, azygos vein; E, esophagus; LMB, left main bronchus; LSCA, left subclavian artery; RA, right atrium; RPA, right pulmonary artery; SVC, superior vena cava. (From Sellke FW, del Nido PJ, Swanson SJ: Sabiston & Spencer Surgery of the Chest, 7th ed. Philadelphia, WB Saunders, 2005.)

CASE 26-7, PART A

You are volunteering as a team doctor for a local high school football team. You watch in horror as a player from the opposing team puts a vicious hit on your team's star running back, Nikolai. The primary point of impact is the lateral aspect of the right knee, which was the leg Nikolai had planted in an attempt to change direction. Nikolai is unwilling to put any weight on his right leg because of the extreme pain. On examination of the knee, you note that an abnormal degree of passive tibial valgus deviation is achievable, and there is a positive McMurray test, as well as a positive anterior drawer sign.

1. **List the structures that Nikolai has injured.**
   Nikolai is suffering from the "unhappy triad" of knee injuries: he has torn his tibial (medial) collateral ligament (MCL), allowing tibial valgus deviation; lateral meniscus with a positive result on a McMurray test; and anterior cruciate ligament (ACL), associated with an anterior drawer sign. Note that the McMurray test can be used to check for both medial and lateral meniscus tears, depending on whether the medial or the lateral meniscus is stabilized by the examiner.

2. **How does the posterior cruciate ligament differ from the anterior cruciate ligament?**

The ACL runs from the posteromedial aspect of the lateral condyle of the femur to the anterior intercondylar area of the tibia. It is weaker than the posterior cruciate ligament (PCL) and it prevents anterior displacement of the tibia. Thus, a torn ACL yields a positive anterior drawer sign: flexing the knee to 90 degrees and pulling the tibia anteriorly under a fixed femur results in the tibia's being pulled out a short distance like a drawer.

The PCL runs from the medial condyle of the femur to the posterior intercondylar area of the tibia, crossing posterior to the ACL. The PCL prevents posterior displacement of the tibia. The most common way to suffer a torn PCL is an impact to the superior tibia with a flexed knee. Consequently, a torn PCL allows the tibia to be displaced posteriorly under a fixed femur, a maneuver known as the posterior drawer sign (Fig. 26-18).

3. **Explain why Nikolai's medial collateral ligament and anterior cruciate ligament tears led to the tear in his lateral meniscus.**

In Nikolai's case, he was hit in the knee from the lateral aspect with his foot planted. The force of the hit abducted his knee joint, rupturing the MCL, and propelled his tibia forward in relation to the femur, rupturing his ACL. Because of the knee abduction, the medial condyle of his femur was essentially lifted off of the medial meniscus, putting the burden of the impact onto the lateral meniscus, which tore in response to shear forces within the joint allowed by his ruptured ACL. It should be noted that the MCL fibers intertwine with those of the medial meniscus, making it possible for chronic damage to the MCL to extend to the medial meniscus. However, in acute injuries, such as Nikolai's, medial meniscus injuries occur only in combination with lateral meniscus injuries.

CASE 26-7, PART A continued:

Nikolai returns to you a year and a half later with issues resulting from another football injury. This past season, he suffered a right fibular neck fracture, and the leg was immobilized for several weeks. Since his cast was removed, he has noticed that his right foot "hangs" and that he must step higher than he did before in order to prevent his toes from dragging on the ground. On physical examination, testing his foot dorsiflexion reveals 5/5 strength on the left and 2/5 strength on the right. In addition, he has reduced sensation over the dorsum of his right foot.

4. **Nikolai's clinical picture suggests injury to what structure?**

The common fibular (or peroneal) nerve is injured. This nerve runs lateral to the fibular neck, coming from just posterior to the fibular head and coursing anterior to the fibular neck, where it divides into the deep and superficial fibular nerves. Owing to its close proximity to the fibular neck, fractures of this structure often injure the common fibular nerve.

5. **How does injury to the common fibular nerve result in footdrop, as seen in Nikolai?**

Footdrop is characterized by difficulty with or an inability to perform dorsiflexion and eversion of the foot, leading to passive plantar flexion and inversion of the foot, especially when walking. Injury to the common fibular nerve is responsible for this dysfunction, because the deep fibular nerve innervates the anterior compartment muscles (tibialis anterior, extensor hallucis longus, extensor digitorum longus, and fibularis tertius) that dorsiflex the foot and the superficial fibular nerve innervates the lateral compartment muscles (fibularis longus and brevis) that evert the foot. Note that the superficial fibular nerve has sensory branches distributed upon the dorsum of the foot and the distal third of the anterior leg. Also note that the fibularis tertius acts to evert the foot and that the actions of all of these muscles have been simplified for this discussion (Fig. 26-19).

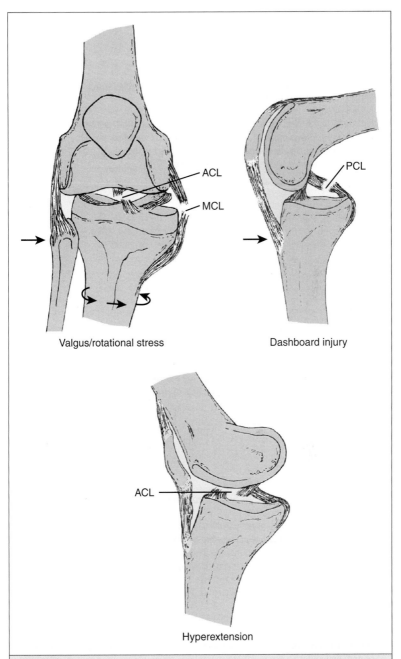

Figure 26-18. Common mechanisms of knee injury. ACL, anterior cruciate ligament; MCL, medial collateral ligament; PCL, posterior cruciate ligament. (From Browner BD, Jupiter JB, Levine AM, et al: Skeletal Trauma: Basic Science, Management, and Reconstruction, 3rd ed. Philadelphia, WB Saunders, 2003.)

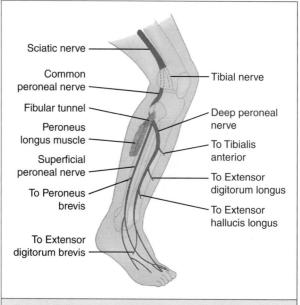

Figure 26-19. Common peroneal nerve, major branches, right leg, anterolateral view. (From Stewart JD: Focal Peripheral Neuropathies, 4th ed. West Vancouver, British Columbia, Canada, JBJ Publishing, 2010, p 473.)

STEP 1 SECRET

Damage to the common peroneal nerve is a favorite on boards. Another favorite is damage to the tibial nerve, which innervates muscles that invert and plantarflex the foot. The tibial nerve is sensory to the sole of the foot.

6. **List the muscles of the posterior compartment of the leg and describe their innervation.**
   The superficial muscle group consists of the gastrocnemius, soleus, and plantaris. This is separated from the deep muscle group by the fibrous transverse intermuscular septum. The deep muscle group includes the popliteus, flexor hallucis longus, flexor digitorum longus, and tibialis posterior. The primary function of the posterior compartment muscles is plantar flexion. They are all innervated by the tibial nerve, which arises just superior to the lateral femoral condyle from the divergence of the two nerves that compose the sciatic nerve (the other being the common fibular nerve).

CASE 26-7, PART A continued:

Nikolai's astonishingly bad luck continues. One year later, he is involved in an automobile accident and suffers a distal left femur fracture, which shears his popliteal artery. He undergoes emergent vascular surgery and his popliteal artery is successfully repaired. However, 4 hours after surgery, Nikolai begins complaining of severe calf pain. On examination, his leg appears pale and his calf is firm. The leg is painful with passive movement and has markedly decreased sensation.

7. **What dreaded vascular surgery complication has Nikolai suffered?**
    Compartment syndrome.

8. **What divides the compartments of the leg?**
    The crural fascia envelops all of the muscles and bones of the leg. The four compartments (anterior, lateral, deep posterior, and superficial posterior) are separated by the anterior, posterior, and transverse intermuscular septa, as well as the interosseous membrane (which connects the tibia and fibula) (Fig. 26-20).

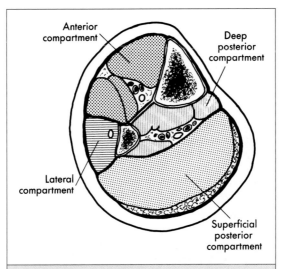

Figure 26-20. Four compartments of the leg: transverse section through middle portion of left leg. (Redrawn from Mubarak SJ, Owen CA: Double incision fasciotomy of the leg. J Bone Joint Surg 59A:184, 1977.)

9. **Describe the major pathophysiologic characteristics of compartment syndrome.**
    The four compartments of the leg are invested with fascia that is highly resistant to stretching. Thus, relatively small volume increases, as would be seen in swelling, result in rapid increases in pressure. Because a compartment represents a closed system, an increase in intracompartmental pressure is directly transmitted to the vasculature, leading first to compression of small, thin-walled vessels. Higher pressures result in compression of progressively larger, thicker-walled vessels. If prolonged, this leads to ischemia and necrosis. In Nikolai's case, his intracompartmental pressure rose because of inflammation and swelling resulting from reperfusion injury.

CASE 26-7, PART B

Beatrice sustains a gunshot wound to the right pelvis. She undergoes emergency surgery to remove the bullet. The surgery is successful, but the attending surgeon admits that some nerve damage was unavoidable during the procedure. Two months later, Beatrice presents to your clinic claiming that the surgery made her right leg shorter than her left leg. To prove this to you, she demonstrates that to keep the foot of her "longer leg" off the ground while walking, she must consciously lift it higher, or she must lean to the right while walking, in effect, using a waddling gait. You note that while her left foot is in the air, her left pelvis sags.

10. **What structure has been injured and how has this led to her awkward gait?**
    Injury to the right superior gluteal nerve has led to paralysis of the gluteus medius and
    gluteus minimus muscles. These muscles abduct the thigh, and when they are not functional, the
    pelvis cannot be stabilized while stepping. While the patient is standing on one foot, the
    contralateral pelvis sags, a characteristic known as the Trendelenburg sign (Fig. 26-21). This is
    definitely a clinical test to know for boards.

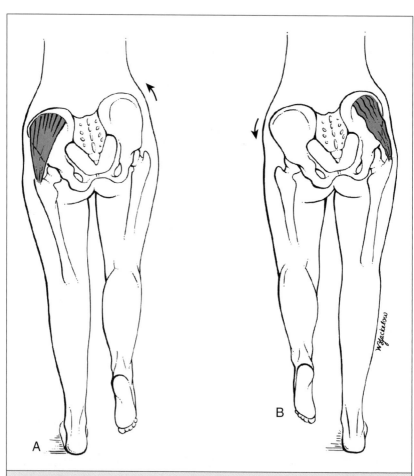

Figure 26-21. Trendelenburg test. **A,** Position of the hips when standing on the normal left leg. Note that
the hip elevates as a result of contraction of the left hip musculature. **B,** Position of the hips when
standing on the abnormal right leg. Note that the left hip falls as a result of lack of adequate contraction
of the right hip muscles. (From Swartz MH: Textbook of Physical Diagnosis, 4th ed. Philadelphia, WB
Saunders, 2001.)

SUMMARY BOX: LOWER EXTREMITY INJURIES ✓

- Note the lower extremity terminology: thigh = hip joint to knee, leg = knee to ankle, foot = ankle to digits.

- The unhappy triad consists of injury to the medial collateral ligament (MCL), anterior cruciate ligament (ACL), and lateral meniscus.

  □ The ACL prevents anterior displacement of the tibia, while the posterior cruciate ligament (PCL) prevents posterior displacement of the tibia.

- The common fibular nerve is often injured in knee injuries or fibular neck fractures.

  □ The common fibular nerve innervates the muscles of foot dorsiflexion and eversion—injury to this nerve results in footdrop.

- The leg is divided into four compartments by unyielding fascia; thus, excessive swelling leads to vascular compression and ischemia (compartment syndrome).

- A functional gluteus medius and gluteus minimus (innervated by the superior gluteal nerve) are necessary for maintaining pelvic stability while walking.

CASE 26-8, PART A

Maureen, a 42-year-old librarian, suffers from Graves' disease and requires a thyroidectomy. She presents to your office 1 month after her surgery with a chief complaint of hoarseness, which she first noticed after her surgery.

1. **What is the differential diagnosis for Maureen's hoarseness?**
   Vocal fold paralysis, laryngitis (infectious or as a result of gastroesophageal reflux disease [GERD]), carcinoma of the vocal folds, nodule of the vocal folds, laryngeal muscle spasm, and idiopathic origin are considerations.

2. **Given the surgical history, which of these diagnoses is most likely and why?**
   Vocal fold paralysis results from injury to the recurrent laryngeal nerve. The two recurrent laryngeal nerves run just posterior to the thyroid gland, and are prone to injury during thyroidectomy.

3. **How does injury to the recurrent laryngeal nerve result in hoarseness?**
   The recurrent laryngeal nerve gives rise to the inferior laryngeal nerve, which innervates all of the intrinsic laryngeal muscles except for one, the cricothyroid muscle. An injury to either of these nerves results in nearly complete vocal cord paralysis on the side of the affected nerve, causing hoarseness. Note that dysfunction of the posterior cricoarytenoid muscle is key in the development of hoarseness, as this is the only muscle that can abduct the vocal folds. Thus, bilateral injury to the recurrent laryngeal nerve can result in dyspnea and stridor, caused by an inability to abduct either vocal fold, which obstructs the airway at the larynx.

STEP 1 SECRET ✓

Be on the lookout for damage to the recurrent laryngeal nerve that results from thyroid surgery. This is a favorite scenario on boards.

4. **Describe the path of the recurrent laryngeal nerve, noting any asymmetries.**
   In the developing embryo, the right and left recurrent laryngeal nerves branch off of the right and left vagus nerves and loop around the fourth aortic arches on their way back into the neck, eventually ending as the inferior laryngeal nerves. The right fourth aortic arch becomes the right subclavian artery, so this is the artery that the right recurrent laryngeal nerve loops around when development is complete. In contrast, the left fourth aortic arch becomes the arch of the aorta, so this structure is what the left recurrent laryngeal nerve loops around when development is complete (Fig. 26-22).

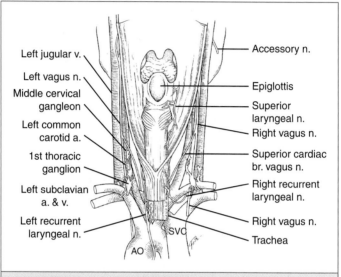

Left jugular v.

Left vagus n.

Middle cervical ganglion

Left common carotid a.

1st thoracic ganglion

Left subclavian a. & v.

Left recurrent laryngeal n.

AO

SVC

Accessory n.

Epiglottis

Superior laryngeal n.

Right vagus n.

Superior cardiac br. vagus n.

Right recurrent laryngeal n.

Right vagus n.

Trachea

Figure 26-22. Diagram of the vagus nerve (cranial nerve X), specifically, its branch, the recurrent laryngeal nerve, and its relationship to the large vessels of the neck. The right and left nerves are not identical, and the recurrent laryngeal nerve branches at the base of the neck on the right and in the thorax on the left. (From Goetz CG: Textbook of Clinical Neurology, 2nd ed. Philadelphia, WB Saunders, 2003.)

5. **Describe the innervation of the lone intrinsic laryngeal muscle not innervated by the recurrent laryngeal nerve: the cricothyroid muscle.**
   The cricothyroid muscle is a tensor of the vocal cords that allows high-pitched phonation. It is innervated by the external laryngeal nerve. Sometimes this nerve can be injured during thyroid surgery as well. This is one of two branches of the superior laryngeal nerve. The other branch is the internal laryngeal nerve, which supplies sensory innervation to the mucous membranes superior to the vocal folds. The superior laryngeal nerve is a direct branch from the vagus nerve.

CASE 26-8, PART B

You are at a fancy restaurant having dinner with your date. Unfortunately, the man at the table next to you begins choking on a piece of steak. You attempt the Heimlich maneuver with no success. You theorize that the piece of steak has entered the larynx and sent the intrinsic laryngeal muscles into spasm, thus tensing the vocal folds and obstructing the airway. As the man loses consciousness, you request a sharp knife from the nearest waitress.

6. **To save this man's life, which structure must you incise? Why?**

The cricothyroid membrane must be cut. This fibrous membrane lies inferior to the thyroid cartilage and superior to the cricoid cartilage, connecting the two structures. Note that the thyroid gland does not overlie the thyroid cartilage, as the bulk of the gland is much more caudal, lying inferior to the cricoid cartilage. Creating an opening in the cricothyroid membrane allows the passage of lifesaving air to bypass the obstruction, because the incision site is inferior to the vocal folds, which are deep to the thyroid cartilage.

7. **Describe the surface anatomy of the neck that allows one to find the cricothyroid membrane.**

The laryngeal prominence (Adam's apple) is the median protrusion of the thyroid cartilage. This lies inferior to the hyoid bone at about the level of C5. By running the fingers inferior to the laryngeal prominence, down to about the level of C6, the arch of the cricoid cartilage can be palpated. The cricothyroid membrane lies just superior to the cricoid cartilage. The incision should be made here, with care not to move too far superiorly, because the thyroid cartilage lies just above. Disruption of the thyroid cartilage could damage the intrinsic laryngeal muscles (Fig. 26-23).

CASE 26-8, PART C

It is Saturday night on your pediatrics rotation and you are covering the obstetrics floor. You enter the room of the next newborn you have prepared to see and find a mother very upset about the fact that her child has two fissures running to his mouth, one from each nostril. On physical examination, you note that the fissures, just lateral to each side of the philtrum, extend into the mouth and meet at the incisive foramen, in essence creating a U-shape from the two nostrils to the incisive foramen.

8. **With what defect(s) has this child been born?**

The child has bilateral cleft lip and cleft primary palate.

9. **Describe the embryologic basis for cleft lip.**

Cleft lip, one of the more common developmental defects, occurs when one or both of the two maxillary processes fail to completely fuse with the corresponding medial nasal process. Note that the two medial nasal processes together make up the intermaxillary segment, the superior portion of which becomes the philtrum.

10. **Describe the embryologic basis for cleft palate.**

Clefts of the *primary palate* occur when the palatal shelves of the maxillary processes fail to fuse with the primary palate, itself formed by the fusion of the maxillary and median nasal processes. If it is bilateral, it results in a U-shaped fissure, with the apex of the U at the incisive foramen (this lies near the three-way fusion point of the primary palate and the two palatal shelves).

Clefts of the *secondary palate* occur when the two palatal shelves fail to fuse at the midline. The nasal septum can be visualized in the middle of the cleft secondary palate (Fig. 26-24).

OTHER IMPORTANT CONCEPTS IN EMBRYOLOGY OF THE FACE AND NECK

11. **Discuss the difference between pharyngeal (branchial) pouches, arches, and clefts.**

The six pharyngeal (branchial) arches consist of a combination of neural crest cells and mesoderm, and play a role in the formation of many structures of the face and neck.

The four pharyngeal pouches lie internally, between the pharyngeal arches, and are lined with foregut endoderm.

The four pharyngeal clefts lie externally, between the pharyngeal arches, and are lined with ectoderm.

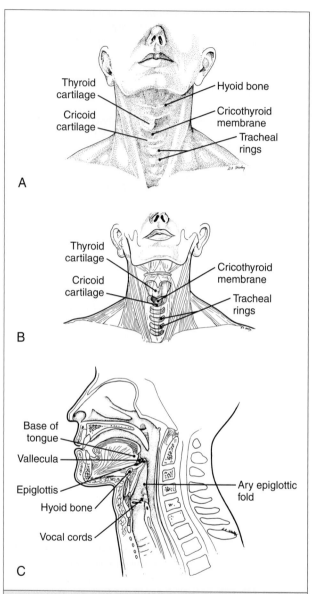

Figure 26-23. Anatomy of the neck. **A,** Surface anatomy of the neck, showing important external landmarks. **B,** Anterior view of the neck, showing various internal structures (overlying superficial skin and structures removed to show cricothyroid membrane). **C,** Lateral view of the neck, showing various structures. (From Roberts JR: Clinical Procedures in Emergency Medicine, 4th ed. Philadelphia, WB Saunders, 2004.)

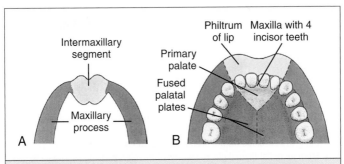

Figure 26-24. A, Schematic drawing of the intermaxillary segment and maxillary processes. **B,** The intermaxillary segment gives rise to the philtrum of the upper lip, the median part of the maxillary bone and its four incisor teeth, and the triangular primary palate. (From Sadler TW: Head and neck embryology. In Sadler TW, Langman J [eds]: Langman's Medical Embryology, 6th ed. Baltimore, Williams & Wilkins, 1990.)

12. In Table 26-5, cover the right column and name the derivatives of each structure listed in the left column.

TABLE 26-5. EMBRYOLOGY OF THE FACE AND NECK

Structure	Derivative(s)
First pouch	Auditory tube and middle ear
Second pouch	Palatine tonsil
Third pouch	Inferior parathyroids and thymus
Fourth pouch	Superior parathyroids and ultimobranchial body (forms thyroid parafollicular C cells)
First arch	Malleus, incus, mandible, maxilla, zygomatic and squamous portion of the temporal bones; muscles of mastication; anterior belly of digastric, mylohyoid, tensor tympani, and tensor veli palatini muscles; innervated by cranial nerves V_2 and V_3
Second arch	Stapes, styloid, most of hyoid bone; muscles of facial expression; stapedius, stylohyoid, and posterior belly of digastric muscle; innervated by cranial nerve VII
Third arch	Greater cornu of hyoid bone, stylopharyngeus muscle; innervated by cranial nerve IX
Fourth and sixth arches	Laryngeal and upper tracheal cartilage; muscles of the soft palate, pharynx, and larynx; striated muscle of esophagus; innervated by cranial nerve X
First cleft	External acoustic meatus
Second/third/fourth cleft	Cervical sinus (eventually becomes obliterated)

STEP 1 SECRET

Embryology in itself is a relatively low-yield subject on boards, but Table 26-5 presents extremely high-yield content. You should expect at least one question on this material.

13. **From where do the parts of the thyroid gland, other than the parafollicular C cells, originate?**

The thyroid gland develops from a proliferation of foregut endoderm at the base of the tongue. From here, the thyroid gland descends through the thyroglossal duct to just inferior to the cricoid cartilage. It remains connected to the foramen cecum via the thyroglossal duct during development. The thyroglossal duct normally degenerates before birth, but the foramen cecum persists, marking the location of the original epithelial proliferation that formed the thyroid.

SUMMARY BOX: NECK ANATOMY AND EMBRYOLOGY

- The recurrent laryngeal nerves lie just deep to the thyroid and are susceptible to injury during thyroid surgery.

  □ These nerves innervate the intrinsic laryngeal muscles except the cricothyroids.

  □ The right recurrent laryngeal ascends from beneath the right subclavian artery.

  □ The left recurrent laryngeal ascends from beneath the aortic arch.

- The external laryngeal nerves, direct branches off the right and left vagus nerves, innervate the cricothyroid muscles.

- The cricothyroid membrane lies inferior to the vocal cords (which are deep to the thyroid cartilage); an airway formed in this membrane can bypass a laryngeal obstruction.

- Cleft lip: Maxillary process fails to fuse with medial nasal process.

- Cleft primary palate: Palatal shelves fail to fuse with the primary palate.

- Cleft secondary palate: Palatal shelves fail to fuse at the midline.

CASE 26-9

Janice, a 20-year-old waitress, presents to the urgent care clinic with severe, sharp, right upper quadrant (RUQ) pain of 6 hours' duration. The pain radiates to her right shoulder, and breathing is moderately painful. She states that she had a mild RUQ ache for a few days, but it didn't bother her and she saw no reason to see a doctor. A urine pregnancy test is negative.

1. **What is the differential diagnosis for Janice's right upper quadrant pain?**

Cholecystitis, choledocholithiasis, cholangitis, peptic ulcer disease, hepatitis, perihepatitis, hepatic abscess or tumor, pyelonephritis, nephrolithiasis, appendicitis, right lower lobe pneumonia, ovarian cysts or tumors, and acute enteritis are possibilities.

CASE 26-9 continued:

Janice's past medical history is unremarkable. However, her sexual history is notable for unprotected sexual intercourse with about 40 different partners over the past 2 years. On physical examination, you note that on palpation, she is experiencing right lower quadrant (RLQ) pain of slightly less severity than her RUQ pain. On pelvic examination, she has exquisite cervical motion tenderness and bilateral adnexal tenderness.

2. **What is the most likely diagnosis?**
   Pelvic inflammatory disease (PID) is most likely.

3. **Name the two most common organisms implicated in pelvic inflammatory disease.**
   Chlamydia trachomatis and *Neisseria gonorrhoeae* are most commonly implicated in PID. Note that rarely PID can be caused by normal vaginal bacterial flora as well as viruses, fungi, and parasites.

4. **How can pelvic inflammatory disease lead to right upper quadrant pain?**
   PID is classically characterized by ascent of bacteria that have infected the vagina and cervix, leading to endometritis, salpingitis, and peritonitis. Peritonitis is possible because the infundibulum of the uterine tubes opens directly into the peritoneal cavity. This means that there is a direct route from the vagina to the peritoneal cavity (via the uterus and uterine tubes) by which bacteria can ascend. In rare cases, this peritonitis can lead to RUQ pain when the offending bacteria reach the liver capsule and cause perihepatitis and inflammation of the right hemidiaphragm. This condition is known as Fitz-Hugh–Curtis syndrome.

5. **Describe how the uterus and ovaries are supported.**
   The cervix is supported anteriorly by the pubocervical ligaments, laterally by the transverse cervical ligaments, and posteriorly by the uterosacral ligaments. The body of an anteverted uterus gains much of its support by resting on the bladder (note that this is not the case in patients with a retroverted uterus). The broad ligament, a double layer of peritoneum, extends laterally from the uterus and functions to support the uterus and all associated structures (note that the mesosalpinx portions of the broad ligament support the uterine tubes), as well as to carry the uterine vasculature. The round ligament, analogous to the spermatic cord, supports the uterine fundus. Each ovary is attached to the uterus via the ovarian ligament, is enveloped by the mesovarium portion of the broad ligament, and is supported laterally by the suspensory ligament of the ovary, which attaches to the lateral pelvic wall and carries the ovarian vasculature (Fig. 26-25).

6. **Can Fitz-Hugh–Curtis syndrome be seen in males?**
   Although PID and Fitz-Hugh–Curtis syndrome classically develop in females through the open connection between the vagina → uterus → uterine tubes → peritoneal cavity, infection can occur through lymphatic, hematogenous, or direct spread from intraperitoneal infections. In males, infections can spread through these routes to the peritoneum and liver capsule, so they also can develop Fitz-Hugh–Curtis syndrome. Note that the lumina of the urethra, ejaculatory duct, vas deferens, epididymis, and seminiferous tubules are not continuous with the peritoneal cavity at any time.

7. **Outline the common drugs used in antimicrobial pharmacotherapy for pelvic inflammatory disease.**
   C. trachomatis and *N. gonorrhoeae* are the most common organisms, but the normal flora of the vagina (e.g., *Gardnerella vaginalis*, *Streptococcus agalactiae*) or gastrointestinal (GI) tract (e.g., *Bacteroides fragilis*, *Peptostreptococcus*, *Escherichia coli*) can play a role in the infection. Infection with multiple organisms is common, so broad-spectrum antibiotics

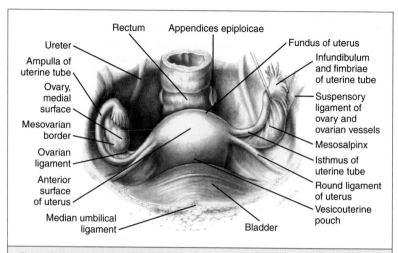

Rectum   Appendices epiploicae

Ureter

Ampulla of uterine tube

Ovary, medial surface

Mesovarian border

Ovarian ligament

Anterior surface of uterus

Median umbilical ligament

Fundus of uterus

Infundibulum and fimbriae of uterine tube

Suspensory ligament of ovary and ovarian vessels

Mesosalpinx

Isthmus of uterine tube

Round ligament of uterus

Vesicouterine pouch

Bladder

Figure 26-25. The organs of the female pelvis. The uterus is surrounded by the bladder anteriorly, the rectum posteriorly, and the folds of the broad ligaments laterally. (Redrawn from Clemente CD: Anatomy: A Regional Atlas of the Human Body. Baltimore-Munich, Urban & Schwarzenberg, 1987.)

are recommended. For mild to moderately severe infections, the recommended regimen is a single intramuscular (IM) dose of a third-generation cephalosporin (such as ceftriaxone or cefoxitin) plus a 14-day course of oral doxycycline and metronidazole. An alternative and equivalent treatment is a single IM dose of ceftriaxone plus high-dose oral azithromycin weekly for 2 weeks. Severe infections (for instance, those associated with tubo-ovarian abscesses) require inpatient treatment with parenteral antibiotics. The two preferred regimens are cefotetan or cefoxitin plus oral or intravenous doxycycline and clindamycin plus gentamicin.

8. In Table 26-6, cover the column on the right and name the abdominal organs in each location.

TABLE 26–6. ABDOMINAL ORGANS	
Location	**Abdominal Organs**
Within the peritoneal cavity	None
	NOTE: The ovaries are exposed to the peritoneal cavity.
Intraperitoneal	Stomach and first part of duodenum
	Liver and gallbladder
	Spleen
	Tail of pancreas
	Jejunum and ileum
	Cecum and appendix
	Transverse and sigmoid colon

TABLE 26–6. ABDOMINAL ORGANS—continued	
Location	**Abdominal Organs**
Secondarily retroperitoneal*	Duodenum: first, second, and third parts
	Ascending and descending colon
	Rectum
	Pancreas: head, neck, and body
Retroperitoneal	Kidneys (plus ureters and adrenal glands)
	Abdominal aorta
	Inferior vena cava

*Note that secondarily retroperitoneal organs develop intraperitoneally (covered by visceral peritoneum) but later move toward the posterior body wall and the retroperitoneal space, leaving only their anterior aspect covered by peritoneum.

SUMMARY BOX: STRUCTURE OF THE FEMALE REPRODUCTIVE SYSTEM AND THE PERITONEUM

- In most cases of pelvic inflammatory disease (PID), bacteria (usually *Chlamydia trachomatis* or *Neisseria gonorrhoeae*) from the vagina pass through the cervix into the uterus and uterine tubes, causing inflammation.

  □ Peritonitis and inflammation in the liver capsule (Fitz-Hugh–Curtis syndrome) can result because the uterine tubes open directly into the peritoneal cavity.

  □ In males, there is no direct connection between the lumen of the genitourinary tract and the peritoneal cavity, so Fitz-Hugh–Curtis syndrome is much more rare.

  □ Antibiotic therapy in PID must include coverage for *C. trachomatis*, *N. gonorrhoeae*, and normal perineal flora (with emphasis on anaerobes).

- The cervix is supported by the pubocervical, transverse cervical, and uterosacral ligaments.

- The uterus is supported by the broad ligament (composed of peritoneum), the round ligaments, and by resting anteriorly on the bladder.

- The ovary is supported by the ovarian ligament, the mesovarium, and the suspensory ligament of the ovary.

- Although the ovaries are exposed to the peritoneal cavity, no viscera actually lie within it.

CASE 26–10, PART A

David, a 64-year-old nurse, suffered an MI 1 month ago. He now presents to the ED with new-onset chest pain that is intermittent and not related to exertion. The pain is severe and is located in the left precordial and retrosternal regions, and it radiates to the neck and back.

1. **What is the differential diagnosis for David's chest pain?**
   Unstable angina, variant (Prinzmetal's) angina, MI, pulmonary embolus, aortic dissection, pericarditis, pleuritis, pneumothorax, pneumonia, costochondritis, rib fracture, anxiety/panic attack, GERD, diffuse esophageal spasm, and peptic ulcer disease are possibilities.

2. **A myocardial infarction in what distribution would be most concerning for damage to the sinoatrial and atrioventricular nodes?**
   Occlusion of the right coronary artery (RCA). The RCA supplies the AV node in nearly 100% of the population via the AV nodal branch, which originates near the origin of the posterior interventricular artery. However, it should be noted that the posterior interventricular artery is a branch of the RCA in 80% of the population and a branch of the circumflex artery in 15% of the population. The remaining 5% have other variations. The sinoatrial (SA) node is supplied by the RCA in 60% of the population via the SA nodal branch, which lies near the origin of the RCA. The SA nodal branch originates from the circumflex artery in the remaining 40%.

3. **Which coronary arteries supply the left ventricle?**
   - *Anterior interventricular*: Shortly after originating from the ascending aorta, the left coronary artery bifurcates. One branch, the anterior interventricular artery, also known as the left anterior descending (LAD) artery, descends in the anterior interventricular groove to the apex. This artery supplies nearly the entire interventricular septum and much of the right ventricle as well.
   - *Circumflex*: The second branch of the bifurcation of the left coronary artery, this artery runs in the AV groove to the posterior side of the heart. It also supplies the left atrium.
   - *Left marginal*: This branch of the circumflex artery descends along the left heart border.
   - *Posterior interventricular*: This artery branches from the RCA, circumflex artery, or both. It descends in the posterior interventricular groove to the apex. It also supplies a small portion of the interventricular septum and part of the right ventricle (Fig. 26-26).

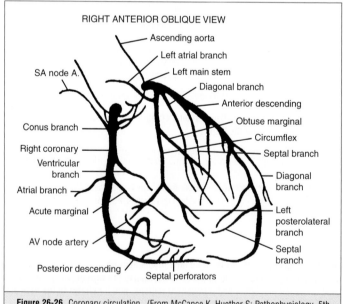

Figure 26-26. Coronary circulation. (From McCance K, Huether S: Pathophysiology, 5th ed. St. Louis, Mosby, 2006.)

4. **If David's chest pain were caused by pleuritis (also known as pleurisy), from which pleural layer would he be sensing pain?**
He would feel pain in the parietal pleura only. In pleuritis, the inflammation involves both pleural layers. Although the visceral pleura lacks sensory innervation and therefore cannot transmit pain sensation, the parietal pleura is exquisitely sensitive to pain because it is abundantly supplied by somatic branches of the intercostal nerves (in the areas bordering the body wall) and the phrenic nerves (in the areas bordering the mediastinum and diaphragm). Because of its differential innervation, referred pain is localized to the body wall for pleuritis in the distribution of the intercostal nerves and to the shoulder and neck for pleuritis in the distribution of the phrenic nerves.

CASE 26-10, PART A continued:

David goes on to say that this chest pain does not feel like the pain that was associated with his heart attack. He has noticed that the pain waxes and wanes with breathing and it is position-dependent: he notes that the pain is least while he sits up and leans forward. On cardiac auscultation, a friction rub is heard.

5. **What is the most likely diagnosis?**
Acute pericarditis is most likely. Weeks to months after a MI, fibrinous pericarditis can occur. This phenomenon is called Dressler's syndrome and is thought to be an autoimmune reaction to novel antigens resulting from cardiac damage, most often in the setting of MI.

6. **If one were to pass a needle from outside the pericardium to the lumen of the left ventricle, through which layers would it pass, in sequence?**
   A. Fibrous pericardium (unyielding, protects heart from acute volume overload; fused with the diaphragm, tunica adventitia of the great vessels, and the posterior sternal surface)
   B. Parietal layer of serous pericardium (fused to the fibrous pericardium)
   C. Pericardial fluid (normally a thin lubricating film; allows the heart to move within the pericardial sac)
   D. Visceral layer of serous pericardium (synonymous with the epicardium; continuous with the parietal layer at the base of the heart)
   E. Myocardium (composed of cardiac muscle)
   F. Endocardium (an endothelial lining; the Purkinje fibers run between this layer and the myocardium)

7. **Enlargement of which chamber of the heart is most likely to cause dysphagia?**
The left atrium, located at the base of the heart, is directly anterior to the esophagus. Marked enlargement of this chamber can lead to compression of the esophagus around the level of T6 through T9.

8. **Enlargement of which chamber of the heart is most likely to cause a parasternal lift?**
A parasternal lift occurs when the right ventricle, which composes the anterior-sternocostal surface of the heart, is enlarged. The elevation is usually seen or felt just to the left of the sternum (i.e., parasternally).

CASE 26-10, PART B

At the end of a long week, you leave the clinic and head to a local movie theater with friends. Soon after settling into your seat to watch *Surf Summer 3: Frosted Tips*, a group of teenagers clamber into the seats directly in front of you. To entertain his buddies before the show, one of the group starts tossing his chewy fruit candies high into the air, catching them in his mouth. Before you can point out the inevitable, one of the candies lands in the boy's mouth just as he is taking a breath, and the gummy giraffe is rapidly out of sight. As the boy coughs, you recall the restaurant fiasco and prepare to start the Heimlich maneuver. However, he immediately begins to breathe, albeit with quite a bit of wheezing and dyspnea.

9. If the candy passed into the bronchial tree, on which side would it most likely be found?
    The right main bronchus is wider and oriented more vertically as compared with the left main bronchus, so it is the more likely site of aspiration.

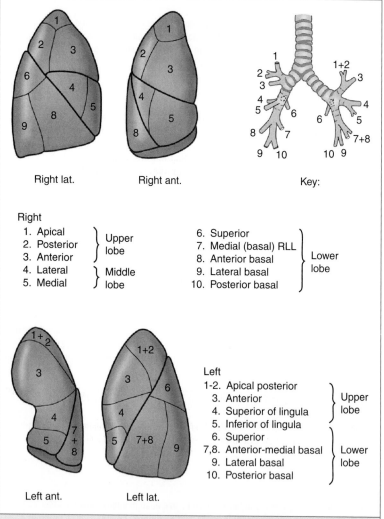

Right lat.   Right ant.   Key:

Right
1. Apical ⎫
2. Posterior ⎬ Upper lobe
3. Anterior ⎭
4. Lateral ⎫ Middle lobe
5. Medial ⎭

6. Superior ⎫
7. Medial (basal) RLL ⎬ Lower lobe
8. Anterior basal ⎪
9. Lateral basal ⎪
10. Posterior basal ⎭

Left
1-2. Apical posterior ⎫
3. Anterior ⎬ Upper lobe
4. Superior of lingula ⎪
5. Inferior of lingula ⎭
6. Superior ⎫
7,8. Anterior-medial basal ⎬ Lower lobe
9. Lateral basal ⎪
10. Posterior basal ⎭

Left ant.   Left lat.

Figure 26-27. Segments of the pulmonary lobes. (Modified from Jackson CL, Huber JF: Correlated applied anatomy of the bronchial tree and lungs with a system of nomenclature. Dis Chest 9:319, 1943.)

10. **Describe the other major asymmetry of the bronchial tree.**
The right main bronchus divides into three lobar bronchi, one for each lobe, whereas the left main bronchus divides into only two, again one for each lobe. The right lung has superior, middle, and inferior lobes. The oblique (major) fissure separates the inferior lobe from the other two lobes and the horizontal (minor) fissure separates the superior lobe from the middle lobe. The left lung has only superior and inferior lobes, separated by the oblique fissure. The inferior portion of the superior lobe of the left lung is called the lingula. It lies adjacent to the heart and is the counterpart of the right middle lobe (Fig. 26-27).

11. **List the four stages in lung development and note whether each is compatible with life.**
    1. *Pseudoglandular period* (weeks 5-18): Formation of the trachea through terminal bronchioles. These structures cannot partake in gas exchange, so birth at this time is incompatible with life.
    2. *Canalicular period* (weeks 16-26): Respiratory vasculature forms and terminal bronchioles give rise to respiratory bronchioles. Survival is rare and can occur only if birth is very late in this period, when there is enough development to allow for adequate gas exchange. Due to neonatal respiratory distress syndrome, intensive care with intubation is necessary, and surfactant must be provided for an extended period.
    3. *Terminal sac period* (weeks 24-36): Formation of terminal sacs (primitive alveoli) and type II alveolar cells (produce surfactant). Chance of survival is good, but if the infant is born early in the period, neonatal respiratory distress syndrome often occurs. Surfactant must be provided until the newborn is able to produce an adequate amount on his own.
    4. *Alveolar period* (week 36 to early childhood): Terminal sacs continue to form and develop into mature alveoli. Chance of survival is excellent.

SUMMARY BOX: CARDIOTHORACIC ANATOMY

- The right coronary artery supplies the atrioventricular (AV) node.

- The right coronary artery supplies the sinoatrial (SA) node in 60% of the population, with the circumflex artery supplying the SA node in the other 40%.

- The anterior interventricular, circumflex, left marginal, and posterior interventricular arteries supply the left ventricle.

  □ The left coronary artery bifurcates into the anterior interventricular and circumflex arteries.

  □ The left marginal artery is a branch of the circumflex artery.

  □ The posterior interventricular artery is a branch of the right coronary in 80% of the population and the circumflex in 15% of the population.

- In pleuritis, although both the visceral and parietal pleurae become inflamed, pain is transmitted only from the parietal pleura because the visceral pleura lacks sensory innervation.

- The outermost fibrous pericardium is fused to the parietal layer of the serous pericardium.

- The parietal and visceral layers of the pericardium are continuous near the base of the heart and contain the pericardial fluid between them.

- The left atrium is the most posterior portion of the heart, lying just anterior to the esophagus.

- The right ventricle is the anterior most portion of the heart, and enlargement can lead to a parasternal lift.

- The right main bronchus is wider and more vertical than the left main bronchus, so an aspirated foreign body is more likely to enter it.

- The three-lobed right lung possesses a middle lobe that corresponds to the lingula of the superior lobe of the left lung, which has only two lobes.

- Because of inadequate respiratory development, approximately 50% of births before 24 weeks of gestation are nonviable.

CHAPTER 27

PATHOLOGY

Nikki Goulet, MD, Thomas A. Brown, MD, and Sonali J. Shah

INSIDER'S GUIDE TO PATHOLOGY FOR THE USMLE STEP 1

You should be aware that the USMLE loves gross anatomy and histopathology images. They *will* show up on your test in the context of second- or third-order questions. Study the HIGH-YIELD images in this chapter (yes, they are all high-yield!) and in the back section of First Aid carefully. Go over them more than once. Pattern recognition is important because you will most likely see slightly different images on your exam.

1. **A 67-year-old white man presented to the emergency department (ED) with worsening dyspnea and cough at night. Physical examination showed jugular venous distention (JVD), bipedal edema, and a liver span of 15 cm. The patient passed away, and a biopsy of the liver is shown in Figure 27-1. What process is shown in the liver tissue? What conditions lead to this process?**
The process shown here is centrilobular hemorrhagic necrosis, otherwise known as "nutmeg liver." The most common causes are right-sided heart failure and left-sided heart failure. Right-sided heart failure leads to increased pressure in the inferior vena cava, which then causes an increased central venous pressure and congestion in the liver. Left-sided heart failure leads to hypoperfusion and ischemia/necrosis of the central lobules (zone 3) first. Zone 3 is affected first because it is the farthest from the oxygenated blood supply (hepatic artery and portal vein) to the liver.

2. **A 62-year-old obese woman with a history of long-standing gastroesophageal reflux disease (GERD) presented to her primary care physician with increasing dysphagia. Her current medications include oral omeprazole 20 mg daily. She undergoes an esophagogastroduodenoscopy (EGD) with biopsy. Her biopsy is shown in Figure 27-2. What disease process is occurring? What is this patient at an increased risk for?**
The patient has metaplasia of the esophagus, otherwise known as Barrett's esophagus. This patient's history of GERD, with consequent chronic acid exposure of the lower esophagus, led to replacement of stratified squamous epithelium (left side) with metaplastic columnar epithelium (right side). These patients are at an increased risk for adenocarcinoma of the esophagus. Although the incidence of esophageal squamous carcinoma was once far greater than that of esophageal adenocarcinoma among Americans, the two are now approximately equal in incidence because of the increasing prevalence of GERD/Barrett's esophagus.

3. **A 45-year-old homeless man, positive for human immunodeficiency virus (HIV), presented to the ED with reported chronic cough, night sweats, and fever. A chest x-ray study was performed and showed apical infiltrates. The patient expired the next day, and a lung biopsy was performed (Fig. 27-3). What was the likely disease that this man suffered from?**

This man likely had reactivation of tuberculosis (TB), evidenced by central caseous necrosis in the biopsy in Figure 27-3 and apical infiltrates on the chest x-ray film. In addition, he has risk factors of homelessness and HIV. Primary disease usually presents with middle or lower lobe infiltrates on chest radiograph while the reactivation form presents with apical infiltrates. Also evident on the biopsy are numerous Langerhans-type giant cells and lymphocytes.

4. **A 35-year-old white woman presents to the ED with acute left lower quadrant abdominal pain that has been sharp and constant for the past 2 hours. She has never had a pain like this before. The pain is a 9/10 and it does not radiate. A pelvic ultrasound is performed and shows a mass in her left ovary. She is taken to the operating room (OR) to have the mass and ovary removed, and the pathologic features are shown in Figure 27-4. What is the most likely diagnosis?**

This patient most likely had torsion of her left ovary due to a teratoma that had developed inside the organ. Most teratomas are benign and contain tissue from all three germ layers. In Figure 27-4, skin, sebaceous glands, fat cells, and a tract of neural tissue (*arrow*) are seen.

5. **A 60-year-old white man with a history of hyperlipidemia and diabetes mellitus type 2 presents to the ED with worsening chest pain and tightness along with shortness of breath (SOB) for the past hour. Aspirin is administered immediately and an electrocardiogram (ECG) is performed that shows ST-segment elevations in leads V_1 to V_5. If this man were to have biopsies taken of his myocardium at this time, they would look similar to those shown in Figure 27-5. Which part of the figure corresponds to the biopsy at 24 hours? At 48 hours? Which cells are most prominent at 24 hours? At 48 hours?**

Figure 27-5A corresponds to the biopsy taken at 24 hours, and Figure 27-5B corresponds to 48 hours. When acute injury occurs, such as an acute myocardial infarction (MI), as described in this question, neutrophils infiltrate the tissue 1 to 3 days after injury (Fig. 27-5A) and then are replaced by monocytes, which peak at 3 to 7 days (Fig. 27-5B) after the initial injury.

STEP 1 SECRET

It is important to know the phases of myocardial injury listed in (Table 27-1)

6. **A 55-year-old white man presented to the ED after suffering severe injuries in a motor vehicle accident. His blood alcohol level at the time of presentation was 300 mg/dL. He had no significant past medical history. Social history revealed that the patient consumed three to four alcoholic beverages per day for the past 10 years. He died in the ED. A section from the liver obtained at autopsy is shown in Figure 27-6. What process was occurring in his liver at the time of death?**

The process occurring in the patient's liver is fatty change (steatosis) from chronic alcohol consumption, as evidenced by the large number of lipid-filled vacuoles (white) shown in

TABLE 27-1. PHASES OF MYOCARDIAL INJURY

Time	Gross Appearance	Light Microscope	Risk
4-24 hours	Dark mottling	Contraction bands, coagulative necrosis	Arrhythmia
1-3 days	Mottling with yellow infarct center	Widespread coagulative necrosis with neutrophil migration	Arrhythmia
3-7 days	Yellow softening with hyperemic border	Macrophage infiltration	Free wall rupture, papillary muscle rupture, intraventricuar septal rupture, cardiac tamponade
10-14 days	Red-gray infarct borders	Well-developed granulation tissue	
2-8 weeks	Gray-white scar	Collagen scar formation	Ventricular aneurysm

Figure 27-6. Alcohol is a hepatotoxin that affects mitochondrial function and therefore prevents the liver from successfully metabolizing certain substances, such as triglycerides, leading to an accumulation in the liver. If this patient had lived and continued to drink the same amount, he might eventually develop cirrhosis of the liver.

7. **A 46-year-old white man presents to his primary care physician with a 1-year history of fatigue, weakness, and arthralgias. His past medical history is significant for diabetes mellitus type 2. On physical examination, his skin is a bronze color and his liver is enlarged. His mother passed away at the age of 70, and her liver biopsy is shown in Figure 27-7. What did this patient's mother pass away from, and what is most likely causing this patient's symptoms?**
The patient's mother suffered from hemochromatosis, which was likely passed on to her son. The biopsy shows rust-brown hemosiderin deposits spread throughout the liver. Hemochromatosis is an autosomal recessive disease that results in increased dietary iron absorption and increased iron release from erythrophagocytosis. Iron deposits are seen mostly in the liver, heart, and endocrine glands (note that deposition in the pancreas can result in diabetes mellitus). Treatment involves phlebotomy (bloodletting).

8. **A 74-year-old woman presents to her primary care physician complaining of constipation and hard stools for the past several weeks. Her complete blood count (CBC) showed a hematocrit (Hct) of 30%. Colonoscopy could not be completed. A computed tomography (CT) scan of the abdomen and pelvis is performed and shows a large mass in the right colon. The patient is taken to the OR to have the mass removed, and a biopsy of the mass is shown in Figure 27-8. What is the diagnosis?**
This patient has an adenocarcinoma in her right colon. In comparison with normal colonic glands, the glands shown in this biopsy are irregular in shape and size. The glands, however, are identifiable in this biopsy, so this would be considered a low-grade adenocarcinoma.

9. **A 60-year-old woman presents to her primary care physician complaining of feeling bloated and full for the past 2 months no matter how much or little she eats. She has no significant past medical history but has a family history positive for hereditary nonpolyposis colon cancer. Her physician refers her to a surgeon, who subsequently orders imaging and operates to remove a mass that was discovered. A biopsy of the mass was done once it was removed, and a preparation of the specimen is shown in Figure 27-9. What disease was discovered in this woman based on the history and histologic features described here? Why was a biopsy not done prior to removal of the tumor?**

    This woman was found to have a papillary serous cystadenocarcinoma in her ovary. Figure 27-9 shows numerous complex papillae that have invaded into the stroma. Genetic mutations contribute to tumor development and include *BRCA1* and *BRCA2*, as well as *MSH2* and *MLH1* mutations found also in hereditary nonpolyposis colon cancer. A biopsy was not done or recommended because of the risk of dissemination of tumor cells into the peritoneal cavity.

10. **A 38-year-old woman is referred by her primary care physician to a surgeon for treatment for a newly palpated, asymptomatic nodule in the left side of her thyroid. An FNA (fine needle aspiration) is performed and the patient is subsequently taken to the OR for a subtotal thyroidectomy. A section of the nodule is shown in Figure 27-10. What is the likely diagnosis? What is the next step in treatment?**

    Based on the patient's young age and pathologic findings of the nodule, the most likely diagnosis is papillary carcinoma. The biopsy shows papillary structures surrounded by nuclei that appear empty and are sometimes referred to as "Orphan Annie eye" nuclei. Papillary carcinoma is the most common type of thyroid cancer and has a very good prognosis. Treatment includes thyroidectomy followed by radioiodine ablation and thyroid-stimulating hormone (TSH) suppression with levothyroxine.

11. **A 77-year-old white man presents to his primary care physician for his annual physical and was found to have a lesion on his forehead (Fig. 27-11A). A biopsy is taken of the lesion and is shown in Figure 27-11B. What type of skin lesion is this? How should this lesion be treated?**

    This patient has a squamous cell carcinoma, which usually presents as a slow-growing nodule that eventually develops into an ulcer as the center becomes necrotic. He is an older man with fair skin who has likely had a high lifetime ultraviolet (UV) exposure, putting him at a greater risk. In this particular biopsy, atypical squamous cells are seen beyond the basement membrane, invading into the dermis. Notice the keratin pearl marked by the arrow in Figure 27-11B. Treatment is based on tumor size and depth of invasion. Some options include cryotherapy and excision with appropriate margins. This type of skin cancer can metastasize to other parts of the body.

12. **A 71-year-old man presents to his primary care physician for the first time in over 10 years with complaints of fatigue and painless lymphadenopathy. On physical examination, swollen supraclavicular, cervical, and submandibular lymph nodes are palpated along with hepatosplenomegaly. His CBC shows lymphocytosis, anemia, and thrombocytopenia. The man's peripheral blood smear is shown in Figure 27-12. What is this man's diagnosis? Should treatment be started?**

    This man has chronic lymphocytic leukemia (CLL) as evidenced by his examination findings, CBC, and peripheral blood smear. His peripheral smear shows small lymphocytes with condensed chromatin and scarce cytoplasm. The characteristic smudge cells are also seen in this smear. This man is now symptomatic, so treatment should begin with chemotherapy. If this man were asymptomatic, he could be observed rather than treated.

13. **A 95-year-old man is brought to the ED for worsening SOB, fever, and productive cough. He is stabilized in the ED and admitted to the hospital. He passes away 3 days later from complications of pneumonia. An autopsy is completed, and a biopsy of his brain is shown in Figure 27-13. What chronic disease did this man likely suffer from based on the biopsy?**

Based on the biopsy, this man most likely was also suffering from Alzheimer's disease at the time of his death. The arrow in Figure 27-13 shows neurofibillary tangles. Also present in most biopsies of Alzheimer's patients are plaques, neuronal loss, and brain atrophy. Pharmacologic treatment includes cholinesterase inhibitors, antidepressants, and antipsychotics if needed.

14. **A 21-year-old woman presents to her gynecologist for her yearly Papanicolaou (Pap) smear. She has been sexually active with three male partners in the past. She has no physical complaints. Her Pap smear is shown in Figure 27-14. What is shown on this Pap smear? What is the next step in management? What is the most likely cause?**

The Pap smear shows a high-grade squamous intraepithelial lesion as evidenced by the reduced amount of cytoplasm in the squamous epithelial cells and the increased nucleus-to-cytoplasm ratio, as well as the hyperchromatic, enlarged nuclei with irregular outlines. The next step in management is a colposcopy to look for any abnormal-appearing areas on the cervix and biopsy them. The most likely cause is human papillomavirus (HPV) 16 or 18. If left untreated, it could develop into cervical cancer.

15. **A 71-year-old man is brought to the ED with an acute exacerbation of congestive heart failure. He has had long-standing left-sided heart failure, atherosclerosis, and hypertension. In the ED, he is unable to be resuscitated. An autopsy is performed, and a gross specimen of his heart is shown in Figure 27-15. What is the most likely cause of his left-sided heart failure based on this figure? What type of heart murmur did this patient likely have?**

The gross specimen shown in Figure 27-15 is the aortic valve with calcific aortic stenosis, which likely contributed to this patient's heart failure. The patient likely had a systolic crescendo-decrescendo murmur heard best at the right upper sternal border that radiated to the carotid arteries.

16. **A 48-year-old woman is referred by her gynecologist to a surgeon for a newly palpated lump in her right breast that was not seen on mammography or ultrasound. On physical examination, the lump is about 1 cm in diameter and palpated in the upper outer quadrant of the right breast. The lump is firm but mobile. The patient undergoes stereotactic biopsy, which reveals the lump to be benign but with the incidental finding shown in Figure 27-16. What is the incidental finding? What is the next step in management?**

The incidental finding is lobular carcinoma in situ (LCIS). The biopsy shows a population of small, rounded cells that do not adhere to one another and fill the lobule. The underlying lobular architecture can still be recognized. The next step in management depends upon the patient's preference. One option would be observation plus tamoxifen for 5 years to decrease the risk of progression to invasive breast cancer; the other option would be bilateral mastectomies, as LCIS is bilateral and found throughout the breast.

17. **A 15-year-old boy's father dies at the age of 50. An autopsy is performed, and the gross colon specimen is shown in Figure 27-17. What does this specimen indicate about a hereditary disorder in this family? What is this boy at risk for developing in the future? What is the treatment for this condition?**

The colon shown in Figure 27-17 has more than 100 polyps, which is the diagnostic criteria for familial adenomatous polyposis (FAP), an autosomal dominant condition caused by germ-line mutations of the APC (adenomatous polyposis coli) tumor suppressor gene. People who have FAP have close to 100% risk of developing colorectal cancer by the age of 40. In FAP, the rectum is always involved. This contrasts with Lynch syndrome, in which the right side of the colon is generally involved. The treatment for FAP is a total proctocolectomy.

18. **A 62-year-old man develops severe chest pain that radiates down his left arm while eating dinner at home. He has a history of angina, hypertension, and diabetes mellitus type 2. He is brought to the ED by ambulance, and upon arrival, he is hemodynamically unstable and in cardiac arrest. He is unable to be resuscitated and he expires 30 minutes later. An autopsy is performed. A heart specimen is shown in Figure 27-18. In which part of the heart did this patient's MI occur? What leads on an ECG would have possibly shown ST-segment elevations or depressions? What artery or arteries supply that part of the heart?**

This patient's MI occurred in the posterolateral portion of the left ventricle, as shown by the discoloration and necrotic area (arrows) in Figure 27-18. The leads on the ECG that would have likely been affected are II, III, and aVF for the posterior portion and I, aVL, and V_6 for the lateral portion. This section of the heart is supplied mostly by the circumflex artery, with some of the posterior portion being supplied by the posterior descending artery off the right coronary artery.

19. **A 63-year-old native Hawaiian woman presents to her primary care physician with worsening dull, aching back pain and fatigue. She has not seen a physician for many years, so no past medical history is available. Her CBC showed a Hct of 31%. Her calcium level was 13.1 mg/dL. Otherwise, her blood work was normal. A bone marrow aspiration was performed and is shown in Figure 27-19. What is this woman's diagnosis? What will be found in her urine?**

This patient has multiple myeloma, which is a hematologic cancer characterized by terminally differentiated plasma cells, infiltration of the bone marrow by plasma cells, and monoclonal immunoglobulin (Ig) in the serum or urine. Patients can have anemia, renal disease, and osteolytic bone disease leading to hypercalcemia. Figure 27-19 shows a plasma cell infiltrate that contain multiple nuclei and droplets containing immunoglobulin in the cytoplasm. A serum/urine electrophoresis and serum free light chain assay should also be performed. M protein in the serum will be found along with light chains in the urine. Treatment involves bone marrow transplantation and bisphosphonates for the osteolytic bone disease.

20. **A 69-year-old white man presents to his primary care physician with a 4-week history of worsening cough productive of blood-tinged sputum, 10-lb weight loss, and SOB. He has a 50-pack-year history of smoking and has not been for a routine check-up for over 8 years. Blood work is normal except for a calcium level of 12.5 mg/dL. Chest radiograph is negative for any obvious acute process. A bronchoscopy with biopsy is performed with the results shown in Figure 27-20. What is this man's diagnosis? Why is his calcium elevated?**

Based on the history and biopsy shown in Figure 27-20, this man has squamous cell lung carcinoma, as indicated by the keratinization seen in the biopsy. Squamous cell carcinoma is more centrally located in the larger bronchi compared with adenocarcinoma, which is more peripheral. Therefore, symptoms normally arise once the tumor is large and obstructive. The calcium is elevated in this patient because squamous cell lung carcinoma is associated with parathyroid hormone–related protein (PTHrP) production, which leads to hypercalcemia.

21. A 26-year-old white man has a 2-week history of fevers that come and go, night sweats, and cervical and supraclavicular lymphadenopathy. His past medical history is significant only for mononucleosis 3 years prior. His CBC shows a hemoglobin level of 11.8 g/dL, white blood cell (WBC) count of 5000 cells/mm³, and a platelet count of 100,000/mm³. A lymph node biopsy is taken and is shown in Figure 27-21. What disease does this man have? What is the name of the cell seen in Figure 27-21?

This man has Hodgkin's lymphoma, which is a hematologic malignancy arising from mature B cells. The biopsy in Figure 27-21 shows a classic Reed-Sternberg cell, which harbors Epstein-Barr virus in many cases. These cells are in the minority in a lymph node effaced by infiltrates of mature lymphocytes, plasma cells, and often eosinophils. In developed countries, there is a bimodal incidence, with the first peak around age 25 and the second after age 50 to 60 years. Symptoms can include night sweats, fevers, and lymphadenopathy. CBC will show decreased hemoglobin, WBCs, and platelets. Treatment includes chemoradiation therapy.

STEP 1 SECRET

Images of Reed-Sternberg cells are commonly shown on boards. Be sure to differentiate these cells from the owl's eye inclusion bodies seen with cytomegalovirus (CMV) infection, which have a single nucleus.

22. A 66-year-old man with a history of diabetes mellitus and many hospital admissions for nausea and vomiting was killed in a drunk driving accident. Upon autopsy, biopsies of various organs were obtained, and one section is shown in Figure 27-22. What chronic disease process did this man suffer from? How is this condition treated? What are the complications?

This man suffered from chronic pancreatitis, likely from chronic alcohol consumption. Figure 27-22 is a pancreas biopsy demonstrating characteristic parenchymal fibrosis and atrophy. Residual islets and ducts can also be seen on the left and right, respectively, along with scattered inflammatory cells. Treatment consists of analgesia, hydration, and alcohol cessation. Potential complications include diabetes mellitus, pancreatic calcifications, malabsorption, narcotic addiction, and pancreatic pseudocysts.

23. A 55-year-old African-American man with a history of GERD presents to his primary care physician with a 10-lb weight loss in the past month, abdominal pain, and dysphagia. He has a 30-pack-year history of smoking. He undergoes an EGD with biopsy the following day, which is shown in Figure 27-23. What is the diagnosis for this patient? What is the next step in treatment?

This patient has gastric carcinoma, intestinal type based on the history and biopsies. In Figure 27-23, malignant cells can be seen forming glands and invading the muscular wall of the stomach. Mucin can also be seen inside the malignant cells. In the United States, proximal gastric cancer is more prevalent and is associated with *Helicobacter pylori*. In areas such as East Asia, Eastern Europe and South America, distal gastric cancers are more prevalent. The next step in treatment is staging, which includes CT scan of the chest, abdomen, and pelvis and endoscopic ultrasound.

24. A 72-year-old African-American man presents to his primary care physician with a 7-week history of worsening cough productive of blood-tinged sputum, 15-lb weight loss, and dyspnea. The patient has a 75-pack-year history of smoking. CBC is within normal limits. A chem 7 reveals a serum sodium of 130 mEq/L but is otherwise normal. Chest x-ray film shows a central mass on the right side. A bronchoscopy and biopsy are performed with the results shown in Figure 27-24. What is this patient's diagnosis? Why is the serum sodium low?

Based on this patient's history and biopsy, he has small cell lung carcinoma. It is usually centrally located near the hilum and is more often metastatic than the non–small cell lung carcinomas. It is also associated with ectopic production of adrenocorticotropic hormone (ACTH) and antidiuretic hormone (ADH), which explains the decreased serum sodium in this patient. Figure 27-24 shows small, round, densely packed cells with scarce cytoplasm and some areas of necrosis. This type of cancer is also frequently referred to as oat cell carcinoma.

Note: Squamous cell carcinoma and small cell carcinoma of the lung are both associated with smoking, but adenocarcinoma is not.

25. A 55-year-old man presents to his primary care physician with a 3-week history of fever that comes and goes, a weight loss of 5 lb, weakness, fatigue, purpura, and paresthesias in his distal upper and lower extremities. His past medical history is significant for diabetes mellitus type 2 and hypertension, both of which are well controlled. A CBC shows Hct of 38%, WBC count of 11,500 cells/mm³, and platelet count of 500,000/mm³. During the wait for the results of other ordered laboratory values, a biopsy is taken of the affected tissue on one of his legs and is shown in Figure 27-25. What is this patient's most likely diagnosis? What is the cause of this disease?

This patient has polyarteritis nodosa, which is caused by immune complex deposition in the walls of medium-sized arteries. Figure 27-25 shows a necrotic vessel wall that is replaced by pink, fibrinoid material. This type of reaction is classified as a type III hypersensitivity reaction. Treatment consists of steroids and disease-modifying antirheumatic drugs (DMARDs).

Note: Polyarteritis nodosa generally affects all visceral vessels except the pulmonary arteries.

26. A 32-year-old man presents to his primary care physician complaining of a lump in his testicle that has been present for the past 2 months and seems to be getting bigger but is not causing him any pain. On physical examination, a hard, painless lump is palpated in one of his testes. Blood work is ordered and shows normal β-hCG (human chorionic gonadotropin) and α-fetoprotein (AFP) levels. The patient undergoes a radical orchiectomy, and a section of the mass is shown in Figure 27-26. What type of testicular mass did this patient have? What is the treatment?

This patient had a seminoma of his testicle as evidenced by the hard, painless mass and the histologic appearance shown in Figure 27-26. Figure 27-26A demonstrates seminoma cells that are divided into classic lobules by septa consisting of fibrous tissue containing lymphocytes and blood vessels. Figure 27-26B shows numerous large seminoma cells that are polyhedral in shape, have clear cytoplasm and well-defined cell borders, and contain distinct nucleoli. Treatment includes radical orchiectomy followed by radiation, as these tumors are highly radiosensitive.

27. A 65-year-old African-American man presents to his primary care physician with a 4-month history of fatigue and dyspnea on exertion. He has no medical conditions that he can recall, and he does not know his family history. On physical examination, he has JVD and bilateral pedal edema that exteds to his knees. His doctor prescribes furosemide, but the patient returns to the office 4 weeks later with no improvement and increased edema. His CBC is normal. A 24-hour urine collection shows 2 g of protein. A tissue biopsy is taken and is shown under polarized light in Figure 27-27. What condition does this man have? What is the cause of his edema?

This patient suffers from amyloidosis. Figure 27-27 shows birefringence of the amyloid deposits. This patient has a systemic process that is evidenced by his edema and JVD. The edema is likely caused by hypoalbuminemia from the amyloid deposits in the kidneys causing nephritic syndrome. In addition, he has deposits in his heart causing a restrictive cardiomyopathy, which leads to high right-sided filling pressures causing edema and JVD.

STEP 1 SECRET

Although fair game on the USMLE, it is relatively low-yield to know the different types of amyloidosis. For this reason, we have chosen not to include this information in this chapter.

28. An 85-year-old man presents to his primary care physician with a 2-week history of what the patient describes as hives on his elbows, knees, and lower abdomen that are pruritic. Yesterday, the patient reports that the hives began to develop into large blisters. A skin biopsy is taken and shown under light microscopy (Fig. 27-28A) and immunofluorescence (Fig. 27-28B). What condition does this man have? Between what layers do the blisters develop?

Based on the biopsy and history, this man has bullous pemphigoid, an autoimmune disease. The reaction is initiated by immunoglobulin G (IgG) autoantibodies to hemidesmosome. On light microscopy, the biopsied tissue shows the beginning of epidermal separation from the dermis, creating a subepidermal space. Also seen are eosinophils, lymphocytes, and neutrophils associated with the destruction. On immunofluorescence, the tissue sample shows characteristic linear deposition of complement along the dermoepidermal junction. In comparison, pemphigus vulgaris involves autoantibodies against desmoglein and results in separation of keratinocytes from the basal layer of the epidermis. On immunofluorescence, pemphigus vulgaris has a fish-net pattern. Pemphigus vulgaris is also typically associated with oral lesions, whereas bullous pemphigoid is not.

29. A 61-year-old white woman is brought to the ED in critical condition following a motor vehicle accident. On physical examination, she has numerous lacerations on her face, with bruising across her chest from the seatbelt, and she is hemodynamically unstable. She also has hyperreflexia of her upper and lower extremities and an upward-going toe reflex. In addition, she has muscle atrophy of her upper and lower extremities. She is unable to be stabilized and dies 45 minutes later. An autopsy is performed, and a section of the patient's spinal cord is shown in Figure 27-29. What disease did this woman suffer from? What is the significance of the neurologic examination findings?

This patient had amyotrophic lateral sclerosis (ALS), which is a neurodegenerative disorder. It involves both the upper and lower motor neurons, which explains the findings of hyperreflexia, the positive Babinski sign (upper motor neuron), and muscle atrophy (lower motor neuron). This section of the spinal cord shows loss of myelinated fibers in the corticospinal tracts.

30. **A 67-year-old white man is brought to the ED from his primary care physician's office with decreased urine output, hemoptysis, fever, lower extremity edema, and SOB. The patient has a 40-pack-year history of smoking. He is stabilized in the ED, and a renal biopsy is performed, which is shown in Figure 27-30. What is this man's underlying diagnosis? What type of antibodies would be found?**
    This man has Goodpasture's syndrome, which is an autoimmune disease that affects the kidneys and lungs. Figure 27-30 demonstrates crescentic glomerulonephritis, a severe end point of Goodpasture syndrome. On fluorescence microscopy, there would be linear IgG and C3 deposits. The disease is caused by autoantibodies to the α-3 chain of type IV collagen, which are found in the lung and in the glomerular basement membrane. This is a rapidly progressing disease that, other than dialysis, is treated with supportive care.

31. **A 68-year-old man presents to his primary care physician with worsening dysphagia and odynophagia. The patient states that he can barely swallow liquids any longer and is now losing weight. His past medical history is significant for hypertension and hyperlipidemia. He has a 75-pack-year history of smoking and has consumed an average of five shots of vodka per day for the past 20 years. His primary care physician sends him to have an EGD with biopsy, which is shown in Figure 27-31. What is this patient's diagnosis? What is the treatment for this disease?**
    Based on this patient's alcohol and smoking history along with the biopsy, he has squamous cell carcinoma of the esophagus. The biopsy shows the carcinoma invading into the submucosa. The treatment of this disease depends on how large the carcinoma is and whether the patient is able to undergo surgery. In most cases, these tumors are unresectable but are responsive to radiation therapy. Management therefore centers on palliative care, including stenting to allow the patient to eat a soft diet.
    Other risk factors for squamous cell carcinoma of the esophagus include achalasia, diverticula, esophageal web, esophagitis, nitrosamines, and family history.

32. **A 32-year-old woman undergoes a kidney transplantation, and 2 weeks after surgery, she develops stomach pain, diarrhea, weight loss, night sweats, and fever. A lymph node biopsy is performed and is shown in Figure 27-32. What did this woman develop? Why did she develop it?**
    This woman developed Burkitt's lymphoma (associated with Epstein-Barr virus) while she was immunosuppressed following her kidney transplant procedure. The biopsy shows a "starry sky" pattern due to the scattered macrophages containing apoptotic fragments (tingible bodies) within a monotonous population of lymphoid cells. Chemotherapy is the mainstay of therapy. The sporadic form of Burkitt's lymphoma is associated with pelvic and abdominal lesions, while the form endemic to Africa (often seeing in young children) is associated with jaw lesions.

33. An 83-year-old white man is brought to his primary care physician by his daughter for a newly discovered skin lesion. The lesion is pearly white (Fig. 27-33A). A biopsy of the lesion is performed (Fig. 27-33B). What type of lesion is this? What is the next step in treatment?

This patient has a basal cell carcinoma, as evidenced by the pearly white gross appearance and the presence of palisading nests of basal cells in the dermis that contain numerous mitotic and apoptotic figures. Basal cell carcinoma is locally invasive and destructive. Treatment involves excision of the lesion and in most cases is curative. Cryotherapy and topical therapies are also options.

34. A 22-year-old woman presents to her primary care physician with complaints of fatigue and dyspnea on exertion for the past 4 weeks. She has no significant past medical history. Her CBC shows Hct of 30%, hemoglobin of 10 g/dL, and platelet count of 350,000/mm^3. Her mean corpuscular volume (MCV) is 70 fL. Her serum iron and ferritin are decreased and total iron-binding capacity (TIBC) is increased. A peripheral blood smear is shown in Figure 27-34. What is this woman's diagnosis? What is the likely cause of this condition in this patient?

This patient has hypochromic microcytic anemia due to iron deficiency. The peripheral blood smear shows pale areas within the red blood cells (RBCs) and thin rims of peripheral hemoglobin. This patient is premenopausal, and therefore, the most likely cause of this condition is blood loss from heavy menses or menorrhagia.

35. A 45-year-old premenopausal obese African-American woman presents to her gynecologist with complaints of menorrhagia and intermenstrual bleeding for the past 4 months. She has never been pregnant, and her age at menarche was 11. Her CBC shows hypochromic microcytic anemia. A uterine biopsy is performed and shown in Figure 27-35. What is the most likely diagnosis? What is the treatment?

This woman has endometrial adenocarcinoma. Adenocarcinoma can be distinguished from hyperplasia by the presence of "back-to-back" glands and stromal invasion. Figure 27-35 shows preserved glandular architecture, making this a well-differentiated tumor. This woman has been exposed to unopposed estrogen, which puts her at an increased risk for developing this disease; this is usually due to the conversion of adrenal androgens by peripheral adipose tissue to estrone in the obese postmenopausal woman whose endometrium is still responsive to estrogen. Treatment includes total abdominal hysterectomy, bilateral salpingo-oophorectomy, and node dissection. She may or may not need chemoradiation.

36. A 59-year-old white man with a history of hypertension and hyperlipidemia presents to the ED with severe chest pain that started 2 hours earlier. It has been constant and radiates down his left arm. On physical examination, he is tachypnic, tachycardic, and diaphoretic. He is given oxygen and aspirin, and an ECG shows ST-segment elevations in leads V_1 to V_4. While in the ED, he goes into cardiac arrest and is unable to be resuscitated. An autopsy is performed, and a section of one of his coronary arteries is shown in Figure 27-36. What was the cause of his MI? What coronary artery was likely affected?

This patient developed an acute thrombosis superimposed on an atherosclerotic plaque with disruption of the fibrous cap, which led to his MI. In Figure 27-36, you can see a break in the fibrous cap and the necrotic, largely lipid core of the plaque (arrow). This plaque is in the left anterior descending artery based on the fact that the ECG shows an anterior MI.

37. **A 14-year-old African-American boy has a history of splenomegaly and undergoes a splenectomy. A section of his spleen is shown in Figure 27-37. What disease does this boy suffer from based on the appearance of his spleen? What vaccines does he need to receive prior to his splenectomy?**

This boy has sickle cell anemia, which causes congestion in the spleen, leading to splenomegaly. The sinusoids that are congested are shown in Figure 27-37. In Figure 27-37, the sinusoids that are congested are darker whereas the pale areas represent fibrosis secondary to previous ischemic damage. Prior to a splenectomy, patients need to be vaccinated for *Streptococcus pneumoniae, Haemophilus influenzae,* and *Neisseria meningitidis,* which are encapsulated organisms normally destroyed by splenic macrophages. These organisms are common causes of sepsis after splenectomy.

38. **An 18-year-old woman presents to her primary care physician with complaints of diarrhea, weight loss (5 lb), and abdominal pain after meals since she started college in the fall (4 months ago). She has not been sick recently other than the symptoms stated and has had no fevers. She is unsure whether her diet has changed at all, but says she now eats a lot of pizza while studying late at night. The physician orders some laboratory tests, and the patient undergoes an intestinal biopsy later that week (Fig. 27-38). What is the most likely cause of this patient's symptoms? What causes this condition?**

This patient is suffering from celiac disease, as evidenced by the atrophy and blunting of villi in her small intestine seen on the biopsy in the figure. Chronic inflammation is also seen in the lamina propria. This is a systemic autoimmune disease triggered by gluten peptides found in wheat, rye, barley, and similar grains. A positive IgA tissue transglutaminase serologic test is suggestive of celiac disease, but a duodenal biopsy is confirmatory.

39. **A 30-year-old woman from the northeastern part of the United States presents to her primary care physician with crampy right lower quadrant abdominal pain that is partially relieved with defecation, nonbloody diarrhea, a weight loss of 10 lb in the past 2 months, and fevers that come and go. On physical examination, there is right lower quadrant tenderness, but no guarding or masses. On rectal examination, numerous perianal skin tags are present, and she has guaiac-positive stool. CBC shows a WBC count of 12,500 cells/mm³ and Hct of 32%. She undergoes a colonoscopy and EGD with biopsy (Fig. 27-39). During the colonoscopy, skip lesions were noted. What condition does this woman have? What are potential complications of this condition?**

This woman has Crohn's disease (CD) as evidenced by the skip lesions, perianal skin tags, and appearance on biopsy. Figure 27-39 shows a deep fissure extending into the muscle wall and lymphocyte aggregates between the mucosa and submucosa. CD involves the mouth to the anus, whereas ulcerative colitis (UC) normally involves the rectum and is continuous. CD is also transmural, but UC involves only the mucosa. Noncaseating granulomas may be found in the intestines of patients with CD, and crypt abscesses are found in those with UC. Peak age at onset of CD is between 15 and 40 years, with another peak between 60 and 80 years. There are a number of potential complications that this woman needs to be monitored for, including extraintestinal manifestations such as arthritis and intestinal complications such as fistulas and primary sclerosing cholangitis. She is also at increased risk for colon cancer, although colon cancer has a stronger association with UC than with CD.

40. **A 45-year-old homeless man is brought to the ED with vomiting and fever. On physical examination, he is disheveled and has track marks on both arms. The rest of his examination is normal except for right upper quadrant abdominal tenderness. His blood work shows a WBC count of 13,000 cells/mm³. Also he**

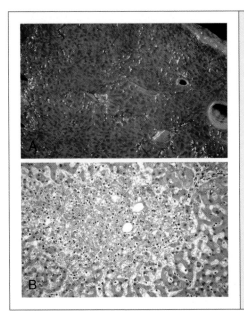

Figure 27-1. (From Kumar V, Fausto N, Abbas A: Robbins and Cotran Pathologic Basis of Disease, 7th ed. Philadelphia, WB Saunders, 2004.)

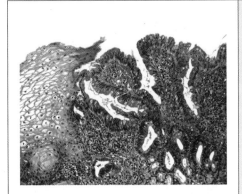

Figure 27-2. (From Kumar V, Fausto N, Abbas A: Robbins and Cotran Pathologic Basis of Disease, 7th ed. Philadelphia, WB Saunders, 2004.)

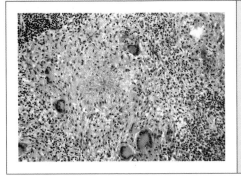

Figure 27-3. (From Kumar V, Fausto N, Abbas A: Robbins and Cotran Pathologic Basis of Disease, 7th ed. Philadelphia, WB Saunders, 2004.)

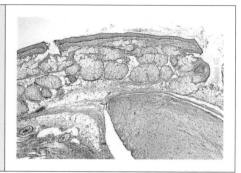

Figure 27-4. (From Kumar V, Fausto N, Abbas A: Robbins and Cotran Pathologic Basis of Disease, 7th ed. Philadelphia, WB Saunders, 2004.)

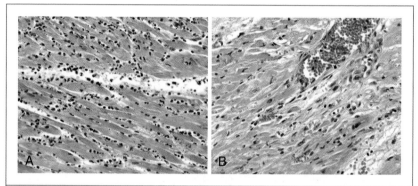

Figure 27-5. (From Kumar V, Fausto N, Abbas A: Robbins and Cotran Pathologic Basis of Disease, 7th ed. Philadelphia, WB Saunders, 2004.)

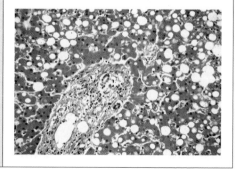

Figure 27-6. (From Kumar V, Fausto N, Abbas A: Robbins and Cotran Pathologic Basis of Disease, 7th ed. Philadelphia, WB Saunders, 2004.)

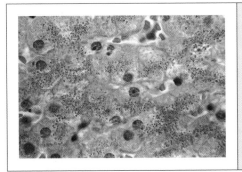

Figure 27-7. (From Kumar V, Fausto N, Abbas A: Robbins and Cotran Pathologic Basis of Disease, 7th ed. Philadelphia, WB Saunders, 2004.)

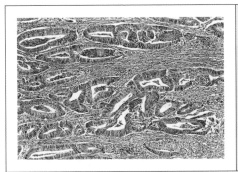

Figure 27-8. (From Kumar V, Fausto N, Abbas A: Robbins and Cotran Pathologic Basis of Disease, 7th ed. Philadelphia, WB Saunders, 2004.)

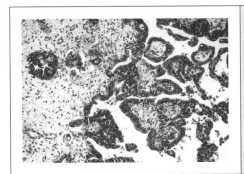

Figure 27-9. (From Kumar V, Fausto N, Abbas A: Robbins and Cotran Pathologic Basis of Disease, 7th ed. Philadelphia, WB Saunders, 2004.)

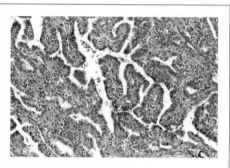

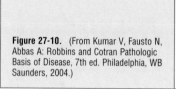

Figure 27-10. (From Kumar V, Fausto N, Abbas A: Robbins and Cotran Pathologic Basis of Disease, 7th ed. Philadelphia, WB Saunders, 2004.)

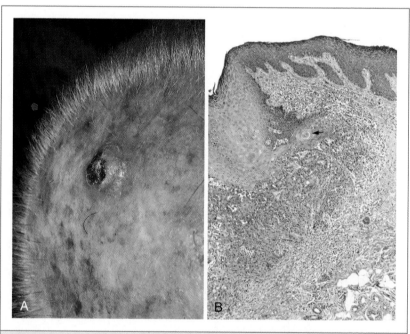

Figure 27-11. (From Kumar V, Fausto N, Abbas A: Robbins and Cotran Pathologic Basis of Disease, 7th ed. Philadelphia, WB Saunders, 2004.)

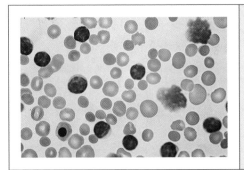

Figure 27-12. (From Kumar V, Fausto N, Abbas A: Robbins and Cotran Pathologic Basis of Disease, 7th ed. Philadelphia, WB Saunders, 2004.)

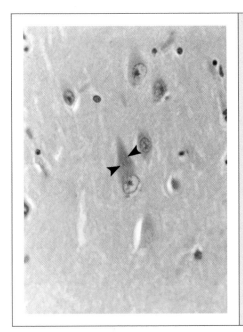

Figure 27-13. (From Kumar V, Fausto N, Abbas A: Robbins and Cotran Pathologic Basis of Disease, 7th ed. Philadelphia, WB Saunders, 2004.)

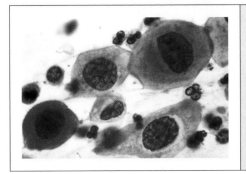

Figure 27-14. (From Kumar V, Fausto N, Abbas A: Robbins and Cotran Pathologic Basis of Disease, 7th ed. Philadelphia, WB Saunders, 2004.)

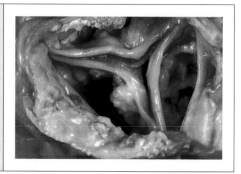

Figure 27-15. (From Kumar V, Fausto N, Abbas A: Robbins and Cotran Pathologic Basis of Disease, 7th ed. Philadelphia, WB Saunders, 2004.)

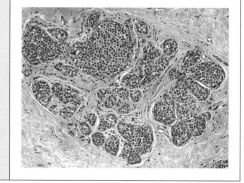

Figure 27-16. (From Kumar V, Fausto N, Abbas A: Robbins and Cotran Pathologic Basis of Disease, 7th ed. Philadelphia, WB Saunders, 2004.)

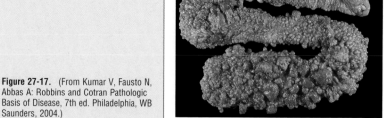

Figure 27-17. (From Kumar V, Fausto N, Abbas A: Robbins and Cotran Pathologic Basis of Disease, 7th ed. Philadelphia, WB Saunders, 2004.)

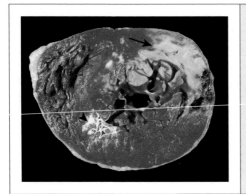

Figure 27-18. (From Kumar V, Fausto N, Abbas A: Robbins and Cotran Pathologic Basis of Disease, 7th ed. Philadelphia, WB Saunders, 2004.)

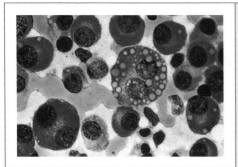

Figure 27-19. (From Kumar V, Fausto N, Abbas A: Robbins and Cotran Pathologic Basis of Disease, 7th ed. Philadelphia, WB Saunders, 2004.)

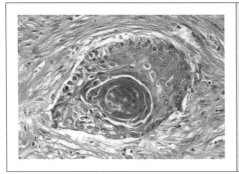

Figure 27-20. (From Kumar V, Fausto N, Abbas A: Robbins and Cotran Pathologic Basis of Disease, 7th ed. Philadelphia, WB Saunders, 2004.)

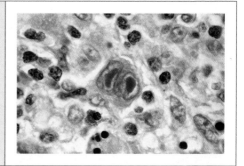

Figure 27-21. (From Kumar V, Fausto N, Abbas A: Robbins and Cotran Pathologic Basis of Disease, 7th ed. Philadelphia, WB Saunders, 2004.)

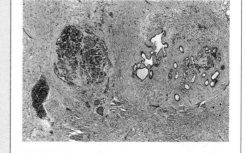

Figure 27-22. (From Kumar V, Fausto N, Abbas A: Robbins and Cotran Pathologic Basis of Disease, 7th ed. Philadelphia, WB Saunders, 2004.)

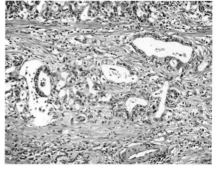

Figure 27-23. (From Kumar V, Fausto N, Abbas A: Robbins and Cotran Pathologic Basis of Disease, 7th ed. Philadelphia, WB Saunders, 2004.)

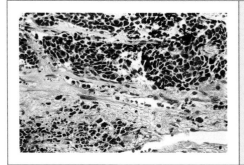

Figure 27-24. (From Kumar V, Fausto N, Abbas A: Robbins and Cotran Pathologic Basis of Disease, 7th ed. Philadelphia, WB Saunders, 2004.)

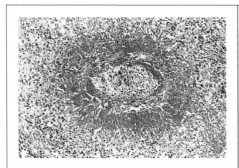

Figure 27-25. (From Kumar V, Fausto N, Abbas A: Robbins and Cotran Pathologic Basis of Disease, 7th ed. Philadelphia, WB Saunders, 2004.)

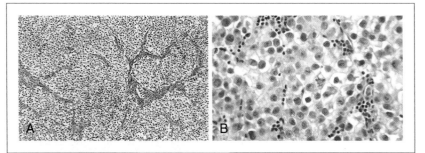

Figure 27-26. (From Kumar V, Fausto N, Abbas A: Robbins and Cotran Pathologic Basis of Disease, 7th ed. Philadelphia, WB Saunders, 2004.)

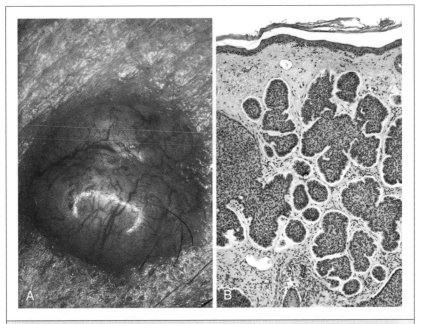

Figure 27-33. (From Kumar V, Fausto N, Abbas A: Robbins and Cotran Pathologic Basis of Disease, 7th ed. Philadelphia, WB Saunders, 2004.)

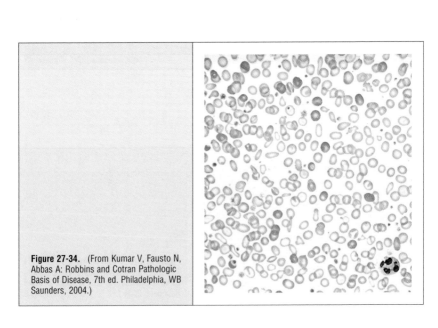

Figure 27-34. (From Kumar V, Fausto N, Abbas A: Robbins and Cotran Pathologic Basis of Disease, 7th ed. Philadelphia, WB Saunders, 2004.)

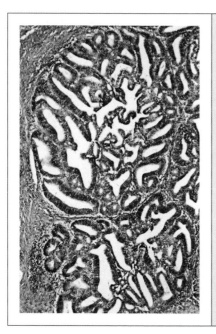

Figure 27-35. (From Kumar V, Fausto N, Abbas A: Robbins and Cotran Pathologic Basis of Disease, 7th ed. Philadelphia, WB Saunders, 2004.)

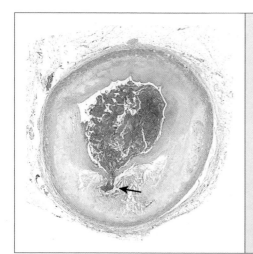

Figure 27-36. (From Kumar V, Fausto N, Abbas A: Robbins and Cotran Pathologic Basis of Disease, 7th ed. Philadelphia, WB Saunders, 2004.)

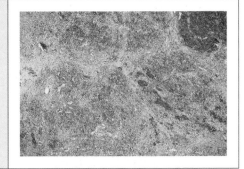

Figure 27-37. (From Kumar V, Fausto N, Abbas A: Robbins and Cotran Pathologic Basis of Disease, 7th ed. Philadelphia, WB Saunders, 2004.)

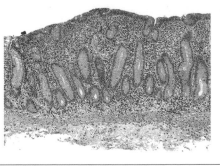

Figure 27-38. (From Kumar V, Fausto N, Abbas A: Robbins and Cotran Pathologic Basis of Disease, 7th ed. Philadelphia, WB Saunders, 2004.)

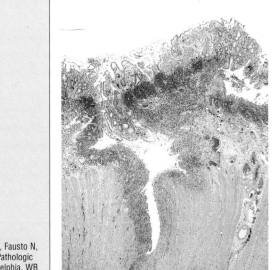

Figure 27-39. (From Kumar V, Fausto N, Abbas A: Robbins and Cotran Pathologic Basis of Disease, 7th ed. Philadelphia, WB Saunders, 2004.)

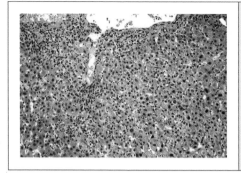

Figure 27-40. (From Kumar V, Fausto N, Abbas A: Robbins and Cotran Pathologic Basis of Disease, 7th ed. Philadelphia, WB Saunders, 2004.)

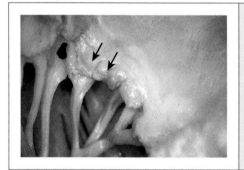

Figure 27-41. (From Kumar V, Fausto N, Abbas A: Robbins and Cotran Pathologic Basis of Disease, 7th ed. Philadelphia, WB Saunders, 2004.)

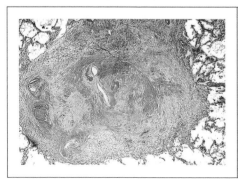

Figure 27-42. (From Kumar V, Fausto N, Abbas A: Robbins and Cotran Pathologic Basis of Disease, 7th ed. Philadelphia, WB Saunders, 2004.)

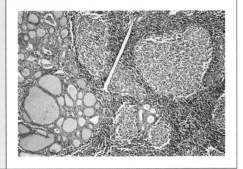

Figure 27-43. (From Kumar V, Fausto N, Abbas A: Robbins and Cotran Pathologic Basis of Disease, 7th ed. Philadelphia, WB Saunders, 2004.)

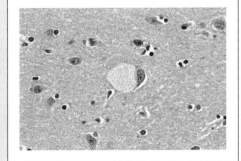

Figure 27-44. (From Kumar V, Fausto N, Abbas A: Robbins and Cotran Pathologic Basis of Disease, 7th ed. Philadelphia, WB Saunders, 2004.)

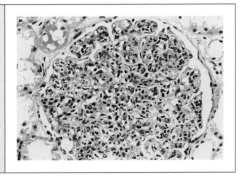

Figure 27-45. (From Kumar V, Fausto N, Abbas A: Robbins and Cotran Pathologic Basis of Disease, 7th ed. Philadelphia, WB Saunders, 2004.)

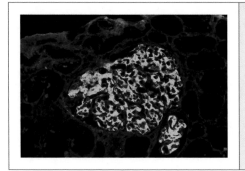

Figure 27-46. (From Kumar V, Fausto N, Abbas A: Robbins and Cotran Pathologic Basis of Disease, 7th ed. Philadelphia, WB Saunders, 2004.)

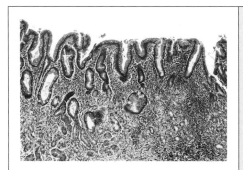

Figure 27-47. (From Kumar V, Fausto N, Abbas A: Robbins and Cotran Pathologic Basis of Disease, 7th ed. Philadelphia, WB Saunders, 2004.)

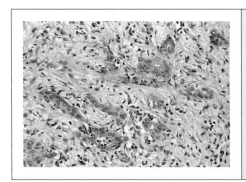

Figure 27-48. (From Kumar V, Fausto N, Abbas A: Robbins and Cotran Pathologic Basis of Disease, 7th ed. Philadelphia, WB Saunders, 2004.)

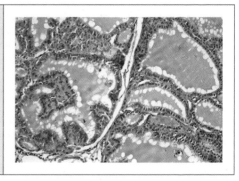

Figure 27-49. (From Kumar V, Fausto N, Abbas A: Robbins and Cotran Pathologic Basis of Disease, 7th ed. Philadelphia, WB Saunders, 2004.)

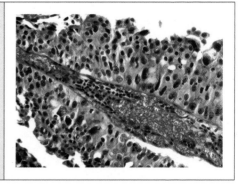

Figure 27-50. (From Kumar V, Fausto N, Abbas A: Robbins and Cotran Pathologic Basis of Disease, 7th ed. Philadelphia, WB Saunders, 2004.)

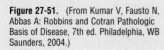

Figure 27-51. (From Kumar V, Fausto N, Abbas A: Robbins and Cotran Pathologic Basis of Disease, 7th ed. Philadelphia, WB Saunders, 2004.)

has a positive serum HBsAg, negative HBsAb, positive HBcAb (IgM), negative HBcAb (IgG), and negative hepatitis C virus (HCV) antibodies. A biopsy of his liver is shown in Figure 27-40. What disease does this man have? How did he most likely acquire it? What are the complications of this disease?

This man has an acute hepatitis B infection based on the serologic features and biopsy. The biopsy shows disruption of lobular architecture along with inflammatory cells in the sinusoids. He most likely acquired it from intravenous drug use. This acute infection may develop into a chronic state, which may lead to complications such as cirrhosis, hepatocellular carcinoma, and liver failure.

Note: Councilman bodies (not singled out in this image) are often seen in association with viral hepatitis. These are eosinophilic hepatocytes undergoing apoptosis secondary to infection.

41. A 35-year-old Hawaiian man presents to his primary care physician for his yearly physical. The only complaint that he has are the arthralgias that he has been having for the past 2 weeks. His past medical history is significant only for numerous episodes of streptococcal pharyngitis as a child. His physical examination is normal except for a new murmur appreciated on cardiac examination. The murmur is a 3/6 pansystolic murmur heard best at the apex, and radiates to his axilla. Upon his death 1 year later in a motor vehicle accident, an autopsy is performed. A gross picture of his heart is shown in Figure 27-41. What was his murmur most likely the result of? What valve was affected? What type of bacteria is responsible for this resulting condition?

His murmur was the result of rheumatic valvulitis that developed from his previous exposures to *Streptococcus* as a child. The valve affected was the mitral valve, as seen in Figure 27-41. The gross section shows acute rheumatic mitral valvulitis, with small vegetations, fibrous thickening, and fusion of the chordae tendineae. The bacteria responsible is group A streptococcus (*Streptococcus pyogenes*).

42. A 70-year-old retired man, who worked in a ceramics manufacturing facility, presents to his primary care physician with worsening dyspnea, which previously occurred only on exertion but now occurs when sitting, and a dry nonproductive cough. His physical examination is normal except for some scattered wheezing on chest auscultation. Chest x-ray study is negative for any masses or acute processes. A lung biopsy is performed and is shown in Figure 27-42. What chronic condition is this man suffering from? What is he at an increased risk of developing?

This man is suffering from silicosis as a result of his occupational exposure in ceramics manufacturing. Figure 27-42 shows collagenous silicotic nodules within the lung. Patients with silicosis may also demonstrate "eggshell calcifications" of local lymph nodes. This patient needs to be followed closely because he is at an increased risk for developing pneumonia, TB, chronic obstructive pulmonary disease (COPD), chronic renal failure, and lung cancer.

43. A 51-year-old woman presents to her primary care physician with weight gain of 10 lb in the last month, along with fatigue, muscle cramps, and constipation. She is still having her usual monthly periods. Her physical examination is significant for bradycardia but is otherwise normal. Her physician orders blood work, and a thyroid biopsy is performed later that week, which is shown in Figure 27-43. What condition is this woman suffering from? What antibodies are associated with this condition?

This woman has Hashimoto's thyroiditis. Her biopsy shows a dense lymphocytic infiltrate in the thyroid parenchyma, along with germinal centers. Her follicular epithelium has undergone Hürthle cell change, with abundant cytoplasm containing numerous mitochondria (this is difficult to appreciate in this image). This is an autoimmune condition with formation of antibodies against thyroid peroxidase or thyroglobin, which causes destruction of the thyroid follicles, resulting in permanent hypothyroidism.

44. **A 4-year-old child presents to the ED with respiratory distress. He had functioned normally at birth until 6 months of age, when his neurologic and physical abilities began to deteriorate. He has been blind and deaf since the age of 2 and has a feeding tube, because he has been unable to swallow for the past year. On physical examination, he is noted to have severe muscle atrophy, and a red spot is seen on his retinas. His respiratory status rapidly declines, and he passes away later that day in the ED. An autopsy is performed, and a biopsy of this patient's brain is shown in Figure 27-44. What disease did this child suffer from? What enzyme is insufficient in this disease?**

This child suffered and died from Tay-Sachs disease, which is an autosomal recessive disorder that results in an insufficient activity of the enzyme hexosaminidase A. Hexosaminidase A catalyzes the biodegradation of gangliosides and is found in lysosomes. Therefore, deficiency in this enzyme results in a buildup of lipids, as seen in the biopsy. The biopsy shows a large neuron with lipid vacuolation.

STEP 1 SECRET

Associate cherry-red spots with Tay-Sachs disease, Niemann-Pick disease, and retinal artery occlusion.

45. **A 44-year-old woman presents to her physician with arthralgias, fatigue, malaise, and fevers. She also notes that within the last week, she has developed a rash on her face that will not go away. A 24-hour urine shows dark, foamy urine with 1 g of protein and some RBCs. Her CBC shows Hct of 32%, WBC count of 3500 cells/mm^3, and platelet count of 95,000/mm^3. A renal biopsy is performed and is shown in Figure 27-45. What systemic disease does this woman have? What will eventually happen to her kidneys?**

This woman has the autoimmune disease systemic lupus erythematosus (SLE), which is affecting her joints, skin, and kidneys. The biopsy shows the diffuse, proliferative type, with increased cellularity in the glomerulus. On immunofluorescence testing (Fig. 27-46), mesangial deposits are seen, as well as possible subendothial and subepithelial deposits. Anti–double-stranded DNA (dsDNA) antibodies found in a patient's serum are highly specific for SLE. Eventually, this patient will suffer from renal failure and will require a kidney transplant.

STEP 1 SECRET

Any time you see nonspecific symptoms in a young to middle-aged woman, consider including systemic lupus erythematosus (SLE) in your differential diagnosis.

46. A 40-year-old woman has chronic back pain secondary to an automobile accident 5 years earlier that has been worsening for the past 3 years. She has no insurance and therefore does not go to see a physician. She presents to the ED with ongoing nausea, reflux, and epigastric pain for the past 2 weeks that is not relieved with omeprazole. An EGD with biopsy is performed and shown in Figure 27-47. A urease test is performed on the biopsy and is negative. What condition is this woman suffering from? What likely caused this condition in this patient? What is another cause for this condition?

Based on the history and biopsy findings this woman is suffering from gastritis that is likely secondary to chronic use of nonsteroidal anti-inflammatory drugs (NSAIDs) for her back pain. On biopsy, some of the gastric mucosal epithelium has been replaced by intestinal metaplasia (upper left in Fig. 27-47) and inflammation (lymphocytes and plasma cells) of the lamina propria (at right in this image) can also be seen. Another common cause of gastritis is *Helicobacter pylori*. In that case, the urease test would have been positive, and treatment would have been eradication with triple or quadruple therapy.

STEP 1 SECRET

The USMLE may occasionally expect you to draw some conclusions about medications that patients are taking based on their histories. The two most common scenarios are those featuring women with chronic pain (in whom you should consider nonsteroidal anti-inflammatory drug [NSAID] use) and bodybuilders (in whom you should consider anabolic steroid use).

47. A 72-year-old man presented to his primary care physician complaining of a weight loss of 10 lb in 1 month and a feeling of discomfort and dull pain in his upper abdomen that has been increasing over the past month. His wife also stated that her husband appears "yellow." He had a 50-pack-year history of smoking but had not had an alcoholic drink in 40 years. He refused any hospital workup and subsequently died 2 months later. Upon autopsy, biopsies of various organs were obtained, and one is shown in Figure 27-48. What disease likely led to this man's death?

This man had pancreatic cancer, as evidenced by the features seen in Figure 27-48, which shows glands that are poorly formed, extensive fibrosis in the stroma, and inflammatory cells. This man's history also points to pancreatic cancer. He was a smoker, which doubles the risk of developing the disease. The tumor was likely in the body or tail of the pancreas because he passed away shortly after he became jaundiced. If the tumor is in the head of the pancreas, obstruction of the common bile duct will occur earlier in the disease process and subsequently will be treated earlier. By the time a tumor in the body or tail causes jaundice, the tumor may be large and widely disseminated.

Note: "Painless jaundice" is a commonly used buzzword for adenocarcinoma of the head of the pancreas.

48. A 30-year-old woman presents to her primary care physician with weight loss, palpitations, and sweating. On physical examination, her thyroid gland feels enlarged diffusely. Blood work is sent, and a biopsy taken is shown in Figure 27-49. What is the likely diagnosis in this patient? What will her TSH and serum free T_4 levels show?

This woman likely has Graves' disease, as determined by the symptoms and biopsy. The biopsy shows hyperplastic thyroid gland with columnar epithelium lining the follicles. This epithelium is reabsorbing colloid, resulting in a scalloped appearance. Her TSH will be low and her free T_4 will be high.

49. **A 54-year-old woman is brought to the ED by ambulance with acute SOB. The patient states (through labored breathing) that she has had restricted breathing for years, but it has been worsening over the past 2 weeks. On physical examination, her point of maximal impulse (PMI) is displaced laterally, dry crackles are heard in the lung bases, and there is swelling of her hands and feet with discoloration of her fingers and toes, which the patient states she has had for many years now. The patient's breathing worsens, she is unable to be resuscitated, and she expires in the ED. Upon autopsy, a skin biopsy is taken and shown in Figure 27-50. What condition did this patient suffer from and ultimately die from? What organs are mainly affected in this disease?**

    This patient suffered from diffuse systemic scleroderma, which is an autoimmune disease. Figure 27-50 shows dense collagen deposition in the dermis of the skin, and the arrow points to an area of inflammation. Besides skin thickening, other organs involved in the diffuse form of the disease include the heart, lungs, kidneys, digestive tract, and joints. Antitopoisomerase I (Scl 70) antibodies are seen in some of the diffuse cases and are associated with an increased risk of interstitial lung disease. Anticentromere antibodies are associated with CREST syndrome.

50. **A 64-year-old white man presents to his primary care physician with complaints of four episodes of hematuria over the past 2 days and increased urinary frequency over the past 2 weeks. He has a past medical history of prostate cancer; he also has diabetes mellitus type 2 and hypertension. He has a 60-pack-year history of smoking, and he reports drinking two shots of vodka per day for the past 20 years. On physical examination, there is no blood in his urethral meatus. He is sent to a urologist, who takes the biopsy shown in Figure 27-51. What disease is this patient likely suffering from? What is the most important risk factor for this disease?**

    This man likely has bladder carcinoma (urothelial neoplasm). In Figure 27-51, a high-grade papillary urothelial carcinoma is shown. Numerous anaplastic cells are seen and contain large, hyperchromatic nuclei. The cells also show no architecture or polarity. The most important risk factor for the development of urothelial neoplasms is smoking. Depending on the extent of the smoking history, it can increase the risk of developing bladder cancer sevenfold.

CHAPTER 28

ECG

Brandon Olivieri, MD, Thomas A. Brown, MD, and Sonali J. Shah

INSIDER'S GUIDE TO ELECTROCARDIOGRAMS (ECGs) FOR THE USMLE STEP 1

Successfully learning to interpret ECGs requires three things: practice, practice, and practice! Fortunately, ECGs on the USMLE are not a high-yield test subject (and, when tested, are generally basic). Reading through this short chapter should be more than sufficient for tackling ECG questions on the USMLE. The most highly tested ECG topics are denoted by the Step 1 Secrets embedded within the chapter. Complex ECG interpretation will become much more important during your clinical years.

1. **An ECG recorded in a 30-year-old healthy woman is shown in Figure 28-1. How would you interpret this ECG?**
   Figure 28-1 shows respiratory sinus arrhythmia, a normal finding. Typically the heart rate increases slightly with inspiration and, due to increased vagal tone, decreases slightly with expiration. Variation of heart rate with the respiratory cycle is believed to increase the efficiency of gas exchange by the lungs.

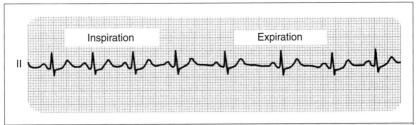

Figure 28-1. Electrocardiogram from 30-year-old healthy woman. (From Goldberger AL: Clinical Electrocardiography: A Simplified Approach, 7th ed. Philadelphia, Mosby, 2006.)

2. **An ECG recorded in a febrile septic patient is shown in Figure 28-2. How would you interpret this ECG?**
   Figure 28-2 shows sinus tachycardia, as might be expected in a febrile septic patient. Each QRS complex is preceded by a P wave, so the rhythm is sinus. The heart rate is also quite elevated at close to 150 beats/min, so this is sinus tachycardia.

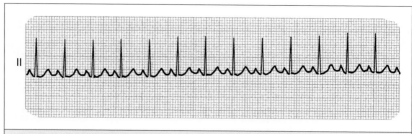

Figure 28-2. Electrocardiogram from febrile septic patient. (From Goldberger AL: Clinical Electrocardiography: A Simplified Approach, 7th ed. Philadelphia, Mosby, 2006.)

3. **An ECG recorded in a healthy middle-aged man after he became dizzy and diaphoretic while having blood drawn is shown in Figure 28-3. How would you interpret this ECG?**
   Figure 28-3 shows a slow heart rate (bradycardia). Each QRS complex is preceded by a P wave, so the rhythm is sinus. Bradycardia is characterized by a heart rate of less than 50 beats/min. A common cause is vagal hyperactivity, as may occur with pain or vomiting, as well as with numerous medications, such as beta blockers.

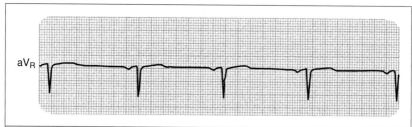

Figure 28-3. Electrocardiogram from middle-aged man after experiencing abrupt onset dizziness. (From Goldberger AL: Clinical Electrocardiography: A Simplified Approach, 7th ed. Philadelphia, Mosby, 2006.)

4. **The patient whose ECG is shown in Figure 28-4 will almost certainly remain asymptomatic throughout life but is at marginally increased risk for sudden cardiac death. How would you interpret this ECG (hint: the arrow is a giveaway)?**
   Wolff-Parkinson-White (WPW) syndrome is characterized by a shortened PR interval and a widened QRS complex with a slurred upstroke (delta wave). Patients with WPW syndrome have an accessory pathway through which action potentials may travel between the atria and ventricles; this is represented by the delta wave on Figure 28-4 (shown by arrow). Unlike the atrioventricular (AV) node, this accessory pathway is unable to slow transmission of action potentials from atria to ventricles. As a result, tachyarrhythmias such as atrial fibrillation can cause marked increase in the rate of ventricular contraction. Such dysrhythmias in WPW patients are dangerous because the resulting ventricular tachycardia can degenerate into potentially fatal ventricular fibrillation.

STEP 1 SECRET

Wolff-Parkinson-White (WPW) syndrome is a USMLE favorite. Not all patients with WPW syndrome are symptomatic, but the condition may lead to supraventricular tachycardia (SVT). The drug of choice for diagnosing and treating SVT is adenosine. You should know the symptoms of adenosine toxicity, which include chest pain, flushing, hypotension, and general patient discomfort.

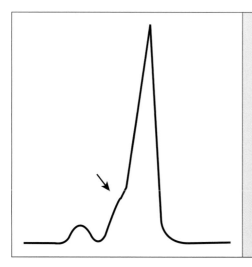

Figure 28-4. Electrocardiogram in asymptomatic adult. (From Ferri F: Practical Guide to the Care of the Medical Patient, 8th ed. Philadelphia, Mosby, 2011.)

5. **The ECG shown in Figure 28-5 comes from a 52-year-old man with chronic obstructive pulmonary disease (COPD) following admission to the hospital with pneumonia. How would you interpret this ECG (hint: look at the p waves)?**
In multifocal atrial tachycardia (MAT), numerous ectopic foci stimulate irregular atrial contraction at a rate of ≥100/min, resulting in morphologically distinct P waves on the ECG. MAT is typically seen in patients with hypoxemia or chronic lung disease.

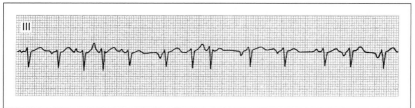

Figure 28-5. Electrocardiogram from COPD patient admitted to hospital with pneumonia. (From Goldberger AL: Clinical Electrocardiography: A Simplified Approach, 7th ed. Philadelphia, Mosby, 2006.)

6. **An ECG recorded in a patient with sudden onset of palpitations and rapid heart rate is shown in Figure 28-6. How would you interpret this ECG (hint: look closely at the rhythm)?**
Figure 28-6 shows atrial fibrillation, characterized by a rapid, irregular ventricular response as well as the absence of P waves. Atrial fibrillation is often seen in patients with a dilated left atrium (as in mitral stenosis or mitral regurgitation). Some patients in atrial fibrillation are asymptomatic, whereas others have severe symptoms, such as palpitations and even syncope. Patients with atrial fibrillation are at increased risk for stroke. This risk can be reduced by patients taking an anticoagulant such as warfarin (Coumadin).

STEP 1 SECRET

Atrial fibrillation is the most common cardiac arrhythmia and is thus the most highly tested arrhythmia on the USMLE. Not only should you be able to recognize the appearance of atrial fibrillation on ECG, but you should know which conditions predispose to atrial fibrillation (e.g., mitral valve stenosis, mitral valve prolapse) and associated symptoms (e.g., palpitations, chest pain, congestive symptoms, exercise intolerance, potential stroke). In addition, recognize the absence of a waves on venous pulse and treatments for atrial fibrillation (rate and rhythm control plus anticoagulation to prevent stroke).

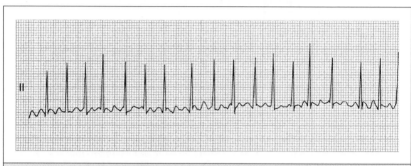

Figure 28-6. Electrocardiogram in patient with sudden onset of palpitations and rapid heart rate. (From Goldberger AL: Clinical Electrocardiography: A Simplified Approach, 7th ed. Philadelphia, Mosby, 2006.)

7. **An ECG in a 38-year-old woman experiencing severe nausea is shown in Figure 28-7. How would you interpret this ECG?**
   Note the slow rate and prolonged PR interval (normal PR interval ≤0.2 second). This represents first-degree AV block, which can occur with increased vagal activity in healthy individuals as well as in elderly patients with dysfunction of the sinoatrial node.

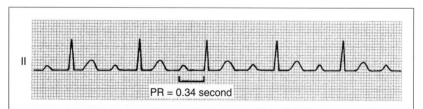

Figure 28-7. Electrocardiogram from healthy 38-year-old woman experiencing nausea. (From Goldberger AL: Clinical Electrocardiography: A Simplified Approach, 7th ed. Philadelphia, Mosby, 2006.)

8. **An ECG recorded in an asymptomatic middle-aged man is shown in Figure 28-8. How would you interpret this ECG? Does he require a pacemaker?**
   Figure 28-8 shows progressive lengthening of the PR interval until a QRS complex is "dropped." This ECG pattern is referred to as Mobitz type I (Wenckebach). Patients with Mobitz type I typically do not require a pacemaker.

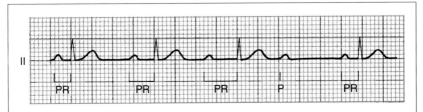

Figure 28-8. Electrocardiogram from middle-aged asymptomatic man. (From Goldberger AL: Clinical Electrocardiography: A Simplified Approach, 7th ed. Philadelphia, Mosby, 2006.)

9. **An ECG recorded in an elderly woman is shown in Figure 28-9. How would you interpret this ECG? Does she require a pacemaker?**
   Figure 28-9 shows Mobitz type II second-degree heart block. Unlike in Mobitz type I, the PR intervals do not progressively increase, but the P waves are not all conducted, resulting in a regular pattern of dropped QRS complexes. Pacemakers are typically placed in patients with Mobitz type II.

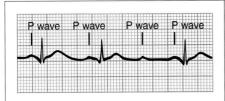

Figure 28-9. Electrocardiogram from an elderly woman. (From Lim EKS, Loke YK, Thompson AM: Medicine and Surgery: An Integrated Textbook. Philadelphia, Churchill Livingstone, 2007.)

10. **An ECG recorded in a 74-year-old man with recurrent syncope is shown in Figure 28-10. How would you interpret this ECG? Would he benefit from a pacemaker?**
    Figure 28-10 shows third-degree (complete) AV block. Note how the P waves and QRS complexes are independent of each other so that the PR intervals are variable and some P waves are "lost" because they fall on the QRS complex or T wave. This patient should receive a pacemaker.

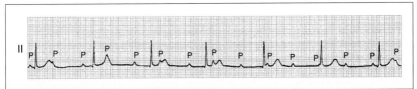

Figure 28-10. Electrocardiogram from an elderly man with recurrent syncope. (From Goldberger AL: Clinical Electrocardiography: A Simplified Approach, 7th ed. Philadelphia, Mosby, 2006.)

STEP 1 SECRET

You should be able to recognize first-, second-, and third-degree atrioventriculat (AV) block for the boards. It is important to know that first-degree AV block and Mobitz type I do not generally require treatment, but third-degree AV block and Mobitz type II (which can progress to third-degree AV block) require immediate pacemaker placement. First-degree AV block is associated with increased vagal tone and can thus be a consequence of digitalis toxicity. Third-degree AV block may be a consequence of Lyme disease.

11. **Figure 28-11 shows an ECG recorded in a 55-year-old man with a history of a massive myocardial infarction 5 years earlier who experiences chest pain just before collapsing. How would you interpret this ECG?**

Figure 28-11 initially shows ventricular tachycardia (note the wide QRS complexes) that in the later part of the rhythm strip degenerates into ventricular fibrillation. Without prompt electrical cardioversion, this is a rapidly fatal rhythm.

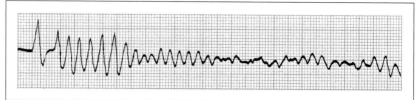

Figure 28-11. Electrocardiogram from a middle-aged man with chest pain who has just collapsed. (From Goldberger AL: Clinical Electrocardiography: A Simplified Approach, 7th ed. Philadelphia, Mosby, 2006.)

12. **An ECG from a middle-aged man started on procainamide for atrial fibrillation is shown in Figure 28-12. How would you interpret this ECG?**

Figure 28-12 shows a type of ventricular tachycardia referred to as torsades de pointes. Note the twisting of the QRS complex around the isoelectric line. The danger of torsades is that it can degenerate into ventricular fibrillation. This potentially fatal dysrhythmia can be triggered by antiarrhythmics such as procainamide, as with this patient.

Monitor lead

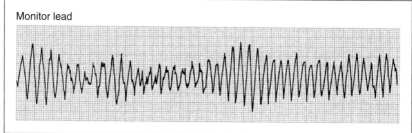

Figure 28-12. Electrocardiogram from a middle-aged man started on the class Ia antiarrhythmic agent procainamide for atrial fibrillation. (From Goldberger AL: Clinical Electrocardiography: A Simplified Approach, 7th ed. Philadelphia, Mosby, 2006.)

STEP 1 SECRET

The USMLE loves torsades de pointes because of its association with class Ia and class III antiarrhythmic toxicity (due to prolonged QT interval). Torsades can also be the result of various congenital ion channel mutations. Jervell and Lange-Nielsen syndrome is a congenital long QT syndrome associated with profound hearing loss.

13. **Figure 28-13 shows an ECG recorded in a 32-year-old otherwise healthy female smoker who takes birth control pills and is experiencing sudden onset of dyspnea. How would you interpret this ECG?**

Note the SI QIII TIII pattern, in which an S wave is seen in lead I, a Q wave in lead III, and inverted T waves in lead III. This pattern is relatively specific for pulmonary embolism but is rarely seen because of its extremely low sensitivity. Nonetheless, it's a pattern you should know for your clinical years.

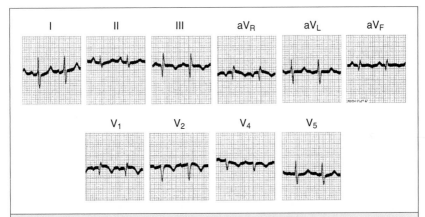

Figure 28-13. SI QIII TIII ECG pattern. (From Goldberger AL: Clinical Electrocardiography: A Simplified Approach, 7th ed. Philadelphia, Mosby, 2006.)

14. **Figure 28-14 shows an ECG recorded in a 52-year-old diabetic smoker who is experiencing sudden onset of chest pain associated with nausea, diaphoresis, and lightheadedness. After he was given something by mouth, his ECG is as shown in Figure 28-14B. What was he given?**
    Figure 28-14A shows an ECG with marked ST-segment depression in lead V_4, representing severe subendocardial ischemia. The patient was given sublingual nitroglycerin, and his symptoms resolved. Figure 28-14B shows normalization of the ST segments.

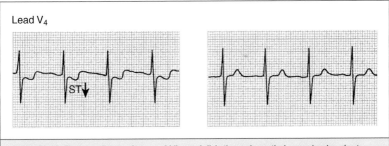

Figure 28-14. Electrocardiogram from a middle-aged diabetic smoker actively experiencing chest pain. (From Goldberger AL: Clinical Electrocardiography: A Simplified Approach, 7th ed. Philadelphia, Mosby, 2006.)

15. **An ECG recorded in a 75-year-old man with a history of coronary artery disease who is experiencing severe substernal chest pressure is shown in Figure 28-15. How would you interpret this ECG?**
    Figure 28-15 shows marked ST-segment elevation in the anterior (V_1-V_3) and lateral (V_4-V_5) leads, indicating an acute anterolateral myocardial infarction.

16. **Figure 28-16 shows an ECG from a 42-year-old obese man who is experiencing severe chest pain. How would you interpret this ECG? For bonus points, which artery is affected?**
    Figure 28-16 shows marked ST-segment elevation in the inferior leads (II, III, aVF), indicating an inferior wall transmural myocardial infarction. The inferior wall is typically supplied by the right coronary artery (RCA).

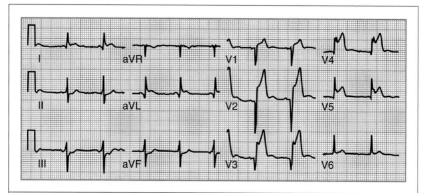

Figure 28-15. Electrocardiogram from an elderly man with a history of coronary artery disease who is actively experiencing chest pain. (From Goldman L, Ausiello DA: Cecil Textbook of Medicine, 23rd ed. Philadelphia, WB Saunders, 2007.)

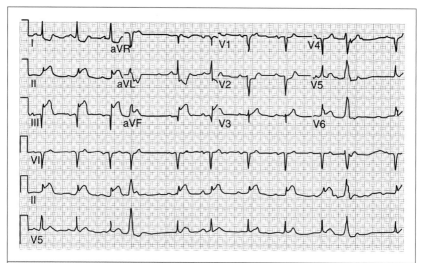

Figure 28-16. Electrocardiogram from an obese middle-aged man actively experiencing chest pain. (From Rakel RE: Textbook of Family Medicine, 7th ed. Philadelphia, WB Saunders, 2007.)

STEP 1 SECRET

Be able to determine which coronary artery is occluded based on ST-segment elevations in various ECG leads. You may also be asked to identify this coronary artery on an angiogram, so practice looking at these images in an anatomy atlas.

INDEX

Note: Page numbers followed by *b* indicate boxes, *f* indicate figures and *t* indicate tables.